Interpretation of the Electrocardiogram in Small Animals

Interpretation of the Electrocardiogram in Small Animals

Nick A. Schroeder, DVM, DACVIM Diplomate, ACVIM (Cardiology)
LeadER Animal Speciality Hospital
Cooper City, FL, USA

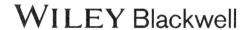

Registered Office
John Wiley & Sons, Inc., 111 River Street, Hoboken, NJ 07030, USA

Editorial Office
111 River Street, Hoboken, NJ 07030, USA

For details of our global editorial offices, customer services, and more information about Wiley products visit us at www.wiley.com.

Wiley also publishes its books in a variety of electronic formats and by print-on-demand. Some content that appears in standard print versions of this book may not be available in other formats.

Library of Congress Cataloging-in-Publication Data

Names: Schroeder, Nick A., 1975- author.
Title: Interpretation of the electrocardiogram in small animals / Nick A.
    Schroeder.
Description: First edition. | Hoboken, NJ : Wiley-Blackwell, 2021. |
    Includes bibliographical references and index.
Identifiers: LCCN 2021015697 (print) | LCCN 2021015698 (ebook) | ISBN
    9781119763055 (cloth) | ISBN 9781119763093 (adobe pdf) | ISBN
    9781119763109 (epub)
Subjects: MESH: Arrhythmias, Cardiac–veterinary |
    Electrocardiography–veterinary | Dog Diseases–diagnosis | Cat
    Diseases–diagnosis
Classification: LCC SF772.58 (print) | LCC SF772.58 (ebook) | NLM SF
    992.C37 | DDC 636.089/61207543–dc23
LC record available at https://lccn.loc.gov/2021015697
LC ebook record available at https://lccn.loc.gov/2021015698

Cover Design: Wiley
Cover Image: © Nick A. Schroeder

Set in 9.5/12.5pt STIXTwoText by Straive, Chennai, India

SKY10027415_060321

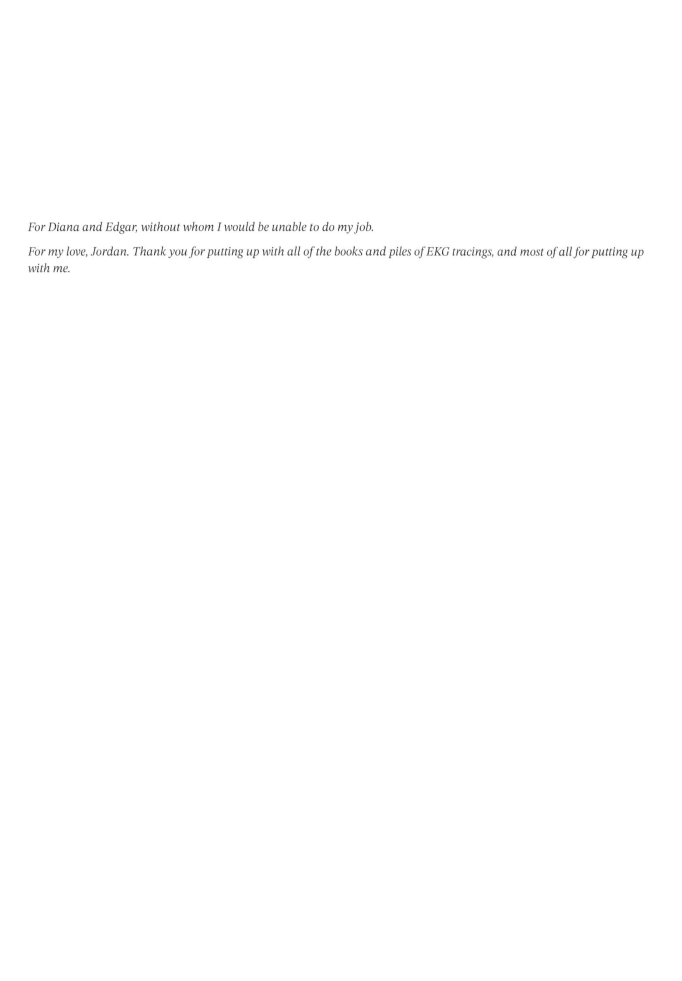

For Diana and Edgar, without whom I would be unable to do my job.

For my love, Jordan. Thank you for putting up with all of the books and piles of EKG tracings, and most of all for putting up with me.

Contents

Abbreviations *xv*
Preface *xvii*
Acknowledgements *xix*
Introduction *xxi*

Part I   The P-QRS-T Complex *1*

1   The P-QRS-T: Basics *3*
Leads *3*
Waveforms/intervals *5*
  P-R interval (P-Ri) *5*
  S-T segment *6*
  Q-T interval (Q-Ti) *6*
Amplitudes *7*
Paper speeds *8*
Mean electrical axis *10*
False poling *12*
Situs inversus *13*
Further reading *15*

2   The P-QRS-T: Some Abnormalities *16*
Right atrial abnormality (P pulmonale) *16*
  P *pseudo*-pulmonale *16*
Left atrial abnormality (P mitrale) *17*
  Interatrial conduction defect *18*
  P *pseudo*-mitrale *19*
Biatrial abnormality/bilateral atrial abnormality (P biatriale) *19*
  P *pseudo*-biatriale *19*
Right ventricular enlargement *19*
Left ventricular enlargement *22*
Biventricular enlargement *23*
Horizontal QRS axis *23*
Vertical QRS axis *24*
Indeterminate QRS axis *24*
Early repolarization *24*
Further reading *26*

3   **The P-QRS-T: Trouble** *27*
     P-R segment changes *27*
     Q-T segment changes *27*
         The prolonged QRS *27*
         Hypokalemia *28*
         Other changes *28*
         Digoxin effects *32*
         Cushing response *34*
         S-T segment elevation/depression *35*
     Low-voltage QRS-T *38*
         Electrical alternans *38*
         Pericarditis *38*
     Further reading *41*

     Part II   Aberrancy *43*

4   **Atrial Aberrancy** *45*
     Interatrial block *45*
     Chung's phenomenon *47*
     Atrial ectopy *47*
     Further reading *54*

5   **Right Bundle Branch Block** *55*
     Incomplete right bundle branch block *55*
     Ashman's phenomenon *55*
     Second-in-the-row anomaly *59*
     Rate-dependent/critical rate BBB *60*
     Complete right bundle branch block *62*
     Further reading *66*

6   **Left Bundle Branch Block** *67*
     Incomplete left bundle branch block *67*
     Rate-dependent/critical rate BBB *67*
     Complete left bundle branch block *68*
     Further reading *76*

7   **Fascicular Blocks** *77*
     Left anterior fascicular block *77*
     Left medial fascicular block *77*
     Left posterior fascicular block *78*
     Bilateral bundle branch block *79*
     Bifascicular block *79*
         Masquerading bundle branch block *80*
     Trifascicular block *81*
     Arborization block *86*
     Further reading *86*

8   **Wide-Complex Supraventricular Tachycardia and Intraventricular Conduction Disturbances** *87*
     Wide-complex supraventricular tachycardias *87*
     Intraventricular conduction disturbances *90*
     Further reading *92*

Part III   Arrhythmias   *93*

Sinoatrial Arrhythmias   *99*
Normal sinus rhythm   *99*
Sinoatrial Bradyarrhythmias   *103*
Sinoatrial Block   *117*
Sick Sinus Syndrome   *123*
Sinoatrial Tachyarrhythmias   *133*
Further Reading   *101*

9   **Sinoatrial Bradyarrhythmias**   *103*
Sinus bradycardia   *103*
Sinus arrhythmia   *105*
   Non-phasic sinus arrhythmia   *105*
   Phasic sinus arrhythmia   *105*
      Respiratory sinus arrhythmia   *105*
      Wandering pacemaker   *105*
      Phasic non-respiratory sinus arrhythmia   *106*
      Ventriculophasic sinus arrhythmia   *108*
Sinus bigeminy   *112*
   Sinoatrial escape-capture bigeminy   *112*
Sinus pause   *114*
Sinus arrest   *114*
Asystole   *114*
Further reading   *116*

10   **Sinoatrial Block**   *117*
Sinoatrial block   *117*
Type I second degree SA block   *117*
Type II second degree SA block   *120*
Further reading   *122*

11   **Sick Sinus Syndrome**   *123*
Sick sinus syndrome   *123*
Overdrive suppression   *123*
Sinus nodal dysfunction   *123*
Bradycardia variant   *126*
Tachycardia-bradycardia variant   *128*
Further reading   *132*

12   **Sinoatrial Tachyarrhythmias**   *133*
Sinus nodal premature systoles   *133*
Sinoatrial reciprocal complexes   *133*
Sinus nodal parasystole   *134*
Sinus tachycardia   *136*
Sinus nodal reentrant tachycardia   *137*
Further reading   *138*

Atrial Arrhythmias *139*
Atrial Bradyarrhythmias *141*
Atrial Tachyarrhythmias *151*
  Atrial Premature Systoles *151*
  Atrial Tachycardia *166*
  Bypass Tract Mediated Supraventricular Tachycardia/Ventricular Pre-excitation Syndromes *175*
  Atrial Flutter *187*
  Atrial Fibrillation *196*

13 Atrial Bradyarrhythmias *141*
Atrial escape beats *141*
  Atrial escape-capture bigeminy *141*
Atrial escape rhythm *141*
Atrial standstill *141*
Further reading *150*

14 Atrial Premature Systoles *151*
Atrial premature complexes *151*
  Right atrial premature complexes *151*
  Left atrial premature complexes *151*
  Multifocal atrial premature complexes *153*
  Resetting *153*
  Resetting with a pause *153*
  Interpolation *154*
  Atrial bigeminy *156*
  Atrial trigeminy *157*
  APCs with aberrancy *157*
    Supernormal excitation *159*
  Non-conducted ("blocked") APCs *159*
Atrial fusion complexes *162*
Atrial reciprocal complexes *162*
Atrial parasystole *163*
Further reading *165*

15 Atrial Tachycardia *166*
Accelerated atrial rhythm *166*
Automatic atrial tachycardia *166*
Intra-atrial reentrant tachycardia *171*
Atrial dissociation *171*
Further reading *174*

16 Bypass Tract–Mediated Macroreentrant Tachycardias/Ventricular Pre-excitation Syndromes *175*
Ventricular pre-excitation and accessory pathways *175*
  RV accessory pathway *176*
  LV accessory pathways *176*
Ventricular fusion *178*
Atrial echo *179*
Atrioventricular reciprocating tachycardia/circus movement tachycardia *179*
Further reading *186*

17 Atrial Flutter *187*
  Atrial flutter *187*
    Type I AFL *187*
    Type II AFL *188*
  Atrioventricular block *193*
  Artifacts *194*
  Further reading *195*

18 Atrial Fibrillation *196*
  Atrial fibrillation *196*
  Aberrancy *201*
    Ashman's phenomenon *201*
  Ventricular ectopics *203*
  Atrioventricular dissociation *204*
  Concealed conduction *207*
  Further reading *209*

  Junctional Arrhythmias *211*
  Junctional Bradyarrhythmias *213*
    Atrioventricular Block *228*
  Junctional Tachyarrhythmias *259*
    Junctional Premature Systoles *259*
    Junctional Tachycardia *270*
  Further Reading *212*

19 Junctional Bradyarrhythmias *213*
  Junctional escape beats *213*
    Junctional escape-capture bigeminy *213*
  Junctional escape rhythm *216*
    Rule of reset *219*
  Reciprocation *219*
  Junctional dissociation *223*
  Ventriculophasic junctional arrhythmia *226*
  Further reading *227*

20 Atrioventricular Block *228*
  Atrioventricular block *228*
  First degree AVB *229*
  Second degree AVB *231*
    Mobitz Type I second degree AVB *231*
      Low-Grade Type I second degree AVB *231*
      2 : 1 Wenckebach *234*
      High-Grade Type I second degree AVB *235*
    Mobitz Type II second degree AVB *240*
      Low-Grade Type II second degree AVB *240*
      2 : 1 Mobitz *240*
      High-Grade Type II second degree AVB *241*
    Block/acceleration dissociation *242*
    Paroxysmal atrioventricular block *247*

Third degree AVB   *248*
   Atrioventricular dissociation   *253*
Ventriculoatrial block   *256*
Exit block   *257*
Further reading   *257*

21   Junctional Premature Systoles   *259*
Junctional premature complexes   *259*
   Resetting   *259*
   Resetting with a pause   *260*
   Interpolation   *260*
   Junctional bigeminy   *262*
   Junctional trigeminy   *262*
   Junctional premature complexes with aberrancy   *262*
   Non-conducted junctional premature complexes   *263*
Concealed conduction   *263*
Atrial fusion   *264*
Junctional reciprocal complexes   *265*
Junctional parasystole   *269*
Further reading   *269*

22   Junctional Tachycardia   *270*
Accelerated junctional rhythm   *270*
   Isorhythmic dissociation   *270*
Automatic junctional tachycardia   *276*
Atrioventricular nodal reentrant tachycardia   *278*
Further reading   *282*

Ventricular Arrhythmias   *283*
Ventricular Bradyarrhythmias   *285*
Ventricular Tachyarrhythmias   *291*
   Ventricular Premature Systoles   *291*
   Ventricular Tachycardia   *319*

23   Ventricular Bradyarrhythmias   *285*
Ventricular escape beats   *285*
   Ventricular escape-capture bigeminy   *287*
Ventricular escape rhythm   *287*
Electromechanical dissociation   *288*
Ventricular asystole   *289*
Further reading   *290*

24   Ventricular Premature Systoles   *291*
Ventricular premature complexes   *291*
   Right ventricular premature complexes   *292*
   Left ventricular premature complexes   *292*
   Compensatory pause   *293*
      The "compensatory-like" pause   *295*

Interpolation   *296*
Post-extraystolic aberrancy   *298*
Ventricular bigeminy   *298*
Rule of bigeminy   *298*
Ventricular trigeminy   *305*
Ventricular quadrigeminy   *306*
Concealed conduction   *309*
Concealed ventricular bigeminy   *309*
Concealed interpolated ventricular bigeminy   *310*
Concealed ventricular trigeminy   *310*
Concealed interpolated ventricular trigeminy   *310*
Ventricular fusion complexes   *311*
Ventriculoatrial conduction and reciprocation   *312*
Atrial fusion   *315*
Ventricular parasystole   *315*
Further reading   *317*

25   **Ventricular Tachycardia, Flutter, and Fibrillation**   *319*
Accelerated idioventricular rhythm   *319*
Atrioventricular dissociation   *321*
Ventriculoatrial association and ventriculoatrial block   *323*
Polymorphic and bidirectional AIVR   *325*
Ventricular tachycardia   *328*
Left ventricular tachycardia   *331*
Fascicular VT   *333*
Bidirectional VT   *333*
Right ventricular tachycardia   *336*
Right ventricular outflow tract-VT   *336*
Bundle branch reentrant VT   *336*
Exit block   *338*
Double tachycardia   *340*
Polymorphic VT   *342*
Torsades de pointes   *342*
Ventricular flutter   *342*
Ventricular fibrillo-flutter/ventricular dissociation   *345*
Ventricular fibrillation   *346*
Further reading   *347*

Part IV   Pacemakers   *349*

26   **Pacemakers: Basics**   *351*
Indications   *351*
Pacemaker polarity   *351*
Modes   *351*
Lead placement   *353*
MEA of the paced QRS   *353*
Further reading   *356*

27   Pacemakers: Some Abnormalities   *357*
Concealed conduction   *357*
Ventriculoatrial conduction   *357*
Paced fusion complexes   *357*
Paced reciprocal complexes   *361*
Further reading   *362*

28   Pacemakers: Trouble   *363*
Undersensing   *363*
 Oversensing   *363*
Failure to capture   *363*
Battery depletion   *367*
Pacemaker-mediated tachycardia   *367*
Pacemaker syndrome   *367*
Further reading   *370*

Index   *371*

Abbreviations

AAR	accelerated atrial rhythm
AAT	automatic atrial tachycardia
AAVNRT	antidromic atrioventricular nodal reentrant tachycardia
AAVRT	antidromic atrioventricular reentrant tachycardia
AF	atrial fibrillation
AFL	atrial flutter
AIJR	accelerated idiojunctional rhythm
AIVR	accelerated idioventricular rhythm
AJR	accelerated junctional rhythm
AJT	automatic junctional tachycardia
Ao	aorta
APC	atrial premature complex
AoV	aortic valve
ARVC	arrhythmogenic right ventricular cardiomyopathy
AS	aortic stenosis or atrial standstill
ASD	atrial septal defect
ATE	arterial thromboembolism
AVB	atrioventricular block
AVN	atrioventricular node
AVR	accelerated ventricular rhythm
AV	atrioventricular or aortic valve
AVSD	atrioventricular septal defect
BAE	biatrial enlargement
bpm	beats-per-minute
BVE	biventricular enlargement
BVF	biventricular failure
CdVC	caudal vena cava
cLBBB	complete left bundle branch block
CKCS	Cavalier King Charles Spaniel
cm	centimeter
CMVDz	chronic mitral valvular disease
cRBBB	complete right bundle branch block
CrVC	cranial vena cava
CS	coronary sinus
CTVDz	chronic tricuspid valvular disease
CVA	cerebrovascular accident
DAVNNT	dual atrioventricular nodal nonreentrant tachycardia
DCM	dilated cardiomyopathy
ECG	electrocardiogram
EKG	electrocardiogram
EMD	electromechanical dissociation
F/S	female spayed
GSD	German Shepherd dog
h	hour
HB	His bundle
HCM	hypertrophic cardiomyopathy
HR	heart rate
IAB	interatrial block
IART	interatrial reentrant tachycardia
IAS	interatrial septum
ICS	intercostal space
iLBBB	incomplete left bundle branch block
iRBBB	incomplete right bundle branch block
IV	intravenous
IVCD	interventricular conduction disturbance
IVS	interventricular septum
JPC	junctional premature complex
LA	left atrium or left arm
LAD	left axis deviation
LAE	left atrial enlargement
LAFB	left anterior fascicular block
LAPC	left atrial premature complex
LAT	left atrial tachycardia
LBB	left bundle branch
LBBB	left bundle branch block
LCHF	left-sided congestive heart failure
LGL	Lown-Ganong-Levine syndrome
LL	left leg
LMFB	left medial fascicular block
LPFB	left posterior fascicular block
LV	left ventricle
LVE	left ventricular enlargement
LVH	left ventricular hypertrophy
LVPC	left ventricular premature complex
LVT	left ventricular tachycardia

M/C	male castrated	RVT	right ventricular tachycardia
MEA	mean electrical axis	PMT	pacemaker-mediated tachycardia
min	minute	PV	pulmonary vein or pulmonary valve
mm	millimeter	s	second
ms	millisecond	SA	sinus arrest
MS	mitral stenosis	SAB	sinoatrial block
mV	millivolt	SAN	sinoatrial node
MV	mitral valve	SANPC	sinoatrial nodal premature complex
MVD	mitral valvular dysplasia	SAS	subaortic stenosis
NSR	normal sinus rhythm	SB	sinus bradycardia
OAVNRT	orthodromic atrioventricular nodal reentrant tachycardia	SCD	sudden cardiac death
		SNRT	sinus nodal reentrant tachycardia
OAVRT	orthodromic atrioventricular reentrant tachycardia	SP	sinus pause
		SR	sinus rhythm
PDA	patent ductus arteriosus	SSS	sick sinus syndrome
PEA	pulseless electrical activity	ST	sinus tachycardia
PHT	pulmonary hypertension	SVPC	supraventricular premature complex
PS	pulmonic stenosis	SVT	supraventricular tachycardia
PTE	pulmonary thromboembolism	TdP	torsades de pointes
PVT	polymorphic ventricular tachycardia	TofF	tetralogy of Fallot
RA	right atrium or right arm	TS	tricuspid stenosis
RAD	right axis deviation	TV	tricuspid valve
RAE	right atrial enlargement	TVD	tricuspid valvular dysplasia
RAPC	right atrial premature complex	VA	ventriculoatrial
RAT	right atrial tachycardia	VAB	ventriculoatrial block
RBB	right bundle branch	VF	ventricular fibrillation
RBBB	right bundle branch block	VFL	ventricular flutter
RCHF	right-sided congestive heart failure	VJA	ventriculophasic junctional arrhythmia
RCM	restrictive cardiomyopathy	VPC	ventricular premature complex
RL	right leg	VPE	ventricular pre-excitation
RSA	respiratory sinus arrhythmia	VSA	ventriculophasic sinus arrhythmia
RVE	right ventricular enlargement	VSD	ventricular septal defect
RV	right ventricle	VT	ventricular tachycardia
RVH	right ventricular hypertrophy	WCT	wide-complex tachycardia
RVOT-VT	right ventricular outflow tract ventricular tachycardia	WPM	wandering pacemaker
		WPW	Wolff-Parkinson-White
RVPC	right ventricular premature complex	y/o	year-old

Preface

The purpose of this work is to provide the reader with an additional reference for interpretation of the electrocardiogram (EKG) in dogs and cats. My goal was to explain EKGs in a simple and straightforward manner utilizing an organization that makes intuitive sense. One of my beloved pastimes is reading books on EKG interpretation and I have accumulated an embarrassing number of them over the years. Of course, I have favorites. If I had to recommend an EKG book for beginners, it would have to be Dubin's **Rapid Interpretation of EKG's**, 6th Edition. The illustrations are impeccable, the language is simple, and the methods used for teaching are genius. At the other end of the spectrum is Pick and Langendorf's **Interpretation of Complex Arrhythmias.** Incomparable in depth, replete with endless ladder diagrams, and brazenly self-aware with alternative interpretations, I never fail to learn something new every single time I pick it up. The very happy middle is Marriot and Conover's **Advanced Concepts in Arrhythmias**, 3rd Edition. Simultaneously easy to read, comprehensive, and full of pearls, this book made my love of EKGs obsessive. Of course, these are books based on human electrocardiography, and we cannot even discuss EKGs in small animals without the influence of the incomparable Tilley's **Essentials of Canine and Feline Electrocardiography**, 3rd Edition as well as the Santilli, Moise, Pariaut, and Perego's more recent beautifully illustrated and brilliant **Electrocardiography of the Dog and Cat**, 2nd Edition. Hopefully, the following will be of some use to veterinary students, veterinarians, interns, residents, specialists, and possibly some of our counterparts in human medicine. If this work contributes in the slightest to the plethora of veterinary information on EKG interpretation in our canine and feline patients, then I will be thrilled.

When trying to come up with an organization, I had a couple of thoughts. Far too many EKG books bounce all over the place and of course the human literature is preoccupied with myocardial ischemia, which is relatively uncommon in dogs and cats. The sheer volume of arrhythmias described in humans dwarfs that of what we know in small animals. Over the years in practice as a veterinary cardiologist, I have come across numerous clinical examples of arrhythmias and other EKG phenomena not yet formally described in small animals. My hope was to include some of these and utilize a simple organization that follows naturally. The reader will have to decide for themselves if I did an adequate job or not. Many authors lament this challenge and I will not belabor the point other than to provide my own perspective.

The easiest thing is to start with the single cardiac cycle as illustrated by surface EKG. From there, it follows to explore variations in the P-QRS-T complex that occur in response to chamber enlargement and hypertrophy as well as electrolyte abnormalities and external influences such as pericardial effusion, body temperature, or neurologic status. Moving on, aberration of the P-QRS-T is discussed since it basically concerns the appearance of the single cycle. Arrhythmias form the bulk of the discussion and sorting out where to discuss certain arrhythmias is not always so clear cut. I opted for a top to bottom, slow to fast approach to the arrhythmias. I followed up with artificial pacemakers. Inevitably, some topics overlap and it can be difficult to decide where, when, and in how much detail should a given concept be discussed. All of the tracings have been taken from real dogs and cats in a clinical setting. All of the illustrations are the work of the author.

If this text accomplishes anything, I hope it encourages the reader to question everything. Without intracardiac EKG/electrophysiologic study, a large part of interpretation of surface EKG is an exercise in deduction. Whenever, things do not make sense, then a reevaluation of assumptions is in order. I assume much of what follows will be clarified, modified, or disproven altogether with time by individuals far more intelligent than I. In the meantime, I hope this helps.

Nick A. Schroeder

Acknowledgements

None of this would be possible without a number of individuals. I would like to thank my mentors: Steve Ettinger, Kirstie Barrett, and Kelly Wessberg; my colleagues in crime: Lyn D'Urso and Scott Forney as well as Lisa DiBernardi, Etienne Côté, and Tacy Rupp. Dr. Thomas Peter at Cedars-Siani occasionally scared me nearly to death and also sometimes made me wish I became an electrophysiologist. I suppose I love dogs and cats just a little too much.

Introduction

Standing on the Shoulders of Geniuses

The following is the result of a combination of studying for the cardiology certifying exam, from my own clinical interest in electrocardiography as well as the admittedly obsessive reading of many far superior original articles and books on the subject. I cannot in any way assume credit for many of the ideas put forward in this text, as I have not yet produced or been involved in original, peer-reviewed scientific articles on all of the subjects discussed. A conceit of my own German heritage, I have deliberately referred to the electrocardiogram with the abbreviation *EKG* (for Einthoven's *elektrokardiogramm* vs. *ECG* – an abbreviation often aurally mistaken for EEG or electroencephalogram). Many original works concerning electrocardiography in small animals (canine and feline) should be regarded with appropriate consideration and include Ettinger and Suter's **Canine Cardiology**, Tilley's **Essentials of Canine and Feline Electrocardiography**, 3rd Edition, Fox/Sisson/Moise's **Cardiology of Small Animals Interpretation and Treatment**, 2nd Edition, Kittleson and Kienle's **Small Animal Cardiovascular Medicine**, 2nd Edition, and Santilli et al.'s **Electrocardiography of the Dog and Cat**, 2nd Edition. To that end, the following is intended as supplemental material, incorporating ideas from the human literature.

This began as a handout for the purposes of teaching veterinarians employed as interns. Many veterinary students feel as though they received a cursory and inadequate instruction in the interpretation of EKGs. The original intent of the following was to explain electrocardiography in a simple, easy-to-understand manner with examples of concepts following the explanations. Clearly, the project had grown in scope, and the following is the result of this. The EKG is an inexpensive screening test for cardiovascular disease. While the sensitivity for chamber enlargement is lacking, specificity is relatively strong. Electrocardiographic monitoring may warn the clinician of electrolyte imbalance, toxicity, shock, etc., and remains the single diagnostic test for cardiac arrhythmias. The perhaps more appropriate term, *dysrhythmia*, is not used for the sake of

historical acceptance of the term *arrhythmia* despite the semantic fact that arrhythmia implies "without rhythm," or atrial and ventricular asystole. The significance of a given arrhythmia tends to be determined by the ventricular rate, subsequent effect on hemodynamics, and the potential for more serious but as yet undocumented arrhythmias. The big questions:

Is this likely to be *a* problem in of itself?
Is this *the* actual problem?
Is this a *consequence* of the real problem?

The importance of accurate EKG interpretation should not be underestimated.

The illustrations in the following are original works of the author. They are intended to help bridge the inevitable gap between the abstract ideas of text and the visceral reality of anatomy. Frequent use of the ladder diagram (Lewis diagram or laddergram) will be seen throughout. It is my fervent opinion that electrocardiography cannot adequately be learned by analyzing the tracing of the EKG alone, and ladder diagrams are invaluable teaching aides. Ladder diagrams provide a visual representation of the EKG that helps to map out the origin, direction, and duration of propagation of the impulse generating complexes on surface EKG. They are very helpful as illustrative tools and helps relate the rather abstract "bumps and squiggles" of the EKG to something more meaningful to the clinician. Several different versions of the ladder diagram may be used, but they all have a fundamental background.

Generally, three tiers are used to represent atrial depolarization (P or P' wave), atrioventricular nodal (AVN) depolarization (usually denoted with a delay), and ventricular depolarization (QRS complex). Importantly, atrial repolarization (Ta wave) and ventricular repolarization (T wave) are not represented graphically on the ladder diagram. The initiation of the complex is denoted by a dot, typically on the very top line of the highest tier if the impulse originates in the sinoatrial (SA) node. Vertical or slanted lines through the given tier will represent the

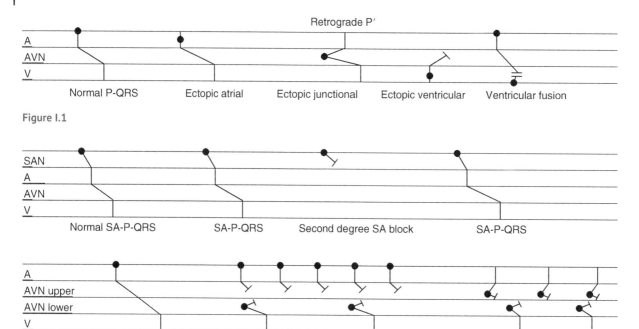

Figure I.1

Figure I.2

respective depolarization events. The more slanted the line, the longer the duration of the given event. Most of the time, the relative duration of atrial and ventricular depolarization is rather fast, so the line may be left vertical for the sake of simplicity. Overtly delayed depolarization, as in what happens during AVN depolarization, is more slanted in keeping with the P-R interval on surface EKG. Ectopic foci are denoted by a dot located within the atrial, AV node or ventricular tiers, respectively. Conduction blockade is denoted by a T-ending. Retrograde conduction may be further emphasized by the placement of an arrow at the end of the impulse. Fusions are marked by T-ending the impulses coming from both origins.

In some situations, it is helpful to add tiers to explain certain arrhythmias. For example, the SA node may be represented by its own tier, making it easier to illustrate SA block. The AVN tier may be divided into an upper nodal level and a lower nodal level/His bundle level.

Attempting to illustrate aberrancy, dual pathways through the AV node and accessory pathways is challenging and may be handled in a few different ways. Aberrancy, whether rate-related or due to permanent bundle branch block may be represented with an inverted "V" in the ventricular tier. Some authors will make a T cut-off midway through the first arm to represent right bundle branch block (RBBB), and through the second to represent left bundle branch block (LBBB). Dual pathways through the AV node may be shown as two differing angled lines through the AVN tier. The steepest angled line represents

depolarization along the "fast pathway" and the shallowest angled line represents depolarization through the "slow pathway." Accessory pathways bypassing the AVN may be illustrated as a dashed line going through the AVN tier.

Ladder diagrams often prove invaluable in teaching EKG interpretation. When faced with a challenging EKG, the clinician can often rely on mapping out the impulses on a ladder diagram. Typically, all atrial depolarizations are noted, then all ventricular depolarizations are noted. Missing P waves hiding within QRS-T complexes may be marched out, provided a regular atrial rhythm. Atrioventricular conduction (or lack thereof) can usually be elucidated from there. If multiple mechanisms may be invoked to explain a certain arrhythmia, ladder diagrams can be particularly useful.

This text is deliberately organized. The single cardiac cycle is evaluated, then aberrancy, which is followed by arrhythmias within the hierarchy of natural pacemakers (SA, atrial, junctional, then ventricular). Bradyarrhythmias are evaluated followed by tachyarrhythmias both in order from mildest to most serious in each section. Finally, we conclude with artificial pacing. Inevitably, any classification system breaks down in the real world, and I am certain better ways to explain the EKG will follow in the future. The distinction of supraventricular tachycardia from ventricular tachycardia based on evidence of an "atrial bridge" or AVN conduction is not made. Some junctional tachycardias (AVN reentrant tachycardia or automatic junctional tachycardia) may not require atrial activation

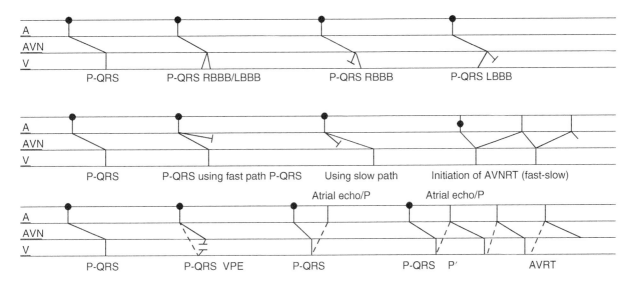

Figure I.3

for perpetuation/maintenance of the arrhythmia. Some atrioventricular reciprocating tachycardias may not involve the atrioventricular node at all (i.e. if two accessory pathways are present). Many ventricular tachycardias have intact ventriculoatrial conduction. It is not the intention of this text to cover older modalities of evaluating the P-QRS-T complex, such as the vectorcardiogram. Similarly, it is beyond the scope of the following to explain intracardiac EKG and electrophysiologic testing, ablation, etc. Signal-averaged EKG and detailed Holter analysis are also not discussed. Surface EKG using standard calibration and paper speed is most commonly used in practice and is thus the focus here. Commonly used antiarrhythmic therapy and effects are discussed when appropriate. Certain phenomena associated with EKG changes in humans are not discussed in detail as canine and feline equivalents have yet to be described and/or are not clinical entities. These include specific myocardial infarction patterns, acute S-T elevation/myocardial infarction, early repolarization abnormality subtypes, specific long Q-T interval syndromes, Brugada syndrome, etc.

Alternate explanations of certain arrhythmias will be presented, when appropriate. Please feel free to contact me regarding other explanations for EKGs presented here. Without the benefit of intracardiac EKG, electrophysiologic testing, etc., many ideas put forth here are unsubstantiated, which should be duly noted by the reader.

Take everything, *EVERYTHING,* you read with a well-deserved grain of salt. Technology and further research will surely contradict some of the ideas brought forth in the following text. My favorite thing to do is try to debunk some antiquated idea or come up with an alternative explanation for electrocardiographic events. The reader is encouraged to do the same. It is human nature to question everything, especially established opinion. Fortunately or not, it is also human nature to organize, pigeon-hole, and generalize phenomena observed in nature. Sometimes, we just need to acknowledge that we do not know everything, and probably not much at all. –NS.

Part I

The P-QRS-T Complex

Interpreting an electrocardiogram (EKG) is a frequently confusing task to the new veterinarian. Some EKGs are very unclear and can really be interpreted in different ways, depending on the cardiologist you talk to. If you look at an EKG the same way, every time, in a systematic manner, you will be able to figure most of them out.

Novice veterinarians often want to be able to glance at an EKG and simply spit out a diagnosis. This is a bad habit and a good way to miss subtle abnormalities. If you take the time to sit down and do everything you are supposed to, there is a much better chance you will figure it out. Before you can determine if an EKG is abnormal or not, you need to know what is normal. This cannot be overstated. First of all, you need to know just what an EKG is. An EKG is a two-dimensional representation of electrical events within the three-dimensional heart that a machine senses from the skin via the use of electrodes and leads. A lead is an electrical perspective. It is like looking at the shadow of something using a light. If you change where the light is, the shadow changes and your perspective changes.

The P-QRS-T complex represents one cardiac cycle. A lot of information may be gleaned from the examination of a single complex. Axis changes, enlargement patterns, and abnormalities secondary to physiologic/metabolic pathology may all manifest on the EKG. Equally as important, it is imperative to remember that a normal EKG does not necessarily exclude serious heart disease. The simple act of calculating a heart rate from the EKG is an oft undervalued skill and gives the clinician critical information regarding the hemodynamic status of the patient in question.

The P-QRS-T: Basics
Leads
Waveforms/intervals
Amplitudes
Paper speeds

Mean electrical axis
False poling
Situs inversus

The P-QRS-T: Some Abnormalities
Right atrial abnormality/P pulmonale
  P pseudo-pulmonale
Left atrial abnormality/P mitrale
  Interatrial conduction defect
  P pseudo-mitrale
Biatrial abnormality/bilateral atrial abnormality/P biatriale
  P pseudo-biatriale
Right ventricular enlargement/hypertrophy
Left ventricular enlargement/hypertrophy
Biventricular enlargement
Horizontal QRS axis
Vertical QRS axis
Indeterminate QRS axis
Early repolarization

The P-QRS-T: Trouble
P-R segment changes
Q-T segment changes
  The prolonged QRS
  Hypokalemia
  Other changes
    Calcium
    Magnesium
    Q-Ti prolongation
    Hypothermia
  Digoxin effects
  Cushing's response
  S-T segment elevation/depression
    Myocardial infarction/ischemic changes
Low-voltage QRS
  Electrical alternans
  Pericarditis

Interpretation of the Electrocardiogram in Small Animals, First Edition. Nick A. Schroeder.
© 2021 John Wiley & Sons Inc. Published 2021 by John Wiley & Sons Inc.

1

The P-QRS-T

Basics

CHAPTER MENU
Leads, 3
Waveforms/intervals, 5
P-R interval (P-Ri), 5
S-T segment, 6
Q-T interval (Q-Ti), 6
Amplitudes, 7
Paper speeds, 8
Mean electrical axis, 10
False poling, 12
Situs inversus, 13

Leads In the frontal plane, that is, the plane that divides the dorsal portion of the animal from the ventral portion, there are six leads that are used to generate an electrocardiogram (EKG, ECG). These are the leads used to create a mean electrical axis (MEA) for the QRS complex. Leads I, II, and III are the bipolar limb leads, and the augmented (unipolar) leads are aVL, aVR, and aVF. The lead attached to the R rear limb (color-coded green) is simply a ground and can really be placed anywhere on the animal. The electrodes may be attached anywhere on the limb, as long as they are positioned approximately equidistant from the heart. The further the leads are placed toward the paws, the greater the chance of baseline artifact from movement. The augmented leads use two of the other leads as one, with the negative pole intermediate between them. Electrodes are placed at the right (R, color-coded white) and left (L, color-coded black) forelimbs and the left rear limb (LL, color-coded red) to get these leads. Leads II, III, and aVF are termed the "inferior" leads (inferior being analogous to caudal in small animals). Leads I and aVL are termed the left lateral leads. The V leads (precordial leads, the left of which are the only ones used with any frequency) are along the horizontal plane – a human term, which is why it is confusing in small animals (the analogue is the transverse plane) – which divides the cranial portion of the animal from the caudal portion. The point at which the QRS complexes change from a rS to Rs pattern (isoelectric RS wave) in the precordial leads is known as the transition zone (normally in V3 or V4).

Lead I: the negative electrode at the R forelimb, the positive electrode is the L forelimb.

Lead II: the negative electrode is at the R forelimb, and the positive electrode is at the L hindlimb.

Lead III: the negative electrode is at the L forelimb, and the positive electrode is at the L hindlimb.

aVR: the negative electrode is between the L forelimb and L hindlimb, and the positive electrode is the R forelimb.

aVL: the negative electrode is between the R forelimb and L hindlimb, and the positive electrode is the L forelimb.

aVF: the negative electrode is between the R forelimb and L forelimb, and the positive electrode is the L hindlimb.

V1 (CV5RL/RV2): the positive electrode is at the R fifth intercostal space (ICS) near the sternum.

> *A Note*: Santilli et al. have proposed a superior location for V1 that more consistently faces the right ventricle (RV) in dogs of all chest conformations. In dolichomorphic (deep-chested) dogs with a vertical heart, V1 at the R fifth intercostal faces the left ventricle (LV) and R waves (not S waves) are seen. In mesomorphic ("normal" chested dogs with a horizontal heart), V1 at the standard location faces the interventricular septum (RS complex). In brachymorphic dogs ("barrel-chested" dogs with a vertical heart), V1 at the fifth ICS gives standard rS complexes and so faces the RV like it should. Thus, the first R ICS at the parasternal

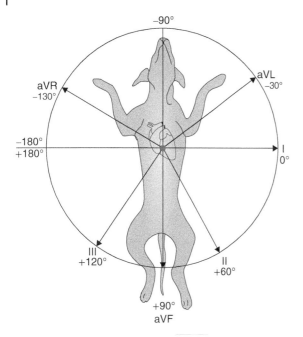

Figure 1.1 Illustration of the limb lead axes in the frontal plane. Lead I is positive at 0 degrees, II is positive at 60 degrees, aVF at 90 degrees, and III at 120 degrees. Lead aVL is positive at −30 degrees and aVR is positive at −130 degrees.

location appears to work best for V1 as it more consistently faces the RV, producing an R/S ratio of <1 and a biphasic P wave. The importance of proper placement of V1 cannot be underestimated, as accurate diagnosis of bundle branch and fascicular blocks of the QRS complex and atrial enlargement patterns is critically dependent on lead positioning.

V2 (CV6LL): the positive electrode is at the L sixth ICS near the sternum.

V3: the positive electrode is placed at the L sixth ICS between V2 and V4.

V4 (CV6LU): the positive electrode is at the L sixth ICS at the costochondral junction.

V5: the positive electrode is at the sixth L ICS above V4, between V4 and V6.

V6: the positive electrode is at the sixth L ICS above V5, between V5 and V7.

V7–V9: in keeping with the same pattern extending to V10.

V10: the positive electrode is at the over the dorsal spinous process of the sixth or seventh thoracic vertebrae.

The negative electrode is the average voltage across leads I, II, and III for the V leads. This is also known as the "V" or Wilson's central terminal, essentially placing the negative pole in the center of the chest. The right precordial leads are designated as RV1-6 and S-T segment elevations in these leads may occur with right ventricular myocardial infarction/ischemia. The left posterior leads (LV7–LV10) may display S-T segment elevations associated with left ventricular

posterior infarction/ischemia. If you had a choice, all you need is three leads in three different axes to get a feel for what is going on:

X plane (frontal): Lead I

Y plane (frontal): Lead aVF

Z plane (horizontal): Lead V10; however, lead V1 typically suffices.

A lead is like looking at the shadow of an object on a wall. If it is at one angle, the shadow may be very long, while at another it may be short. If you are looking at it from an entirely different angle, the shadow may point the other way. If you think about EKGs this way, they tend to make a little more sense. The baseline is termed "isoelectric" and without atrial fibrillation, artifact, rapid heart rates, or ventricular fibrillation, the baseline should return to the isoelectric level following each series of deflections that constitute one cycle or heartbeat. If a deflection moves up from the baseline, it is moving toward the positive electrode in whatever lead you are looking at. If the deflection moves

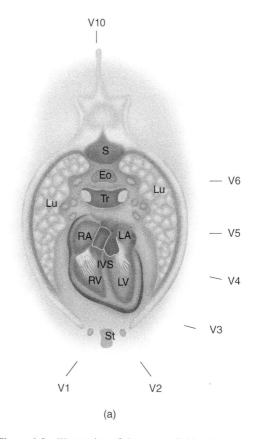

(a)

Figure 1.2a Illustration of the precordial lead axes in the horizontal plane: transverse section at the level of the sixth ICS. Lead V1 is positive to the R of midline and V2–V6 are positive to the left. V10 is situated at the dorsal spinous process, and leads V7–V9 are omitted. **S**: spine, **Eo**: esophagus, **Lu**: lung, **Tr**: trachea, **RA**: right atrium, **LA**: left atrium: **RV**: right ventricle, **LV**: left ventricle, **IVS**: interventricular septum, **St**: sternum.

Figure 1.2b Illustration of the placement of the precordial leads along the sixth ICS. The position of lead V1 at the R fifth ICS near the sternum may be better placed at the first ICS on the right.

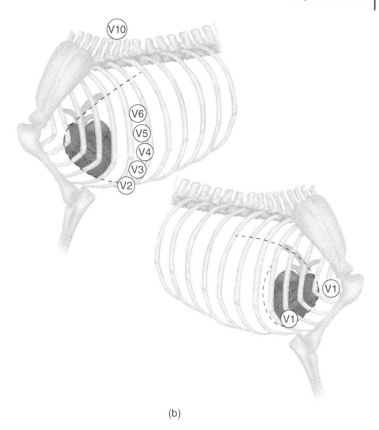

(b)

down from the baseline, it moves toward the negative electrode in that lead. Strong deflections have greater amplitude (positivity or negativity) than weak deflections. What makes up one cycle of a heartbeat? Here are some definitions.

Waveforms/intervals
The waveforms and intervals/segments make up the pattern seen on surface EKG. Commonly identified waveforms are in bold and commonly assessed intervals are italicized. Some of the waveforms are not normally evident or present, and the QRS complex itself is assessed as a complex of waveforms and also evaluated for duration though not referred to as a specific interval per se.

P wave: atrial depolarization. The entire P wave is the summation of the right and left atrial (LA) depolarizations. The first half is right atrial (RA) depolarization and the last half is LA depolarization. Depolarization is mediated initially by sodium channels. The normal MEA for the P wave in dogs is −18 to +90 degrees (0 to +90 degrees in the cat).

P' wave: Atrial depolarization originating at or above the level of the atrioventricular (AV) node, usually ectopic atrial or junctional, but outside the sinus node. A P' wave has a different morphology than that of the normal sinus P wave and can occur after the QRS if retrograde/ventriculoatrial conduction is present.

Ta wave (also known as the Tp wave): Atrial repolarization may be seen in P-R segment or S-T segment, opposite in polarity of the P wave, associated with RA enlargement, hypoxia, and electrolyte imbalances, and is usually too low in amplitude to be detected in the P-R interval or buried in the QRS complexes. The Ta wave may be seen in second/third degree AV block as it is no longer obscured by an intervening QRS complex.

P-Ta segment: From the beginning of the P wave to the end of the Ta wave. This may be elevated with atrial infarction, leading to P-R elevation if the Ta wave is buried within the QRS complex, aka "PQ elevation." Depression of P-R segment may occur with elevated sympathetic tone.

P-R interval **(P-Ri)** From the beginning of the P wave to the start of the Q wave (or the R wave if no Q wave is present), the P-Ri represents the delay of the impulse through the AV node. This delay is mediated via slower L-type calcium channels. The P-Ri is normally constant and of a certain duration (0.13 second or less in dogs, 0.06 second or less in cats). If the P-Ri is consistently short (0.03 second or less), then an accessory pathway or retention of rapid juvenile AV nodal conduction is present. If the P-Ri is prolonged, first degree AV block is present. If two distinct P-R intervals are present, then dual AV nodal physiology is suggested. If a predictable and progressive prolongation before a second degree AV block (P wave without associated QRS complex) occurs, then a Type I second degree AV block is present. If the P-R intervals are completely variable (i.e. no P-Ri is the same as another without any discernable pattern), then AV dissociation is present.

Q wave: First negative deflection after the P wave before a positive deflection. The Q wave represents the initial rightward interventricular septal wall depolarization.

q wave: If less than 0.5 mV in amplitude.

Delta wave: This is a slurring of the upstroke of the R wave, associated with a short P-R interval and ventricular pre-excitation syndromes. The presence of a delta wave indicates the presence an accessory pathway bypassing the AV node.

R wave: The first positive deflection after a negative, actually with or without a Q wave preceding. The R wave represents the endocardial to epicardial depolarization of the ventricles.

r wave: If less than 0.5 mV in amplitude.

S wave: The first negative deflection after the R wave. The S wave represents the final apical to basilar depolarization of the ventricles.

s wave: If less than 0.5 mV in amplitude.

QRS complex: Represents ventricular depolarization. The order of depolarization of the IVS, endocardium to epicardium, then apicobasilar directions correspond to the EKG deflections of Q, R, and S waves, respectively. The QRS complex itself is a summation of right and left ventricular (RV, LV) depolarizations. Given that the LV is normally the more massive of the two chambers, the vector of the LV dominates that of the RV. The QRS complex is initiated by sodium channels. Most of the time, it is more correctly termed qRs given the relative amplitudes of the different waves. The MEA of the QRS complex is normally between +40 and +100 degrees in the dog and between 0 and +160 degrees in the cat.

Intrinsicoid deflection (R peak time): This is the interval from the beginning of the QRS complex to the beginning of the descending branch. Practically, this means from the start of the QRS with or without a q wave to the peak of the R wave (or s/S wave if no R wave present). This interval is used in humans and measured from the precordial leads. The intrinsicoid deflection represents depolarization from the endocardium to the epicardium. Prolongation may occur secondary to ventricular hypertrophy or conduction delay. Normal times for small animals are yet to be definitively established.

S-T segment From the end of the S wave to the start of the T wave, indicating that all regions of the ventricle are depolarized. The S-T segment should be isoelectric, but may be slurred or coved, and significant elevations or depressions from the baseline may indicate myocardial ischemia/infarction or hypoxia.

QS wave: Negative deflection without a positive.

q' wave: The first positive deflection after a positive.

r' wave: The next positive deflection after the S wave before returning to baseline (before the T).

s' wave: The next negative deflection after the S wave before returning to baseline (before the T).

J point: Where the S wave just returns to the baseline, may be elevated or depressed along with S-T segment changes.

Osborn wave: Also known as the J wave, the Osborn wave is a hump where the QRS complex joins the S-T segment and is commonly seen in severe hypothermia along with bradycardia, prolonged P-Ri, QRS duration, and Q-Ti.

Epsilon wave: May be seen in association with arrhythmogenic right ventricular cardiomyopathy, and is best seen in V1 and V2 (occasionally V1–V4). The epsilon wave is a deflection seen within the S-T segment as late potentials (little wiggles) caused by postexcitation of the myocytes in the RV.

Q-T interval (Q-Ti) From the onset of the QRS complex to the end of the T wave, this is the period of ventricular action potential duration and is potassium or sodium channel dependent. The Q-Ti is shorter with a higher HR and longer with a slower HR and is often corrected for the HR (termed QTc interval). Normally from 0.14 to 0.22 second in dogs and up to 0.16 second in cats.

T wave: Ventricular repolarization; technically occurs from the onset of the QRS complex and continues through the end of the T wave. The T wave is not caused by a propagated wave and should be approximately $\frac{1}{4}$ the amplitude of the R wave, positive in V1 and negative in V10 (mediated via potassium channels). The MEA of the T wave in dogs and cats is generally not calculated as its axis may be concordant or discordant with the MEA of the QRS and may vary even within individuals, essentially rendering the calculation irrelevant.

U wave: A deflection following the T wave usually in the same direction as the T wave. The U wave was previously attributed to m cells (ventricular myocytes located in the midmyocardium with very long action potentials), and has been also theorized to result from repolarization of Purkinje fibers and potentials formed during isovolumetric relaxation. U waves are associated with long Q-T syndromes (LQTS), hypokalemia, and bradycardia. U waves may be mistaken for non-conducted sinus or ectopic atrial beats.

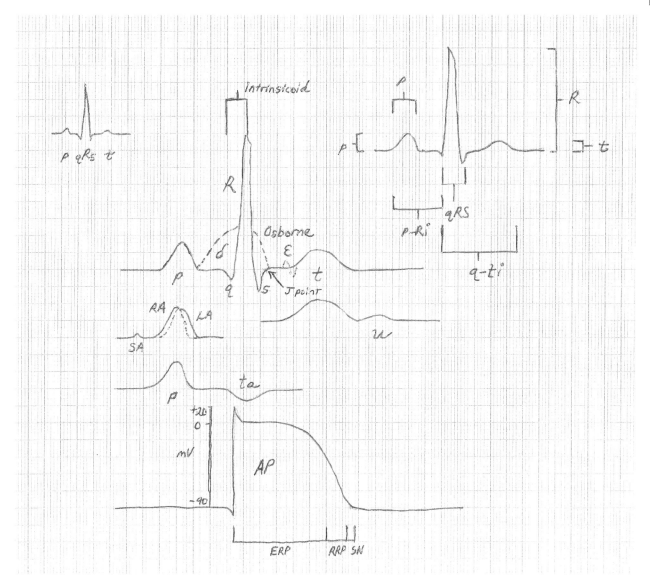

Figure 1.3 Illustration of the waveforms and intervals. **P**: p wave, **q**: q wave, **R**: R wave, **s**: s wave, **t**: t wave, **qRs**: QRS complex, **δ**: delta wave, **ε**: epsilon wave, **SA**: sinoatrial depolarization, **RA**: right atrial depolarization, **LA**: left atrial depolarization, **ta**: Ta wave, **u**: U wave, **P-Ri**: P-R interval, **q-Ti**: Q-T interval, **AP**: action potential, **ERP**: effective refractory period (absolute refractory period), **RRP**: relative refractory period, **SN**: supernormal period.

Amplitudes

How tall (positive) or deep (negative) is termed the amplitude of a wave. As measured from the baseline, a positive wave is deflected upward, and means the impulse is directed toward the positive pole in that lead at that instant. A negative wave is deflected downward and means the impulse is directed toward the negative pole in that lead at that instant. We measure the amplitude of a wave in millivolts. A calibration mark is typically created by the machine immediately before a tracing and tells us the scale. By convention, one centimeter on the strip (one large box) equals one millivolt (1 cm/mV or 10 mm/mV).

Just remember to check the sensitivity prior to measuring the amplitudes, so the measurement is correct. The amplitude of a wave is measured from the baseline (zero voltage, isoelectric line) to the most positive or negative point.

1 cm/mV (10 mm/mV) is standard.

0.5 cm/mV (5 mm/mV) or half-sensitivity makes the complexes smaller.

2 cm/mV (20 mm/mV) or double-sensitivity makes the complexes taller.

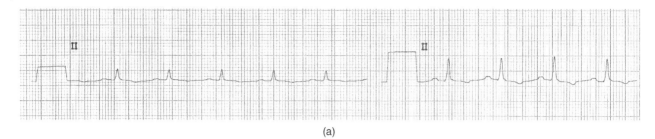

(a)

Figure 1.4a Paper speed 50 mm/s, lead II, canine. Comparison of half-sensitivity to full-sensitivity. Note the calibration marks. Both are 1 cm wide indicating a consistent paper speed of 50 mm/s. The first has an amplitude of 0.5 cm tall corresponding to **0.5 cm/mV**, and the second has an amplitude of 1 cm indicating **1 cm/mV**. Note all waveforms have the same duration, but the second set of waveforms is twice as tall. Lower sensitivity makes the waveforms more difficult to tell apart.

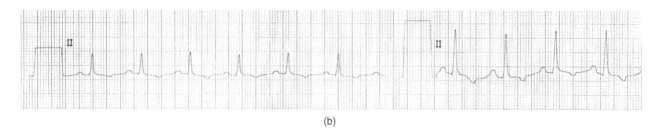

(b)

Figure 1.4b Paper speed 50 mm/s, lead II, same dog. Comparison of full-sensitivity to double-sensitivity. Again, note the calibration marks. Their widths are the same at 1 cm, alerting the examiner that the paper speed is 50 mm/s. The first has an amplitude of 1 cm (**1 cm/mV**), and the second has an amplitude of 2 cm (**2 cm/mV**), so the complexes are again now twice as tall. Higher sensitivity exaggerates the complexes and makes it easier to measure *amplitudes*, but it does amplify any underlying baseline artifact as well. The QRS complexes are all approximately *0.8* mV.

Paper speeds The duration of a wave refers to the total time it takes to return to baseline and is a function of how fast the paper speed is. The heart rate may be calculated a few different ways. If the rhythm is perfectly regular, then instantaneous heart rates (i.e. using an R-R interval) can be calculated. If the rhythm is irregular, then a longer duration of time should be used (i.e. 3–6 seconds).

At 25 mm/s: Standard for humans – 1 small box is 0.04 second and 1 big box is 0.2 second
   1500/# of small boxes in one R-R interval = bpm
   300/# of big boxes in one R-R interval = bpm
   # of beats in one pen length (approximately 30 big boxes or 6 seconds) × 10 = bpm
So at 100 bpm, there should be 15 little boxes (or 3 big boxes) between R waves.

   Quick and Dirty: At 25 mm/s, if you find an R wave on a bold line on the EKG paper, and the next R wave is 1 big box away, the HR is 300 bpm. If the next R wave is 2 big boxes away, the HR is 150 bpm. If the next R wave is 3 big boxes away, the HR is 100 bpm. If the next R wave is 4 boxes away, the HR is 75 bpm. If the next R wave is 5 boxes away, the HR is 60 bpm. If the next R wave is 6 boxes away, the HR is 50 bpm. "1-2-3-4-5-6 is 300-150-100-75-60-50 bpm."

50 mm/s: Is standard for small animals – 1 small box is 0.02 second and 1 big box is 0.1 second
   3000/# of small boxes in one R-R interval = bpm
   600/# of big boxes in one R-R interval = bpm
   # of beats in one pen (approximately 30 big boxes or 3 seconds) length × 20 = bpm
So at 100 bpm, there should be 30 little boxes (or 6 big boxes) between R waves.

It is best to evaluate the EKG in the following manner. However it is done, it is best to do it systematically in the same manner every time.

Rate: Is the rate normal or abnormal? Too fast? Too slow? Calculate the HR.

Rhythm: Regular or irregular? Regularly irregular ("allorhythmia" – or a regularity within an irregularity, most often respiratory sinus arrhythmia, premature beats with consistent pauses?), irregularly irregular (atrial fibrillation? frequent and multifocal premature beats?). *Too regular* (pacemaker, ectopic tachycardia)?

P waves?: Present? Not present? (look in other leads, consider atrial fibrillation, atrial standstill).

P for every QRS?: If not, consider premature beats.

QRS for every P?: If not, consider AV block.

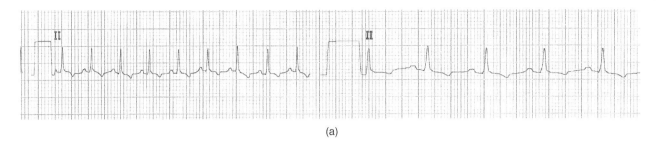

(a)

Figure 1.5a Amplitude 1 cm/mV, lead II, canine. Comparison of paper speeds. Note the calibration marks preceding the recordings. Both are at the same amplitude of 1 cm, indicating 1 cm/mV. The first is only 0.5 cm wide, alerting the examiner that the paper speed is **25 mm/s**. The second is 1 cm wide, indicating the paper speed is now **50 mm/s**. The faster paper speed stretches out the waveforms, making the measurement of *intervals* easier. The R waves are nearly 4 big boxes apart at 50 mm/s, indicating the heart rate is just over *150* bpm.

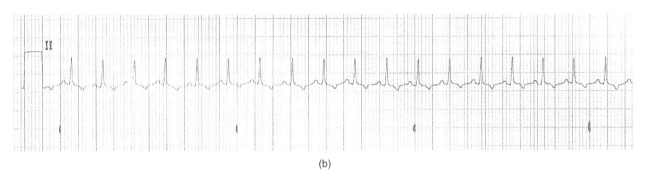

(b)

Figure 1.5b Amplitude 1 cm/mV, paper speed 25 mm/s, lead II, same dog. More accurate calculation of the heart rate can be made by counting the number of complexes in a 6 second period. Thirty big boxes are counted out and 17 complexes are counted within this interval. The heart rate is therefore calculated as 17×10 or *170* bpm.

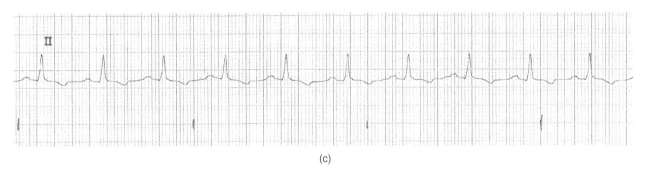

(c)

Figure 1.5c Amplitude 1 cm/mV, paper speed 50 mm/s, lead II, same dog. Calculation of the heart rate is calculated as nine complexes within a 3 second period or $9 \times 20 = 180$ bpm. Given the very regular rhythm, a more accurate estimation of heart rate is calculated as: 3000/18 little boxes between R waves or *167* bpm. Practically speaking, the difference between 167, 170, and 180 bpm is clinically unimportant.

Measurements: Any RA or LA abnormalities, right or left ventricular enlargement, bilateral atrial enlargement, or biventricular enlargement?

P MEA: Is it normal or abnormal? Consistent with sinus focus, R or L atrial focus, junctional/retrograde conduction?

QRS MEA: Is it normal or abnormal? Right axis deviation (RAD) or left axis deviation (LAD)? Extreme axis deviation?

Q-Ti: Is it normal? Prolonged/shortened QRS complex or S-T segment? S-T segment deviations?

Arrhythmias and conduction abnormalities will be discussed elsewhere. Never forget the importance of independently calculating the atrial and ventricular heart rates, though keep in mind that the ventricular rate has more hemodynamic importance. Remember when interpreting the heart rate, ask yourself if it is appropriate for the given situation? Dogs that are healthy may have a phasic respiratory sinus arrhythmia, and nervous cats in the exam room usually have sinus tachycardia. If the heart rate is inappropriate for the situation, consider pathologic states. Remember that common things occur commonly. Never forget this.

Mean electrical axis The MEA of the QRS reflects the main vector of ventricular depolarization, and the MEA of the P wave similarly describes the vector of the atrial depolarization. Ventricular enlargement or ectopy may change the MEA of the ventricles, and atrial enlargement or ectopy may alter the axis and appearance of the P wave.

The MEA of the QRS complex can be a tricky thing for new veterinarians to deal with, and it is really not all that difficult. However, you need more than one lead to determine the MEA. There are two easy ways to determine the MEA. The thing to realize is that the circle in the frontal plane is arbitrarily 0 degrees at lead I (straight to the patient's L) and proceeds +180 degrees clockwise (caudally) and −180 degrees counterclockwise (cranially).

Lead I: 0 degrees
Lead II: +60 degrees
Lead aVF: +90 degrees
Lead III: +120 degrees
Lead aVL: −30 degrees
Lead aVR: −160 degrees

If you find the most isoelectric lead (the one with the positive and the negative deflections approximately equal to each other, RS or rs complexes) and go 90 degrees in the direction of the most positive leads, this will give you the MEA. Another method is to use two leads that are perpendicular to each other (i.e. lead I and aVF or lead II and aVL), count the positive and the negative units of amplitude (small boxes) in one complex of each lead on the EKG and count out the number of units from the center of the circle along that lead equal to the number you came up with (e.g. +10 added to −5 boxes results in a net +5 boxes). Drawing a line perpendicular to that lead at that level of units and do it with the other lead you are looking at. Find where those lines intersect on each lead, and where they bisect gives you the MEA. Another easy way to figure out which quadrant the mean QRS vector resides in is to check leads I and aVF, which are perpendicular to each other. If the QRS complex in lead I is positive, then the mean QRS is between −90 and +90 degrees. If the QRS complex in lead I is negative, then the mean QRS is between +90 and −90 degrees. If the QRS complex in lead aVF is positive, then the mean QRS vector is between 0 and +180 degrees. If the QRS complex lead aVF is negative, then the mean QRS vector is between 0 and −180 degrees. Checking the axis of the QRS in these two leads quickly tells you which quadrant the MEA of the QRS is located in.

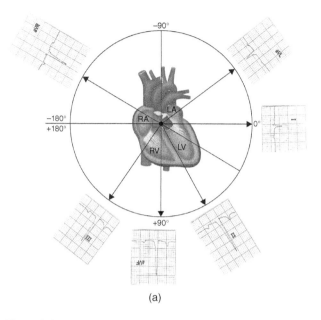

(a)

Figure 1.6a Illustration of the limb leads with superimposed EKG from a normal canine. The angle of the tracing reflects the direction of the positive pole in each lead.

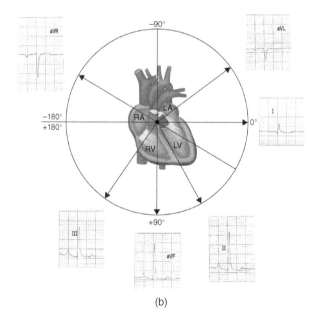

(b)

Figure 1.6b Illustration of the limb leads with superimposed EKG from the same dog. Here, the angles are situated normally. We know the MEA here is likely closest to aVF, given the R waves have the greatest magnitude in that lead. We also know the MEA must be between 0 and +90 degrees, given that the QRS complexes are positive in leads I and aVF. Lead I is most isoelectric and going 90 degrees in the direction of the most positive leads puts the MEA close to +90 degrees.

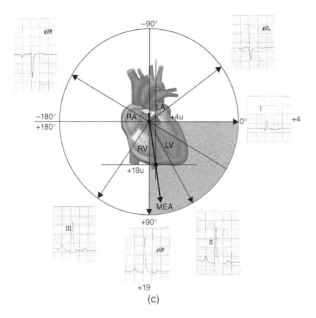

(c)

Figure 1.6c Illustration of the limb leads with superimposed EKG from the same dog. Calculation of the MEA is made using leads I and aVF. In lead I, the R wave is 4 little boxes tall in amplitude. Four units toward the positive pole in lead I are counted out. In lead aVF, the R wave is 19 small boxes tall in amplitude. Nineteen boxes are counted out toward the positive pole. Where perpendicular lines to each lead at their respective levels intersect is where the MEA of the QRS is. In this case, the MEA is approximately +80 degrees.

Left axis deviation suggests left ventricular enlargement, hypertrophy, or aberrancy and RAD suggests right ventricular enlargement, hypertrophy, or aberrancy. If the mean QRS vector lies between 0 and −90 degrees, LAD is present. If the mean QRS vector lies between 90 and +180 degrees, RAD is present. If the mean QRS vector lies between +180 and −90 degrees, extreme axis deviation ("no man's land") is present.

Normal dogs have a MEA of +40 to +100 degrees.
    LAD if the MEA < +40 degrees
    RAD if the MEA > +103 degrees
Normal cats have a much wider MEA of 0 to +160 degrees.
    LAD if the MEA <0 degrees
    RAD if the MEA > +160 degrees

> ***Quick and Dirty***: Find the lead with the most positive QRS, and the MEA is likely close to that. If the QRS is positive (upright) in leads II, III, and aVF (the inferiors), then the axis is probably normal. The P waves should be positive in lead I and negative in lead aVR. This indicates that atrial depolarization began from a superior position on the right, consistent with an impulse generated anatomically within the sinoatrial node in the right atrium. The leads are likely on correctly if the P waves are oriented normally.

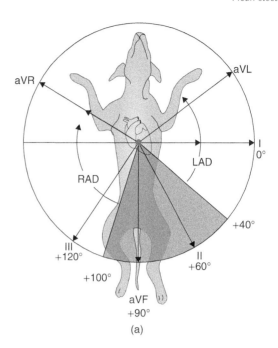

(a)

Figure 1.7a Illustration of the canine normal mean electrical axis of the QRS. The normal MEA ranges between +40 and +100 degrees. As such, the QRS complexes should be positive in I and aVF if the MEA is between 0 and +90 degrees. Most of the time, lead II provides the tallest amplitude QRS complexes, which is why it is commonly used as a monitoring lead. The QRS complexes should always be negative in aVR and aVL if the MEA is within normal limits and are usually positive in the inferiors (II, III, and aVF).

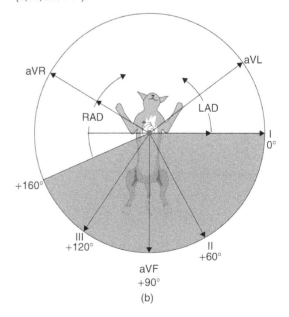

(b)

Figure 1.7b Illustration of the feline normal mean electrical axis of the QRS. The normal MEA in the cat is wider and ranges between 0 and +160 degrees. As such, the QRS complexes should be positive in I and aVF if the MEA is between 0 and +90 degrees. The QRS complexes should be negative if aVR and aVL and positive in the inferiors (II, III, and aVF) if the MEA is within normal limits.

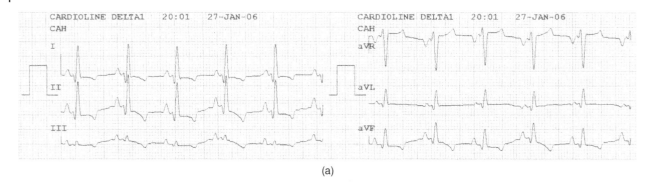

(a)

Figure 1.8a Paper speed 50 mm/s, 1 cm/mV, full EKG, canine. **Normal sinus rhythm** (NSR). This is a **normal** EKG with a **normal** MEA. The P waves are positive in I and aVF, and negative in aVR, indicating a normal P wave axis. The QRS complexes are positive in I, II, III, aVF (and aVL).

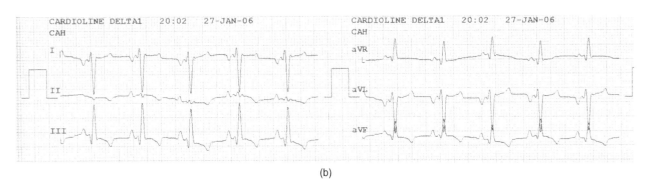

(b)

Figure 1.8b Paper speed 50 mm/s, 1 cm/mV, full EKG, same dog. **False poling** (the leads are placed incorrectly). The clue is that the P wave MEA is abnormal. The P waves are positive in aVR and negative in lead I, which over 99%of the time indicates false poling (less than 1% of the time in humans indicates atrial ectopy or *situs inversus* – see below). The **RA** (white) and **LA** (black) electrodes have been *switched*. This essentially switches aVR and aVL, turns lead II into lead III, lead III into lead I, and inverts lead I. This is the most common error in lead placement, a pattern that mimics **situs inversus**.

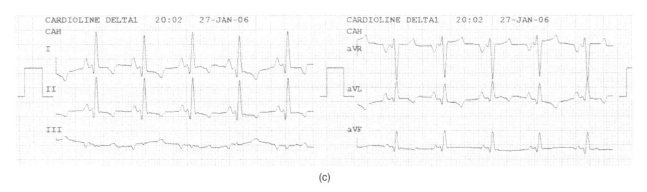

(c)

Figure 1.8c Paper speed 50 mm/s, 1 cm/mV, full EKG, same dog. False poling. The **LA** (black) and **LL** (red) electrodes have been *switched*. Leads I and aVR look normal in this case, so looking at the P waves in these leads is not helpful. The clue here is that there appears to be L axis deviation with a MEA of approximately +30 degrees, and the P waves are *negative* in lead III. P waves should be positive in I, II, and aVF, negative in aVR, and are usually positive in III (but can be negative). This dog has no other EKG criteria consistent with LVH (normal amplitude and duration of the QRS complexes) that would otherwise support a left axis deviation. Switching the LA and LL electrodes effectively inverts lead III, reverses aVL and aVF, and reverses I and II.

False poling When the leads are incorrectly applied to the animal, this is termed false poling. The most common error is switching the left and right forelimb leads, which simulates situs inversus (see below). Always verify correct placement of the leads prior to recording an EKG.

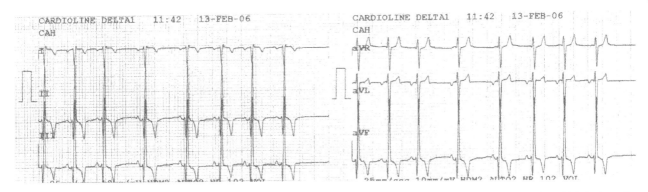

Figure 1.9a Paper speed 25 mm/s, 1 cm/mV, full EKG, canine with **situs inversus**. The P waves are *negative* in lead I, which is the only situation in which this would be a "normal" and expected finding, since this patient's heart and internal organs are reversed or the "mirror image" of normal. In cases of situs inversus, the SAN is in the "RA" which is *anatomically* on the left side of the body, so the P waves are directed from L to R, and would thus be negative in lead I. Note that aVL has negatively oriented P waves, and the QRS complexes in I are negative from RAD. Despite the fact that these are *abnormal* findings on surface EKG, this pattern is *normal* for a patient with situs inversus.

Figure 1.9b Ventrodorsal radiograph from the same dog. **Situs inversus**. The standard view shows a mirror image of normal with the cardiac apex and gastric fundus is on the right.

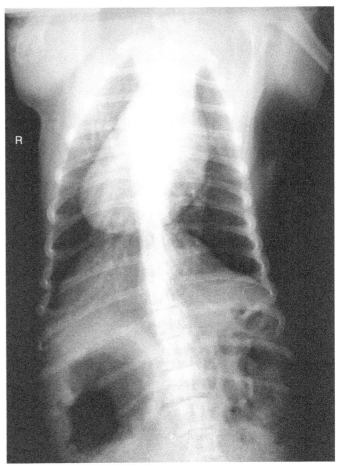

Situs inversus

This is a very rare condition where the internal organs are reversed (mirror image) from normal. Dextrocardia is present so the apex of the heart will be on the right and the right atrium/sinus node is anatomically located on the left. Situs inversus therefore creates a unique EKG pattern with negative P waves (provided sinus rhythm) in lead I. The MEA of the QRS will be slightly deviated to the right. Dextropositioning of the heart, as what can happen in isolation or association with severe left ventricular enlargement may show some minor axis shift of the QRS, but sinus P waves should still be positive in lead I. Situs inversus is commonly misdiagnosed from false poling of the limb leads on EKG or mislabeled thoracic radiographs.

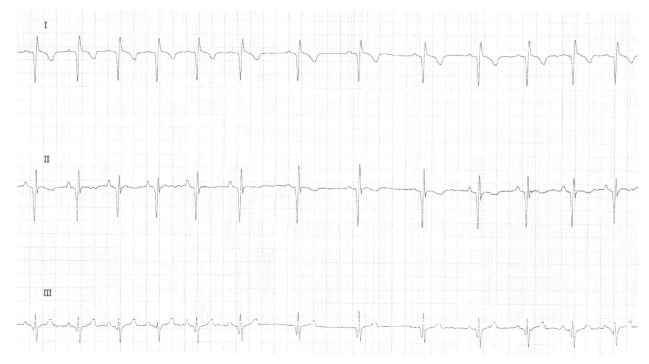

Figure 1.10a Paper speed 50 mm/s, 1 cm/mV, leads I, II, III, canine with isolated **dextropositioning**. A right axis deviation of the QRS is apparent with S waves in leads I and II and an s wave in III. Note the P waves are still positive in lead I, indicated a normal R to L P wave axis.

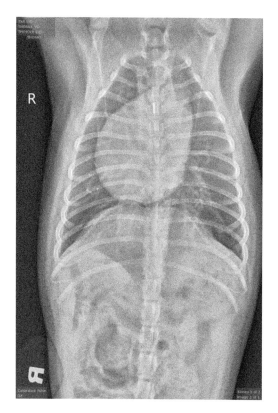

Figure 1.10b Ventrodorsal radiograph from the same dog. **Isolated dextropostioning**. The cardiac apex is deviated to the R hemithorax and the gastric fundus is on the left. This dog had otherwise cardiac anatomy evident on echocardiography, albeit with malpositioning of the cardiac apex to the right.

Further reading

Chou, T. and Helm, R. (1965). The pseudo P pulmonale. *Circulation* 32: 96–105.

Dubin, D. (2000). *Rapid Interpretation of EKG's*, 6e. Cover Inc.

Gertsch, M. (2004). *The ECG: A Two-Step Approach to Diagnosis*. Springer.

Hurst, J.W. (1998). Naming of the waves in the ECG, with a brief account of their genesis. *Circulation* 98: 1937–1942.

Kittleson, M.D. and Kienle, R.D. (1998). *Small Animal Cardiovascular Medicine*. Mosby.

Macfarlane, P.W., Van Oosterom, A., Pahlm, O., Kligfield, P. et al. (2011). *Comprehnsive Electrocardiology*, 2nd Ed., Springer.

Santilli, R., Sydney Moïse, N., Pariaut, R., and Perego, M. (2018). *Electrocardiography of the Dog and Cat: Diagnosis of Arrhythmias*, 2e. Edna.

Tilley, L.P. (1992). *Essentials of Canine and Feline Electrocardiography*, 3e. Lippincott Williams & Wilkins.

2

The P-QRS-T

Some Abnormalities

CHAPTER MENU

Right atrial abnormality (P pulmonale), 16
  P *pseudo*-pulmonale, 16
Left atrial abnormality (P mitrale), 17
  Interatrial conduction defect, 18
  P *pseudo*-mitrale, 19
Biatrial abnormality/bilateral atrial abnormality (P biatriale), 19
  P *pseudo*-biatriale, 19
Right ventricular enlargement, 19
Left ventricular enlargement, 22
Biventricular enlargement, 23
Horizontal QRS axis, 23
Vertical QRS axis, 24
Indeterminate QRS axis, 24
Early repolarization, 24

Right atrial abnormality (P pulmonale)

"P pulmonale": Think of this as "P" for "peaked" or tall P waves. P wave >0.4 mV in dogs, >0.2 mV in cats ±, tall, slender, peaked P waves ± slight depression of the baseline following the P wave (Ta wave). The P wave is the summation of both the right atrial (RA) and left atrial (LA) depolarizations. The MEA for the R atrial vector is more inferiorly directed and occurs just before the L atrial depolarization. Thus, the P waves get taller in the inferior leads when the R atrial vector predominates secondary to RAE. A large, positive initial deflection in V1 is characteristic. The P wave in V1 is normally biphasic, with an initial positive component from the RA and a terminal negative component from the LA. P pulmonale is a specific, but insensitive indicator of RAE. The Ta wave is usually more prominent, and resultant P-R segment depression may be seen, especially if sympathetic tone is high (i.e. tachycardia). An increased negative (terminal) portion of the P wave in VI may occasionally occur and is thought to be secondary to an extremely large right atrium with extension of the auricle to the left of midline. This may con-fused with "P pseudo-pulmonale" (see below). The term "P congenitale" has been coined for so-called "gothic" P waves where the amplitude in lead I exceeds that of the amplitude in lead III (P pulmonale with left axis deviation of the P wave vector).

P *pseudo*-pulmonale Increased P wave amplitude may alternatively be the result of an anatomically enlarged left atrium with the resulting P wave vector directed more posteriorly and inferiorly than it is to the left, mimicking P pulmonale. This results in tall P waves in II and aVF with slight notching, the greater hump of which is due to activation of the enlarged left atrium. Lead V1 will show increased amplitude of the negative terminal portion of the P wave (normally biphasic in V1 with a positive initial portion from the RA and a negative terminal portion from the LA). Echocardiography will confirm severe left atrial enlargement (LAE) with normal (or near normal) RA dimensions. This is not uncommon in dogs with chronic mitral valvular disease (CMVDz) and severe LAE. If the P waves are tall, but the

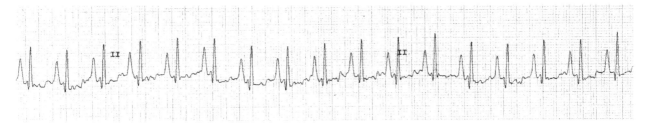

Figure 2.1 Paper speed 50 mm/s, 1 cm/mV, lead II, canine, sinus tachycardia, **P pulmonale**. The P waves are very tall at 0.8 mV.

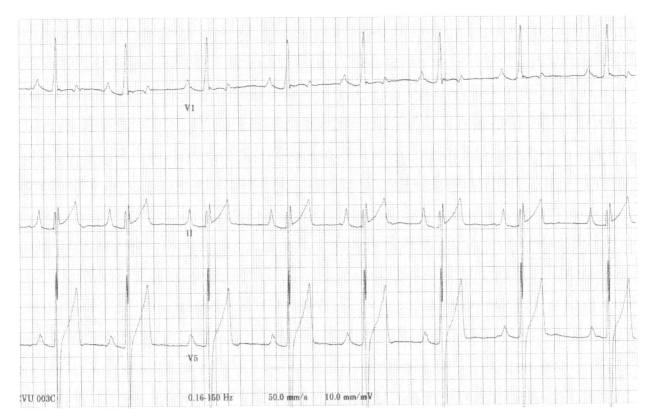

Figure 2.2 Paper speed 50 mm/s, 1 cm/mV, leads V1, II, and V5, canine with severe tricuspid dysplasia/Ebstein's type anomaly. Sinus rhythm, **P pulmonale**, extreme right axis deviation. The P waves are approximately 0.7 mV in height, and severe RA enlargement was present in this patient. Note the strongly positive P wave in V1, confirming the tall P waves in lead II are secondary to RAE.

rest of the EKG (and physical exam, signalment, etc.) fits with left-sided disease, chances are good that the reason why is LAE. Other causes of increased P wave amplitude reported in people in the absence of RAE include hypokalemia, increased sympathetic tone (shifting the pacemaker to a more superior focus within the sinoatrial node/SAN associated with sinus tachycardia), hyperinflated lungs/flattened diaphragm, or asthenic habitus (physically thin/underweight).

Left atrial abnormality (P mitrale) "P mitrale": Think of this as "M" for "M-shaped" P waves but they are also prolonged in duration. P waves >40 ms in dogs, >35 ms in cats, bifid P waves present in I, II, aVR, aVF, with diphasic P waves in aVL and III. A large negative P wave in V1 is expected. Remember notching of the P wave can be normal unless the P wave is also wide. The L atrial vector is normally directed laterally to the left. Since the L atrial depolarization occurs after the R atrial depolarization, a

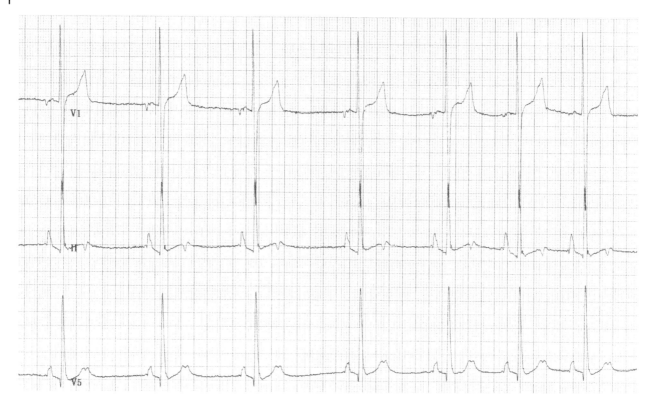

Figure 2.3 Paper speed 50 mm/s, 1 cm/mV, leads V1, II, and V5, canine. Sinus arrhythmia, **P pseudo-pulmonale**. The P waves are tall (0.5–0.6 mV) in lead II; *however,* the terminal (negative) portion of the P wave in VI is accentuated, and tall R waves in II and V5 are suggestive of LV enlargement. The right atrium was normal sized in this miniature poodle with advanced chronic mitral valvular disease (CMVDz) and echocardiographically confirmed severe LA and LV enlargement. In this case, the tall P waves were secondary to L atrial enlargement.

predominating vector of the L atrium will tend to prolong the P wave duration. P mitrale is a specific, but insensitive indicator of LAE and may more often occur at least in humans from interatrial block. This may be confused with "P pseudo-mitrale" (see below).

Interatrial conduction defect Excessive P wave pro-longation/severe P mitrale is known as interatrial block. The distinction between P mitrale, interatrial and intra-atrial block has been unclear in the medical literature with the terms often used (erroneously?) interchange-ably. More often, prolonged P waves may result from so-called first degree interatrial block and are associated with LAE. Exactly when P mitrale constitutes intera-trial block has not been clearly defined in dogs and cats. Interatrial/intra-atrial block is discussed in more detail in Chapter 4.

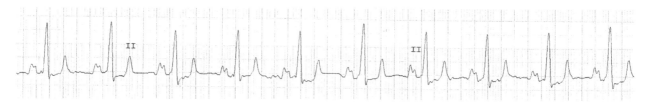

Figure 2.4 Paper speed 50 mm/s, 1 cm/mV, lead II, canine, Sinus rhythm, **P mitrale**. The P waves are wide (almost 0.08 second) as well as notched.

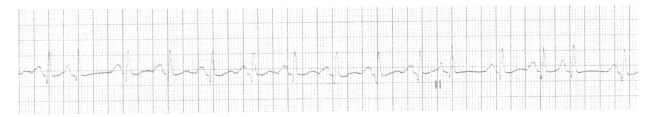

Figure 2.5 Paper speed 50 mm/s, 1 cm/mV, lead II, feline with severe cardiomyopathy and left atrial enlargement. **P-mitrale** with P wave duration of approximately 0.06 second. Intermittent supraventricular premature beats are also present.

P pseudo-mitrale Prolonged P wave duration may conversely be the result of an anatomically enlarged right atrium. This results in a P wave that is >0.04 second and <0.4 mV, exactly mimicking P mitrale. Lead V1 may be biphasic and the positive initial component may be more prominent. Echocardiography will confirm normal LA dimensions and RAE, which must be marked to increase the P wave duration. Isolated interatrial block is a rule out. If the P waves are wide, but the rest of the EKG (and physical exam, signalment, etc.) fits with right-sided disease, then chances are good that the underlying reason is actually RAE. This is a rare manifestation of RAE on surface EKG.

> *A Note:* Cor pulmonale is a term applied to a group of diseases in which right ventricular hypertrophy (RVH) occurs with or without congestive heart failure (CHF) as a result of pulmonary disease, or, more generally speaking, RVH secondary to pulmonary vascular or pulmonary disease, regardless of the etiology. (Think heartworm disease or pulmonary hypertension.) These conditions may result in EKG evidence of RV/RA hypertrophy or enlargement, but is not a specific EKG term per se.

Biatrial abnormality/bilateral atrial abnormality (P biatriale)

"P biatriale": P wave >0.4 mV dog (0.2 mV cat), P >0.04 second, with notching often present. This pattern is surprisingly uncommon despite the incidence of bivalvular disease/biatrial enlargement with myxomatous degeneration of the atrioventricular (AV) valves or biatrial enlargement in cats with cardiomyopathy. Basically, the P waves are both tall and wide. This may be confused with "P pseudo-biatriale" (see below).

P pseudo-biatriale This pattern is present if EKG criteria for P biatriale are met and structurally only LA (most commonly or rarely only RA) enlargement is evident on further testing (echocardiography). P pseudo-biatriale may actually be more common than true P biatriale in practice. The term "P tricuspidale" has been coined to describe the biatrial enlargement pattern where the peak for the RA vector exceeds that of the LA.

Right ventricular enlargement

Technically, three of the following: S wave in V2 >0.8 mV, MEA > +103 degrees (>+ cat)/clockwise, S wave in V4 >0.7 mV, S wave in I >0.05 mV, R/S ratio in V4 <0.87 mV, S wave in II >0.35 mV, S waves in I, II, III (so-called S1-S2-S3 pattern), aVF, + in V10 (except in Chihuahuas), W-shaped QRS in V10. Mild QRS prolongation is common, but excessive QRS prolongation is more suggestive of interventricular conduction disturbance, right bundle branch block, or

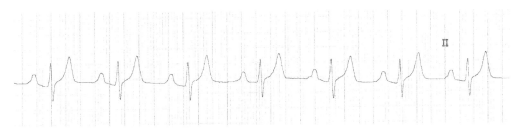

Figure 2.6 Paper speed 50 mm/s, 1 cm/mV, lead II, canine with severe pulmonary arterial hypertension and cor pulmonale. **P pseudo-mitrale**. The P wave duration is 0.07 second and the P wave amplitude is within normal limits. The MEA was indeterminate with rs complexes in all limb leads. This dog had severe right atrial enlargement with normal left atrial dimensions confirmed on echocardiography.

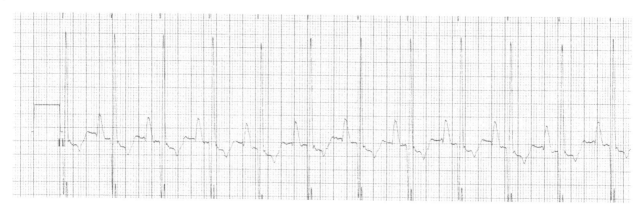

Figure 2.7 Paper speed 50 mm/s, 1 cm/mV, lead II, canine. Sinus rhythm, **P biatriale**. The P waves are 0.8 mV in amplitude, and 0.06 second in duration. LVH is also present with tall R waves. The deep Q waves are suggestive of right ventricular enlargement as well.

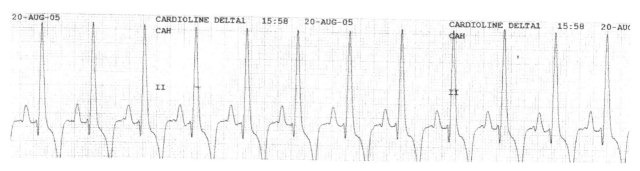

Figure 2.8 Paper speed 50 mm/s, 1 cm/mV, lead II, canine. Sinus rhythm, **bilateral atrial enlargement**. The P waves are 0.5 mV in amplitude and 0.06 second in duration. LVH is also present with tall R waves and QRS complexes of prolonged duration.

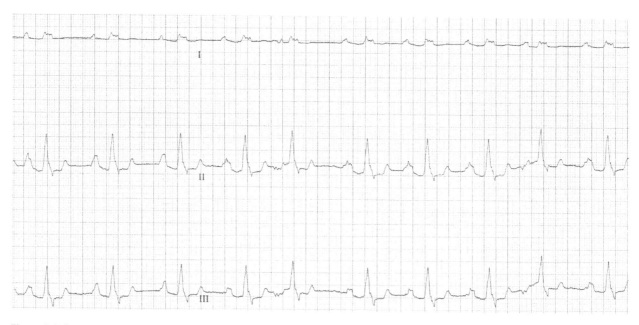

Figure 2.9 Paper speed 50 mm/s, 1 cm/mV, leads I, II, and III, canine. Sinus rhythm, interatrial block, **BAE**. *Extreme* prolongation of the P wave duration (approximately 0.1 second) occurs in this patient with multiple congenital heart defects, including pulmonic stenosis and tricuspid dysplasia. Marked right atrial and moderate left atrial enlargement was present in this patient who presented for supraventricular tachycardia and collapse. The P waves are also tall, have bizarre notching, and are predominantly positive in V1. The fifth and ninth complexes are supraventricular premature beats. The QRS complexes are mildly prolonged, likely from an interventricular conduction defect.

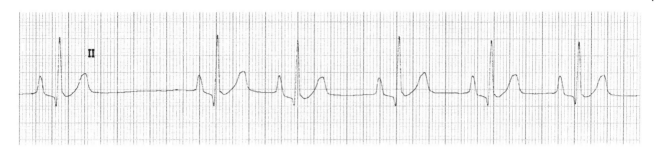

Figure 2.10 Paper speed 50 mm/S, 1 cm/mV, lead II, canine. **P pseudo-biatriale with LAE**. This dog had severe CMVDz, with echocardiographically confirmed severe left atrial enlargement and normal right atrial dimensions. The P waves are prolonged at 0.05 second and increased in amplitude at 0.5 mV consistent with P-biatriale based on EKG criteria.

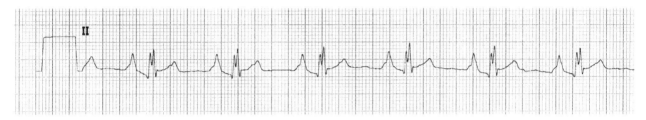

Figure 2.11 Paper speed 50 mm/s, 1 cm/mV, lead II, canine. **P pseudo-biatriale with RAE**. This dog actually had tricuspid dysplasia with massive right atrial enlargement evident on echo with normal left atrial dimensions. The P wave amplitude is 0.6 mV and the duration 0.08 second consistent with biatrial enlargement based on EKG criteria. Dogs with tricuspid dysplasia not uncommonly have very tall P waves often referred to as "Himalayan P waves." The QRS complexes are splintered (qrsR's) which is commonly associated with tricuspid dysplasia.

a left ventricular origin of the QRS. These patterns are specific, but insensitive indicators of RVE. In general, severe concentric RVH (i.e. from pulmonic stenosis or pulmonary hypertension) produces more profound right axis shifts and prolongation of the QRS than does eccentric hypertrophy (enlargement) of the right ventricle (from tricuspid dysplasia, acquired chronic tricuspid valvular disease, or right ventricular cardiomyopathy).

A Note: Isolated minor right axis deviation may also be caused by a left posterior fascicular block or an incomplete right bundle branch block. Bifascicular block (right bundle branch block with concurrent left posterior fascicular block) may prolong the QRS in addition to causing an R axis shift (see Chapter 7). Complete right bundle branch block typically deviates the terminal portion of the QRS to the right and markedly prolongs the QRS duration (see Chapter 5).

Another Note: True S1-S2-S3 has S waves =/> R waves in leads I, II, and III, the S2 > S3 and is rare. Usually the S wave is still less than that of the R wave in lead I. If the R/S ratio + 1, then the MEA is indeterminate. If left axis deviation, then the S3 will be > S2.

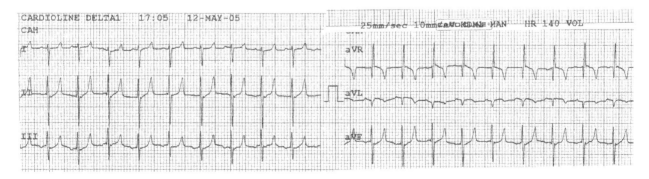

Figure 2.12 Paper speed 25 mm/s, 0.5 cm/mV, canine, sinus rhythm with **S1-S2-S3 pattern** with S waves in aVF and right axis deviation of the QRS.

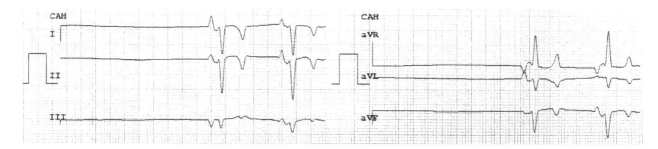

Figure 2.13 Paper speed 50 m/s, 1 cm/mV, syncopal Chihuahua with severe pulmonic stenosis. Severe **R axis deviation** is apparent. The P waves are normally oriented (positive in I and negative in aVR). The QRS complexes are negative in the inferiors and positive in aVR. The MEA is approximately minus 160–170 degrees. The long pause evident before the beats seen may be partially responsible for syncope. This Chihuahua also had 1.5 mV S wave in V4 and a negatively oriented QRS in V10.

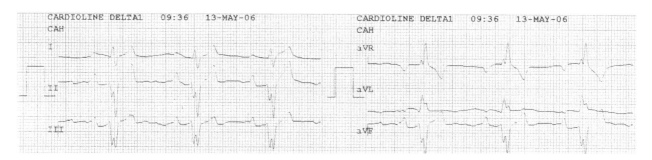

Figure 2.14 Paper speed 50 mm/s, 1 cm/mV, full EKG. Canine with severe pulmonic stenosis. Sinus rhythm, severe **R axis deviation**, with mild prolongation of the QRS complexes (rsr'S' in lead II) likely from an intraventricular conduction disturbance.

Left ventricular enlargement In dogs greater than two years of age, dolicomorphics and large breeds, the R wave is generally in excess of 3 mV in II and aVF. In dogs over two years of age and small breeds, the R wave >2.5 mV in II, III, aVF, it is >3 mV in V4, and the R wave >2.5 mV in V2. In cats, the R wave exceeds 0.9 mV in II and is over 1 mV in V4. In small-to-medium breed dogs, the QRS exceeds 0.05 second in duration. In large breed dogs, the QRS is over 0.06 second. In cats, the QRS exceeds 0.04 second in duration. Excessive QRS prolongation

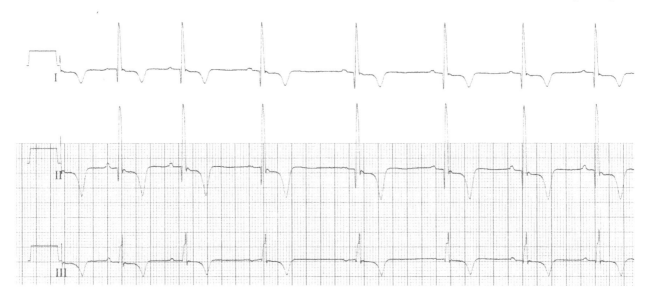

Figure 2.15 Paper speed 50 mm/s, 0.5 cm/mV, lead I, II, III, Cairn terrier with hypertrophic cardiomyopathy (HCM), **LVH** with R waves approximately 5.8 mV in lead II. The Q-Ti is a little long, and there are deep, negative T waves. Respiratory sinus arrhythmia with a wandering pacemaker is present.

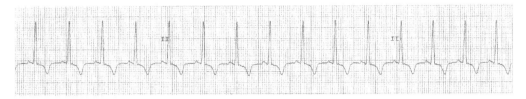

Figure 2.16 Paper speed 50 mm/s, 1 cm/mV, lead II, feline, sinus rhythm, **LVH** with R waves approximately 1.8 mV.

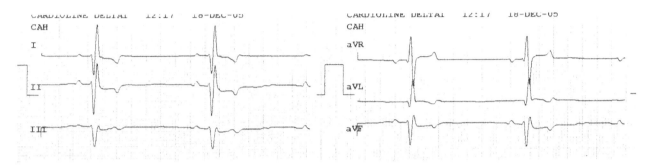

Figure 2.17 Paper speed 50 mm/s, 1 cm/mV, lead II, canine, sinus rhythm, **L axis deviation**. The MEA is approximately −70 degrees.

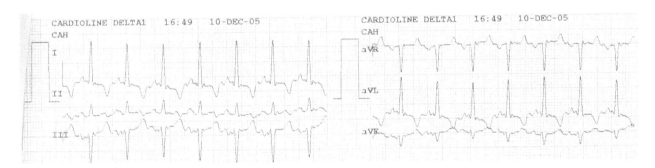

Figure 2.18 Paper speed 50 mm/s, 2 cm/mV, full EKG, Maine Coon cat with severe HCM. Sinus rhythm with **left axis deviation** is present. The MEA is approximately −5 degrees.

suggests interventricular conduction disturbance, left bundle branch block, or a right ventricular origin of the QRS. The S-T segment may sag into the T wave and the T wave may be increased in amplitude. The MEA is less than +40 degrees in dogs and less than 0 degrees in cats. In general, severe concentric LVH (from hypertrophic cardiomyopathy, chronic systemic hypertension, or aortic stenosis) produces more profound left axis shift and prolongation of the QRS than does eccentric hypertrophy (enlargement) of the left ventricle (from patent ductus arteriosus, ventricular septal defect, acquired CMVDz, or dilated cardiomyopathy).

> *A Note*: Isolated left anterior fascicular block or incomplete left bundle branch block may also cause left axis deviation of the QRS, and bifascicular block (right bundle branch block with concurrent left anterior fascicular block) may also prolong the QRS in association with a L axis shift (see Chapter 7). Complete left bundle branch block markedly prolongs the QRS and commonly deviates it to the left (see Chapter 6).

Biventricular enlargement Precordial leads show changes for both RVE (deep S waves in V4, V2) and LVE (tall R waves in V4, V2) on EKG with R axis deviation. LVH with tall R waves, a prolonged QRS in V2, a normal EKG with cardiomegaly on thoracic radiographs, and deep Q waves in I, II, III, aVF with LVH criteria can also be consistent with BVE. Concomitant EKG criteria for L and R atrial enlargement are not uncommon. A big ventricle is usually associated with a big atrium.

Horizontal QRS axis Also known as a "horizontal heart," this is really an electrical phenomenon and thought to occur in people as the heart lies horizontally in the chest. A common pattern in obese humans, this may more common in mesomorphic dogs. Technically, the mean axis is close to 0 degrees (minor left axis deviation) in the frontal plane, leads I and aVL will have a predominately upright qR pattern, and II, III, and aVF will show rS or RS patterns.

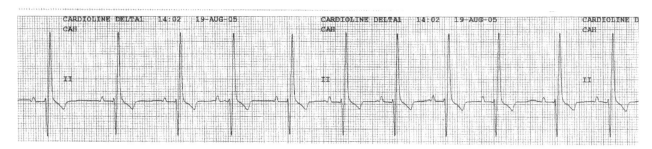

Figure 2.19 Paper speed 25 mm/s, 1 cm/mV, lead II, canine, sinus arrhythmia, the R waves are a little variable, but approximately 3.5–4 mV suggestive of LVH and deep Q waves suggest RVH consistent with **BVE**.

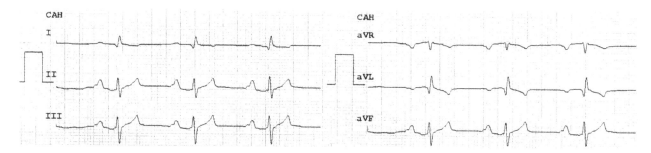

Figure 2.20 Paper speed 50 mm/s, 1 cm/mV, canine, sinus rhythm, **horizontal heart pattern** with P mitrale. The MEA is approximately 0 degrees, and the P waves are wide and notched (p mitrale).

Vertical QRS axis Also known as a "vertical heart." Common in physically thin people, the heart is vertical, but in animals it is actually "layed down" along the sternum, often seen in elderly cats. When the MEA is closer to 90 degrees (inferior and rightward axis deviation) in the frontal plane, the QRS in leads II, III, and aVF will be mainly upright with a qR pattern. Lead I will be isoelectric with a qRS/qrs pattern.

Indeterminate QRS axis An indeterminate axis occurs when all six extremity leads (I, II, III, aVR, aVL, and aVF) show biphasic QR/qr or RS/rs patterns. This means all the leads are isoelectric (regardless of amplitude, though often mildly decreased), and the mean QRS vector is perpendicular to the frontal plane. An indeterminate axis may be normal or pathologic. The precordial leads should be examined for evidence of a normal (or abnormal) axis. This may include a shift in the transition zone (normally V3 or V4) and/or increased amplitude of QRS complexes in precordials leads facing either the right or left ventricles.

Early repolarization Abnormalities of repolarization typically involve prolongation or shortening of the Q-T interval (see Chapter 3). If the Q-Ti is within normal limits, then a possible repolarization abnormality is a so-called early repolarization. This occurs when the S-T segment immediately slopes into the T wave from the J-point without a return to zero voltage and thus may simulate S-T segment elevation/depression. The following down/upstroke of the T wave is steep. Early repolarization abnormality is a common occurrence in asymptomatic athletic male humans and is an important distinction from myocardial infarction patterns. Whether this occurs to a clinical degree in small animals is undetermined at this time. We would expect this pattern in certain athletic breeds such as Greyhounds, but thus far it has not been formally described. In fact, "early repolarization" appears to be benign as well as fairly ubiquitous in small animals, so it is significant insofar as the pattern may be confused with S-T segment elevation/depression.

Figure 2.21 Paper speed 25 mm/s, 1 cm/mV, full EKG, canine. Sinus rhythm, **vertical heart** pattern. The MEA is approximately 90 degrees, excluding fascicular block.

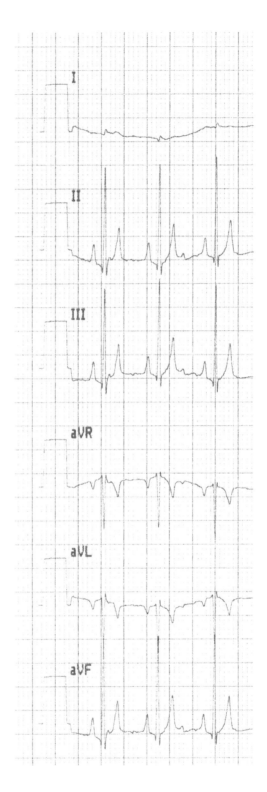

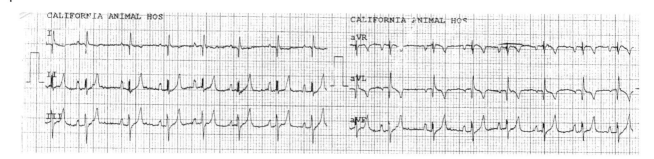

Figure 2.22 Paper speed 25 mm/s, 1 cm/mV, full EKG, canine. **Indeterminate QRS axis**. All limb leads have biphasic patterns and are essentially isoelectric.

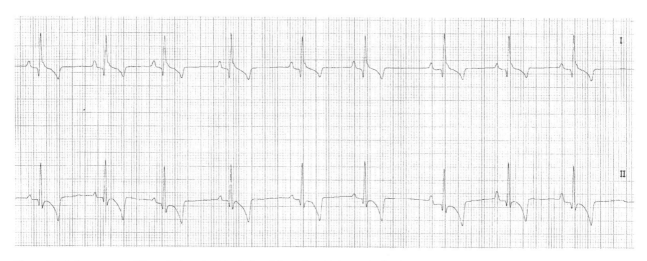

Figure 2.23 Paper speed 50 mm/s, 1 cm/mV, leads I and II, canine. **Early repolarization** with sinus arrhythmia. The Q-Ti is within normal limits and the S-T segment slopes right into the peak of the T wave consistent with early repolarization. This particular dog was not an overtly athletic breed, so the significance of this finding is uncertain.

Further reading

Batchvarov, V.N. (2015). The syndrome of inter-atrial conduction block. *Eur. Cardiol. Rev.* 10 (2): 74–75.

Bayes de Luna, A., Baranchuk, A., LAE, R. et al. (2017). Diagnosis of interatrial block. *J. Geriatr. Cardiol.* 14: 161–165.

Bradley, S.M. and Marriot, M.A. (Dec 1956). Intra-atrial block. *Circulation* XIV.

Chou, T. and Helm, R.A. (1965). The Pseudo P Pulmonale. *Circulation* 32: 96–105.

Chugh, S.N. (2012). *Textbook of Clinical Electrocardiography for Postgraduates, Residents and Practicing Clinicians*, 3e. Jaypee Brother Medical Publishers Ltd.

Marriott, H.J. (1998). *Pearls & Pitfalls in Electrocardiography, Pithy Practical Pointers*, 2e. Williams & Wilkins.

Santilli, R., Sydney Moïse, N., Pariaut, R. and Perego, M. (2018). *Electrocardiography of the Dog and Cat: Diagnosis of Arrhythmias*, 2e. Edna.

Sternic, E.B. et al. (2018). Split P waves: marker of extreme intraatrial delay. *EP Eurpoace* 20 (4): 603.

Surawicz, B. and Knilans, T.K. (2001). *Chou's Electrocardiography in Clinical Practice: Adult and Pediatric*, 5e. Saunders.

3

The P-QRS-T

Trouble

CHAPTER MENU

P-R segment changes, 27
Q-T segment changes, 27
   The prolonged QRS, 27
   Hypokalemia, 28
   Other changes, 28
   Digoxin effects, 32
   Cushing response, 34
   S-T segment elevation/depression, 35
Low-voltage QRS-T, 38
   Electrical alternans, 38
   Pericarditis, 38

P-R segment changes P-R segment depression commonly occurs in association with sinus tachycardia as the negative Ta wave comes out of the QRS complex and closer to the P wave (see Chapter 12). P-R segment elevation may occur in response to atrial infarction in humans, and naturally occurring atrial infarction is apparently exceedingly rare or a nonentity in small animals. A short P-Ri may occur from sinus tachycardia or from the presence of an accessory pathway bypassing the atrioventricular node (see Chapter 16). A prolonged P-Ri may occur from first degree atrioventricular block (see Chapter 20).

Q-T segment changes Changes may occur in the QRS-T segment that signals the clinician to some underlying problem. These include prolongation of the QRS complex, Q-T interval prolongation or shortening, amplitude decrease of the QRS-T complex, coving of the Q-T segment, elevation/depression of the Q-T segment, widening/amplitude changes of the T wave, and the presence of U waves. These changes may be associated with ventricular arrhythmias, accessory pathways, bundle branch blocks, ventricular enlargement, atrial standstill, electrolyte imbalance, hypothermia, drug toxicity, infarction/myocardial ischemia, neurological disorders, and pericardial effusion/pericarditis.

The prolonged QRS When the QRS complex is prolonged for whatever reason, S-T segment changes typically follow with some prolongation of the Q-Ti and T wave changes. The more prolonged the QRS, the more likely the T wave axis becomes opposite that of the QRS complex with a large amplitude and longer duration (a prolonged ventricular depolarization causes an abnormal and prolonged ventricular repolarization). QRS complex prolongation may occur with a ventricular origin of the QRS or a supraventricular origin.

Most commonly, an abnormally prolonged QRS complex is secondary to a **ventricular origin**. Usually, the QRS is prolonged to >0.10 second in the dog, >0.06 second in the cat, is often marked by atrioventricular dissociation (AVD) with compensatory pauses or interpolation and associated with precordial concordance. Uncommonly, prolongation of the QRS may occur due to the presence of an accessory pathway that bypasses the AV node. The resulting QRS is often a fusion, and how prolonged the QRS becomes dependent on how much activation of the ventricular myocardium occurs via the accessory pathway vs. that occurring across the AVN and normal His-Purkinje system (see Chapter 16).

Less often, an abnormally prolonged QRS complex may be *supraventricular* in origin, and three basic causes may be at play. Pre-existent **bundle branch block** (BBB) will lead

---

to a typical pattern in V1 (normal to L axis in the frontal plane for LBBB, and R axis for RBBB, incomplete BBB may minimally prolong the QRS as do fascicular blocks), and interventricular conduction disturbances (IVCDs) may show bizarre notching without a typical BBB pattern in V1 (see Chapters 6–8). These are uncommon.

Ventricular enlargement may also cause prolongation of the QRS. Patients with left ventricular enlargement tend to have a normal to left axis deviation with tall R waves, whereas right ventricular enlargement may result in a normal to right axis shift with deep S waves. Typically, the degree of prolongation is rather modest, with the QRS ranging from 0.06 to 0.08 second QRS in canines. This may be a relatively common cause of QRS prolongation (see previous descriptions in Chapter 2).

Atrial standstill from **hyperkalemia** (in which the QRS may be markedly prolonged if severe) with sinoventricular rhythm is an uncommon cause of prolongation of the QRS complex. The EKG shows characteristic and reversible changes when serum potassium levels elevate. These are bradycardia, prolonged QRS duration, prolonged Q-T interval, decreased P wave amplitude, prolonged P-R interval, and tall, spiked T waves (>25% of QRS total amplitude). The atria are more sensitive to the effects of elevated serum potassium. The SA node and the ventricular myocardium retain their ability to depolarize until very high levels of hyperkalemia are reached. When the P waves disappear

completely, there is still conduction from the SA node to the AV node and ventricles, and the apparent atrial standstill creates the slow rhythm properly termed "sinoventricular rhythm." Sinoventricular rhythm is easily confused with persistent atrial standstill, which has complete lack of P waves and a slow ventricular escape rhythm due to atrial myocarditis or muscular dystrophy (also see Chapter 13). Hyperkalemia is commonly associated with an Addisonian crisis or severe uremia in the dog, whereas in the male cat it is associated with urethral obstruction or severe uremic crises from oliguric/anuric renal failure. Importantly, all of the classic EKG features associated with hyperkalemia may or may not be present in individuals even with severe hyperkalemia.

Hypokalemia The EKG shows characteristic changes when serum potassium levels fall. These are prolonged Q-T interval, depressed S-T segment, decreased T wave amplitude, a wide/tall QRS complex (if severe hypokalemia), and rarely increased P wave amplitude. Hypokalemia may be encountered in association with diabetic ketoacidosis (DKA) and albuterol toxicity, and concomitant hypomagnesemia is not uncommon.

Other changes Electrolyte changes apart from those associated with potassium and other physiologic issues may affect the Q-T segment. Hypercalcemia tends to shorten the Q-T interval (S-T segment portion due to

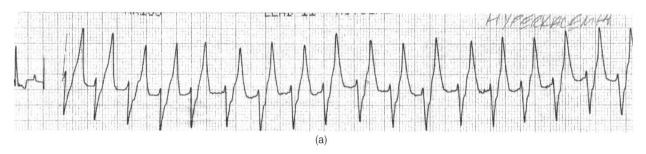

(a)

Figure 3.1a Paper speed 25 mm/s, 1 cm/mV, lead II, feline urethral obstruction, potassium >9 (around 12 mEq/l), pH 7.051, **sinoventricular rhythm**. No P waves are apparent, the QRS complexes are wide and negative with very tall, peaked T waves.

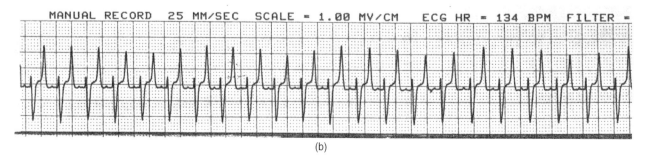

(b)

Figure 3.1b Paper speed 25 mm/s, 1 cm/mV, lead II, same cat, potassium now around 8.0 mEq/l, pH 7.019, administered bicarbonate, P waves just beginning to be visible and the distinction between the deep, wide S wave and the tall, peaked T wave is apparent.

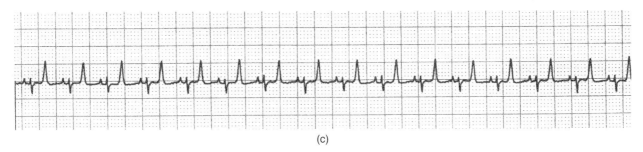

(c)

Figure 3.1c Paper speed 25 mm/s, 1 cm/mV, lead II, same cat, following unblocking, the P waves are obvious, and the tall, peaked T waves still apparent.

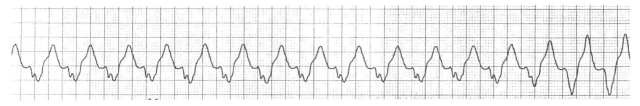

Figure 3.2 Paper speed 50 mm/s, 1 cm/mV, lead II, feline with severe hyperkalemia due to urethral obstruction. **Sinoventricular rhythm**. No P waves are evident, the QRS complexes are wide and bizarre with positive T waves, and by the end of the strip the EKG appears more "sine wave" in appearance. This patient is severely compromised, and a sine-wave appearance to the EKG is frequently preterminal.

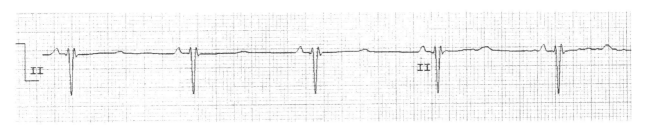

Figure 3.3 Paper speed 50 mm/s, 1 cm/mV, lead II, feline, sinus bradycardia with severe **Q-T interval prolongation** (0.34 second) in this severely dehydrated and weak cat in chronic renal failure suggestive of hypokalemia. There is also marked bradycardia and an L anterior fascicular block giving rise to the deep S waves. Note the relatively tall P waves despite the bradycardia.

shortening of phase 2 of the action potential or AP), and if severe, one may see decreased T wave amplitudes, ± notching or inversion of the T waves, and high take off of the S-T segment in V1 and V2 simulating ischemia. Long Q-T intervals may be seen with hypocalcemia (prolongation of phase 2, S-T segment). The EKG triad of peaked T waves (from hyperkalemia), Q-T interval prolongation (from hypocalcemia), and LVH (tall R waves from systemic hypertension) is strongly suggestive of chronic renal failure. Severe hypermagnesemia can cause AV intraventricular conduction disturbances, culminating in third degree AVB and cardiac arrest, but specific and consistent changes to the QRS appear to be lacking. Hypomagnesemia is associated with hypokalemia or hypocalcemia, can potentiate certain digitalis toxic arrhythmias, and plays a role in the pathogenesis and treatment of acquired long Q-T(U) syndromes and torsades de pointes

(TdP). Congenital long Q-Ti prolongation with associated syncope and sudden death has been described in a family of English Springer Spaniels (KCNQ1 mutation similar to human LQTS 1) but has not formally been described in cats. Congenital short Q-Ti syndrome associated with sudden death in humans has not been described in small animals. Increased dispersion of refractoriness, a substrate for ventricular arrhythmia, can be exacerbated by long-short sequences, bradycardia, and T wave alternans. Hypothermia may lead to bradycardia, long Q-Ti, and so-called Osborn waves (J waves), which are positive "camel hump"-like deflections on the initial portion of the S-T segment that may be evident in the inferior and precordial leads. Post-extrasystolic T wave changes may transiently be seen for a beat or two and is attributed to asynchronous depolarization associated with changes in cycle length.

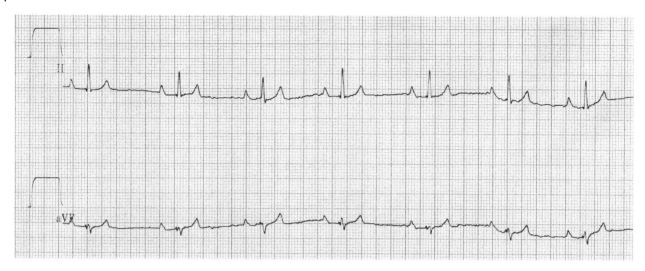

Figure 3.4 Paper speed 50 mm/s, 1 cm/mV, leads II and aVF, canine with **hypercalcemia** (serum calcium > 15.3 mg/dl). The Q-Ti is mildly shortened at 0.16 second and T wave changes are not evident.

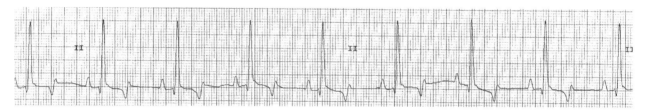

Figure 3.5 Paper speed 50 mm/s, 1 cm/mV, lead II, canine with acute onset of seizures and uremia. The R waves are tall suggestive of LVH from chronic hypertension, the Q-T interval is long from **hypocalcemia** (approximately 0.63 ionized calcium mg/dl), and here the T waves are biphasic, perhaps from hyperkalemia (approximately 7.1 mEq/l). These findings are consistent with chronic renal failure.

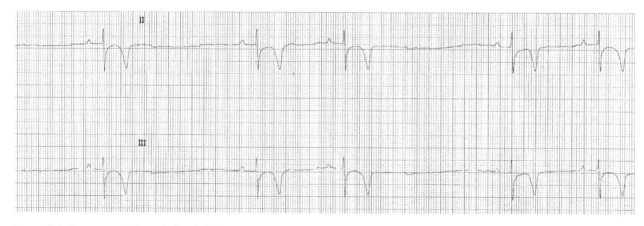

Figure 3.6 Paper speed 50 mm/s, 1 cm/mV, leads II and III, F/S Miniature Schnauzer with atrioventricular valvular disease and history of lymphoma. The Q-Ti is prolonged at 0.26 second with deep T waves and early repolarization. Sinus bradycardia/arrhythmia with possible sinoatrial block suggests underlying sick sinus syndrome. The Q-Ti is excessively prolonged considering the relatively mild bradycardia, the electrolytes were normal, no neurologic deficits were noted, and the patient was normothermic but hypotensive. Perhaps this dog has a congenital **repolarization abnormality/long Q-Ti**.

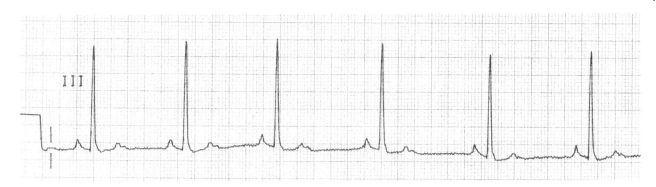

Figure 3.7 Paper speed 50 mm/s, 1 cm/mV, lead III, canine, sinus rhythm. The R waves are tall at 3 mV, suggestive of LVH, the Q-T interval is 0.26 second, and there are **U waves**, small positive deflections following the T waves.

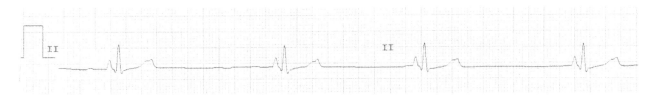

Figure 3.8 Paper speed 50 mm/s, 1 cm/mV, lead II, canine. Sinus bradycardia, **long Q-Ti**, and **U waves**.

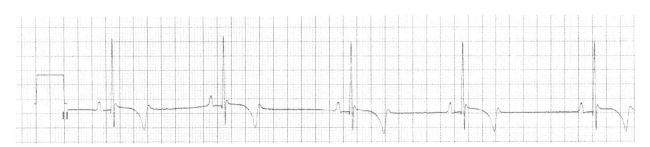

Figure 3.9 Paper speed 50 mm/s, 1 cm/mV, lead II, canine with *Bufo marinus* intoxication. The secretions of the parotid gland of the marine toad contain neurotoxin as well as digitalis-like glycosides. Many cardiac arrhythmias may be seen with acute toxicosis, in addition to neurologic seizures. Typical of glycoside toxicosis, the Q-Ti is markedly prolonged, and the T waves are deep with a scooped-out downstroke similar to that seen with the Cushing response (see below). Type I second degree sinoatrial block accounts for the pauses.

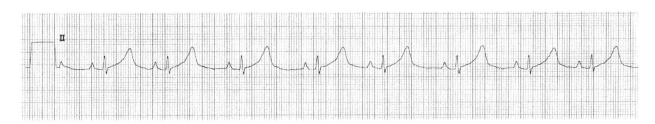

Figure 3.10 Paper speed 50 mm/s, 1 cm/mV, lead II, feline. **Long Q-T interval**, sinus bradycardia. The Q-Ti is 0.28 second. This cat had a normal serum potassium level and very tall T waves.

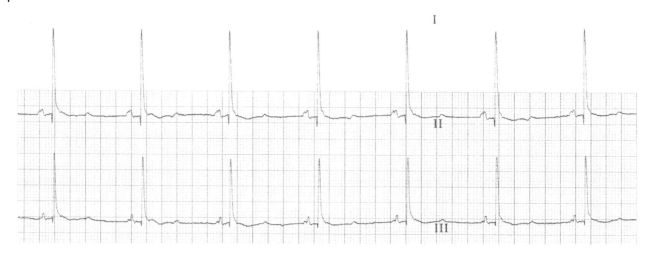

Figure 3.11 Paper speed 50 mm/s, 1 cm/mV, leads II and III, Chihuahua with advanced chronic mitral valvular disease (CMVDz), left atrial enlargement, acute/severe renal failure, hypotension, and hypothermia. **Long Q-T intervals** are present with a distinct hump in the initial portion of the S-T segment in the inferior leads (II, III, and aVF, which is not shown). Best seen in the precordial leads, this is termed a "camel hump," **J** or **Osborn wave**, commonly seen with hypothermia. Tall R waves in this patient are suggestive of LV enlargement.

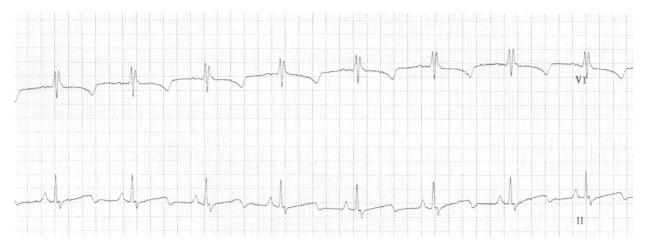

Figure 3.12 Paper speed 50 mm/s, 2 cm/mV, leads V1 and II, hypothermic (95.4 F) feline with pyothorax under anesthesia. Sinus bradycardia, markedly **prolonged Q-T interval**, and **J (Osborn) waves**.

Digoxin effects Classically, patients suffering from digoxin toxicity may not only display a variety of arrhythmias (usually sinoatrial block, atrioventricular block, ventricular premature complexes, accelerated idioventricular/idiofascicular or idiojunctional rhythms, excessively slow ventricular rate response in atrial fibrillation), but may also show characteristic changes on the QRS-T complex itself. The "digoxin effect" results in an S-T segment that is often depressed with a coving of the waveform into the T wave. This results in the appearance of a so-called "Salvador Dali sign" (reversed-tick, hockey-stick, hammock sign, sagging). The Q-Ti may be short and a prolonged P-Ri (first degree atrioventricular block) can be present. The T waves may be diphasic, inverted, or flattened and U waves may be more prominent. Importantly, the effects of digoxin on the QRS complex itself may or *may not* be associated with actual toxicity. Anorexia, vomiting, and diarrhea and/or the development of any new arrhythmia suggest toxicity and warrant discontinuation of the drug or at least a dosage reduction.

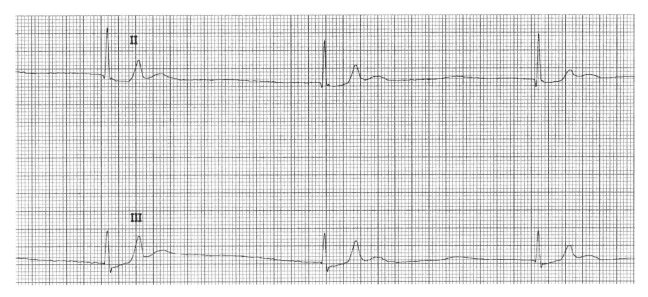

Figure 3.13 Paper speed 50 mm/s, 1 cm/mV, canine with sick sinus syndrome (SSS). HR 46 bpm. Atrial standstill and junctional escape rhythm. The Q-T/Ui is approximately 0.40 second, and prominent **U waves** are visualized following the T waves. No atrial activity is recorded (atrial standstill vs. prolonged sinus arrest), and the QRS complexes are narrow/upright at a rate consistent with that of a junctional escape (or accelerated septal/bundle of His focus/ventricular escape focus).

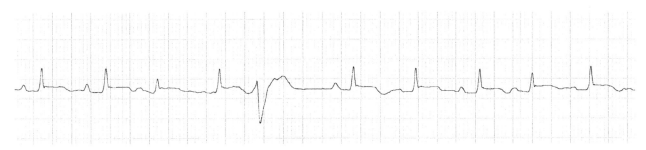

Figure 3.14 Paper speed 50 mm/s, 1 cm/mV, feline. The third beat, seventh and ninth complexes are supraventricular premature beats with minor aberrancy and the fifth is a ventricular premature beat. The **post-extrasystolic beats** show altered, more negative T waves. The S-T segment is mildly elevated suggestive of ischemia and the Q-Ti is mildly prolonged.

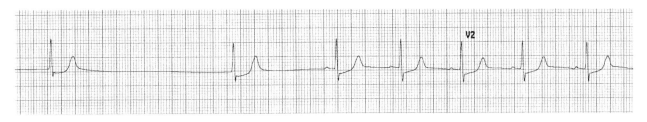

Figure 3.15 Paper speed 50 mm/s, 1 cm/mV, canine with suspected **digoxin toxicity**. Sinus arrhythmia with wandering pacemaker. The S-T segment is mildly depressed with coving into the T wave commonly seen with digoxin administration.

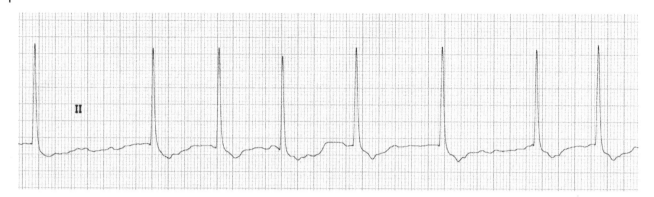

Figure 3.16 Paper speed 50 mm/s, 1 cm/mV, lead II, canine on digoxin and diltiazem for chronic atrial fibrillation with azotemia. The S-T segment is coved consistent with **digitalis effect** and the heart rate is a bit low 100 bpm.

Cushing response Most commonly, this occurs due to a compensatory mechanism responding to pathologic elevations in intracranial pressure from intracranial bleeding (cerebrovascular accident or CVA). Intracranial hypertension results in decreased cerebral blood flow. The local carbon dioxide accumulation that results is sensed in the vasomotor area of the brain and triggers a massive sympathetic discharge. This causes peripheral vasoconstriction, causing marked elevations in mean arterial pressure which then maintains the cerebral perfusion pressure. Baroreceptors sense the hypertension and cause reflex bradycardia. The point is, if you see a patient with bradycardia and hypertension with altered mentation, suspect high intracranial pressures and treat appropriately and aggressively.

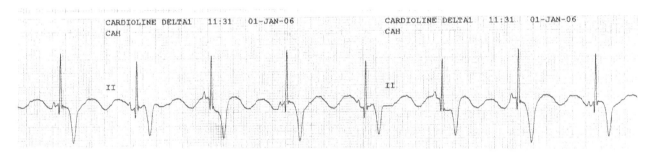

Figure 3.17 Paper speed 25 mm/s, 1 cm/mV, lead II, canine that sustained head injuries from impact with a car. **Cushing response**. Bradycardia with a HR of approximately 50 bpm is present with markedly deep T waves is evident. This patient had peripheral hypertension and altered mentation likely due to cerebral contusions. The undulating baseline seen here was secondary to respiratory excursions.

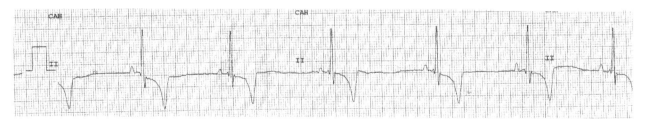

Figure 3.18 Paper speed 50 mm/s, 1 cm/mV, lead II, canine. **Cushing response**. Interestingly, the same markedly deep T waves are present in this hypertensive, bradycardic patient with altered mentation. This is a common EKG abnormality described in humans as a **"CVA T wave pattern"** associated with cerebrovascular accidents (CVAs), particularly *subarachnoid hemorrhage*, with a diffuse and widely splayed appearance to the T wave with marked Q-T interval prolongation. Dogs, however, tend to have intraparenchymal or subdural hemorrhages with intracranial bleeding.

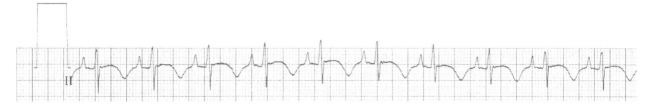

Figure 3.19 Paper speed 50 mm/s, 1 cm/mV, lead II, arrested feline with hypertension. A cerebrovascular accident likely occurred in this patient, as sinus bradycardia, long QT intervals are present, and deep, wide T waves are evident.

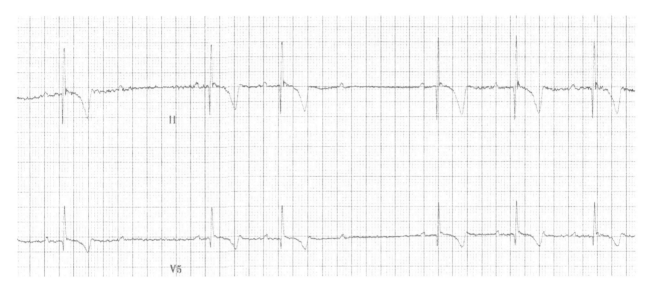

Figure 3.20 Paper speed 50 mm/s, 1 cm/mV, leads II and V5, canine with severe systemic hypertension and a head tilt. **CVA T waves** with first degree and Type I second degree AVB secondary to pathologically elevated vagal tone secondary to presumed intracranial bleeding.

S-T segment elevation/depression In humans (depending on the pattern) associated with myocardial hypoxia (usually ischemic). Depending on the EKG pattern, the likely site of infarction can be determined. Since veterinary patients rarely have coronary atherosclerosis/infarction, S-T segment changes are usually nonspecific and just indicate myocardial hypoxia. T wave inversion is an important

clue to ischemia in people; however, in dogs and cats, the T wave axis is generally unimportant.

J-point: The exact point at which the wave of ventricular depolarization just completes its passage through the heart, point at the end of the QRS, all parts of the ventricles depolarized, including both damaged and normal parts, even the current of injury disappears at this

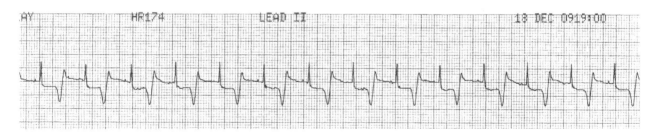

Figure 3.21 Paper speed 25 mm/s, 1 cm/mV, lead II, feline with severe **S-T segment depression and Q-T interval prolongation**, the patient was severely flea anemic and arrested shortly after this strip. The P waves are very small, but positive, and the T waves are deep and negative.

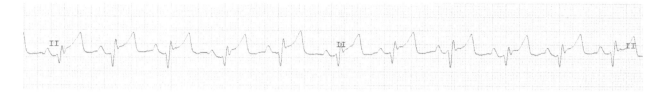

Figure 3.22 Paper speed 50 mm/s, 1 cm/mV, lead II, canine with large heart-based mass. **S-T segment elevation**.

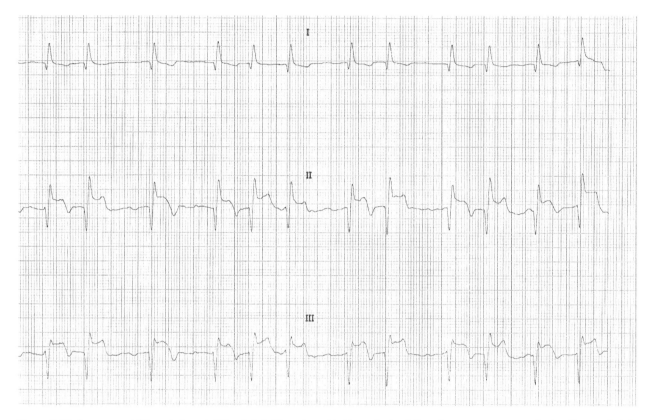

Figure 3.23 Paper speed 50 mm/s, 1 cm/mV, leads I, II, III, canine with biventricular failure from myxomatous valvular disease. Atrial fibrillation with moderate ventricular rate response and severe **S-T segment elevation** in the inferiors. No P waves are evident, and the supraventricular rhythm is irregularly irregular, consistent with atrial fibrillation. This patient was nonambulatory, hypotensive, and was euthanized shortly after this strip. Whether the S-T segment elevation was secondary to myocardial hypoxia vs. a posterior wall infarction was not determined.

point. The potential of the EKG at this instant is at zero voltage.

> ***Take Home Point:*** We usually think of zero voltage at the level of the P-R interval or the baseline level between QRS complexes. This is INCORRECT. "S-T segment depression" is more correctly representative of P-R segment elevation, and "S-T segment elevation" represents P-R segment depression.

The voltage of the current of injury in each lead is the difference between the level of the T-P segment and the actual zero voltage potential, identified at the J-point. Plotting these differences on their respective leads on the hexagonal reference system allows the clinician to presumptively identify the injured area of the ventricles in the frontal plane. Similarly, the chest leads can be used to identify the injured area in the horizontal plane. The negative end of the mean vector calculated points to the permanently depolarized, "injured" myocardium. Generally, transmural ischemia causes S-T segment elevation, and subendocardial ischemia causes S-T segment depression. The R precordials must be examined to screen for the rare right ventricular (RV) infarction. Early repolarization abnormalities classically described in young, athletic human males may cause mild S-T segment elevation and prominent J waves with a rapid upstroke into the T wave and may confuse the examiner with infarction or pericarditis (see Chapter 2). A canine or feline equivalent of Brugada syndrome (RBBB associated with S-T segment elevation in V1–V3 with sudden death in humans) has yet to be described.

Acute Anterior Wall Infarction: V2 should show intense S-T segment elevation from a wide current of injury pattern, indicating an anterior region of ischemia. Lead I should show S-T segment elevation (negative potential) from the current of injury. Lead III should show S-T segment depression (positive potential) from the current of injury. Therefore, the negative end of the vector of the current of injury should point to the left ventricle (LV) and the positive end should point to the RV. This occurs with occlusion of the anterior descending branch of the L circumflex artery (LAD or paraconal artery in veterinary medicine).

Posterior Wall Infarction: V2 should show intense S-T segment depression from a wide current of injury pattern, indicating a posterior region of ischemia. If leads II and III show S-T segment elevation, the mean vector of the current of injury points apically.

Old Recovered Myocardial Infarction: Usually a Q wave develops at the beginning of the QRS in lead I due to loss of muscle mass in the anterior wall of the LV. Usually a Q wave develops at the beginning of the QRS in lead III due to loss of muscle mass in the posteroapical part of the LV. Decreased (or low) voltage QRS may occur due to widespread muscle mass loss. The QRS may be prolonged from conduction block.

T wave Changes: Remember, the T waves are only stable in V1 and V10 in the dog. When conduction of depolarization through the ventricles is greatly delayed, the T wave is almost always opposite in polarity to the mean QRS polarity (T wave inversion). This is because the refractory periods of the RV and LV are similar. This is also the reason why the T waves are opposite in polarity of the QRS in right or left BBB, ventricular premature complexes, or aberrantly conducted supraventricular premature complexes. Mild ischemia may result in T wave changes; biphasic T waves may appear. Hyperacute marked T wave amplitude increase occurs within minutes of MI and last a few hours. The T waves then tend to decrease in amplitude, inverting in the leads facing the ischemic area. S-T segment changes tend to resolve in one to two days, at which time Q waves appear.

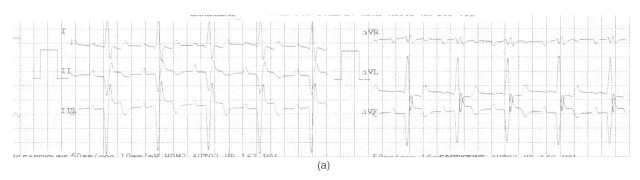

(a)

Figure 3.24a Paper speed 50 mm/s, 1 cm/mV, full EKG. Doberman with very large infiltrative mass of the RV, LV apex, and IVS. **S-T segment elevation** in the inferior leads creates a current of injury pattern, the negative pole of which points to an apical region of ischemia.

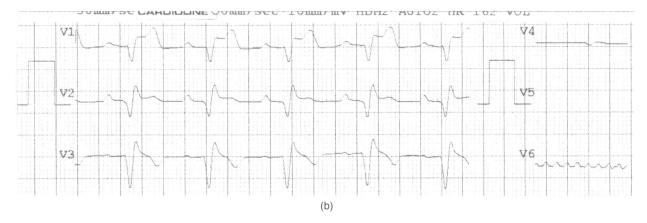

(b)

Figure 3.24b Paper speed 50 mm/s, 1 cm/mV, precordial leads, the same dog. "V2" is actually V5 and "V3" is actually V10. The current of injury pattern here is wide, with S-T segment elevation most prominent in VI, the negative pole of which points to an anterior (ventral in the dog) region of ischemia.

Low-voltage QRS-T Classically associated with pericardial effusion, a low-amplitude QRS-T complex may also be associated with a large thoracic cavity, obesity, and pleural effusion – all the result of the insulating effects of fluid, air, and/or adipose tissue. Low-voltage QRS complexes may also be produced from hypovolemia, hemoconcentration/polycythemia, or be idiopathic in origin. Conversely, high-voltage QRS complexes may not only occur with ventricular enlargement, but also be the result of anemia. These changes are secondary to changes in blood resistivity. Low-voltage QRS complexes may also be the result of large amounts of intrathoracic fat, the short-circuiting effects of pericardial/pleural effusion and pneumothorax, or myxedema coma with severe hypothyroidism.

Electrical alternans Total QRS-T alternans occurs when the amplitude of the QRS complex (and to a less obvious extent, the T wave amplitude) alternates regularly on a beat-to-beat basis. Less commonly, it may be phasic over a series of beats, usually the result of respiratory variation. This may be subtle or quite dramatic and is highly associated with pericardial effusion, though it may be seen during some tachyarrhythmias and occasionally with changes in intracardiac blood volume (Brody effect, so-called **pseudo-electrical alternans**). The phenomenon when secondary to pericardial effusion is due to the swinging motion of the heart within the fluid-filled pericardium and often produces very small QRS complexes. Low-voltage QRS in combination with sinus tachycardia is probably the most common EKG manifestation of pericardial effusion in reality. Electrical alternans in association with pericardial effusion has been shown to be rate-dependent and most likely to occur at relatively normal heart rates of 90–144 bpm in dogs. P wave alternans is difficult to detect (>10% variation) due to normally low P wave amplitudes, and it may be seen with alpha-antagonist administration. Isolated T wave alternans may herald ventricular tachyarrhythmias and is associated with prolongation of the Q-T interval. Pseudo-electrical alternans associated with supraventricular tachycardia, while suggestive of atrioventricular reentrant tachycardia, may be seen during sinus tachycardia, other supraventricular tachycardias, atrial fibrillation, or ventricular tachycardias as well as even during sinus arrhythmia. While electrical alternans associated with pericardial effusion commonly produces pulsus paradoxus (phasic increasing intensity of palpable pulses during expiration), pulse deficits are common during pseudo-electrical alternans with tachycardia.

Pericarditis Pericarditis is typically associated with some degree of pericardial effusion and may be an underlying occult cause of so-called "idiopathic hemopericardium." These cases may or may not be associated with a cardiac mass, *Bartonella* or *Leishmania* infection. Long-term

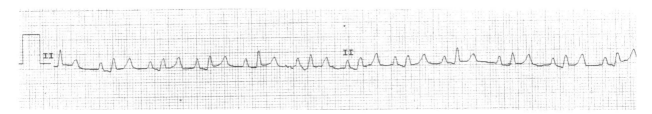

Figure 3.25 Paper speed 25 mm/s, 1 cm/mV, lead II, obese Husky, sinus rhythm with **low-voltage QRS complexes**. Large amounts of intrathoracic (or intrapericardial) fat can cause the QRS complexes to become small, as can pericardial effusion. The R waves are only approximately 0.4 mV in this large-breed dog.

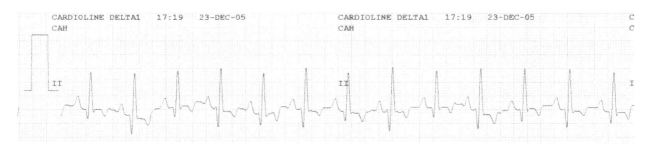

Figure 3.26 Paper speed 50 mm/s, 2 cm/mV, lead II, Old English Sheepdog with a large volume of pericardial effusion. Sinus tachycardia with small (low voltage) QRS complexes are present (R waves less than 1 mV in amplitude in a large dog) with **electrical alternans**.

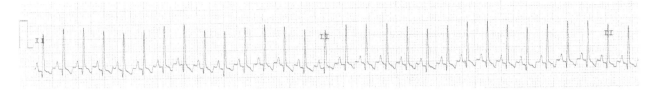

Figure 3.27 Paper speed 25 mm/s, 1 cm/mV, lead II, canine with pericardial effusion. Sinus tachycardia with **phasic electrical alternans** that occurs gradually over a number of beats is evident. The R wave amplitude gradually increases and decreases (vs. on a beat-to-beat basis) as the heart swings in the fluid-filled pericardium.

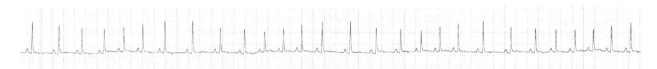

Figure 3.28 Paper speed 25 mm/s, 1 cm/mV, lead I, canine. **Phasic pseudo-electrical alternans** coincident with respiratory phase during sinus arrhythmia. During inspiration, the sinus rate increases and the QRS amplitude decreases. This is likely due to a combination of the Brody effect along with changes in forelimb lead distance that occurs with chest excursion. The larger the inspiration, the further the electrodes may shift in position (especially if they are closer to the elbows) and the smaller the ventricular volume as cycle length decreases leaving less time for ventricular filling. This patient had no pericardial effusion.

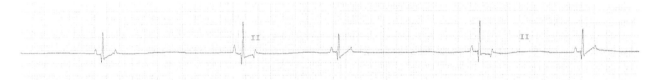

Figure 3.29 Paper speed 25 mm/s, 1 cm/mV, lead II, canine sedated with medetomidine, BP 130 mmHg. Sinus **bradycardia** and **pseudo-electrical alternans**. Every other beat displays alternation of the P-QRS-T amplitude, with biphasic T waves apparent on the higher-amplitude beats. These alternations were not the result of respiratory excursions (a rule out, especially for phasic electrical alternans). Electrical alternans has been reported in association with xylazine administration, another alpha-blocker and is presumed to be secondary to changes in autonomic influences on depolarization in the heart. Alternations in the P-R interval and P wave amplitudes are also present, albeit subtly. These changes may be attributed to the so-called **Brody effect**, in which variation of the R wave amplitude is seen in association with changes in intracardiac blood volume. Here, the beats terminating long cycle lengths have taller R waves, possibly due to increased filling of the ventricle from a relatively longer diastole. This patient had no pericardial effusion.

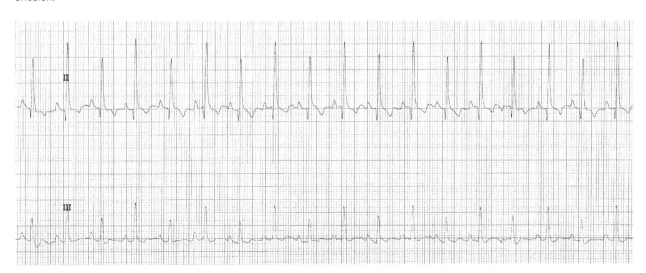

Figure 3.30 Paper speed 50 mm/s, 1 cm/mV, lead I, canine. Sinus **tachycardia** and **pseudo-electrical alternans**. Every-other-beat displays marked alternation of the QRS amplitude by 0.6 mV. Mitral valvular disease in this patient resulted in an enlarged L heart, and this patient was in heart failure without pericardial effusion. Congestive heart failure may result in sinus tachycardia and QRS alternans.

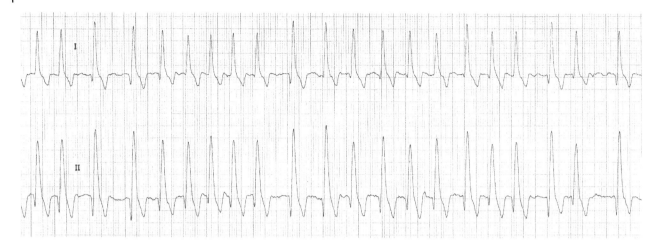

Figure 3.31 Paper speed 50 mm/s, 1 cm/mV, leads I and II, Great Dane with dilated cardiomyopathy. **Atrial fibrillation and pseudo-electrical alternans**. P waves are absent and the ventricular response is irregularly irregular consistent with atrial fibrillation. The QRS complexes are mildly prolonged from left ventricular enlargement. There is conspicuous alternation of the QRS amplitudes (up to 0.5 mV change) as a direct function of cycle length consistent with the **Brody effect**. Longer cycle lengths permit more time for ventricular filling, resulting in a QRS of greater amplitude.

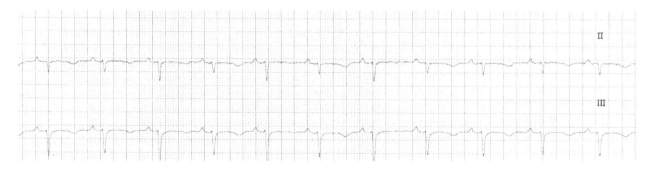

Figure 3.32 Paper speed 50 mm/s, 1 cm/mV, feline with severe renal failure. Sinus bradycardia, LAD (LAFB pattern), long Q-Ti (0.26 second), and intermittent **QRS-T pseudo-electrical alternans**. Though the long Q-Ti is suggestive of hypokalemia or hypocalcemia, the electrolytes in this patient happened to be within normal limits. The QRS-T complexes alternate in amplitude for the first half of the strip, then remain stable in size for the last four beats. T wave alternans in association with bradycardia and LQTi predisposes patients to a potentially lethal form of polymorphic ventricular tachycardia known as torsades de pointes.

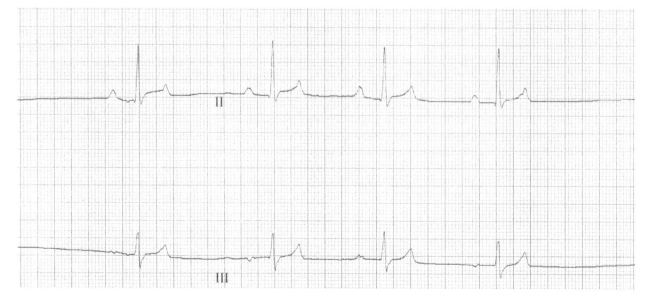

Figure 3.33 Paper speed 50 mm/s, 1 cm/mV, leads II and III, canine sedated with medetomidine. Sinus arrhythmia, first degree AV block (P-Ri 0.14 second), and **P wave alternans**. The P wave change morphology on a beat-to-beat basis. This is likely secondary to the autonomic changes induced by medetomidine.

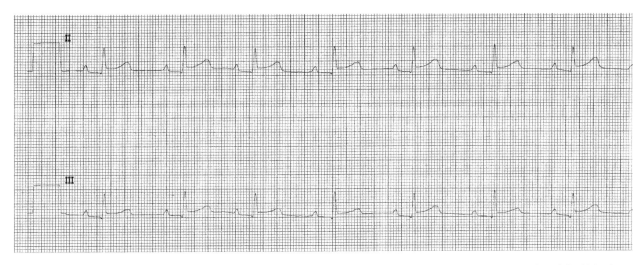

Figure 3.34 Paper speed 50 mm/s, 1 cm/mV, leads II and III, canine with pericardial effusion. **S-T segment elevation** (0.2 mV) in the inferior leads. Electrical alternans is not evident and this patient is not overtly tachycardic (HR 109 bpm). The S-T segment elevation suggests myocardial ischemia and some degree of concurrent pericarditis is commonly associated with pericardial effusion.

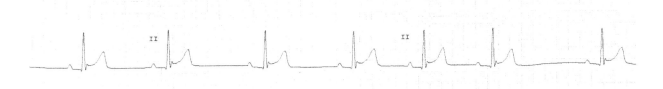

Figure 3.35 Paper speed 50 mm/s, 1 cm/mV, lead II, canine with notable **S-T segment elevation.** This patient had pericardial effusion secondary to a right atrial mass. S-T segment elevation is likely secondary to epicardial inflammation.

pericarditis may result in severe fibrosing (constrictive and/or constrictive-effusive pericarditis). Acute pericarditis in humans may produce a characteristic appearance of the QRS in V1. This has been referred to as the "stork leg sign" given the appearance. The T-P segment may slope slightly from higher at the J-point to lower at the Q/R wave, leading to an undulating baseline which may give the appearance of P-R depression and S-T segment elevation (so-called Spodick's sign). Most often, EKG changes associated with pericarditis in dogs is attributed to pericardial effusion (sinus tachycardia, low-voltage QRS, electrical alternans) and in many cases some degree of S-T segment elevation.

Further reading

Bové, C.M. (2010). ECG of the month. *JAVMA* 237 (5): 509–511.

Brugada, J., Brugada, P., and Brugada, R. (1999). The syndrome of right bundle branch block ST segment elevation in V1 to V3 and sudden death – The Brugada syndrome. *Europace* 1: 156–166.

Braunwald, E., Zipes, D., and Libby, P. (2001). *Heart Disease: A Textbook of Cardiovascular Medicine*, 6e. Saunders.

Chung, E.K. (1972). Digitalis intoxication. *Postgrad. Med. J.* 48: 163–179.

Kittleson, M.D. and Kienle, R.D. (1998). *Small Animal Cardiovascular Medicine*. Mosby.

Levine, H.D., Lown, B., and Streeper, R.B. (1952). The clinical significance of Postextrasystolic T-wave changes. *Circulation* VI: 538–548.

Marriott, H.J. (1998). *Pearls & Pitfalls in Electrocardiography, Pithy Practical Pointers*, 2e. Williams & Wilkins.

Mendes, R.G.G. and Evora, P.R.B. (1999). Atrial infarction is a unique and often unrecognized clinical entity. *Arq. Bras. Cardiol.* 72 (3): 338–342.

Omar, H.R. and Camporesi, E.M. (2017). Pseudoelectrical alternans during supraventricular tachycardia. *Turk J. Emerg. Med.* 17 (1): 32–33.

Romito, G.I., Côté, E., and Domenench, O. (2013). ECG of the month. *JAVMA* 243 (8): 1108–1110.

Saelinger, C.A., Estrada, A.H., and Maisenbacher, H.W. III, (2008). ECG of the month. *JAVMA* 233 (2): 231–233.

Santilli, R., Sydney Moïse, N., Pariaut, R., and Perego, (2018). *Electrocardiography of the Dog and Cat: Diagnosis of Arrhythmias*, 2e. Edna.

Scheinman, M. (2016). *Electrophysiology Clinics. Interpretation of Complex Arrhythmias: A Case-Based Approach*, vol. 8. No.1. Elsevier.

Surawicz, B. and Knilans, T.K. (2001). *Chou's Electrocardiography in Clinical Practice: Adult and Pediatric*, 5e. Saunders.

Van Mieghem, C. et al. (2004). The clinical value of the ECG in Noncardiac conditions. *Chest* 125: 1561–1576.

Ware, W.A. et al. (2015). Sudden death associated with QT interval prolongation and KCNQ1 Gen mutation in a family of English Springer Spaniels. *J. Vet. Intern. Med.* 29 (2): 561–568.

Weintraub, B.M. and McHenry, L.C. (1974). Cardiac abnormalities in subarachnoid hemorrhage: a resume. *Stroke* 5.

Part II

Aberrancy

Normal myocardial tissue may conduct normally or abnormally. Abnormal depolarization of myocardial tissue typically results in some abnormality of morphology of the resulting complex and commonly prolongs depolarization of the affected tissue. The atria are capable of being conducted aberrantly as are the ventricles. Aberrant atrial depolarization results in an abnormal P wave morphology, whereas aberrant ventricular depolarization results in abnormal QRS morphology, often with prolonged duration and secondary S-T segment changes. Bundle branch blocks (BBBs) are supraventricular (usually sinoatrial) beats that are conducted with aberration. Generally, this means there is a P wave in front of a strange-looking, prolonged/widened QRS complex. Beats conducted with BBB are frequently confused with ventricular arrhythmias and often cause unnecessary alarm. The term "bundle branch" refers to one of the branches coming off the common bundle from the AV node that branch to the right or left ventricles and are part of the specialized conduction system that allow for normally rapid and coordinated ventricular depolarization. The right bundle branch (considered to be one fascicle) services the right ventricle, and the left bundle branch services the left ventricle which also subdivides into anterior and posterior fascicles. The fascicular division may really be only an electrical phenomenon as there is wide variation on exact branching of the left bundle seen in both people and animals. Bear that in mind. The left bundle branch may be trifascicular with anterior, medial, and posterior divisions, or may have diffuse branching.

Bundle branch blocks may be functional (i.e. ventricular in origin or supraventricular conducted with aberrancy), transient, and even rate-dependent. Some authors reserve the term "aberrancy" for rate-related/transient conduction abnormalities. Permanent bundle branch block results in BBB of all supraventricular beats. Bundle branch blocks, even if "complete," may simply be due to extreme conduction delay in the affected branch, allowing for transseptal activation from the functional branch and does not imply a complete anatomic transection of the branch in question. Incomplete BBBs may produce axis deviation and mild QRS prolongation and represent the mildest "degree" of BBB. Incomplete BBB has been referred to as "1st degree BBB," intermittent BBB as "2nd degree BBB" (with 2:1, Wenckebach and Mobitz varieties), and permanent or complete BBB as "3rd degree BBB." An ectopic ventricular beat (ventricular premature complex/VPC, accelerated focus or ventricular escape complex) occurring in the same ventricle with an otherwise blocked bundle at the right time may actually normalize/narrow the QRS duration. Wenckebach periodicity in a bundle branch may produce group beating with progressive worsening of conduction, typically involving a normal QRS for the first cycle in each sequence, followed by worsening incomplete BBB in the next cycle(s) and terminated by a cycle with complete BBB. Wenckebach (Type I) periodicity rarely affects the His bundle or distal bundle branches, which more commonly is characterized by Mobitz (Type II) block in which failure of conduction is random. Uncommonly, alternating patterns of BBB may occur (i.e. during trifascicular block), typically secondary to concealed transseptal conduction, though other mechanisms may be at work. Supraventricular tachycardia with pre-existent BBB may mimic ventricular tachycardia. Ventricular conduction delay may also result from nonspecific intraventricular conduction disturbances that do not display classic BBB patterns. By themselves, BBBs may cause no significant hemodynamic compromise or warrant specific therapy. However, they can represent an electrical manifestation of underlying cardiac disease, especially in cases of deceleration-dependent BBB, left BBB, bi/trifascicular blocks, and interventricular conduction disturbances. Therefore, identification of a BBB should warrant further testing (radiographs, echocardiography, etc.).

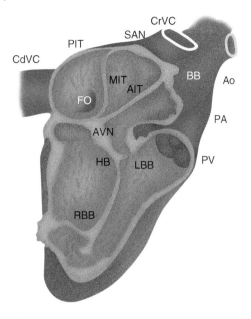

Figure AI.1 Illustration of the conduction system of the heart, right atrium and right ventricle opened. **CrVC**: cranial vena cava, **CdVC**: caudal vena cava, **FO**: fossa ovalis, **SAN**: sinoatrial node, **AIT**: anterior internodal tract, **MIT**: middle internodal tract, **PIT**: posterior internodal tract, **BB**: Bachman's bundle, **Ao**: aorta, **PA**: pulmonary artery, **PV**: pulmonary valve, **AVN**: atrioventricular node, **HB**: His bundle, **LBB**: left bundle branch, **RBB**: right bundle branch, **TV**: tricuspid valve.

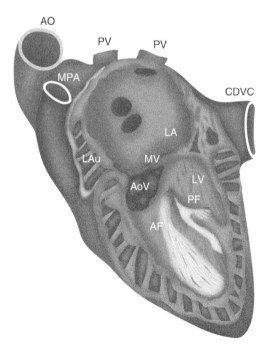

Figure AI.2 Illustration of the conduction system of the heart, left atrium and left ventricle opened. **Ao**: aorta, **MPA**: main pulmonary artery, **PV**: pulmonary vein, **LAu**: left auricle, **LA**: left atrium, **MV**: mitral valve, **CdVC**: caudal vena cava, **AoV**: aortic valve, **LV**: left ventricle, **AF**: anterior fascicle of the left bundle branch, **PF**: posterior fascicle of the left bundle branch.

Atrial Aberrancy

Interatrial/intra-atrial block
Chung's phenomenon
Atrial ectopy

Right Bundle Branch Block

Incomplete bundle branch block
Ashman's phenomenon/Second-in-the-row anomaly
Phase 4 deceleration-dependent and intermittent bundle branch block
Complete right bundle branch block

Left Bundle Branch Block

Incomplete left bundle branch block
Phase 3 acceleration-dependent and intermittent bundle branch block
Complete left bundle branch block

Fascicular Blocks

Left anterior fascicular block
Left medial fascicular block
Left posterior fascicular block
Bifascicular block
  Masquerading bundle branch block
Trifascicular block
Arborization block

Wide-Complex Supraventricular Tachycardia /Intraventricular Conduction Disturbances

Wide-complex supraventricular tachycardia
Intraventricular conduction disturbances

4

Atrial Aberrancy

CHAPTER MENU
Interatrial block, 45
Chung's phenomenon, 47
Atrial ectopy, 47

The atria are capable of aberrant conduction, just as the ventricles are. Changes in morphology and/or duration of the P wave constitute aberrancy of atrial depolarization. These changes may be transient (second degree interatrial block, Chung's phenomenon, atrial fusion) or permanent (first and third degree interatrial block). Interatrial block may be divided into three degrees similar to that seen with sinoatrial, atrioventricular, ventriculoatrial, bundle branch, and exit blocks. If the atria are depolarized prematurely, the following sinus beat may be aberrantly conducted (Chung's phenomenon) or the focus is temporarily displaced to an ectopic atrial center. Interatrial/intra-atrial block may be the result of atrial enlargement or atrial fibrosis/myocarditis while Chung's phenomenon and atrial fusion are rate-dependent.

Interatrial block

P mitrale (prolongation of the P wave) is also considered a manifestation of atrial aberrancy and mild prolongation has been termed first degree interatrial block (partial interatrial block). First degree interatrial block leads to mild and persistent P wave prolongation (>0.06 second in dogs, >0.05 second in cats) often with associated notching. Separation of the R atrial and L atrial depolarization is more evident when L atrial enlargement is present leading to the notching. Since P mitrale is associated with left atrial enlargement (which generally does not go away), this EKG phenomenon leads to permanent prolongation of the P wave (see Chapter 2).

Intermittent prolongation of the P wave has been termed second degree interatrial block. The differentiation of Type I (Wenckebach) and II second degree (Mobitz) IAB has not been described in small animals and likely difficult if not impossible to differentiate on surface EKG. Theoretically, Type I should have progressive prolongation of the P wave and Type II should have random/intermittent prolongation. Brief induction of second degree interatrial block has been implicated as a cause of Chung's phenomenon following premature beats. Atrial ectopy and fusion must be excluded by demonstrating a lack of at least intermittent premature or late ectopic atrial beats. Wandering pacemaker accounting for changes in P wave morphology can generally be ruled out by a conspicuous absence of concurrent respiratory or phasic sinus arrhythmia.

Markedly and permanently prolonged/diphasic P waves in the inferiors leads (split P waves) has been termed third degree interatrial block (advanced interatrial block or intra-atrial block). Intra-atrial block is assumed when the R and L atria depolarize separately leading to two distinct P waves preceding single supraventricular QRS complexes and is the result of complete block in Bachmann's bundle. The LA depolarization is actually retrograde so the "second P wave" will be negative as left atrial activation proceeds from a caudoventral to superiodorsal direction. The normal atrial repolarization (Ta wave) should be excluded. The presence of abnormally prolonged P′ waves (of ectopic atrial foci) or F waves (of atrial

Interpretation of the Electrocardiogram in Small Animals, First Edition. Nick A. Schroeder.
© 2021 John Wiley & Sons Inc. Published 2021 by John Wiley & Sons Inc.

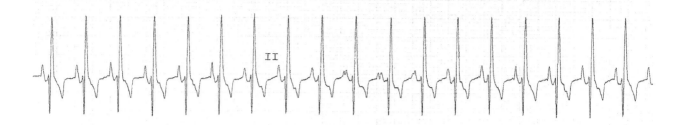

Figure 4.1 Paper speed 25 mm/s, 1 cm/mV, lead II, canine, sinus rhythm, intermittent P mitrale (**second degree interatrial block**). The P waves are 0.04 ms on average and vary up to 0.08 second. Atrial ectopy and fusion should be excluded. The lack of obvious atrial premature beats and regular atrial rhythm here supports this interpretation.

flutter) with notching/splintering or coarse atrial fibrillation may indicate an interatrial conduction defect/block in the absence of sinus rhythm. Historically, the term "complete intra-atrial block" had been used to describe completely dissociated left and right atrial depolarizations (*atrial dissociation*, see Chapter 15), as well as being interchangeable with IAB, leading to some confusion. For these reasons, the term "3rd degree IAB" is preferable. These patients are considered at risk for atrial tachyarrhythmias including atrial fibrillation (Bayés syndrome) given associated underlying left atrial enlargement and atrial fibrosis.

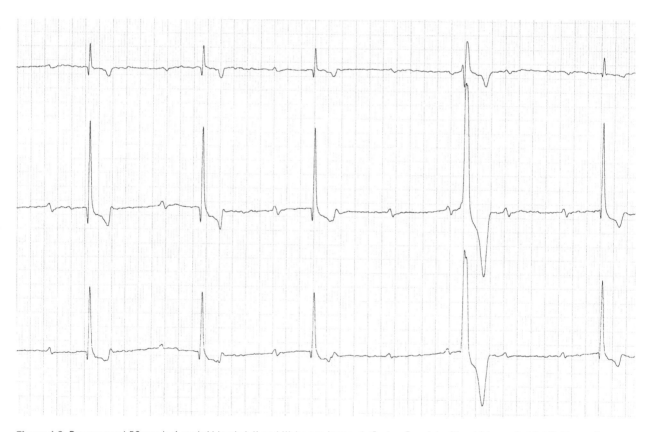

Figure 4.2 Paper speed 50 mm/s, 1 cm/mV, leads I, II and III (top to bottom). Cocker Spaniel with a history of atrial flutter and high-grade AV block. R/O **third degree interatrial block**. Sinus rhythm, marked first degree AVB (P-Ri 0.30 second) and high-grade AVB (Type II second degree) with the pause following the second QRS (capture) terminated by escape rhythm (R/O junctional by rate with deceleration-dependent left bundle branch block). The P waves are markedly prolonged (at least 0.09 second) and diphasic as the left atrium is depolarized in a retrograde manner. The Ta waves are actually positive and low amplitude at 0.05 mV.

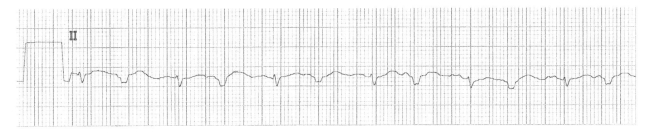

Figure 4.3 Paper speed 50 mm/s, 1 cm/mV, lead II, feline with cardiomyopathy. Ventricular bigeminy (1 : 1 extrasystole). Every-other-beat is a ventricular premature complex. The sinus beats have markedly prolonged P waves (0.06 second) that are notched with nearly separated left and right atrial depolarizations suggestive of **third degree interatrial block**.

Chung's phenomenon The atria may be conducted aberrantly following ectopic beats. The post-extrasystolic P wave may be of altered morphology following atrial premature complexes (APCs), ventricular premature complexes (VPCs), or ectopic escape beats with ventriculoatrial conduction, and this has been termed Chung's phenomenon. This is analogous to post-extrasystolic aberrancy of the QRS following VPCs (see Chapter 24) and may be the result of transient second degree interatrial block.

Atrial ectopy It has been demonstrated in isolated rabbit atria that post-extrasystolic supraventricular beats with altered P wave morphology may actually be **ectopic atrial beats** (atrial escape complexes-see Chapter 13), which can actually persist for a few beats before the SAN takes over again. If the "aberrant" post-extrasystolic P wave occurs after an exact normal sinus P-P interval (i.e. perfect resetting), aberrant atrial conduction is favored.

If the P′-post-extrasystolic P interval is longer (i.e. reset with a pause), the post-extrasystolic beat may more likely be ectopic atrial in origin. **Atrial fusion** may also explain some of these beats if the P′-P interval equals the P-P interval. If the post-extrasystolic beat has a P′ wave with morphology intermediate between that of the sinus P wave and the ectopic, or if an atrial escape has intermediate P′ wave morphology between sinus and ectopic atrial, atrial fusion is a real possibility.

While theoretically possible, Chung's phenomenon seems unlikely in most circumstances, whether it results from initiating ectopic supraventricular or ventricular foci. Minimal alterations in P′ waves and even less obvious changes in post-extrasystolic P wave morphology have been demonstrated in dogs following atrial pacing at a variety of coupling intervals. During ectopic atrial or junctional tachycardia, atrial flutter, or ventricular tachycardia with VA conduction, variable P′ morphology during the tachycardia is generally unheard of. This would be

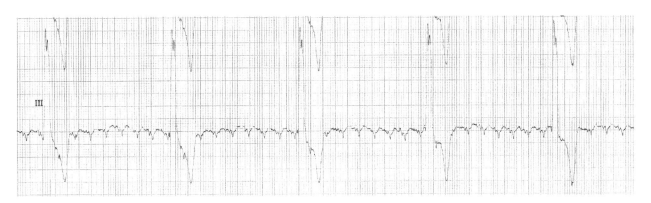

Figure 4.4 Paper speed 50 mm/s, 1 cm/mV, lead III, Cocker Spaniel. Atrial flutter, high grade or third degree atrioventricular block, suspected **interatrial block** and ventricular escape rhythm. The F waves are prolonged at 0.07 second with bizarre notching suggestive of an interatrial conduction defect.

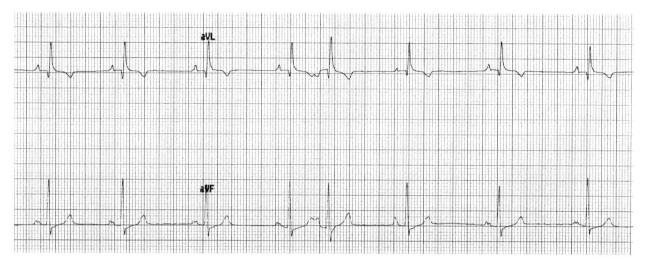

Figure 4.5 Paper speed 50 mm/s, 1 cm/mV, leads aVL and aVF, canine. The fifth complex is a SVPC (likely septal APC), which resets the rhythm and is followed by an apparent sinus beat with altered P wave morphology consistent with **Chung's phenomenon**. The APC resets with a P′-Pi equal to that of the underlying P-Pi. The following sinus P waves resume normal morphology.

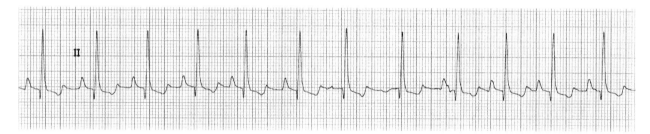

Figure 4.6 Paper speed 50 mm/s, 1 cm/mV, lead I, canine. The seventh complex is an APC that resets. The following eighth and ninth complexes have altered P wave morphology consistent with **Chung's phenomenon**. It is tempting to simply diagnose multifocal APCs; however, the eighth and ninth complexes do not vary in rate at all from the underlying sinus rate which follows and consecutive atrial fusions in rhythm with the sinus nodal discharge is unlikely.

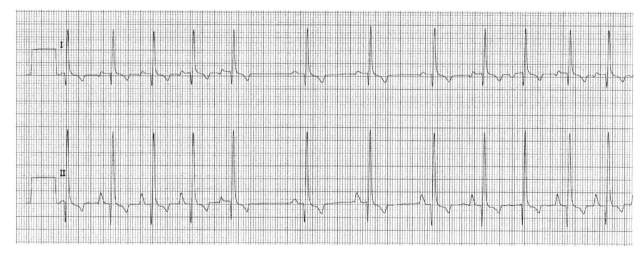

Figure 4.7 Paper speed 50 mm/s, 1 cm/mV, leads I and II, canine. The fifth beat is an APC that resets with a pause. The post-extrasystolic beat has altered P wave morphology, but likely is **ectopic atrial**. Beat #10 appears to be an **atrial fusion**.

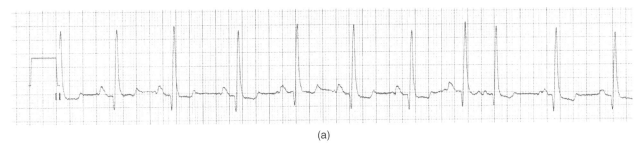

(a)

Figure 4.8a Paper speed 50 mm/s, 1 cm/mV, lead II, canine. The eighth complex is premature and resets the rhythm consistent with an APC, the ninth (post-extrasystolic) complex has a sinus P wave of altered morphology seemingly consistent with **Chung's phenomenon** since the APC resets and the P′-Pi is equal to the P-Pi.

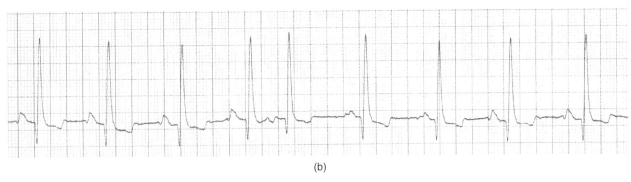

(b)

Figure 4.8b Paper speed 50 mm/s, 1 cm/mV, lead II, same dog. Another APC (fifth complex) occurs, but this time is followed by two supraventricular beats with altered P wave morphology. It seems unlikely that partial refractoriness of the atrial myocardium could persist for this length of time following the APC, and that these beats are more likely **ectopic atrial** in origin. The APC caused a brief **transition of a pacemaker** via concealed conduction by transiently suppressing the sinus node, allowing the ectopic focus to capture the heart for two beats.

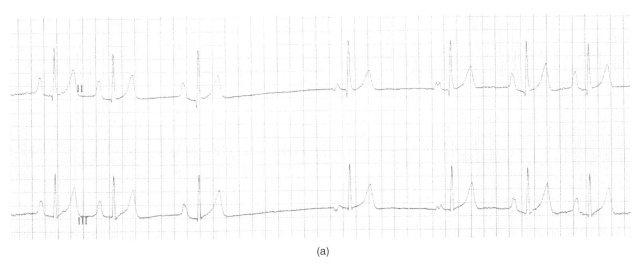

(a)

Figure 4.9a Paper speed 50 mm/s, 1 cm/mV, leads II and III, canine with CMVDz. **Atrial escape beat** with possible **post-extrasystolic aberrancy** vs. **ectopic atrial beat**. A pause in the rhythm elicits an ectopic atrial *escape* beat (#4). The fifth complex has altered P wave morphology suggestive of a Chung's phenomenon-type post-extrasystolic aberration. The fifth beat is likely ectopic atrial from another focus given the different P′ morphology and the fact that it occurs at such a *long* cycle length following the ectopic atrial escape beat, making it unlikely for partial atrial refractoriness to have persisted this length of time to cause aberrant atrial conduction. Alternatively, the atrial escape beat (#4) may simply be an **atrial fusion** between the sinus and ectopic atrial focus.

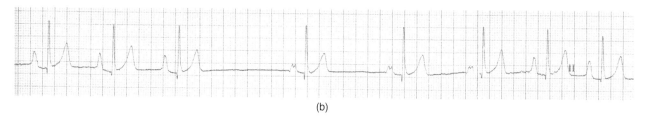

(b)

Figure 4.9b Paper speed 50 mm/s, 1 cm/mV, lead II, same dog. **Ectopic atrial escape rhythm**. A pause after the third beat elicits a three-beat run of atrial escape rhythm, confirming that the above "post-extrasystolic aberrant P wave" is really ectopic atrial. Note that the P′ morphology is identical to that of the fifth beat in the above strip. While this patient may have had two ectopic atrial escape foci, atrial fusion is still a possible explanation of the second P′ morphology (beat #4 in the first strip).

expected if rapid stimulation of the atria occurred, and at least on the second-in-the-row beat of an ectopic tachycardia (in which the ventricular complex may variably become aberrant if supraventricular in origin). That said, Chung's phenomenon appears to be occasionally a valid concept, albeit perhaps more likely at relatively slow cycle lengths with associated longer relative refractory periods of atrial myocardial cells as seen in humans.

Take Home Message: Chung's phenomenon causes changes of the post-extrasystolic P wave and may confuse the examiner with multifocal SVPCs. Post-extrasystolic displacement of the pacemaker and atrial fusion also result in changes in P wave morphology. While these EKG phenomena are interesting, they tend to be only clinically important insofar as are the frequency and origin of the initiating ectopic premature beats.

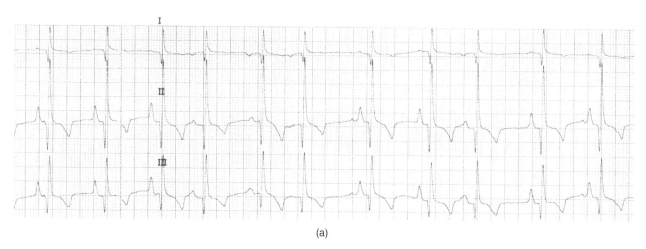

(a)

Figure 4.10a Paper speed 50 mm/s, 1 cm/mV, leads I, II, III, canine. The fourth beat is an APC (likely left atrial since the P′ is negative in lead I), resets the rhythm, and is followed by a beat with an altered P′ morphology possibly aberrant due to Chung's phenomenon. The sixth and ninth beats are APCs with post-extrasystolic sinus captures with P waves of normal morphology. The fifth complex is most likely an **atrial fusion beat** (see below).

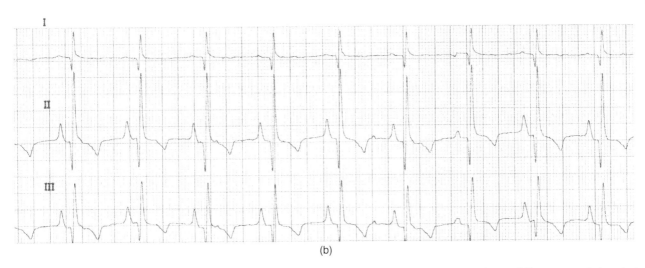

(b)

Figure 4.10b Paper speed 50 mm/s, 1 cm/mV, leads I, II, III, same dog. The seventh complex has an abnormal P′ wave morphology but is neither early nor late. This indicates an **atrial fusion beat**. When a supraventricular premature beat (ectopic atrial or junctional) fires simultaneously with the sinoatrial node, the resulting P′ wave is intermediate between that of the sinus and ectopic foci. This confirms that the post-extrasystolic aberrant P′ wave in the above strip is likely the result of atrial fusion as well, rather than from Chung's phenomenon per se.

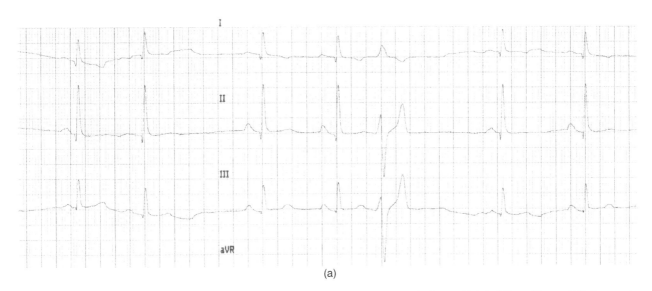

(a)

Figure 4.11a Paper speed 50 mm/s, 1 cm/mV, leads I, II, III, canine. The first complex is sinus, which is followed by an APC that resets with a pause. The fifth complex is a **VPC** and is followed by a supraventricular complex that is *suspicious* of **Chung's phenomenon** (beat #7, note the altered P′ morphology). However, this beat is most likely **ectopic atrial** (see below).

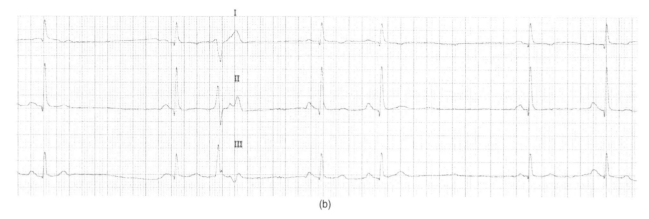

(b)

Figure 4.11b Paper speed 50 mm/s, 1 cm/mV, leads I, II, III, same dog. The first two supraventricular beats are **ectopic atrial** (note the negative/isoelectric P′ in I). The third complex is a VPC with clear evidence of **VA conduction** (note the retrograde P′ within the S-T segment). The following beat (#4) is sinus with a normal P wave configuration. If this dog had "aberrant post-extrasystolic conduction" of the atria, we would certainly not be surprised if this occurred following a VPC with VA conduction for one beat. In this case, the pacemaker is displaced from the ectopic atrial focus back to the sinus node by the VPC. Given the *persistence* of ectopic atrial rhythm in this dog, it is unlikely that temporary partial refractoriness of the atrial tissue is causing altered P wave morphology.

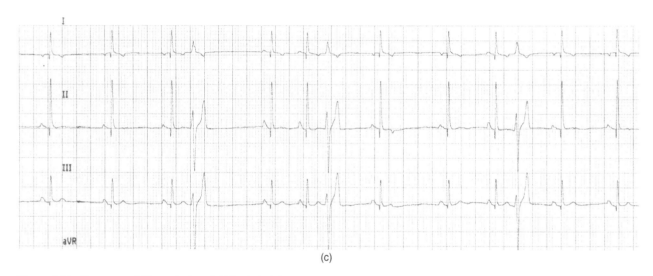

(c)

Figure 4.11c Paper speed 25 mm/s, 1 cm/mV, leads I, II, III, same dog. The first three complexes are ectopic atrial (**atrial "escape" rhythm,** since the cycle length is longer than that of the sinus cycle length). The fourth complex is a VPC, which displaces the pacemaker back to the sinus node. The seventh complex is another VPC that displaces the pacemaker back to the ectopic atrial focus. The sinus node captures again (beat #10), and then a VPC again displaces the pacemaker to the ectopic atrial focus. Note the inverted P′ waves of the ectopic atrial pacemaker in lead I. The VPCs in this dog likely have **VA conduction** since the pacemaker is typically displaced (concealed conduction). The retrograde P′ waves are not evident here, but likely hiding in the T waves.

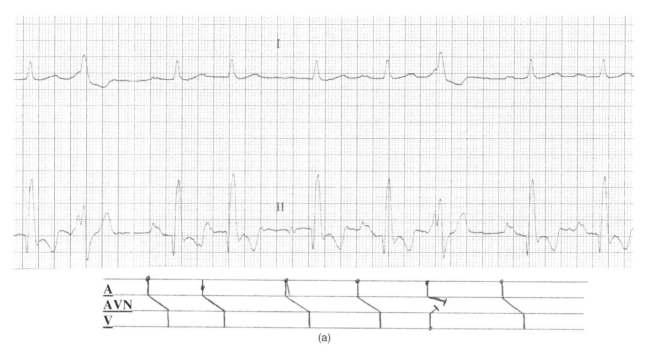

(a)

Figure 4.12a Paper speed 50 mm/s, 1 cm/mV, leads I and II, canine. The second complex is a VPC. The fourth complex is an APC, and the post-extrasystolic P wave has altered morphology consistent with **Chung's phenomenon**. Note the post-extrasystolic P′-P interval appears to exactly match that of the underlying sinus P-P interval.

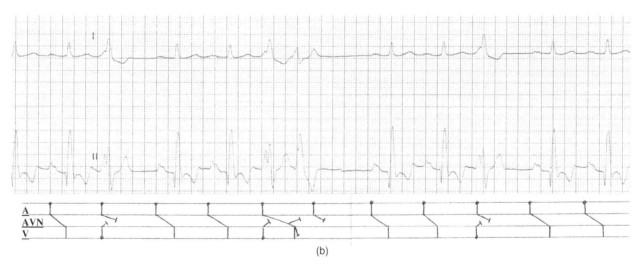

(b)

Figure 4.12b Paper speed 50 mm/s, 1 cm/mV, leads I and II, same dog. **Ventricular trigeminy with post-extrasystolic aberration of the QRS mimicking a ventricular couplet and aborted concealed atrial reentry**. The ladder diagram illustrates the mechanism. The first and third VPCs (RBBB, likely LV origin) create typical compensatory pauses. The second VPC is actually interpolated, prolongs the following P-R interval and the following QRS is of LBBB aberration (likely since the left bundle is still refractory from the preceding VPC). **P-mitrale/interatrial block** is also present with P wave duration of 0.09 second and notching.

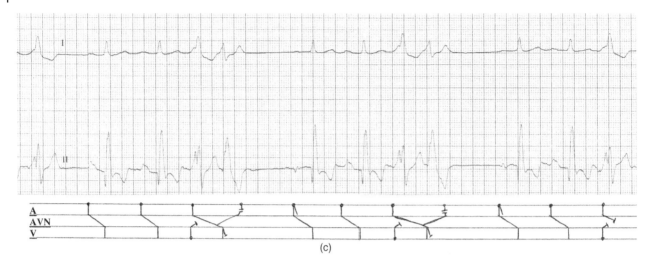

(c)

Figure 4.12c Paper speed 50 mm/s 1 cm/mV, leads I and II, same dog. **Ventricular trigeminy, post-extrasystolic aberration of the QRS mimicking a ventricular couplet and concealed atrial reentry.** The 6th and 10th beats have altered P wave morphology consistent with Chung's phenomenon. This implies that atrial reentry from the preceding complex must have succeeded to some degree, whether it was an atrial fusion, as depicted here, or retrograde atrial/sinus echo is not known.

Further reading

Almeida, G.L.G., de Almeida, M.B., de Mattos, A.V. et al. Intermittent advanced Bachmann's bundle block in a boxer dog. *Acta Sci. Vet.* 38 (4): 439–442.

Bayés de Luna, A. et al. (2015). The diagnosis and clinical implications of interatrial block. *Eur. Cardiol. Rev.* 10 (1): 54–59.

Bayes de Luna, A. et al. (2017). Diagnosis of interatrial block. *J. Geriatr. Cardiol.* 14: 161–165.

Bonke, F.I., Bouman, L.N., and Schopman, F.J.G. (1971). Effect of and early atrial premature beat on activity of the sinoatrial node and atrial rhythm in the rabbit. *Circ.Res.* 29: 704–712.

Bradley, S.M. and Marriott, J.I. (1956). Intra-Atrial Block. *Circulation* XIV.

Chhabra, L. et al. (2014). Interatrial block in the modern era. *Curr. Cardiol. Rev.* 10 (3): 181–189.

Fisch, C. and Knoebel, S.B. (2000). *Electrocardiography of Clinical Arrhythmias.* Futura Publishing Co.

Probst, P. et al. (1973). Investigation of atrial aberration as a cause of altered P wave contour. *Am. Heart J.* 86 (4): 516–522.

Surawicz, B. and Knilans, T.K. (2001). *Chou's Electrocardiography in Clinical Practice: Adult and Pediatric*, 5e. Saunders.

5

Right Bundle Branch Block

CHAPTER MENU

Incomplete right bundle branch block, 55
Ashman's phenomenon, 55
Second-in-the-row anomaly, 59
Rate-dependent/critical rate BBB, 60
Complete right bundle branch block, 62

Incomplete right bundle branch block It results in slightly smaller R waves with S waves in I, II, III, and aVF without prolongation of the QRS complex, can occur with disruption of the right ventricular (RV) moderator band, focal hypertrophy of the right ventricular free wall (RVFW) or right ventricular outflow tract (RVOT), and mimics right axis deviation (RAD). The normal r′ in VI is attributed to normal terminal depolarization of the crista supraventricularis, proximal septum, and base of the heart. With iRBBB, lead V1 will show rSr′ QRS complexes, the typical variation of which has an r amplitude >r′ amplitude and has been referred to as "1st degree RBBB" or Type A iRBBB. Another variation in which the r′>r has been referred to as "2nd degree RBBB" or Type B iRBBB (though it is more appropriate to refer to intermittent RBBB as second degree). Incomplete RBBB produces mild RAD and may mimic left posterior fascicular block (see Chapters 2 and 7). Right ventricular enlargement and hypertrophy should technically be excluded by echocardiography.

Ashman's phenomenon It is a form of aberrancy that is associated with changing cycle (R-R interval) lengths on refractoriness. The duration of the refractory period is dependent on the length of the cycle immediately preceding it. The longer the preceding cycle, the longer the refractory period, and vice versa. Thus, if the HR is fairly regular, a sudden prolongation in cycle length may result in aberration. At lower heart rates, the RBB has a longer refractory period than the LBB, so aberration is usually of RBBB (though LBBB or atypical BBB patterns may be seen). Ashman's phenomenon is characterized by a relatively long cycle immediately preceding the cycle terminated by

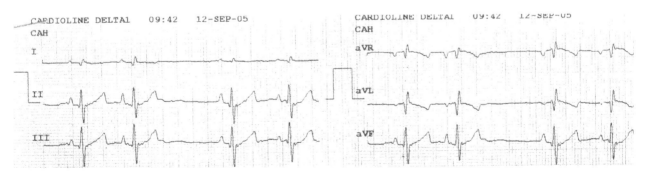

Figure 5.1 Paper speed 50 mm/s, 1 cm/mV, young Bischon with right ventricular volume overload due to an atrial septal defect. **Incomplete RBBB**. The QRS duration is normal and S waves are present in II, III, and aVF. The **MEA is indeterminate**, as all the leads are isoelectric. Perhaps overload of the RV disrupted the moderator band.

Interpretation of the Electrocardiogram in Small Animals, First Edition. Nick A. Schroeder.
© 2021 John Wiley & Sons Inc. Published 2021 by John Wiley & Sons Inc.

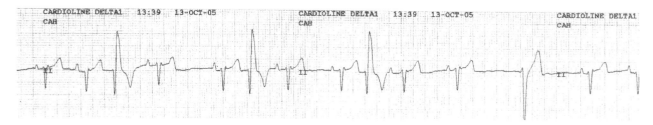

Figure 5.2 Paper speed 50 mm/s, 1 cm/mV, lead II, canine. **Incomplete RBBB** and right ventricular premature complexes (**RVPCs**, conducted with LBBB-like morphology). The third complex is a RVPC that *resets*. The interval between the third and fourth complexes equals the R-R interval. The sixth and ninth complexes are interpolated RVPCs and cause P-R interval prolongation of the post-extrasystolic beats, indicating concealed retrograde VA conduction (partial penetration of the VPC into the AV node). A pause follows the 11th complex and is terminated by an LV escape complex with RBBB morphology. This strip highlights the difference between *resetting* and *interpolation* and the difference between sinus complexes with RBBB and VPCs. It also demonstrates the difference between ventricular *premature* complexes and ventricular *escape* complexes. This dog had a MEA of approximately −120 degrees, so extreme RAD is present. The QRS duration is normal. Therefore, an incomplete RBBB *may* be present, but the R waves should be a little more prominent.

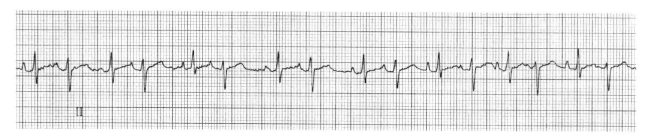

Figure 5.3 Paper speed 50 mm/s, 1 cm/mV, lead II, feline. Sinus rhythm, atrial bigeminy. Every-other-beat is an atrial premature complex that is conducted with and conducted with an **incomplete RBBB**. This is evidenced by resetting of the rhythm and the P′ waves that precede the premature beats.

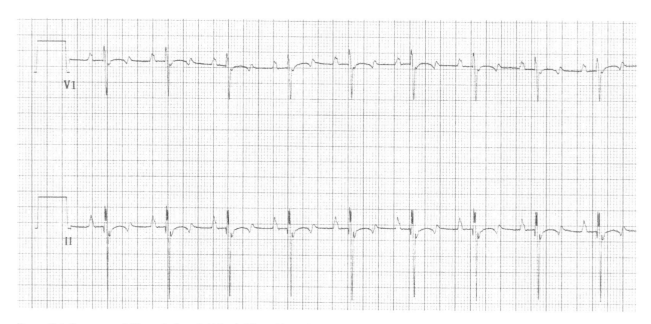

Figure 5.4 Paper speed 50 mm/s, 1 cm/mV, leads V1 and II, canine. **Incomplete RBBB** (Type A or first degree iRBBB). Note the rSr′ complex in V1 with the r >r′. This is the most common variant in humans with iRBBB.

Figure 5.5 Paper speed 50 mm/s, 1 cm/mV, full EKG, canine. **Incomplete RBBB**. This dog had a structurally normal heart.

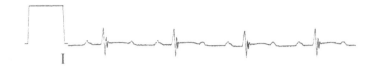

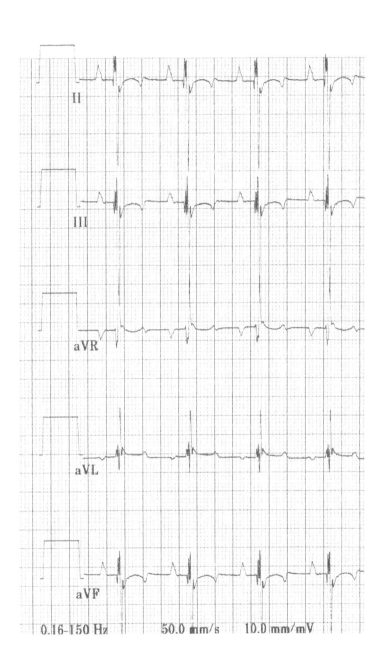

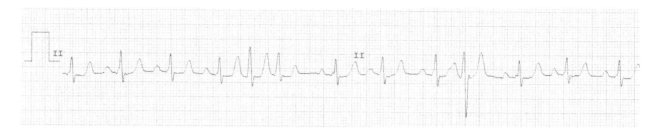

Figure 5.6 Paper speed 50 mm/s, 1 cm/mV, lead II, canine, the fifth and sixth complexes are APCs that reset the rhythm. The 10th complex is an APC conducted with an (incomplete) **RBBB** pattern and *resets* the rhythm. The cycle preceding the APC is slightly longer than normal, making this an example of **Ashman's phenomenon**. The P wave of the post-extrasystolic beat (#7) following the couplet of APCs is different than the normal P wave and is thus an example of **Chung's phenomenon**. This is from aberrant *atrial conduction* caused by the APC (see below).

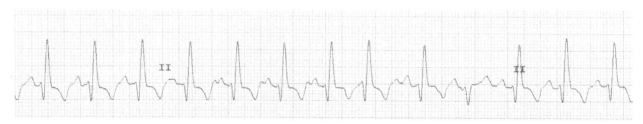

Figure 5.7 Paper speed 50 mm/s, 1 cm/mV, lead II, canine with SAS. The eighth complex is an APC that resets. The 10th complex is sinus and conducted with RBBB morphology. This is secondary to the long-short sequence induced by the pause created by the APC, and another example of **Ashman's phenomenon**.

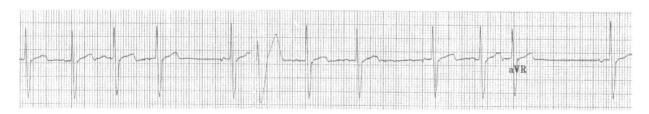

Figure 5.8 Paper speed 50 mm/s, 0.5 cm/mV, lead aVR, canine with chronic mitral valvular disease (CMVDz). A pause in the sinus rhythm after the fourth complex is followed by another sinus beat, then an aberrant supraventricular premature beat with RBBB morphology from **Ashman's phenomenon**. The aberrant APC resets the sinus rhythm. The 11th complex is another APC, but is of normal morphology as it follows a short cycle.

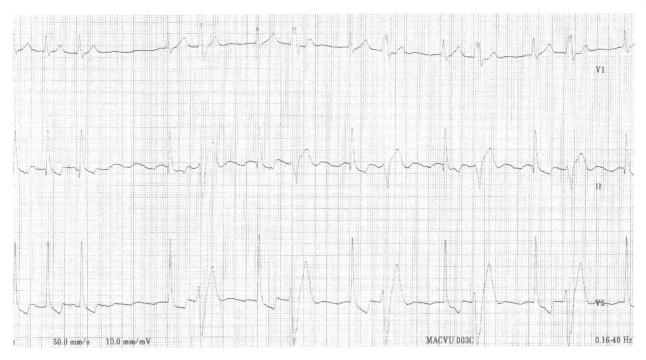

Figure 5.9 Paper speed 50 mm/s, 1 cm/mV, leads V1, II and V5, canine. **Atrial flutter, alternating 2:1 and 4:1 conduction with RBBB aberrancy mimicking ventricular bigeminy**. The regularly undulating baseline is characteristic of atrial flutter. A long pause in conduction creates a long-short cycle sequence precipitating RBBB on the short cycles. This dog was being treated with digoxin and to mistake these for VPCs could cause the clinician to stop the drug when it may really help.

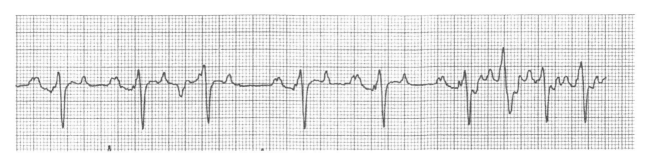

Figure 5.10 Paper speed 50 mm/s, 1 cm/mV, lead II, 2 y/o Pitt Bull with Tetralogy of Fallot. R axis deviation is present, as well as P mitrale. The third complex is an APC with a negative P′ that resets the rhythm. The seventh beat is premature, aberrantly conducted (RBBB pattern), preceded by a negative P′ wave (within the S-T segment of the previous beat) and is the **second-in-the-row** of a supraventricular tachycardia.

the aberrant QRS (a so-called "long-short sequence"), the aberrant QRS is of RBBB morphology, a non-compensatory pause follows the aberrant QRS, and there is irregular coupling of the aberrant QRS. Importantly, RBBB from Ashman's phenomenon may mimic ventricular ectopy. This is especially the case during atrial fibrillation and atrial flutter, when sudden changes in cycle length commonly occur. In patients being treated with digoxin for atrial flutter, alternating 2:1 and 4:1 conduction may develop, and RBBB on beats following shorter cycle lengths may simulate ventricular bigeminy (1:1 extrasystole). The clinician is warned not to mistake this as a sign of digoxin toxicity and discontinue the drug prematurely.

Second-in-the-row anomaly The second complex in a row of a run of rapid beats is most likely to display RBBB aberration. This is because the second beat is the one that ends a relatively short cycle and is preceded by a relatively long cycle, and the right bundle branch has a longer refractory period than the left bundle branch. The action potential duration (and hence, the relative refractory period) is directly related to the cardiac cycle, accounting for the aberrancy. This is an Ashman's type aberration. Occasionally, the second beat will display other forms of aberrancy, including incomplete RBBB, fascicular blocks, etc., and this depends on the relative prolongation of action potential duration of the various branches. A rule

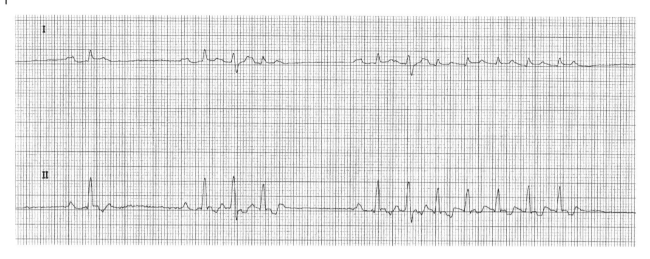

Figure 5.11 Paper speed 50 mm/s, 1 cm/mV, leads I and II, canine. Atrial echoes (retrograde P′ waves follow the QRS complex) indicate the presence of a retrogradely conducting accessory pathway. Short runs of SVT (orthodromic atrioventricular reciprocating tachycardia) display RBBB aberrancy on the second complex (beats #3 and #6).

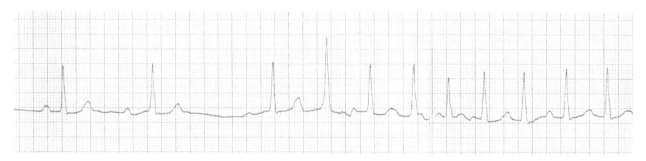

Figure 5.12 Paper speed 50 mm/s, 1 cm/mV, lead II, canine. The fourth complex is aberrantly conducted and the second-in-the-row of a supraventricular tachycardia. Note the long-short cycle that precedes aberration (in this case a left *medial* fascicular block-pattern). The P′ is inapparent in this case.

out is a ventricular premature complex (VPC) that initiates atrioventricular reciprocating tachycardia. If the abnormal beat is preceded by a P′ wave at a believable/physiologic P′-Ri, then aberration is favored (even if a typical rsR′ in V1 is not present and the morphology of the QRS is ambiguous). A VPC is favored if no P′ is visible or the P′-Ri is unphysiologically short. Occasionally, the distinction on surface EKG is impossible.

Rate-dependent/critical rate BBB

Rate-dependent BBB occurs when BBB comes and goes with changes in the HR. In deceleration-dependent (bradycardia-dependent, diastolic, or phase four of the action potential) block, conduction delay happens when the HR falls below a critical level and is less common than acceleration-dependent (tachycardia-dependent, phase 3) block. The critical rate is the rate at which BBB develops during acceleration or disappears during deceleration. Deceleration-dependent block typically results in RBBB.

Once BBB is established, the actual cycle for the blocked bundle does not begin until approximately halfway through the QRS complex. The cycle during deceleration (from the beginning of one QRS complex to the beginning of the next QRS complex) must be longer than the "critical" cycle during acceleration. This may occur following extrasystoles. Criteria for diagnosis of a bradycardia-dependent RBBB include: the P-R interval of the aberrantly conducted beats should be plausible/within-normal-limits for that patient, atrial fibrillation/flutter is not present, aberration must occur repeatably on more than one beat, incomplete bilateral BBB should be excluded, and supernormal conduction cannot apply to the normally conducted beats. Rule outs include fortuitously timed left-ventricular escape beats (conducting with a RBBB-like morphology) and are suspected when the apparent P-R interval is too short and the escape interval is plausible for that associated with a ventricular escape focus. Right BBB may be acceleration-dependent and is not uncommon given that

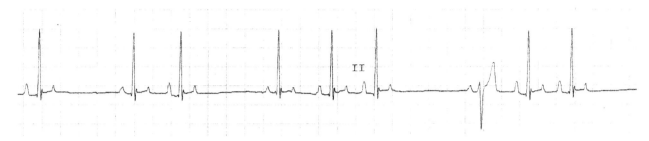

Figure 5.13 Paper speed 25 mm/s, 1 cm/mV, lead II, canine. Phase 4 (**deceleration-dependent RBBB**) aberration is seen following a pause created by a sinus arrhythmia. A wandering pacemaker is also present, as the P wave morphology varies.

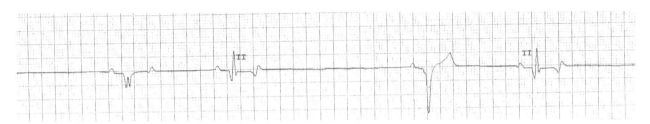

Figure 5.14 Paper speed 50 mm/s, 1 cm/mV, lead II, canine, **alternating RBBB**. A sinus pause occurs after the second beat, which is then followed by an aberrantly conducted sinus beat (RBBB). This is referred to as **deceleration-dependent BBB**. Every other complex was conducted aberrantly in this patient, and the complexes following the pauses were the aberrantly conducted ones. Variable degrees of aberrancy are evident as the first complex has a QRS with a slightly different morphology. Alternatively, the "aberrant" beats may simply represent variable degrees of fusion with left ventricular escape foci elicited by the pauses. Given that the P-R intervals appear to remain constant, ventricular fusion seems less likely.

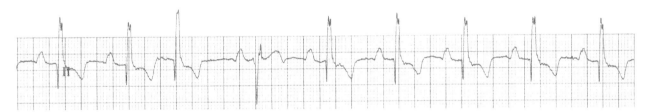

Figure 5.15 Paper speed 50 mm/s, 1 cm/mV, lead II, canine, **post-extrasystolic deceleration-dependent aberrancy**. The third complex is an APC. This causes the pause that is terminated by a sinus beat with an incomplete RBBB. This could also be referred to as a "short-long sequence" (vs. a long-short sequence/Ashman's). The sudden decrease in rate caused by the pause resulted in aberrancy of the next sinus beat.

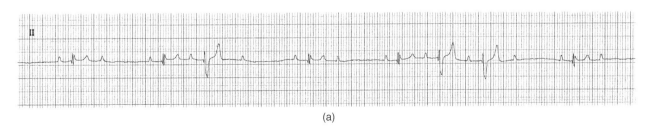

(a)

Figure 5.16a Paper speed 25 mm/s, 1 cm/mV, lead II, canine. **Wenckebach periodicity in the RBB.** Ventriculophasic sinus arrhythmia with gradual onset of RBBB, progressing from iRBBB to cRBBB and finally an AV block. First degree AVB is also present with progressive P-Ri prolongation prior to failure of conduction consistent with Type I second degree AVB/Wenckebach periodicity. This may be a bilateral BBB or trifascicular block.

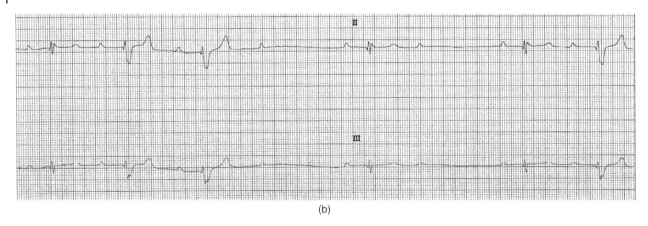

Figure 5.16b Paper speed 50 mm/s, 1 cm/mV, leads II and III, same dog. The P-Ri progresses from 0.20 to 0.22 second and the QRS duration from 0.06 to 0.10 second over the Wenckebach period.

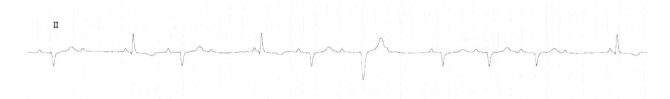

Figure 5.17 Paper speed 50 mm/s, 1 cm/mV, lead II, feline. Possible **Wenckebach periodicity in the RBB**. The first complex is conducted (incomplete RBBB), followed by AV block and an escape beat (positive QRS), and the sequence repeats. The sixth complex conducts with a longer P-Ri and the simultaneously prolongs to a complete RBBB, suggestive of Wenckebach periodicity in the BB. A typical Wenckebach period follows with culmination in an AV block. The escape beats happen to be preceded by P waves, but are not conducted.

the refractory period for the RBB is normally longer than that of the LBB.

Second degree RBBB occurs when RBBB is intermittent and not necessarily rate-related. This can be further subdivided into Type I (Wenckebach) and Type II (Mobitz) second degree RBBB. With Type I second degree RBBB, incomplete RBBB may progress over a sequence of complexes to complete RBBB. Typically, a normally conducted QRS will be followed by one with incomplete RBBB, which is then followed by a QRS displaying complete RBBB. Occasionally, this phenomenon may be associated with pre-existent BBB and/or AV block. If first degree AVB is noted on conducted complexes in association with second degree BBB, then "trifascicular" block is present (so diffuse conduction system disease may be inferred even if Wenckebach periodicity is evident) and pacing may be indicated. Type II second degree RBBB (Mobitz) occurs when the complete RBBB displayed on conducted complexes is not only intermittent, but random and not rate-related or associated with incomplete RBBB and/or first degree AVB. Type II second degree RBBB is often seen with bilateral BBB (sinus rhythm with cLBBB with sudden second degree AVB indicative of intermittent conduction

blockade in the RBB) or trifascicular block (bifascicular block with L anterior and posterior fascicular block).

Complete right bundle branch block

It is characterized on surface EKG by deep and wide S waves in leads I, II, III, and aVF with tall R waves in lead aVR. The QRS complexes are wide and bizarre-looking, like ventricular complexes, but are not early or late and are preceded by P waves. The QRS is >0.08 second (0.06 second for cats), R axis deviation, QRS + in aVR, aVL, CV5RL (V1, RV2) ± M-shaped, S waves large and wide in I, II, III, aVF, L precordials, S wave, or W-shaped QRS in V10. The MEA is usually deviated to the right (RAD). Right bundle branch block may be persistent/permanent (third degree RBBB) or transient and rate-related (second degree RBBB). It is not often associated with structural heart disease and thus may be a benign and incidental finding. If RBBB occurs in conjunction with bilateral BBB (alternating R and LBBB) or trifascicular block (RBBB + intermittent left anterior and left posterior fascicular block), then pacing may be warranted.

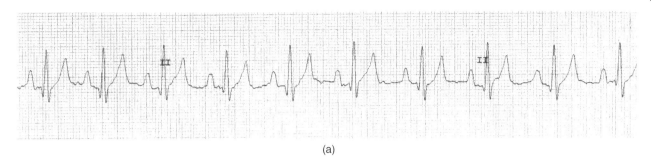

(a)

Figure 5.18a Paper speed 50 mm/s, 1 cm/mV, lead II, canine with a small R atrial hemangiosarcoma and history of pericardial effusion. Sinus rhythm.

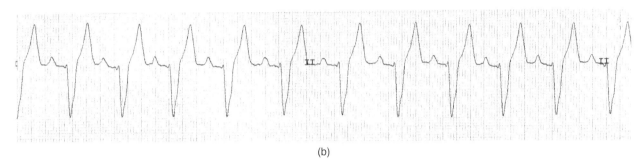

(b)

Figure 5.18b Paper speed 50 mm/s, 1 cm/mV, lead II, the same dog develops **complete RBBB** with deep, wide S waves as the expanding tumor presumably destroys the RBB.

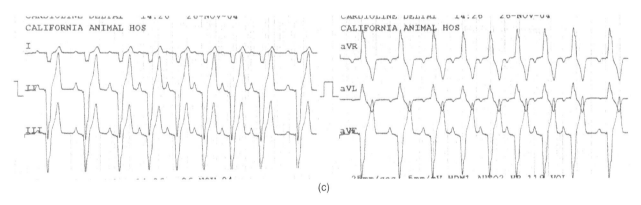

(c)

Figure 5.18c Paper speed 25 mm/s, 0.5 cm/mV, same patient, full EKG.

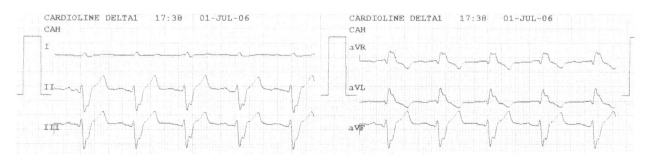

Figure 5.19 Paper speed 50 mm/s, 2 cm/mV, full EKG, feline with **complete RBBB**.

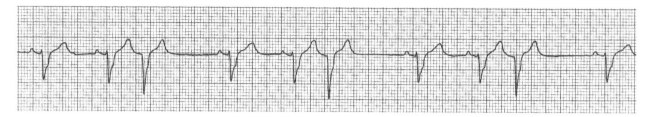

Figure 5.20 Paper speed 50 mm/s, 1 cm/mV, lead II, feline, **complete RBBB** and **ventricular trigeminy**. Every third complex is a LVPC followed by a compensatory pause. Note the similarity between the aberrantly conducted sinus beats and the ventricular beats.

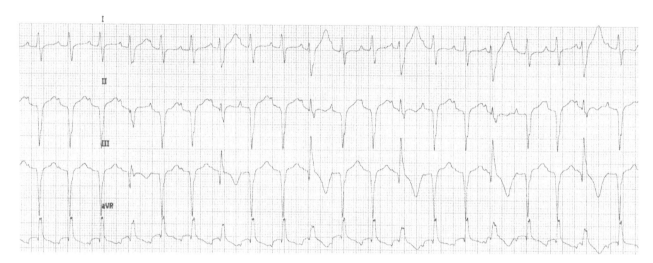

Figure 5.21 Paper speed 50 mm/s, 1 cm/mV, leads I, II, III, avR, feline with hyperthyroidism. **Complete RBBB**, sinus tachycardia, and ventricular trigeminy. Here, the VPCs are likely originating in the left anterior fascicle/radiation, as they are conducted with a RBBB/LPFB pattern. The 4th, 7th, 10th, 13th, 16th, and 19th complexes are the VPCs. The P-R′ intervals are variable and the beats are followed by compensatory pauses consistent with VPCs.

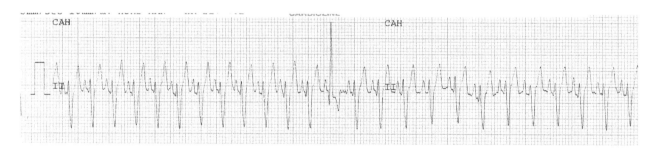

Figure 5.22 Paper speed 25 mm/s, 1 cm/mV, lead II, canine. Sinus tachycardia with **RBBB**. The 13th complex is normally conducted, illustrating the difference between normal and aberrant conduction. The fact that this patient is capable of normal conduction suggests that the BBB is rate-dependent; however, the normally conducted beat is neither early nor late, offering the examiner no clues. Perhaps this complex is a fusion beat occurring between the sinus impulse and a VPC from the right ventricle. If the P-R′ interval were shorter than the P-R interval of the rest of the beats, this would support a ventricular fusion; however, at this paper speed it is too close to call.

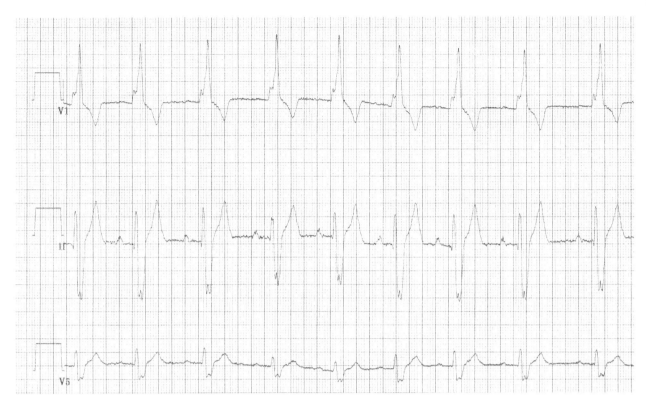

Figure 5.23 Paper speed 50 mm/s, 1 cm/mV, leads V1, II, and V5, canine. **Complete RBBB**. Note the positive and delayed intrinsicoid deflection in V1.

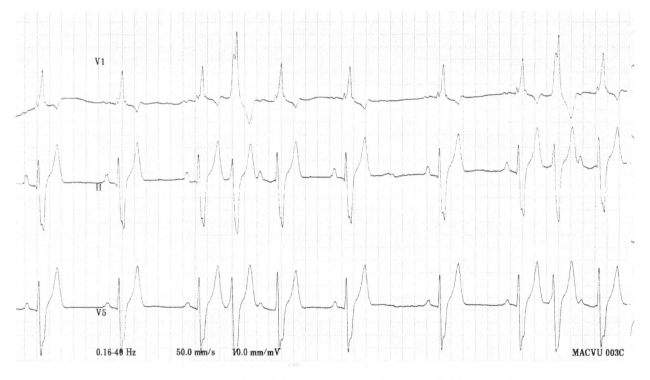

Figure 5.24 Paper speed 50 mm/s, 1 cm/mV, leads V1, II, V5, asymptomatic canine. The underlying rhythm is sinus arrhythmia. The QRS complexes display complete **RBBB**, the fourth and ninth complexes are LVPCs that have a RBBB-like morphology, confusing the examiner with SVPCs. Careful examination of the complexes in V1 reveal a markedly different QRS morphology, and these beats are interpolated and post-extrasystolic P-Ri prolongation is evident, making these premature beats more likely to be ventricular in origin.

Patients with a pre-existent RBBB having RV ectopic beats (escape, accelerated, or prematures) with fusion may actually have paradoxical narrowing of the QRS due to simultaneous activation of the ventricles. The LV is activated over the normal His-Purkinje system and the RV is depolarized by the ectopic focus. This transiently shortens the QRS duration. The degree of narrowing depends on the timing of the ectopic beat. Mild fusion results in an incomplete RBBB pattern and perfectly timed fusions result in a normal QRS duration.

Right BBB is most accurately diagnosed by examining the precordial leads in addition to the horizontal leads. The "intrinsicoid deflection" (ventricular activation time) is measured from the onset of the QRS to the summit. Lead I should show a wide S wave. V1 shows a late intrinsicoid deflection, an M-shaped QRS (rSR′ variant), and sometimes a wide R or qR wave. V6 shows a wide S wave and early intrinsicoid deflection. The net septal depolarization vector is the first deflection of the QRS, and the leftward vector of this is contributed to by the right bundle, which is lost in RBBB. Thus, the rightward vector is unopposed, which usually predominates anyway, so there is still an R wave in V1. The LVFW is depolarized via the left bundle, resulting in a large leftward vector that is unopposed. The wave of excitation then begins to depolarize the RVFW later, producing a large unopposed vector because the LV has already been depolarized. Typically, the T wave will be opposite in polarity of the QRS with slurring of the S-T segment. Right BBB may be confused with ventricular ectopics originating from the LV.

Further reading

Achen, S.E., Saunders, A.B., and Miller, M.W. (2008). ECG of the month. *JAVMA* 232 (5): 684–686.

Johns, S.M., Stern, J.A., and Nelson, O.L. (2011). ECG of the month. *JAVMA* 238 (8): 982–984.

MacGregor, J.M. (2002). ECG of the month. *JAVMA* 221 (6).

MacGregor, J.M. and Morisson, K. (2002). ECG of the month. *JAVMA* 221 (6).

Marriot, J.L. (1998). *Pearls & Pitfalls in Electrocardiography: Pithy Practical Pointers*, 2e. Williams & Wilkins.

Marriot, H.J.L. and Conover, M.B. (1998). *Advanced Concepts in Arrhythmias*, 3e. Mosby.

Massumi, R.A. (1968). Bradycardia-dependent bundle-branch block: a critique and proposed criteria. *Circulation* 38: 1066–1073.

Surawicz, B. and Knilans, T.K. (2001). *Chou's Electrocardiography in Clinical Practice: Adult and Pediatric*, 5e. Saunders.

Thomason, J.D., Thomason, S.S., Fallaw, T. et al. (2015). ECG of the month. *JAVMA* 246 (9): 962–964.

6

Left Bundle Branch Block

CHAPTER MENU
Incomplete left bundle branch block, 67
Rate-dependent/critical rate BBB, 67
Complete left bundle branch block, 68

Incomplete left bundle branch block This results in a QRS that is wider than normal but of duration less than that associated with complete L bundle branch block (BBB), is associated with the left ventricular hypertrophy (LVH) pattern, and may be associated with rate-dependent BBB and ventricular fusion complexes. The QRS axis may be normal and if deviated to the left may be confused with left ventricular enlargement or left anterior fascicular block (see Chapters 2 and 7). Left ventricular hypertrophy or enlargement should technically be excluded via echocardiography.

Rate-dependent/critical rate BBB Acceleration-dependent aberration (Phase 3 block) may occur because the ventricle is being depolarized during its relative refractory period. First, as the heart rate (HR) increases, the refractory period decreases in duration, and normal conduction tends to be preserved. As the HR decreases, the refractory period increases in duration. Thus, the HR has to slow down more than would be expected to reestablish the normal intraventricular conduction in acceleration-dependent BBB. A very premature supraventricular premature beat occurring during Phase 3 of the action potential of the previous beat may result in aberrant conduction of the extrasystole. This can be physiologic (or functional) if the impulse is early enough to reach the fiber during electrical systole of the preceding beat (when the membrane potential is still reduced) and is common. So-called "linking" can perpetuate BBB from concealed transseptal conduction from the opposite bundle. Phase 3 aberration may occur pathologically if the electrical

systolic period is abnormally prolonged beyond the action potential duration or the Q-T interval, and the affected fascicle is stimulated at a relatively rapid rate. Because the right bundle branch has a longer refractory period normally, rate-dependent BBB usually results in RBBB (Ashman's phenomenon). Rate-dependent BBB may be associated with incomplete to complete LBBB, depending on the relative degree of acceleration (i.e. the shorter the R-R interval, the more prolonged the QRS complex), is associated with a prolonged refractory period of the LBB, which exceeds the duration of that of the RBB at short cycle lengths. Rate-dependent LBBB may be unmasked by pauses in the rhythm precipitated by premature beats. Deceleration-dependent LBBB appears to be quite rare.

Second degree LBBB occurs when LBBB is intermittent and is not always rate-related. This can be further subdivided into Type I (Wenckebach) and Type II (Mobitz) second degree LBBB. With Type I second degree LBBB, incomplete LBBB may progress over a sequence of complexes to complete LBBB. Typically, a normally conducted QRS will be followed by one with incomplete LBBB, which is then followed by a QRS displaying complete LBBB, and this may be rate-related to some extent. Occasionally, this phenomenon may be associated with pre-existent BBB and/or AV block. If first degree AVB is noted on conducted complexes in association with second degree BBB, then "trifascicular" block is present, diffuse conduction system disease may be inferred (even if Wenckebach periodicity is evident), and pacing may be indicated. Type II second degree LBBB (Mobitz) occurs when the complete LBBB displayed on conducted complexes is not only intermittent,

Interpretation of the Electrocardiogram in Small Animals, First Edition. Nick A. Schroeder.
© 2021 John Wiley & Sons Inc. Published 2021 by John Wiley & Sons Inc.

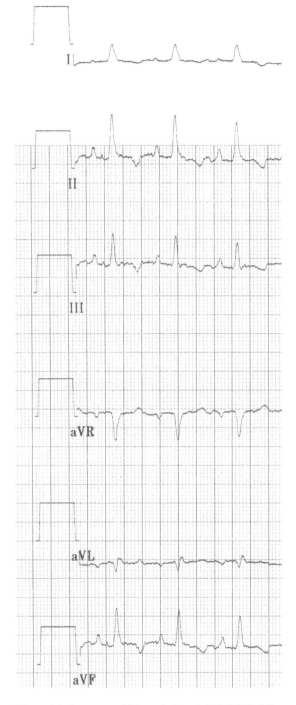

Figure 6.1 Paper speed 50 mm/s, 1 cm/mV, full EKG, feline. **Incomplete LBBB**. The MEA is normal, and the QRS complexes are mildly prolonged at 0.06 second. Note that the T waves are opposite in polarity of the main QRS vector in all leads, similar to that seen with complete LBBB.

but also random and not rate-related, associated with incomplete LBBB or first degree AVB. Type II second degree LBBB is commonly implicated in bilateral bundle branch block (sinus rhythm with cRBBB with sudden second degree AVB indicating conduction blockade in the LBB) or trifascicular block (both the L anterior and posterior fascicles of the LBB). Gradual onset of BBB over a series of beats is distinguished from the gradual onset of ventricular fusion by an accelerated idioventricular rhythm by failure of the P-R intervals to shorten. They will either remain constant or increase in duration with the onset of BBB aberration.

Complete left bundle branch block This is characterized on surface EKG by tall and wide S waves in leads I, II, III, and aVL, and marked by wide, bizarre QRS complexes, resembling ventricular complexes, but are not early/late and are preceded by P waves at a believable P-R interval, provided sinus rhythm. The QRS is >0.08 second (0.06 second in cats), QRS wide and + in I, II, III, aVF, L precordials, QRS inverted in aVR and R precordials. Q waves are often absent. The MEA can be normal or deviated to the left. If the axis is deviated far enough to the left, LBBB may masquerade as RBBB if the QRS complexes end up negative in lead II. This may be from incomplete LBBB + L anterior fascicular block. Left BBB with R axis deviation is suggestive of dilated cardiomyopathy. Left BBB may be persistent/permanent or transient and rate-related. Boxer dogs with arrhythmogenic cardiomyopathy typically have ventricular arrhythmias with a LBBB-like pattern. Pacemakers have leads typically placed in the RV apex, so the paced beats tend to be wide and conducted with a LBBB pattern. Isolated LBBB in the absence of structural heart disease almost never occurs and is thus rarely benign. If LBBB is complete and present on all supraventricular conducted complexes, then it is considered to be third degree LBBB.

> ***Take Home Message***: If LBBB is diagnosed, the patient is assumed to have serious heart disease! It can be associated with LVH, LV myocardial disease, and diffuse degenerative conductive system disease (i.e. concurrent sinoatrial block, atrioventricular block, bilateral bundle branch block).

Patients with a pre-existent LBBB having LV ectopic beats (escape, accelerated, or prematures) with fusion may actually have paradoxical narrowing of the QRS due to simultaneous activation of the ventricles. The RV is activated over the normal His-Purkinje system and the LV is depolarized via the ectopic focus. This transiently normalizes the QRS duration. Mild fusion results in an incomplete LBBB pattern and perfectly timed fusions result in a normal QRS duration.

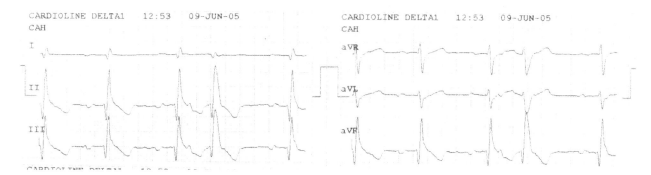

Figure 6.2 Paper speed 25 mm/s, 1 cm/mV, canine, the fourth complex is premature and conducted with aberrancy (**LBBB**) and *resets* the rhythm consistent with an APC. The P′ of the APC is in the S-T segment of the previous complex. The long P′-R interval is also suggestive that this beat is actually an APC. This is an example of Phase 3 (acceleration-dependent) LBBB. This patient was a Boxer, and RVPCs are quite common in this breed. These premature beats are unlikely to be ventricular in origin in this case, however, because the rhythm is reset by the premature beat.

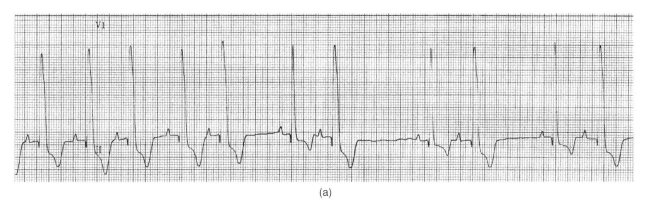

(a)

Figure 6.3a Paper speed 50 mm/s, 1 cm/mV, lead II, canine. **Rate-dependent LBBB**. Sinus rhythm with pauses (R/O sinoatrial block) with obvious narrowing of the QRS complex following a long R-R interval. Interestingly, the bigeminal rhythm that ensues (likely from 3 : 2 sinoatrial block) showcases normal QRS conduction on the first complex *and* first degree AVB with LBBB on the second complex in each pair secondary to the short P-Pi.

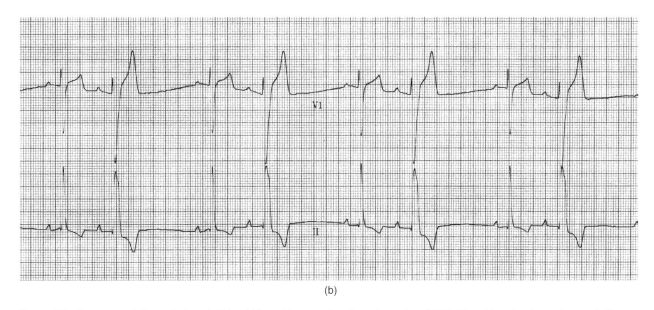

(b)

Figure 6.3b Paper speed 50 mm/s, 1 cm/mV, lead V1 and II, same dog. Rate-dependent LBBB. Sinus bigeminy (secondary to 3 : 2 sinoatrial block). The second complex in each pair has LBBB aberration due to a short R-Ri. The P-Ri interval alternates as well. Note the deep broad S waves in V1 and broad R waves in II characteristic of LBBB.

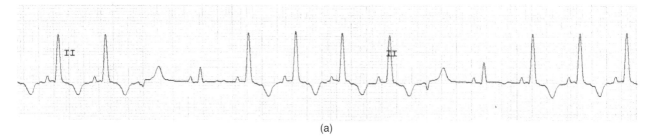

(a)

Figure 6.4a Paper speed 50 mm/s, 1 cm/mV, lead II, feline. LBBB is present in beats 1, 2, 5, 6, 7, 8, 11, 12, and 13. The 3rd and 9th complexes are VPCs. The 4th and 10th complexes (post-extrasystolic) are normal in duration. This is an example *of* **post-extrasystolic revelation of rate-dependent BBB**. The pauses created by the VPCs allow better interventricular conduction of the post-extrasystolic beats. At a faster HR (approximately 200 bpm), this cat manifested LBBB. This cat had significant structural heart disease.

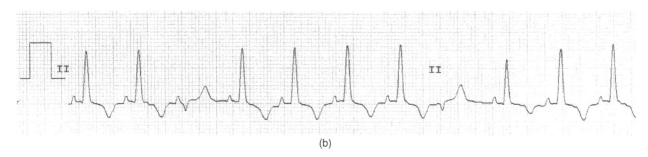

(b)

Figure 6.4b Paper speed 50 mm/s, 1 cm/mV, lead II, same cat. The third complex is a VPC and the next sinus beat is conducted with LBBB. The eighth complex is another VPC that results in **incomplete LBBB** of the post-extrasystolic beat (ninth complex). The interventricular conduction is better than on the rest of the beats, but not quite normal as in the above strip. The more premature the VPC is, the higher the likelihood of improved conduction on the post-extrasystolic beat. The first VPC here has a longer R-R' interval and the post-extrasystolic beat still has **cLBBB**. The second VPC is a little earlier (shorter R-R'i), and the extra time gives the left bundle a chance to become only partially refractory, leading to the incomplete LBBB on the post-extrasystolic beat.

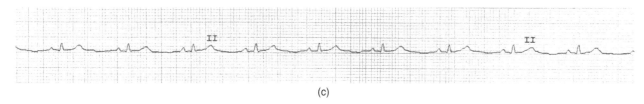

(c)

Figure 6.4c Paper speed 50 mm/s, 1 cm/mV, lead II, same cat after atenolol administration. NSR with a HR of approximately 150 bpm. The LBBB has completely resolved.

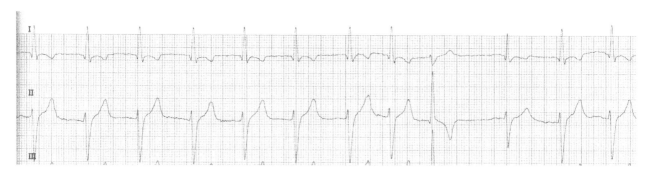

Figure 6.5 Paper speed 50 mm/s, 1 cm/mV, leads I and II, feline. Atrial fibrillation, **LBBB masquerading as RBBB** due to axis deviation. The ninth complex is a VPC, which is followed by a compensatory-like pause. The **post-extrasystolic beat** has a narrower complex (**incomplete LBBB**) from better intraventricular conduction induced by the pause from the VPC.

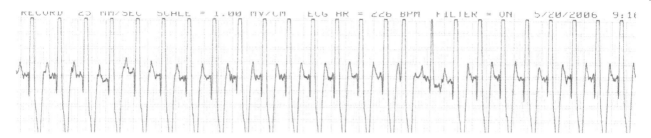

Figure 6.6 Paper speed 25 mm/s, 1 cm/mV, lead II, canine with congestive heart failure and pulmonary hypertension. LBBB and sinus tachycardia. The 16th complex is an APC with LBBB aberration, and the complex that follows is of normal duration, suggesting the LBBB here is **rate-dependent**. The amplitude is set too high on this strip, and the R and T waves go off the strip. This was initially confused with VT by the rDVM; however, P waves clearly precede each beat (save for the APC).

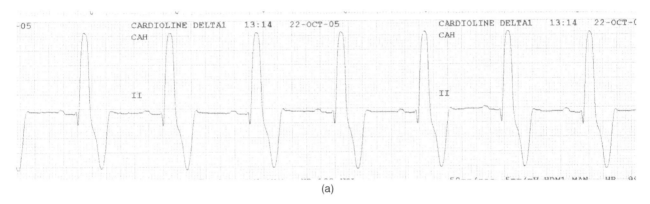

(a)

Figure 6.7a Paper speed 50 mm/s, 0.5 cm/mV, lead II, canine. **LBBB** is persistent in this dog. The QRS complexes are very wide at 0.12 second in duration.

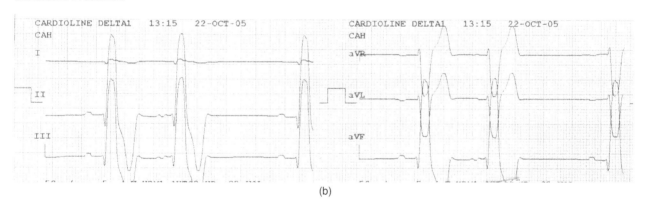

(b)

Figure 6.7b Paper speed 50 mm/s, 0.5 cm/mV, lead II, same dog, full EKG. The second complex is an APC which resets the rhythm.

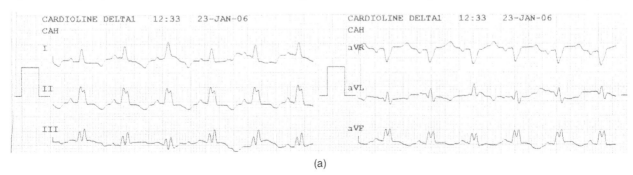

(a)

Figure 6.8a Paper speed 50 mm/s, 1 cm/mV, feline, full EKG. **Complete LBBB**. The QRS complexes are positive in I, II, III, and aVF (and L precordials – not shown).

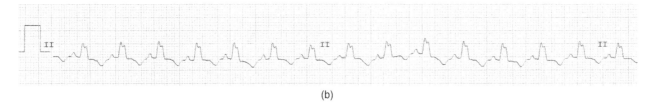

(b)

Figure 6.8b Paper speed 50 mm/s, 1 cm/mV, lead II, same cat. The QRS duration is prolonged at approximately 0.08 second and has a distinctive notch on the downstroke of the S wave. P waves are clearly seen preceding all QRS complexes, indicating sinus rhythm.

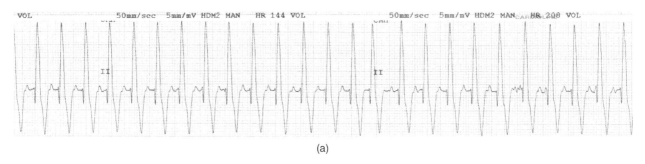

(a)

Figure 6.9a Paper speed 25 mm/s, 0 5 cm/mV, lead II, canine. **LBBB** and sinus tachycardia. The 15th complex is an APC with LBBB aberration.

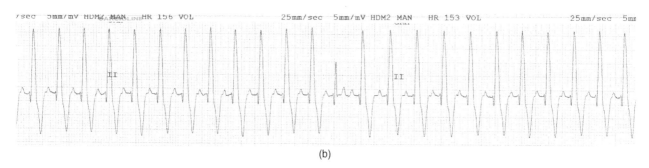

(b)

Figure 6.9b Paper speed 25 mm/s, 0.5 cm/mV, lead II, same dog. The 13th complex is normally conducted, illustrating the marked difference between normal conduction and aberrant conduction. Perhaps this beat is a **ventricular fusion** with a fortuitously timed VPC from the left ventricle. If the P-R' interval was shorter than that of the P-R interval of the rest of the beats, this would support a diagnosis of ventricular fusion. At this paper speed, however, it is difficult to be certain.

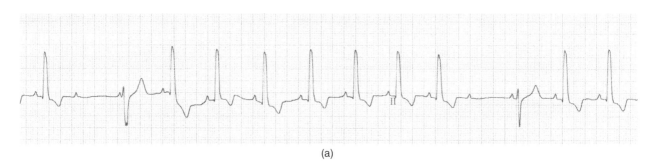

(a)

Figure 6.10a Paper speed 50 mm/s, 1 cm/mV, lead II, feline. SR with HR of 120 bpm. Complete LBBB. Intermittent Type II second degree AVB results in pauses that elicit ventricular escapes. In this case, the ventricular escape complexes have a RBBB-like morphology, consistent with a left ventricular origin. The 10th QRS complex shows a paradoxically **narrowed QRS** due to fusion of the supraventricular focus initiated by the sinus P wave with a LBBB and a fortuitously timed LV originating spontaneous focus resulting in near-simultaneous activation of the RV and the LV, narrowing the QRS complex, albeit with axis deviation.

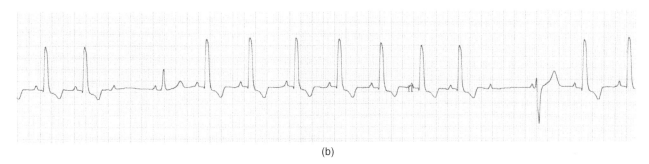

(b)

Figure 6.10b Paper speed 50 mm/s, 1 cm/mV, lead II, same cat. The first two sinus complexes are followed by a non-conducted P wave, which is terminated by a ventricular fusion with near-normal QRS duration/configuration due to the mechanism as described above. Note the near-normal P-R' interval. The 11th QRS complex is a ventricular escape from the LV (RBBB-like configuration) with little to no ventricular fusion and a prolonged QRS complex. The Type II second degree AVB (Mobitz) here likely occurs to bilateral BBB with intermittent block in the RBB.

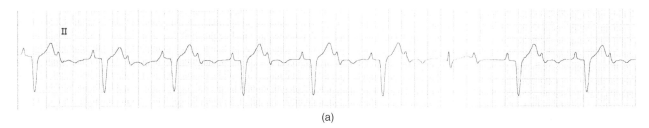

(a)

Figure 6.11a Paper speed 50 mm/s, 1 cm/mV, lead II, feline. Sinus rhythm, **cLBBB masquerading as RBBB** from R axis deviation, ventricular bigeminy. The VPCs are not apparent at first glance, and it is tempting to call this 2 : 1 AVB (suggestive of bilateral BBB). The VPCs are superimposed on the P wave immediately following the QRS complexes of the sinus beats, and the T waves of the VPCs are negative. The 13th complex is a ventricular fusion with **narrowing** of the QRS consistent with a VPC originating from the left ventricle.

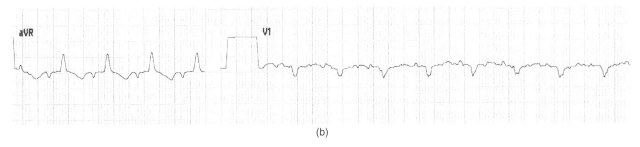

(b)

Figure 6.11b Paper speed 50 mm/s, 1 cm/mV, leads aVR, V1. Same cat. Sinus rhythm, cLBBB. Note the QRS complexes are negative in V1 consistent with LBBB.

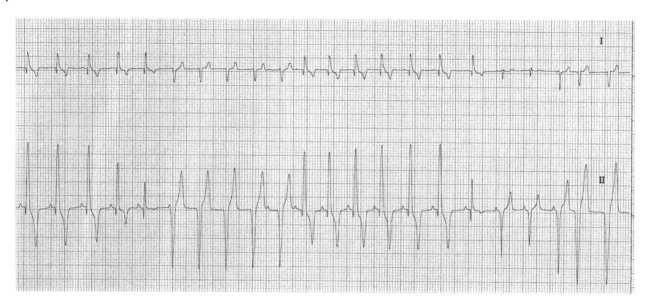

Figure 6.12 Paper speed 50 mm/s, 0.5 cm/mV, leads I and II, canine with hepatic neoplasia. Sinus arrhythmia, cLBBB, incomplete AVD secondary to usurpation by AIVR of LV origin, ventricular fusions with **normalized QRS duration**. The first three complexes are sinus in origin conducted with LBBB. The 4th, 5th, 17th–19th complexes are ventricular fusions with narrowing of the QRS due to fortuitous timing of the LV ectopics. It is tempting for the clinician to label the narrow complexes as sinus captures with gradual alternation of axes of the AIVR, but careful inspection of the P-R intervals reveals AV association during LBBB (constant P-Ri despite variable P-Pi) and AV dissociation (variable P-Ri/R-Pi) during AIVR.

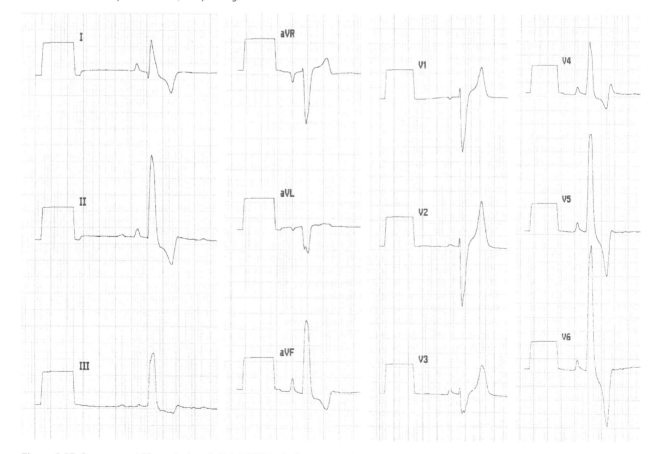

Figure 6.13 Paper speed 50 mm/s, 1 cm/mV, full EKG including precordials, canine. **Sinus rhythm, cLBBB** Note the normal QRS axis in the limb leads and negative complexes in VI with delayed intrisicoid and positive complexes in V6.

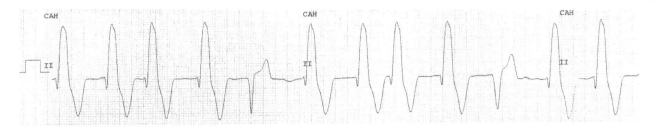

Figure 6.14 Paper speed 50 mm/s, 0.5 cm/mV, lead II, canine. **Complete LBBB**, atrial fibrillation and right ventricular premature complexes with fusion. P waves are absent, and the ventricular rhythm is irregularly irregular consistent with atrial fibrillation. The QRS complexes are markedly prolonged from underlying LBBB. The fifth complex is a fortuitously timed VPC originating from the left ventricle (RBBB-like morphology), which *normalizes* the QRS duration as it merges with the supraventricular impulse that activates the RBB. The 10th complex has less of a degree of fusion with a longer QRS duration as a result.

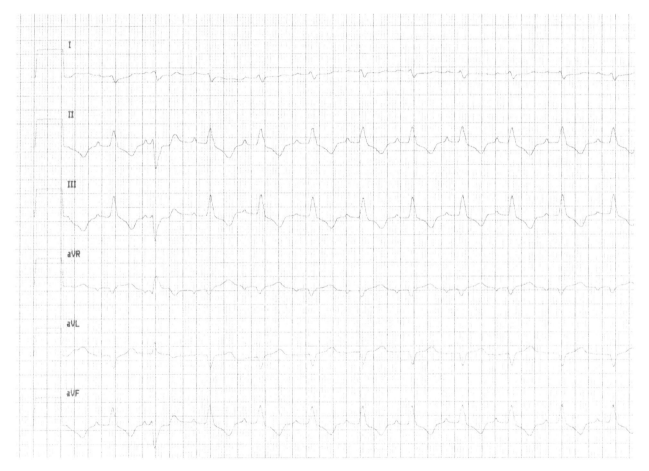

Figure 6.15 Paper speed 50 mm/s, 1 cm/mV, full EKG, cat with severe hypotension, DCM and systolic failure. **Complete LBBB**. The second complex is a VPC. Note the concurrent first degree AVB (long P-Ri). Conduction system disorders are quite common in cats with systolic failure.

Left bundle branch block is most accurately diagnosed by examining the precordial leads in addition to the limb leads. Lead I shows a monophasic R wave, no Q wave or wide, notched rR' waves. Lead V1 shows a qS or rS pattern, and V6 shows a monophasic R wave, no Q or wide, notched rR' waves with a late intrinsicoid deflection. The asynchronous activation of the ventricles increases the QRS duration, making the QRS complexes wide. The abnormal initial vector results in loss of "normal" septal forces (absence of a q wave in I, aVL and V6). Late activation of the left ventricle, prolongation of the dominant, leftward vector, and progression of the middle and terminal forces lead to positive and wide R waves in the left lateral leads. The S-T segment and T wave vectors are opposite in polarity of the QRS with slurring of the S-T segment into the T wave from a secondary repolarization abnormality. Left BBB may be confused with ventricular ectopics originating in the RV.

Further reading

Fisch, C. and Miles, W.M. (1982). Deceleration-dependent left bundle branch block: a spectrum of bundle branch conduction delay. *Circulation* 65: 1029–1032.

Marriott, H.J.L. (1998). *Pearls & Pitfalls in Electrocardiography: Pithy Practical Pointers*, 2e. William & Wilkins.

Marriott, H.J.L. and Conover, M.B. (1998). *Advanced Concepts in Arrhythmias*, 3e. Mosby.

Mulz, J.M. and Schrope, D.P. (2009). ECG of the month. *JAVMA* 235 (1): 35–36.

Nakamura, R.K. and Zimmerman, S.A. (2012). ECG of the month. *JAVMA* 241 (4), 15: 433–434.

Surawicz, B. and Knilans, T.K. (2001). *Chou's Electrocardiography in Clinical Practice: Adult and Pediatric*, 5e. Saunders.

Toaldo, M.B., Diana A, Sgreccia G et al. ECG of the month, *JAVMA*, Vo 240, No. 12, 2012, p 1419–1421

Tou, S.P., DeFrancesco, T.C., and Keene, B.W. (2011). ECG of the month. *JAVMA* 239 (1): 55–57.

Vessel, H. and Lowen, G. (1963). Electrocardiogram of the month: Normal intraventricular conduction following post-extrasystolic pause in bundle branch block; with critical rate phenomenon. *Chest* 43 (1): 94–96.

7

Fascicular Blocks

CHAPTER MENU

Left anterior fascicular block, 77
Left medial fascicular block, 77
Left posterior fascicular block, 78
Bilateral bundle branch block, 79
Bifascicular block, 79
   Masquerading bundle branch block, 80
Trifascicular block, 81
Arborization block, 86

Remember, these proposed examples of the hemiblocks and bifascicular blocks are based on human criteria. The exact branching of the specialized Purkinje cell bundles in animals (and humans, for that matter) is in reality highly variable. Consequently, we may identify a pattern consistent with a hemiblock in our patients, but remember it is a pattern and not necessarily reflective of discrete conduction blockade in a simple trifascicular branching system, since that just may not exist. The left bundle may branch into anterior, middle, and posterior fascicles or diffuse branching may be present. First, second and third degree blocks can occur in the His bundle, R and L bundle branches. That said, take the following with a well-deserved grain of salt.

Left anterior fascicular block
Left anterior fascicular block (LAFB) (may be referred to as left anterior hemiblock) is a common finding in cats with cardiomyopathy, particularly hypertrophic cardiomyopathy/HCM (usually explained by simple left axis deviation/LAD), but also may be seen in hyperkalemia and myocardial infarction. It is more technically correct to refer to LAFB as a "LAFB pattern" or simply "LAD," in cats with HCM. Causes of LAD should technically be excluded. Left axis deviation alone has no direct relationship to left ventricular hypertrophy and may be attributed to degenerative disease of the conduction system, sclerosis of the left side of the ossa chordis (cardiac skeleton), or myocardial

fibrosis – which is what occurs in cats with HCM. Left anterior fascicular block is characterized by normal to slightly prolonged QRS, marked L axis shift with small Q waves, and tall R waves in I and aVL and deep S waves in II, III, and aVF. Proposed electrocardiographic criteria in humans for LAFB include aVR and aVL end in an R wave and that the peak of the terminal R wave in aVR occur later than the peak of the terminal R wave in aVL, due to the terminal forces directed superiorly and in a counterclockwise direction. The pattern of LAFB may occur in patients with AVSDs (atrioventricular septal defects, endocardial cushion defects) and is due to pre-excitation of the posterobasal region of the LV from the abnormal anatomical structure of the conduction system. It may also occur with isolated ostium primum atrial septal defects or be secondary to WPW/VPE (Wolff-Parkinson-White, ventricular pre-excitation). Rarely, Left anterior fascicular block may be associated with intermittent Mobitz Type I or II block.

Left medial fascicular block
Left medial fascicular block, (LMFB) (left septal fascicular block) is occasionally evoked to explain the slightly aberrant and taller QRS complexes occasionally associated with supraventricular premature beats. If a patient actually has three main fascicular divisions of the left bundle branch, a block in the so-called medial fascicle may cause the axis of the QRS to be slightly deviated in the direction of

Interpretation of the Electrocardiogram in Small Animals, First Edition. Nick A. Schroeder.
© 2021 John Wiley & Sons Inc. Published 2021 by John Wiley & Sons Inc.

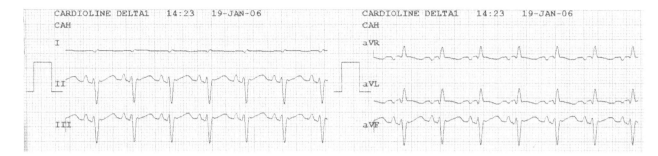

Figure 7.1 Paper speed 50 mm/s, 1 cm/mV, feline, **LAFB**. Leads II, III, and aVF have deep S waves. Left axis deviation is present with a MEA of approximately −90 degrees making lead I isoelectric.

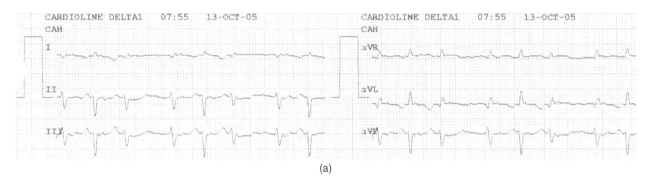

(a)

Figure 7.2a Paper speed 50 mm/s, 2 cm/mV, feline. **LAFB** and what appears to be atrial trigeminy. This cat had a history of supraventricular tachycardia. The second, fifth, and eighth complexes of each strip are premature beats, which seem to be interpolated and mildly aberrant. Alternatively, the premature beats may be fascicular, and the post-extrasystolic beats could be re-entrant or echo beats.

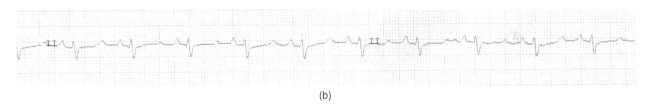

(b)

Figure 7.2b Paper speed 50 mm/s, 2 cm/mV, lead II, same cat in sinus rhythm.

the blocked fascicle. This would be expected to make the QRS more parallel with lead II, potentially resulting in a slightly taller QRS complex in lead II. Proposed criteria for LMFB in human medicine include the loss of the septal q waves (if present), absence of septal infarction, complete or incomplete LBBB and ventricular pre-excitation, no more than 10 ms prolongation of the QRS, normal intrinsicoid deflection time (ventricular activation time) in leads V5-6, aVL, and aVF, no slurring or notching on the upstroke of the R wave in leads I and V5-6, and little change in the frontal QRS MEA. This is obviously not something provable without invasive testing and is essentially clinically irrelevant aside from possibly confusing the examiner with ventricular ectopy.

Left posterior fascicular block Left posterior fascicular block (LPFB, may be referred to as left posterior hemiblock) is characterized by abnormal RAD due to unbalanced late forces of depolarization being deviated caudally and to the right. In humans, this means a QRS MEA of > =110 degrees; if young age, extensive anterior/lateral or inferior infarction, right ventricular hypertrophy (RVH), and asthenic habitus (causes of physiologic or pathologic right axis deviation) are excluded. Left posterior fascicular block is characterized by a positive QRS in II, III, and aVF and negative QRS in lead I (qR pattern in I and aVL and tall R waves in II, III, and aVF). Often, there is a slurred R downstroke in III, aVF, and V6, with mild QRS prolongation. Kittleson noted that experimentally induced LPFB has not changed the MEA or terminal forces

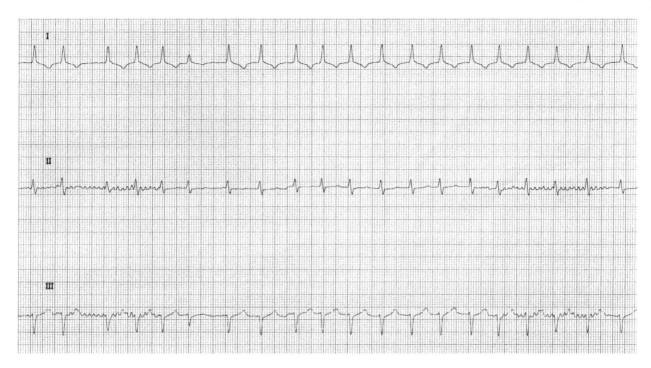

Figure 7.3 Paper speed 50 mm/s, 1 cm/mV, leads I, II, III, feline with dilated cardiomyopathy. Atrial fibrillation is present with no discernable P waves and an irregularly irregular apparently supraventricular rhythm. **Left anterior fascicular block** of the QRS complexes is evident and baseline purring artifact is intermittently apparent.

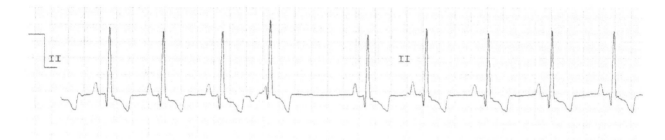

Figure 7.4 Paper speed 50 mm/s, 1 cm/mV, lead II, canine. The fourth beat is a supraventricular premature beat (junctional premature beat vs. low ectopic atrial premature beat), and the QRS complex is slightly taller than the sinus QRS complexes, suggestive of a functional **left medial fascicular block**.

in the dog. Right axis deviation secondary to right ventricular enlargement should be excluded. Rarely, intermittent LPFB may occur with Mobitz Type I or II block in the LPF.

Bilateral bundle branch block Bilateral BBB (block in both the RBB and the LBB), if complete, causes AV conduction to fail, resulting in third-degree AVB. Ventricular escape rhythm must rescue the heart if asystole is protracted. If this phenomenon is transient, then the term third degree AVB is inappropriate (since AV conduction is at least intermittently possible) and either the term paroxysmal AVB or transient ventricular asystole is used. This occurs when a patient with complete BBB of

one branch suddenly develops second degree AVB (usually Mobitz) in the contralateral bundle branch, which often persists for more than one sinoatrial discharge (high-grade block). Escape rhythms may rescue the heart before conduction resumes.

Bifascicular block It occurs when a patient with complete RBBB has coexistent LAFB or LPFB, and it has also been referred to as bilateral bifascicular block. Basically, the first portion of the QRS displays either LAFB or LPFB and the terminal portion results from RBBB. Thus, the limb leads display fascicular block with abnormal prolongation while the pattern is RBBB in the precordials.

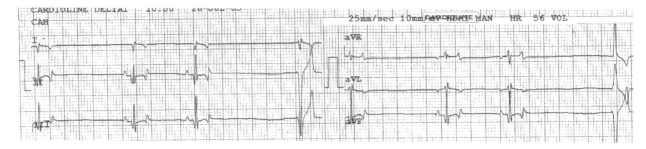

Figure 7.5 Paper speed 25 mm/s, 1 cm/mV, full EKG, canine, *possible* **LPFB**. Here, the MEA is approximately 110 degrees or so. Lead aVL has an rS pattern, and qR pattern is seen in II, III, and aVF. A pause after the third complex is terminated by a ventricular escape beat. Simple RAD could explain this EKG as well.

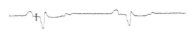

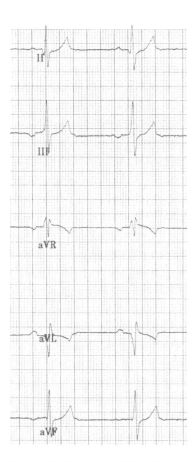

Figure 7.6 Paper speed 50 mm/s, 1 cm/mV, full EKG, canine. Possible **LPFB**. Note the RAD past 110 degrees.

This underscores the importance to note the "pre-blocked QRS axis" in the frontal plane. This is the mean electrical axis of the intrinsicoid deflection. In the presence of RBBB, a pre-blocked left axis shift is consistent with LAFB and a right axis shift is suggestive of LPFB. Tilley stated that RBBB + LAFB results in QRS duration of 0.06 second or greater; marked LAD (usu. > −60 degrees); wide and deep S waves in I, II, III, aVF, V4; tall R waves and small q waves in I and aVL; QRS in V4 with a wide rsR' or RSR' pattern that is often M-shaped. Kittleson also noted that experimentally disrupting the LAF in dogs with pre-existing RBBB resulted in very minor changes to the already rightward-oriented MEA. Bifascicular block can result in "masquerading BBB," since the QRS axis in the limb leads is discordant from the precordial axis. Since LAFB + LPFB involves two fascicles, complete LBBB has also been referred to as a bifascicular block (though not bilateral per se). Supraventricular premature complexes may be conducted with aberrancy, and if bifascicular, RBBB+LAFB is much more common since the LAF has a longer refractory period than the LPF. The RBB has the longest refractory period of the fascicles normally.

Masquerading bundle branch block It results in a widened QRS complex, is the result of abnormal axis deviation in the presence of a BBB, and can be from a specific form of bifascicular block. The end result is often a LBBB pattern in the limb leads with a RBBB pattern in the precordial leads. Alternatively, if a LBBB occurs with a QRS axis deviated far enough to the L, the QRS will be negative in lead II, confusing the examiner with a RBBB. Abnormal chest conformation (asthenic habitus) with a RBBB or a congenital defect involving RVH may also produce such a pattern. Bifascicular block with RBBB+LAFB associated with LVH or fibrosis in the anterolateral LV wall produces this pattern as well. So-called "standard masquerading BBB" is present when RBBB+LAFB occurs and S wave is absent in lead I, and "precordial masquerading BBB"

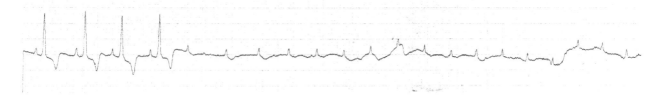

Figure 7.7 Paper speed 25 mm/s, 1 cm/mV, lead II, feline, *transient ventricular asystole* from paroxysmal AV block. The conducted QRS complexes have a LBBB morphology, suggestive that the AVB is secondary to **bilateral BBB**. Complete failure of conduction to the ventricles occurs following the fifth P wave. This resulted in syncope in this patient. Third degree AVB is *not* present, as conduction is possible through the AVN, as evidenced by the first four complexes.

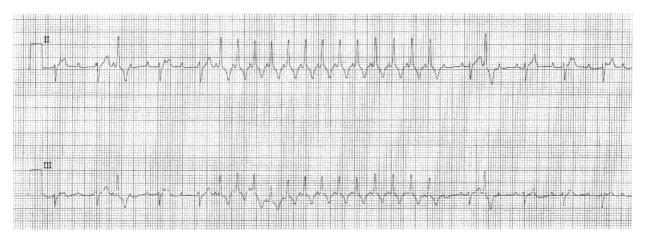

Figure 7.8 Paper speed 25 mm/s, 1 cm/mV, lead II, feline. **Bilateral BBB.** Incomplete (second degree, Mobitz/Type II, high grade) AV block with LV escape rhythm. Initially, the ventricular rate is 96 bpm, with occasional supraventricular capture. The sixth ventricular complex is a sinus capture followed by sinus rhythm/cLBBB, which is abruptly terminated by an AV block, followed by a single ventricular escape, another sinus capture, and then ventricular escape rhythm. The abrupt AVB in the presence of cLBBB suggests Mobitz periodicity in the contralateral RBBB and intermittent failure of conduction to the ventricles consistent with bilateral BBB.

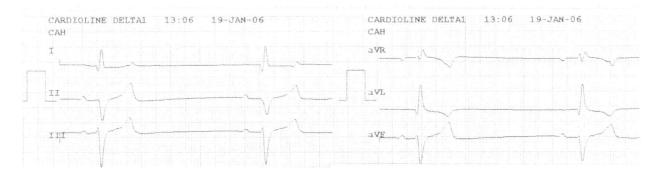

Figure 7.9 Paper speed 50 mm/s, 1 cm/mV, German Shepherd with a structurally normal heart. **Bifascicular block** (**RBBB** *and* **LAFB**). Leads II, III, and aVF have deep S waves. The peak of the terminal R wave in aVR occurs just after the peak of the terminal R wave in aVL as well. Left axis deviation is present (MEA approximately −60 degrees). The QRS duration is prolonged at 0.08 second. A wide rsR' or RSR' (often M-shaped) in V1 would complete the criteria for both RBBB and LAFB.

occurs when the S wave is absent from V5 to V6, but V1 still displays typical RBBB in both scenarios. This is why the precordial leads need to be investigated if a BBB is diagnosed, given that LBBB generally has a worse prognosis than RBBB.

Trifascicular block (RBBB + LAFB + LPFB), a cause of transient high-grade AVB/transient ventricular asystole (if incomplete), is suggested when a patient with bifascicular block without impaired AV conduction suddenly develops a prolonged P-R interval or higher

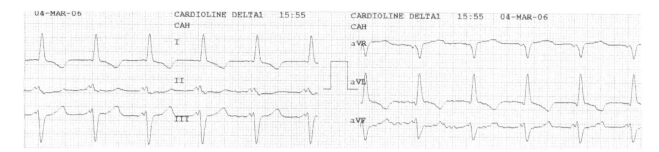

Figure 7.10 Paper speed 50 mm/s, 1 cm/mV, full EKG, feline. **Bifascicular block** (**RBBB** *and* **LAFB**), rule-out **masquerading BBB** (**RBBB + LAD**). The P-R interval is extremely short in this patient (approximately 0.03 second) secondary to ventricular pre-excitation (LGL syndrome). The QRS duration is wide at approximately 0.06 second. Left axis deviation is present as well. This patient had significant structural heart disease, so RBBB + LAD alone could explain this pattern.

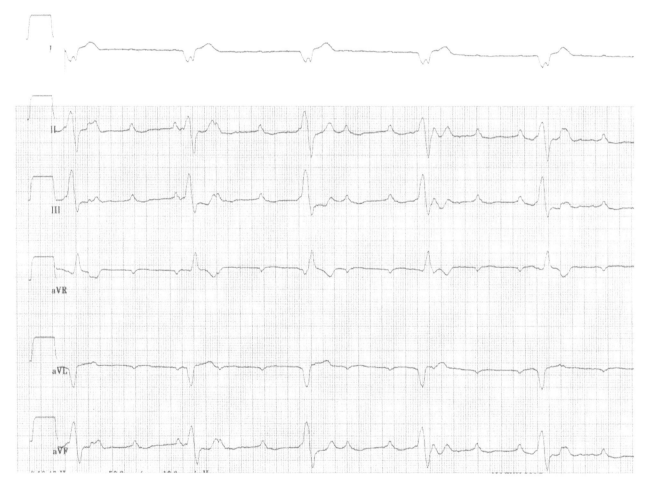

Figure 7.11 Paper speed 50 mm/s, 1 cm/mV, full EKG, canine. Third degree AVB, sinus rhythm of the atria, junctional escape rhythm of the ventricles (HR: 66 bpm), **bifascicular block** (RBBB+LPFB). Note the atypical RBBB + RAD. A R/O would include an accelerated ventricular focus from the L anterior fascicle. The QRS complexes are markedly prolonged, which would fit better with a ventricular origin; however, the rate is more suggestive of a junctional origin.

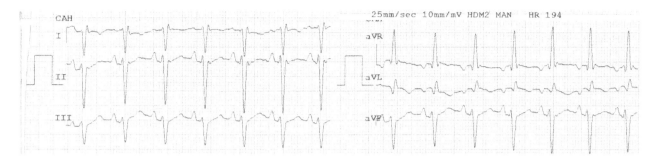

Figure 7.12 Paper speed 50 mm/s, 1 cm/mV, cat with AV canal defect. **Masquerading BBB (RBBB and LAD, r/o LAFB + extreme RAD)**. Leads II, III, and aVF have deep and wide S waves. The QRS duration is slightly prolonged at 0.06 second. Marked LAD with a MEA of approximately −130 degrees (or extreme RAD of −230 degrees) is present. RBBB + LAFB produces a MEA with LAD beyond −45 degrees, and RBBB + LPFB produces a MEA to the right of +120 degrees. Alternatively, this EKG may simply represent LAFB + RVH, which produces extreme RAD, and the increased duration of the QRS may be from LVH in this cat with confirmed RVH and LVH on echocardiography secondary to an atrioventricular canal defect. Left axis deviation/LAFB pattern of the QRS is common in patient with an atrioventricular canal defect (endocardial cushion defect, atrioventricular septal defect or AVSD).

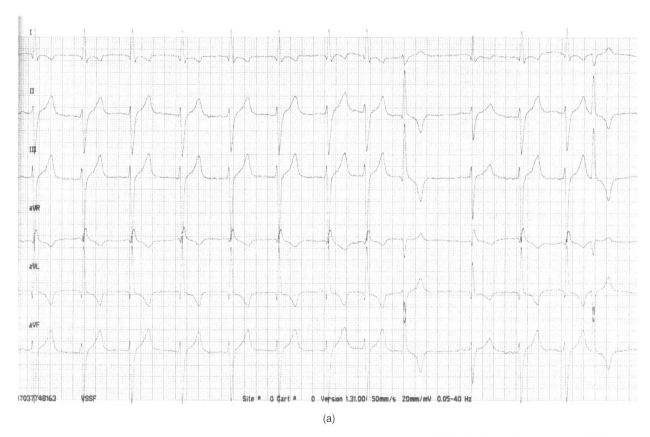

(a)

Figure 7.13a Paper speed 50 mm/s, 1 cm/mV, full EKG (limb leads), feline. *Masquerading BBB*. **Atrial fibrillation, complete LBBB masquerading as RBBB due to severe LAD**. The 9th and 13th complexes are VPCs. The 10th complex may be a fusion beat as it is slightly narrower than the normal supraventricular complexes, and the VPCs have a RBBB/LPFB morphology, consistent with a focus in the left anterior fascicle or radiation. VPCs arising on the opposite side of a blocked bundle may fuse with a supraventricular beat occurring simultaneously, normalizing the QRS to some extent. The compensatory-like pause following the ninth complex may alternatively have allowed for better intraventricular conduction (provided the BBB is rate-dependent), which may be more likely in this scenario, given the narrower complex only occurs following the pause.

V1

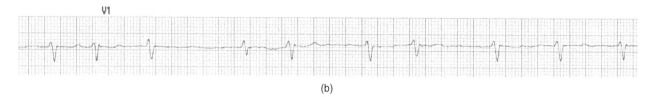

(b)

Figure 7.13b Paper speed 50 mm/s, 1 cm/mV, lead V1, same cat. The complexes have deep and broad S waves consistent with LBBB. The third complex is a VPC.

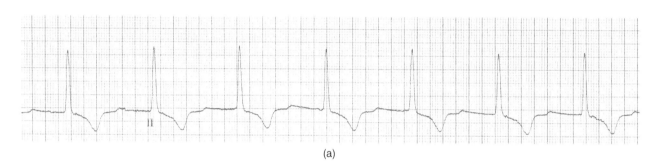

(a)

Figure 7.14a Paper speed 50 mm/s, 1 cm/mV, lead II, feline with history of high-grade AVB and ventricular escape rhythm. Severe first degree AVB is present with a P-R interval of approximately 0.26 second! The HR here is approximately 90 bpm. This cat was severely hypotensive, hypothermic, and had CHF from a combination of bradycardia and HCM. Left BBB in sinus rhythm is suggestive of transient **bilateral BBB** (RBBB + LBBB) leading to AVB and ventricular escape. **Trifascicular block** is therefore suggested. Long AV nodal conduction time just confirms diffuse conduction system disease.

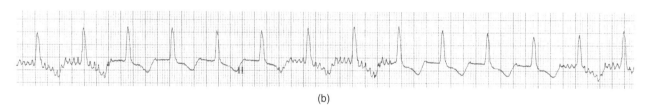

(b)

Figure 7.14b Paper speed 50 mm/s, 1 cm/mV, lead II, same cat after rewarming and dobutamine infusion. The P-R interval is still long but shortened at approximately 0.12 second. The HR has increased to approximately 176 bpm. Purring artifact is seen as an intermittently rapidly undulating baseline.

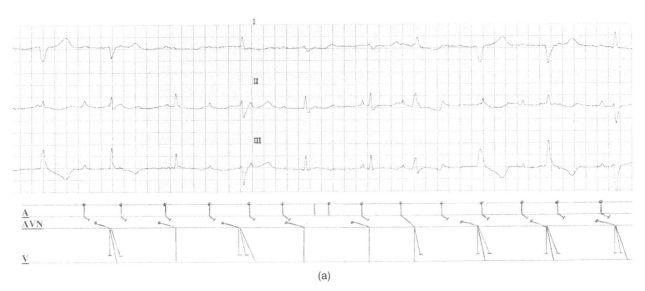

(a)

Figure 7.15a Paper speed 50 mm/s, 1 cm/mV, leads I, II, III, feline. Incomplete AV dissociation is present from high-grade AV block. Sinus rhythm of the atria is present with an atrial rate of approximately 176 bpm. Escape rhythm with a ventricular rate approximately 130 bpm is in control of the ventricles. The underlying escape rhythm appears to be *reset* by sinus captures, suggesting a junctional escape focus by the Rule of reset. Alternating aberrancy of the junctional escapes is occurring as well. The first QRS complex has a RBBB+LPFB pattern (RAD) with conduction along the L anterior fascicle/radiation. The second QRS (as diagrammed) appears to be conducted with slightly less aberration, suggestive of an incomplete block in the left posterior fascicle. The third is normally conducted. The fourth is conducted with a RBBB+LAFB pattern (LAD). The fifth complex is again normally conducted but possibly followed by an atrial echo. Alternatively, the next sinus beat may be reentering the atria, resetting the sinus node at a new interval. The only sinus capture (complex #7) is conducted with an incomplete LBBB. The following beats are conducted with a RBBB+LPFB, and the last beat is conducted with RBBB+LAFB. The varied conduction blocks are certainly rate-related to some degree, and the alternating fascicular blocks in the presence of high-grade AV block are suggestive of **trifascicular block**.

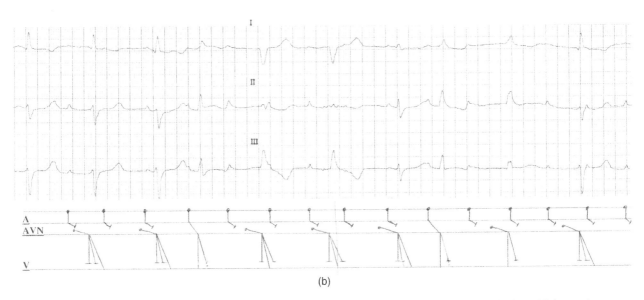

(b)

Figure 7.15b Paper speed 50 mm/s, 1 cm/mV, leads I, II, III, same cat. Two sinus captures here reset the rhythm with incomplete or complete LBBB aberration and have a consistent P-R interval (0.10 second, the same as in the above strip). The junctional escapes alternate with RBBB+LAFB at the beginning, and RBBB+LPFB at the end. The sixth complex has an apparent incomplete block in the left anterior fascicle.

degree AVB. The first degree AVB may actually occur in the intact fascicle below the level of the AVN itself. Mobitz Type II second degree BBB commonly manifests as intermittent/incomplete trifascicular block. If trifascicular block is complete, then third degree AVB is present and ventricular escape rhythm must ensue if the patient is to survive.

Arborization block It is the slowed conduction in the distal His-Purkinje system (terminal ramifications), is associated with peri-infarction patterns, tends to markedly widen the QRS complex and can be seen in severe end-stage heart disease associated with refractory congestive heart failure. It is questionable whether or not this phenomenon occurs in dogs as experimental infarction failed to alter morphologies of Purkinje spikes, and nonspecific intraventricular conduction disturbances associated with advanced myocardial fibrosis in canine dilated cardiomyopathy or other advanced structural heart disease may account for such a QRS pattern (see Chapter 8).

Further reading

Choudhary, D., Namboodri, N., and Tharakan, J.A. (2014). A case of 'Masquerading' bundle branch block: a forgotten concept. *Indian Heart J.* 66 (1): 139–140.

Elizari, M., Baranchuk, A., and Chiale, P. (2013). Masquerading bundle branch block: a variety of right bundle branch block with left anterior fascicular block. *Expert. Rev. Cardiovasc. Ther.* https://doi.org/10.1586/erc.12.142.

Kittleson, M.D. and Kienle, R.D. (1998). *Small Animal Cardiovascular Medicine*. Mosby.

Marriot, H.J.L. and Conover, M.B. (1998). *Advanced Concepts in Arrhythmias*, 3e. Mosby.

MacAlpin, R.N. (2003). Left septal fascicular block: myth or reality? *Indian Pacing Elecrophysiol. J.* 3 (3): 157–177.

Nelson, W.P., Marriott, H.J.L., and Schocken, D.D. (2007). *Concepts & Cautions in Electrocardiography*. MedInfo Inc.

Tilley, L.P. (1992). *Essentials of Canine and Feline Electrocardiography: Interpretation and Treatment*, 3e. Lippincott Williams & Wilkins, Lea & Febiger.

Surawicz, B. and Knilans, T.K. (2001). *Chou's Electrocardiography in Clinical Practice: Adult and Pediatric*, 5e. Saunders.

Watt, T.B. and Pruitt, R.D. (1972). Focal lesions in the canine bundle of his: their effect on ventricular excitation. *Circ. Res.* XXXI: 531–545.

Unger, P., Lesser, M.E., Kugel, V.H., and Lev, M. (1958). The concept of "masquerading" bundle-branch block: an electrocardiographic-pathologic correlation. *Circulation* 17: 397–409.

8

Wide-Complex Supraventricular Tachycardia and Intraventricular Conduction Disturbances

---

CHAPTER MENU

Wide-complex supraventricular tachycardias, 87
Intraventricular conduction disturbances, 90

Wide-complex supraventricular tachycardias

Occasionally, a supraventricular tachycardia (SVT) will have QRS complexes that are prolonged in duration, confusing the examiner with ventricular tachycardia (VT). Fortunately, wide-complex tachycardia (WCT, aka wide QRS tachycardia/WQRST) secondary to SVT is relatively uncommon in veterinary patients. When it does occur, the most common cause is a pre-existing bundle branch block aberration (LBBB or RBBB). If sinus complexes are noted before or after the SVT with typical patterns of BBB aberration and the tachycardia has the same QRS pattern/configuration, then SVT is the likely diagnosis. It should be noted, however, that BBB aberration can develop during SVT for functional or rate-related reasons and the QRS is of normal duration in sinus rhythm. Often, the aberrancy is transient and conduction normalizes over time. Rarely, a bundle branch will experience "fatigue" during a tachycardia with late-developing aberrancy. Extremely wide QRS complexes with atypical BBB patterns, atrioventricular dissociation, fusion and capture beats, precordial concordance, etc., favor a diagnosis of VT. Other causes of a wide-complex tachycardia include SVT with pre-existing abnormal QRS (usually patients with underlying structural heart disease – i.e. left ventricular hypertrophy, congenital lesions), widened QRS secondary to drug administration, or electrolyte abnormalities and ventricular pacing (pacemaker-mediated tachycardia). Again, these have wide QRS complexes in sinus rhythm and during SVT. Rare (and not or rarely reported in veterinary patients) causes of wide-complex SVT include antidromic atrioventricular reciprocating tachycardia, circus movement tachycardia with two accessory pathways, and atrial fibrillation or flutter with pre-excitation. Transient post-tachycardia BBB

in sinus rhythm may develop from overdrive suppression following a VT.

Of utmost importance is to remember that VT is a far more common cause of a WCT than is SVT. Lead II is terrible for the differentiation of VT from SVT as QS complexes may be present in SVT/LBBB, SVT/RBBB, and in VT from the right or left ventricles. Lead V1 is much better. Supraventricular tachycardia is commonly regular, but so is VT and VT is not uncommonly well-tolerated by the patient. As a side-note, when human physicians are presented with a patient with WCT, an affirmative answer to the following two questions predicts VT regardless of morphology on surface EKG with great accuracy:

Did you recently suffer from myocardial infarction?

Did you have symptoms due to tachycardia only after myocardial infarction?

When in doubt, procainamide is a reasonable choice for converting wide-complex tachycardia of unknown origin, as it may work for either SVT or VT. If the patient is a Boxer, Doberman Pinscher, or Bulldog, VT should be suspected. Giant breed dogs presenting for tachyarrhythmia, especially if the rhythm is irregular are suspected to have atrial fibrillation until proven otherwise.

> ***A Note:*** Unexpected narrowing of the QRS complexes may occasionally be encountered. If the QRS complexes are narrower during tachycardia than in baseline EKG in which the complexes are wide, this suggests VT from a septal focus, activating the ventricles nearly simultaneously. Transient narrowing may occur if fortuitous ventricular fusion occurs. A ventricular premature complex (VPC) arising from a ventricle with a pre-existent BBB or ventricular enlargement may create narrow fusion beats. Ventricular premature complexes fusing with ventricular escape

Interpretation of the Electrocardiogram in Small Animals, First Edition. Nick A. Schroeder.
© 2021 John Wiley & Sons Inc. Published 2021 by John Wiley & Sons Inc.

complexes from the opposite ventricle, left ventricular premature complexes fusing with right ventricular paced beats, supernormality of atrial premature complexes with pre-existent BBB and VPCs from the same ventricle with an accessory pathway may also create unexpectedly narrow QRS complexes. Examples are provided in relevant chapters.

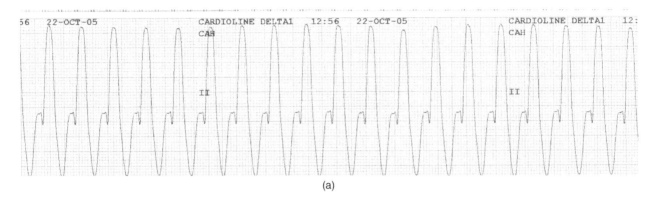

(a)

Figure 8.1a Paper speed 50 mm/s, 0.5 cm/mV, lead II, 15 y/o Standard Poodle. **SVT** with **LBBB**. The HR is approximately 200 bpm. No P waves are visualized marching through the complexes (which would otherwise suggest VT). P′ waves are presumably lost within the T waves.

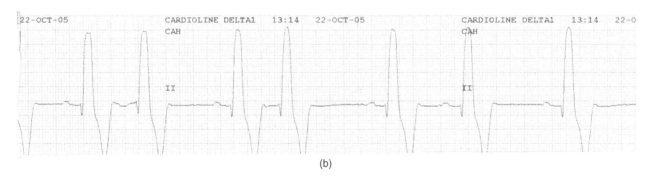

(b)

Figure 8.1b Paper speed 50 mm/s, 0.5 cm/mV, lead II, same dog after a precordial thump restored a sinus rhythm. The sinus complexes are clearly conducted with a LBBB. The first half of the strip showed atrial bigeminy (the second and fourth complexes are atrial premature complexes/APCs that reset the rhythm). Supraventricular tachycardia conducted with BBB is an imposter of VT and it is easy to see why based on the first strip.

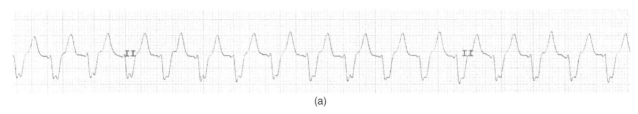

(a)

Figure 8.2a Paper speed 50 mm/s, 2 cm/mV, lead II, cat with **SVT** and **RBBB**. This is a wide-complex tachycardia with a heart rate of approximately 272 bpm. P′ waves are not obvious on this strip.

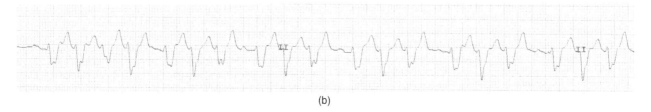

(b)

Figure 8.2b Paper speed 50 mm/s, 2 cm/mV, lead II, same cat. Here, triplets and couplets of APCs follow sinus beats. The premature beats alternate in degrees of aberrancy.

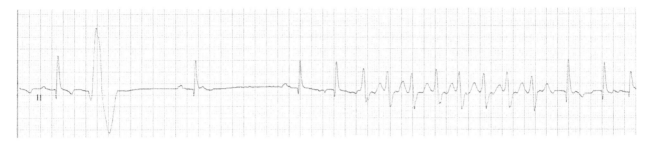

Figure 8.3 Paper speed 50 mm/s, 1 cm/mV, lead II, canine. The second complex is a VPC. The fifth complex is an APC initiating a run of SVT. **RBBB** develops with the sixth complex and persists until the rate slows down enough for normal intraventricular conduction to resume.

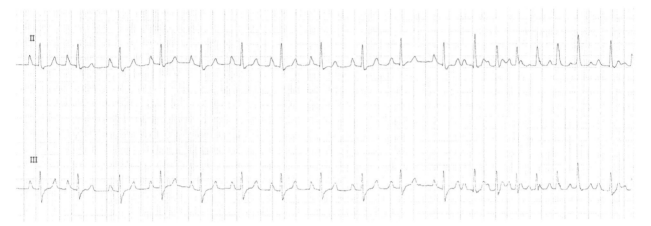

Figure 8.4 Paper speed 50 mm/s, 1 cm/mV, leads II and III, canine. Sinus rhythm followed by a run of **atrial tachycardia** with mild **aberrancy**.

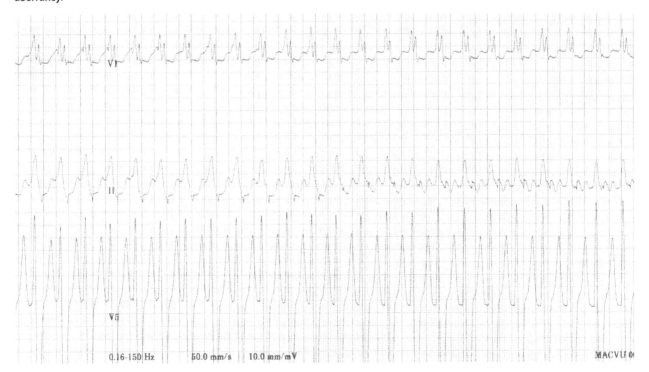

Figure 8.5 Paper speed 50 mm/s, 1 cm/mV, leads V1, II, and V5, canine. **Wide-complex tachycardia**. At the beginning, the QRS complexes are widened; however, as the rate slows, the complexes normalize in duration, indicative of rate-dependent aberrancy. This patient had atrial flutter.

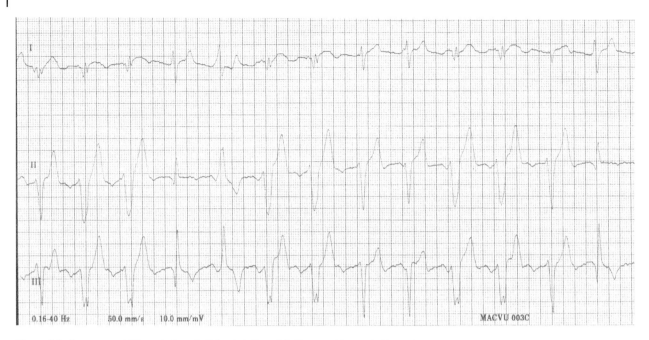

Figure 8.6 Paper speed 50 mm/s, 1 cm/mV, leads I, II, and II. Bernese Mountain Dog with Type I Typical (counterclockwise) AFL. **Rate-dependent bundle-branch block aberration**. The ventricular rate is constant throughout the record. Incomplete RBBB on the 1st, 8th, 9th, and 12th complexes. Complete RBBB appears on the 2nd, 3rd, 6th, 7th, 10th, and 11th complexes. The 4th and 13th complexes are normally conducted, and the 5th complex has an incomplete LBBB morphology. The baseline is undulating regularly from the AFL.

Intraventricular conduction disturbances

Occasionally, the QRS complex itself may be notched and odd-looking in morphology atypical of that associated with BBB or fascicular blocks. Splintered QRS complexes are common in association with tricuspid dysplasia (TVDysplasia). Patients with Ebstein's anomaly in particular may have abnormal QRS complexes with nearly two distinct QRS complexes and is the result of RBBB with delayed activation of the atrialized portion of the right ventricle. Deep, wide, and notched Q waves are not uncommon in patients with ventricular septal defects (VSDs). Microscopic intramural myocardial infarction (MIMI) in association with chronic mitral valvular disease

(CMVDz) and dilated cardiomyopathy may generate a notch or slur on the downstroke of the R wave. A notch briefly reverses polarity, whereas a slur does not. Slurs are often due to QRS projection, and if located on the upstroke of a R wave, may mimic the delta wave of ventricular pre-excitation (which is excluded by a normal P-Ri). True intraventricular conduction disturbances are associated with at least a mildly prolonged QRS complex. If the QRS is normal in duration, then notches are typically the result of projection. These changes are nonspecific, but identification of intraventricular conduction disturbances may prompt further diagnostics such as thoracic radiography and echocardiography.

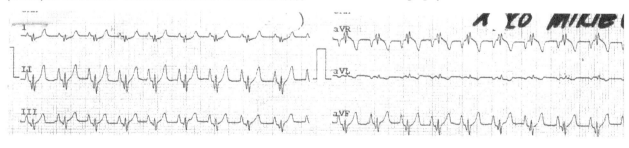

Figure 8.7 Paper speed 50 mm/s, 1 cm/mV, lead II, canine with a ventricular septal defect. Small QRS complexes are present with deep Q waves.

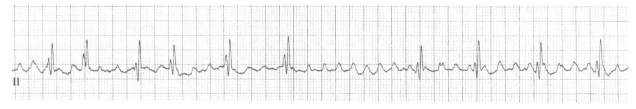

Figure 8.8 Paper speed 50 mm/s, 1 cm/mV, lead II, canine with tricuspid valvular dysplasia of the Ebstein's-type anomaly. Type II atrial flutter. The QRS complexes are splintered (rsR') secondary to an **intraventricular conduction disturbance**.

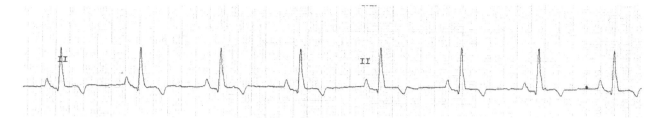

Figure 8.9 Paper speed 50 mm/s, 1 cm/mV, lead II, canine with chronic mitral valvular disease. The **slur** on the downstroke of the R wave is suggestive of **MIMI**. The QRS complexes are mildly prolonged at 0.06 second.

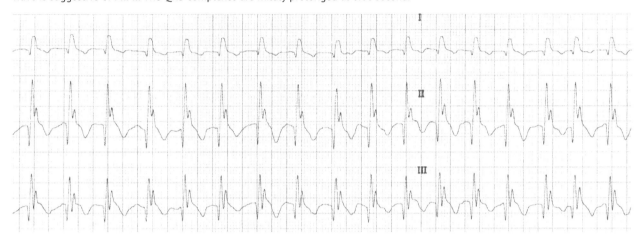

Figure 8.10 Paper speed 50 mm/s, 1 cm/mV, lead II, canine. **Atrial fibrillation with intraventricular conduction disturbance (IVCD)**. The QRS complexes are mildly prolonged at 0.08 second, and the inferior leads have a qRsr' morphology. This patient had atypical QRS patterns in the precordial leads, so a BBB is ruled out. The wide-complex tachycardia here could easily be confused with VT; however, the irregularly irregular rhythm without obvious P waves is indicative of atrial fibrillation. The rapid ventricular rate response makes picking out the subtle R-R variability difficult.

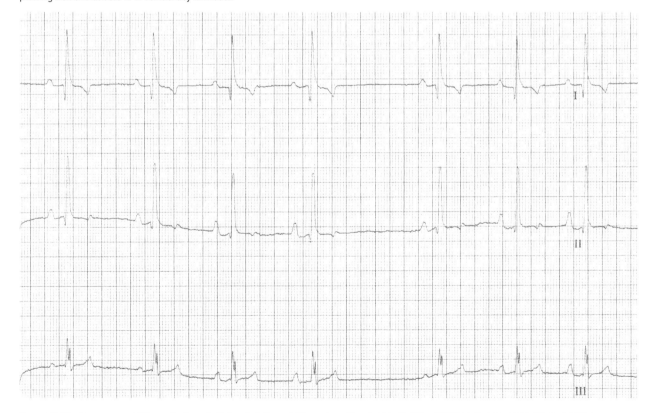

Figure 8.11 Paper speed 50 mm/s, 1 cm/mV, leads I, II, and III, canine. Sinus arrhythmia, **notching** due to projections mimics an intraventricular conduction disturbance in lead III. Note that the complexes are not overtly prolonged at 0.05 second.

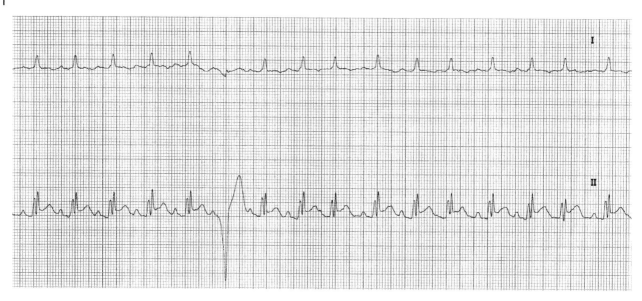

Figure 8.12 Paper speed 50 mm/s, 1 cm/mV, leads I and II, feline. Sinus rhythm with **IVCD**/splintered QRS. The fifth complex is a VPC. The QRS complexes are splintered with rR' complexes, prolonged at 0.06 second and have a pattern not typical of that associated with a BBB.

Further reading

Braunwald, E., Zipes, D., and Libby, P. (2001). *Heart Disease: A Textbook of Cardiovascular Medicine*, 6e. Saunders.

Ettinger, S.J. and Suter, P.F. (1970). *Canine Cardiology*. W.B. Saunders Company.

Fisch, C. and Knoebel, S.B. (2000). *Electrocardiography of Clinical Arrhythmias*. Futurama Publishing Co.

Marriott, H.J.L. (1998). *Pearls & Pitfalls in Electrocardiography: Pithy Practical Pointers*, 2e. William & Wilkins.

Marriott, H.J.L. and Conover, M.B. (1998). *Advanced Concepts in Arrhythmias*, 3e. Mosby.

Part III

Arrhythmias

Arrhythmias are often generated by three basic mechanisms: reentry, abnormal automaticity, and triggered activity. Blockade of conduction and concealed conduction may also cause an irregular rhythm on surface EKG. If the P-R (or R-P') interval is constant, then the atrial and ventricular depolarizations can generally be assumed to be related as a cause and effect, implying sinus rhythm with the sinus node in charge of the ventricles (or ventricular rhythm with ventriculoatrial conduction). In the absence of atrioventricular or ventriculoatrial block, the fastest pacemaker will control the heart. Though an irregular rhythm is the hallmark of an arrhythmia, a regular rhythm may be produced by an arrhythmia. Reentry is dependent on the presence of dual pathways, slowing or asynchrony of conduction, unidirectional block, and recovery of excitability. Abnormal automaticity may be normal or abnormal. Normal enhanced automaticity occurs with elevated sympathetic tone and most commonly manifests as sinus tachycardia. Abnormal automaticity results when latent escape foci become more rapid, competing with the dominant pacemaker. Triggered activity is dependent on repolarization abnormalities and may cause early or late afterdepolarizations. Conduction blockade results in such arrhythmias as sinoatrial block, interatrial block, atrioventricular block (antegrade and retrograde/ventriculoatrial block), bundle branch blocks, and exit blocks. These are generally divided into three degrees. A first-degree block is present when conduction still occurs but is abnormally prolonged. This is only evident on surface EKG with atrioventricular block (antegrade or retrograde) and to a lesser extent with interatrial and bundle branch block. A second degree block occurs when conduction is intermittent and is subdivided into Type I (Wenckebach) and Type II (Mobitz) blocks. Type I is characterized by group beating and conduction delay that progresses to a conduction blockade. A 2 : 1 block causes every-other impulse to fail to conduct (two impulses for one propagation). Type II is marked by random and intermittent conduction block. A third degree block results in complete failure of conduction and is only evident on surface EKG with atrioventricular block (AVB) and complete bundle branch block. The terms block and nonconduction are often used interchangeably. However, it is important to understand the connotations of both terms. Nonconduction is generally considered to be physiologic/functional, and block is usually thought of as pathologic. Of course, there are exceptions (i.e. non-conducted premature beats may be pathologic and even a high-grade Type I sinoatrial or atrioventricular block is considered physiologic). Concealed conduction may be deduced from surface EKG and is inferred if conduction fails to appear when otherwise expected resulting in unexpected pauses or delay of conduction.

When confronted with a patient with an arrhythmia, the first thing the clinician must assess is the physical state of the animal and the heart rate. If the patient appears stable, is normotensive, and the heart rate is within normal limits, then the arrhythmia is highly unlikely to be life-threatening. Therefore, immediate intervention is probably unwarranted. Seriously slow or very rapid heart rates and sudden onset of asystole are more likely to be associated with symptoms such as weakness, collapse, or syncope and thus need immediate attention. On the other hand, some arrhythmias, even if alone are hemodynamically insignificant, may be harbingers of more malignant rhythms and warrant preemptive intervention. Changes in autonomic tone may predispose to or worsen many arrhythmias, and these secondary arrhythmias typically will resolve on their own following appropriate therapy for underlying causes. The Heisenberg uncertainty principle is important to keep in mind when evaluating patients with arrhythmias. The very act of observation (i.e. restraining an animal to obtain an EKG or the application of a Holter monitor) may influence the results of the test. Stressed animals being held down tend to have elevated sympathetic tone, which may exacerbate certain arrhythmias (i.e. premature beats or tachycardia) making them appear clinically more important than they really are. The clinician should also

Interpretation of the Electrocardiogram in Small Animals, First Edition. Nick A. Schroeder.
© 2021 John Wiley & Sons Inc. Published 2021 by John Wiley & Sons Inc.

remember Ockham's Razor: essentials ought not to be multiplied. This basic scientific precept means that "all things being equal, the simplest explanation tends to be the right one." Do not assume some crazy or tricky phenomenon is at work just because you read about it once. Adding tiers of complexity lowers the probability of truth. What appears to be a normal sinus rhythm could conceivably be interpreted as sinus rhythm of the atria, accelerated idiojunctional rhythm of the ventricles, and isorhythmic dissociation with synchrony where the P waves fortuitously precede the QRS complexes. However, sinus rhythm is common and therefore more probable, whereas isorhythmic dissociation is not. Common things occur commonly.

Some terminology is helpful to review when discussing arrhythmias in general. Standstill, arrest, or asystole denotes prolonged periods without apparent depolarization or myocardial contraction. Ectopy generally refers to foci originating outside of the sinoatrial node. Subsidiary pacemakers outside of the sinus node that may take over by default when sinoatrial discharge fails (or is "at fault") are termed escape foci and are "late." Acceleration of these ectopic centers may compete for control with the sinus node, and "transition of a pacemaker" from sinus to ectopic origin and fusion complexes that occur "on time" are common in these situations. Ectopic beats that occur sooner than expected considering the underlying rhythm produce so-called premature systoles/complexes (extrasystoles), and capture beats are similarly "early." A capture is a supraventricular interruption of atrioventricular dissociation, most often sinus in origin. Parasystole occurs when two foci control depolarization, variable coupling intervals are present, and fusions occur due to simultaneous activation. The predominant rhythm is usually sinus and the ectopic focus is protected by entrance block, but this may be modulated. Tachycardias generally outpace the sinus node altogether. Flutter causes rapid but coordinated depolarization, results from a macroreentry circuit, and is limited to the atrial or ventricular myocardia, though sinoatrial and junctional (atrioventricular) reentry are nodal equivalents. Fibrillation results from microreentry and causes uncoordinated and rapid depolarization of the atria or ventricles. In the absence of an accessory pathway bypassing the atrioventricular node, atrial fibrillation is normally held in some degree of check by the atrioventricular node, preventing ventricular fibrillation.

Premature systoles (premature beats/complexes, extrasystoles) are classified according to the specific cardiac tissue of origin. The differentiation of supraventricular vs. ventricular premature complexes (VPCs) is important, as clinical management may be affected. Supraventricular premature complexes (SVPCs, PSVCs, supraventricular extrasystoles) are ectopic early beats that originate at or above the level of the AV node. These typically have a "supraventricular" QRS complex that is usually (or nearly) identical to that of the QRS of a normal sinus beat. Rarely, they may be conducted with aberrancy and may not have an obviously associated P′ wave, making them difficult or impossible to distinguish from VPCs. Supraventricular premature complexes include sinoatrial, atrial, and junctional premature complexes. The more premature the SVPC is, the more likely the P′-Ri will be prolonged (functional first degree AVB). Occasionally, SVPCs will fail to conduct to the ventricles (functional second degree AVB) due to excessive prematurity with the ectopic impulse finding the AVN/His bundle tissue physiologically refractory to propagation. In the presence of a pre-existent bundle branch block, SVPCs may rarely conduct with a normal (or near-normal) QRS duration from supernormal conduction. Premature activation of the atria may also occur secondary to reciprocation, and parasystolic foci may be seen. Fusion with the sinus node or other ectopic atrial rhythm may occur (in which case multifocal SVPCs cannot always be excluded). If SVPCs are single/unifocal/rare, then their clinical significance is minimal. However, if SVPCs are frequent and especially if multifocal, they may be a harbinger for supraventricular tachycardia (SVT) or atrial fibrillation, warranting therapeutic intervention. Ventricular premature complexes are usually characterized by a wide QRS with atrioventricular dissociation. The site of origin of ectopy may be suspected based on the morphology of the QRS complex and mean electrical axis. Fusion within the ventricular myocardium is commonly associated with VPCs and should not be confused with polymorphism. The clinician should be aware that sometimes SVPCs may have a prolonged QRS and occasionally VPCs may have ventriculoatrial conduction. Learning how premature beats are likely to behave can make it easier for the examiner to correctly identify the site of origin despite an ambiguous waveform on EKG.

Ratios are commonly used in reference to conduction/block and premature beats. Block may occur at the sinoatrial, atrioventricular (junctional) levels, at the level of the bundle branches, and also may occur with localized exit block or retrograde (ventriculoatrial block) through the atrioventricular node or in accessory pathways. When discussing conduction, the numerator refers to the number of initiating impulses and the denominator represents the number of resulting conductions. During AVB, the atrial rate is usually from the sinus node, though ectopic rhythms may initiate conduction as well, and the ventricular rate is always the result. The denominator is how many impulses are blocked out of a certain number of atrial depolarizations (numerator). When discussing ratios in relation to conduction blockade, it is critical for the interpreter to explicitly state whether the ratio refers to conduction or block. For example, if 4 atrial depolarizations only result in one ventricular response, then 4 : 1 conduction (4 P waves for every 1 QRS) or 4 : 3 AVB (3 out of every 4 P waves are blocked) is present. Rapid atrial rhythms may have 2 : 1 conduction (two atrial depolarizations for every one ventricular response). The terms are interchangeable in 2 : 1 conduction/block (every-other-atrial depolarization produces a ventricular depolarization). The closer the numerator and denominator are in this situation during tachycardia confers a more rapid ventricular rate response and thus a more potentially dangerous situation requiring intervention. An atrial flutter with an atrial rate of 400 bpm with 1 : 1 conduction is bad and likely produces hypotension/syncope since the ventricular rate is also 400 bpm, but 1 : 4 conduction is probably well-tolerated as the ventricular rate is only 100 bpm. A 3 : 1 AVB (3 : 2 conduction) is considered low-grade and well-tolerated while 5 : 4 AVB (5 : 1 conduction) in the setting of sinus rhythm constitutes a high grade of block and likely associated with symptoms referable to the resulting bradycardia. In this situation, the wider the disparity between the numerator and denominator (conduction ratio), the higher grade of block and the greater the chance of an unacceptably low ventricular rate response.

When premature beats occur with pattern/regularity, ratios may be used as well. In this case, the numerator refers to the number of supraventricular (usually sinus) beats, and the denominator refers to the number of ectopic beats. Premature beats may display 1 : 1 extrasystole (bigeminy, every-other-beat is premature), 2 : 1 extrasystole or 1 : 2 extrasystole produces trigeminy, and 3 : 1, 1 : 3, or 2 : 2 extrasystole produces quadrigeminy. When discussing prematurity, the higher the denominator, the more ectopic premature beats vs. supraventricular beats there are. A 2 : 1 extrasystole is less worrisome than a 1 : 2, 1 : 3, or 1 : 4 extrasystole. A couplet is two ectopic complexes in a row. A triplet is three ectopic complexes in a row. Couplets and triplets of premature beats (1 : 2 and 1 : 3 extrasystole) are more likely associated with non-sustained or sustained tachycardia and require therapy. A run is more than three ectopic complexes in a row. A salvo is a run of less than eight ectopic complexes in a row. A paroxysm is a run of more than eight consecutive ectopic complexes (hence the term paroxysmal VT or SVT). Sustained tachycardias (greater than 30 seconds in duration) or incessant tachycardias (>50% of the day) of any origin may not only predispose the patient to hemodynamic collapse and sudden cardiac death, but also may predispose to tachycardia-induced cardiomyopathy (TICM). Though ratios are useful for describing conduction/block and premature beats, the resulting ventricular rate is the most important factor for the animal.

Arrhythmias may have secondary effects on the EKG. Premature beats in particular may have effects on the post-extrasystolic cycle, including the induction of some degree of block. These include aberration of the P wave (Chung's phenomenon/intra-atrial block) or displacement of the pacemaker. Aberration (functional bundle branch block) of the QRS complex may occur. Occasionally, a taller than normal QRS complex may be seen secondary to the Brody effect: increased ventricular filling from post-extrasystolic potentiation caused by the pause. Post-extrasystolic first degree AVB causing P-R interval prolongation may occur following interpolated extrasystoles. Transient second degree AVB with nonconduction of the post-extrasystolic P wave results in the compensatory pause. Revelation of rate-dependent bundle branch block may result in a normalized QRS duration. Transient T wave changes have been reported in humans but appear to be rare in small animals.

The clinician ought to be able to differentiate supraventricular from ventricular tachycardias. Aside from sinus tachycardia, atrial fibrillation, and atrial flutter, there are other supraventricular tachyarrhythmias (SVTs) that you need to be aware of. Supraventricular tachycardias are commonly divided by AV nodal involvement, automatic or reentrant types, and by R-P′ interval. If the P′ wave is closer to the preceding QRS than to the next QRS so the R-P′ interval is less than or equal to 50% of the R-R interval, the SVT is termed a short R-P′ SVT. If the P′ wave is closer to the next QRS complex with the R-P′ interval greater than 50% of the R-R interval, it is classified as a long R-P′ SVT. Sudden onset and offset are characteristic of reentrant SVTs, and automatic SVTs are usually gradual onset and offset. Importantly, reentrant tachycardias may be interrupted or initiated by an extrasystole, rely on delayed atrioventricular conduction, and resume when atrioventricular conduction achieves a critical value. If a vagal maneuver terminates SVT, it is likely to be atrioventricular nodal reentrant tachycardia, orthodromic atrioventricular reentrant tachycardia, or sinus nodal reentrant tachycardia. Vagal maneuvers include carotid sinus massage and ocular pressure (no more than 5 seconds at a time, as ventricular fibrillation may result from aggressive vagal maneuvers during SVTs). Usually, SVT will have narrow, upright QRS complexes in the inferior leads. The terms orthodromic and antidromic are also important here. Orthodromic physiology results in SVT using the AV node in the normal direction (i.e. from the atrial side to the ventricular side). Antidromic physiology results in ventriculoatrial conduction with impulses going from the ventricular side to the atrial side, retrogradely (the wrong way) through the AV node. Ventricular tachycardias are usually characterized by a wide QRS complex with atrioventricular dissociation, but ventriculoatrial association may occur. Ventricular tachycardias tend to be more life-threatening and associated with sudden cardiac death, which underscores the importance of early diagnosis. Bear in mind that wide-complex SVT and narrow-complex VT do occur. The differentiation of aberrancy from ventricular ectopy can be clinically challenging.

Additional terms in reference to arrhythmias are helpful to review and include atrioventricular dissociation, allorhythmia, and interference (thwarts). Atrioventricular dissociation is a general term that refers to the independent electrical activity of the atria and ventricles and may be incomplete or complete. Four basic causes of atrioventricular dissociation are AVB, sinus bradycardia, acceleration, and pause-producers (usually premature beats). Quite often, combinations of these will conspire to result in atrioventricular dissociation. Allorhythmias are repeated arrhythmic sequences. These may be caused by Wenckebach periodicity, reciprocation, or bigeminal/trigeminal rhythms. In the absence of premature beats or reciprocation, if two cycle lengths are present, it may be helpful to assume the shorter is the basic cycle length and that something has happened to force lengthening of the longer one. Interference may be the result of normal escape foci or usurpation by an accelerated focus and often thwarts the expected sequence of events. These may include interruption of Wenckebach periods in atrioventricular or sinoatrial block with junctional escapes, escapes thwarting captures, disruption of escape rhythm by premature beats or captures, simultaneous activation (fusions), and functional/physiologic AVB from tachycardia or acceleration.

Marriot and Conover have described some basic causes of arrhythmias in general, and a review here is helpful:

1) *Premature complexes*: these include extrasystoles, parasystole, capture beats, reciprocal beats, better conduction that interrupts poorer conduction, supernormal conduction during AVB, and resumption of rhythm following inapparent bigeminy.

2) *Unexpected pauses*: these include non-conducted supraventricular premature complexes, second degree atrioventricular and sinoatrial block, sinus pauses/arrests in sick sinus syndrome, concealed conduction, concealed junctional premature complexes, and pauses induced by artificial pacemakers.

3) *Tachycardias*: tachycardias originating in or requiring the sinus node, the atria, or the atrioventricular junction are termed supraventricular tachycardias while those originating/perpetuated in the ventricles are called ventricular tachycardias.

4) *Bradycardias*: these may originate in the sinus node, the atria, the junction, or the ventricles and include sinus bradycardia, sinoatrial block, non-conducted atrial bigeminy, AVB, junctional and ventricular escapes.

5) *Bigeminal rhythms*: pairs of beats separated by pauses may be produced by many things including extrasystoles, parasystole, 3:2 conduction including escape-capture bigeminy ("reversed bigeminy"), escape-echo bigeminy, reciprocal beating, dual atrioventricular nodal conduction and fortuitous pairing in sinus arrhythmia and atrial fibrillation.

6) *Group beating*: groups of beats separated by pauses with an increase in ventricular rate prior to the pause includes sinus rhythm or SVT with Wenckebach periods, atrial flutter with 2:1 filtering in the upper atrioventricular node and Wenckebach periodicity in the lower atrioventricular node, sinus rhythm with two or more extrasystoles in a row, recurrent bursts of supraventricular or ventricular tachycardia, and 2:1 interpolated extrasystole.

7) *Absolute ventricular arrhythmia*: is produced most commonly by atrial fibrillation, but also by atrial flutter with variable atrioventricular conduction, Type II atrial flutter, multifocal atrial tachycardia, wandering pacemaker with multifocal extrasystoles, and mixed ventricular rhythms.

8) *Regular non-sinus rhythms at normal heart rates*: these include accelerated and paced rhythms.

Many arrhythmias initially appear complex and rapid diagnosis may be challenging. Sorting out "who's who" (which deflections represent P waves, QRS complexes, and T waves) and "who's married to whom" (which P waves are conducted to the ventricles or which QRS complexes are associated with retrograde P′ waves from ventriculoatrial conduction) may not be so easy since relative anterograde and retrograde conduction times may vary in certain situations. Most of the time on surface EKG, the QRS complex is the largest deflection (has the greatest amplitude), followed by the T wave and then the P wave. P waves may be hiding in QRS complexes or S-T segments, especially during tachyarrhythmias. Alternative leads should be explored if P waves are not readily identified. Notches and perturbations of the S-T segment suggest superimposed atrial activity. The presence of P waves (whether sinus, ectopic, retrograde, etc.) excludes atrial fibrillation and atrial standstill, just as the presence of QRS complexes excludes ventricular fibrillation and asystole. The QRS complexes may be of low amplitude (especially in cats), and which deflections represent P waves versus T waves may not be clear. Sometimes, atrial activity is easier to ascertain in a lead where the QRS complexes are nearly isoelectric (the so-called haystack principle – look for your needle in the smallest haystack whenever possible). P waves may or may not be related to the QRS complexes; however, the T waves always are. T waves always follow a single morphology

QRS at a constant interval. Prolonged QRS complexes typically have prolonged and abnormal T waves from repolarization abnormalities. So-called "sore thumbs" or breaks in the rhythm frequently are the best places to sort out what is going on with a given arrhythmia. Walking the rhythm backward from these breaks can be helpful and a ladder diagram is often invaluable. Once the P waves are identified and a P-P interval is established, those hiding within complexes can be ferreted out as sinus rhythms are often regular. Always reevaluate your assumptions if things do not make sense. For every "rule" there are always (and often multiple) exceptions. Patterns are helpful, but occasionally unreliable. Mimics/impostors, thwarts, and artifacts may all conspire to confound the clinician.

If you analyze EKGs systematically, the same way, every time, chances are you will come to the correct diagnosis. The heart has mechanisms to prevent an excessive ventricular rate response (physiologic block) and backup systems (tiered escape foci) to ensure that oxygen demands are met in response to any given situation. The body is thus wonderfully designed to avoid failure and meet demand. When these systems are compromised or end up detrimental for whatever reason, failure ensues. This is where the clinician comes in.

The Sinus Node

Bradyarrhythmias
   Bradycardia
   Arrhythmia
   Escape
   Arrest/asystole
   Block
   Sick sinus node
Tachyarrhythmias
   Premature Systole
   Parasystole
   Tachycardia
   Reentry

The Atria

Bradyarrhythmias
   Escape
   Standstill
Tachyarrhythmias
   Premature systole
   Parasystole
   Acceleration
   Tachycardia
   Reentry
   Flutter
   Fibrillation

The Junction

Bradyarrhythmias
   Escape
   Block
Tachyarrhythmias
   Premature systole
   Parasystole
   Acceleration
   Tachycardia
   Reentry

The Ventricles

Bradyarrhythmias
   Escape
   Asystole
Tachyarrhythmias
   Premature systole
   Parasystole
   Reentry
   Acceleration
   Tachycardia
   Flutter
   Fibrillation

Further Reading

Fisch, C. and Knoebel, S.B. (2000). *Electrocardiography of Clinical Arrhythmias*. Futurama Publishing Co.

Marriott, H.J. (1998). *Pearls & Pitfalls in Electrocardiography, Pithy Practical Pointers*, 2e. Williams & Wilkins.

Marriot, H.J.L. and Conover, M.B. (1998). *Advanced Concepts in Arrhythmias*, 3e. Mosby.

Nelson, W.P., Marriott, H.J.L., and Schocken, D.D. (2007). *Concepts & Cautions in Electrocardiography*. MedInfo Inc.

Pick, A. and Langendorf, R. (1979). *Interpretation of Complex Arrhythmias*. Lea & Febiger.

Surawicz, B. and Knilans, T.K. (2001). *Chou's Electrocardiography in Clinical Practice: Adult and Pediatric*, 5e. Saunders.

Sinoatrial Arrhythmias

The normal sinus node is anatomically located in a superioposterior location (craniodorsal) and laterally within the right atrium. It is an almond-shaped structure that is within the junction of the cranial vena cava and the right atrium (provided situs solitus). Specialized conduction tissue connects the sinoatrial and atrioventricular nodes (internodal tracts). Sinus nodal depolarization is electrocardiographically silent on surface EKG, but the resulting atrial depolarization is characteristic. As such, the electrocardiographic manifestation of sinus nodal discharge is the "normal" P wave morphology. The mean electrical axis in the frontal plane of the normal P wave is −15 to +110 degrees in the dog and 0 to +160 degrees in the cat, resulting in an "eccentric antegrade" but normal activation of the atria (generally proceeding right-to-left, and cranial to caudal/superior-to-inferior). Thus, the P waves should be positive in lead I and negative in aVR. The sinus node cells typically have the fastest rate of diastolic Phase 4 depolarization, so the sinus node normally dominates (or is "in charge" of) the heart rate, suppressing subsidiary pacemakers in the atrial myocardium, junctional tissues and Purkinje fibers of the ventricles. Normal sinus nodal rates may range from 60 to 180+ bpm in the dog and 140 to 220+ bpm in the cat. At sinus rates below 160 bpm, sinus arrhythmia from variations in autonomic tone typically prevail in the dog and in sedentary cats at home. The normal sinus rhythm in dogs and cats must be defined prior to any description of an arrhythmia.

Normal sinus rhythm (NSR) A normal sinus rhythm is characterized by regular supraventricular QRS complexes at a normal rate, all preceded by sinus P waves with a normal P-R interval, normal amplitudes and intervals for the species, etc. Thus, there is a P for every Q wave, and a Q for every P wave, and so the atrial rate equals the ventricular rate. If any abnormalities are present and the underlying rhythm is sinus in origin, the proper term is "sinus rhythm with…(whatever abnormalities)." The point is, one should not offer an interpretation stating

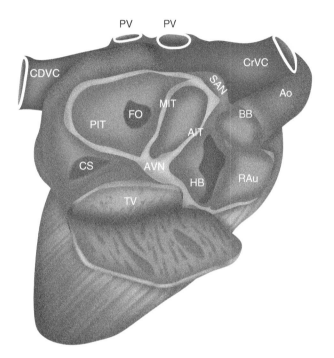

Figure SAI.1 Illustration of the anatomical location of the sinoatrial node. **CdVC**: caudal vena cava, **CrVC**: cranial vena cava, **SAN**: sinoatrial node, **BB**: Bachman's bundle, **AIT**: anterior internodal tract, **MIT**: middle internodal tract, **PIT**: posterior internodal tract, **FO**: fossa ovalis, **CS**: coronary sinus, **TV**: tricuspid valve, **HB**: His bundle, **Ao**: aorta, **RAu**: right auricle.

"normal sinus rhythm with frequent supraventricular premature beats," but rather "sinus rhythm with frequent supraventricular beats" or some pertinent alternative.

The sinus nodal discharge is most often irregular and tends to be associated with normal heart rates or bradyarrhythmias. Most commonly, this "sinus arrhythmia" is denoted by a greater than 20% variation in cycle length, is usually secondary to respiratory variation, but may be non-respiratory in nature. Since multiple discreet centers within the sinus node itself may compete for control, the term "wandering pacemaker" may be misleading given that the center usually abruptly changes from one area to the next. If the heart rate is relatively rapid, the focus tends to shift toward a more cranial location, resulting in P wave

Interpretation of the Electrocardiogram in Small Animals, First Edition. Nick A. Schroeder.
© 2021 John Wiley & Sons Inc. Published 2021 by John Wiley & Sons Inc.

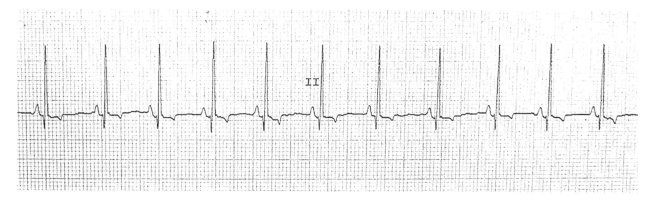

Figure SAI.2 Paper speed 25 mm/s, 1 cm/mV, lead II, canine, NSR.

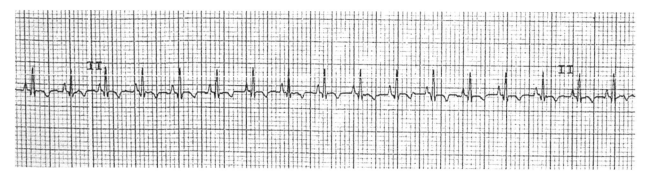

Figure SAI.3 Paper speed 25 mm/s, 1 cm/mV, lead II, feline, NSR.

with a more inferior axis, and when the heart rate is slower, the P wave may shift to a more caudal region within the sinoatrial node. These shifts tend to be sudden, and the P wave morphology thus may abruptly change. As long as the P wave axis and rate are within normal limits for the species and the atrial rate is within the range of normal, then it can be presumed that the atria are controlled by the sinus node.

Exit and entrance block may occur associated with sinus nodal discharge. Exit block (sinoatrial block) is typified by a predictable pattern of P wave (and subsequent QRS) appearance on surface EKG, whereas entrance block is evidenced by interpolation of supraventricular premature complexes or ventricular premature complexes with ventriculoatrial conduction. Most ectopic atrial impulses and those arising from ventricles and junction with ventriculoatrial conduction penetrate the sinoatrial node, resetting the rhythm. Sinoatrial dissociation ("double sinus rhythms"/two or more foci within the sinoatrial node with entrance block) is expected to be extremely rare, probably associated with tachyarrhythmias and likely indistinguishable on surface EKG from atrial dissociation with a right atrial focus. Sinus rhythms are not considered to ever really be "accelerated," and "inappropriate sinus tachycardia" (persistent sinus tachycardia with no obvious underlying physiologic cause) is apparently not a clinical entity in small animals. Atrioventricular dissociation in the absence of atrioventricular block is not a feature associated with sinoatrial arrhythmias in general.

Sinoatrial Bradyarrhythmias

Sinus bradycardia
Sinus arrhythmia
   Non-phasic sinus arrhythmia
   Phasic sinus arrhythmia
      Respiratory sinus arrhythmia
         Wandering pacemaker
      Non-respiratory sinus arrhythmia
      Ventriculophasic sinus arrhythmia
Sinus bigeminy
   Sinoatrial escape-capture bigeminy
Sinus pause
Sinus arrest
Asystole

Sinoatrial Block

Second degree sinoatrial block
   Type I (Wenckebach)
   Type II (Mobitz)

Sick Sinus Syndrome
Overdrive suppression
Sinus nodal dysfunction
Bradycardia variant
Tachycardia–bradycardia variant

Sinoatrial Tachyarrhythmias
Sinoatrial premature systoles
Sinoatrial reciprocal complexes
Sinoatrial parasystole
Sinus tachycardia
Sinus nodal reentrant tachycardia

Further Reading

Santilli, R., Moïse, S., Pariaut, R., and Perego, M. (2018). *Electrocardiography of the Dog and Cat: Diagnosis of Arrhythmias*, 2e. Edna.

9

Sinoatrial Bradyarrhythmias

CHAPTER MENU

Sinus bradycardia, 103
Sinus arrhythmia, 105
   Non-phasic sinus arrhythmia, 105
   Phasic sinus arrhythmia, 105
      Respiratory sinus arrhythmia, 105
      Wandering pacemaker, 105
      Phasic non-respiratory sinus arrhythmia, 106
      Ventriculophasic sinus arrhythmia, 108
Sinus bigeminy, 112
   Sinoatrial escape-capture bigeminy, 112
Sinus pause, 114
Sinus arrest, 114
Asystole, 114

Sinoatrial bradyarrhythmias can be generally divided into sinus bradycardia and sinus arrhythmias, which may be further subdivided into non-phasic and phasic sinus arrhythmias. Sinus bradycardia tends to be regular. Sinus arrhythmia is included in this section even though it is normal in the dog and cat and generally associated with a normal heart rate overall (HR) because of periodic and relative bradycardia. Non-phasic sinus arrhythmia has an irregular rhythm unrelated to respiratory variation whereas phasic sinus arrhythmia varies according to changes in autonomic tone, often associated with respiratory variation (respiratory sinus arrhythmia/RSA) or ventricular systole (ventriculophasic sinus arrhythmia/VSA). Sinus pauses and arrests are denoted by unexpected pauses in the sinoatrial rhythm. Sinus escape beats (technically captures) may be elicited by such pauses, and if occurring in a predictable pattern may result in escape-capture bigeminy. Sinus arrests may precipitate escape beats from subsidiary pacemakers in the atria, atrioventricular junction or ventricles and may be associated with elevated parasympathetic tone or pathologic disease within the sinus node itself (sick sinus syndrome/SSS). Prolonged sinus arrest results in asystole.

Sinus bradycardia This is characterized by a slower than normal HR, with a regular supraventricular rhythm, normal sinus P waves preceding the QRS complexes at a consistent P-Ri and no evidence of second or higher degree of atrioventricular block, etc. Sinus bradycardia may result from excessive parasympathetic tone, intoxication with parasympathomimetics, electrolyte disturbances (specifically hyperkalemia), or rarely from sinus nodal disease. Non-conducted atrial bigeminy or 2:1 atrioventricular block with VSA may masquerade as sinus bradycardia, so check the T waves for any irregular bumps suggestive of superimposed atrial activity. Junctional or ventricular escapes may be seen if the sinus bradycardia is slow enough, provided the subsidiary pacemakers are unsuppressed, and intermittent atrioventricular dissociation (AVD) may occur by default.

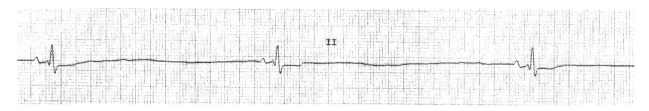

Figure 9.1 Paper speed 50 mm/s, 1 cm/mV, lead II, canine, **sinus bradycardia**. The heart rate is approximately 39 bpm. This patient had occasional episodes of lethargy associated with bradycardia of unknown etiology (suspected toxicity). No subsidiary pacemakers here capture the rhythm despite the very low heart rate.

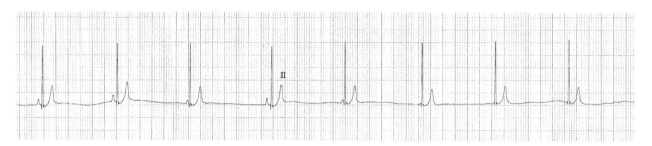

Figure 9.2 Paper speed 25 mm/s, 1 cm/mV, lead II, canine. **Sinus bradycardia** (HR 50 bpm) interrupted by junctional escapes and atrioventricular dissociation by default. The first two complexes are sinus conducted, followed by a junctional escape beat, then a sinus capture. Atrioventricular dissociation ensues and the sinus P waves are likely superimposed on junctional QRS complexes (isorhythmic dissociation). Retrograde capture of the atria by the junctional focus is not evident. The primary rhythm disturbance here is **sinus bradycardia**. The junctional beats and AVD are secondary. Junctional escape rhythm in dogs ranges from 40 to 80 bpm.

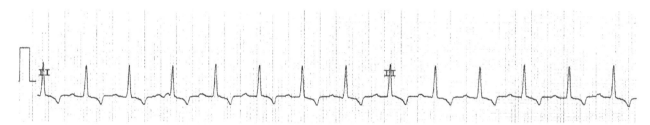

Figure 9.3 Paper speed 25 mm/s, 1 cm/mV, lead II, 20 y/o cat with hyperkalemia, congestive heart failure, hyperthyroidism, and pulmonary carcinoma. **Sinus bradycardia** is present with a HR of approximately 107 bpm. The bradycardia is likely secondary to the elevated potassium.

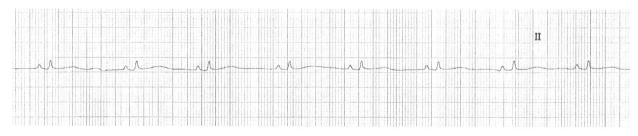

Figure 9.4 Paper speed 50 mm/s, 1 cm/mV, lead II, feline with a history of congestive heart failure. **Sinus bradycardia**. The heart rate is approximately 100 bpm and the Q-T interval is long at 0.24 second. Junctional escape rhythms in cats are frequently in the 100–140 bpm range, suggesting subsidiary escapes are similarly depressed in rate as is the sinus node.

Sinus arrhythmia

A sinus arrhythmia is an irregular rhythm (P-Pi variation >20%) of sinus origin and may be non-phasic or phasic. Non-phasic arrhythmias have random variation whereas phasic arrhythmias have a predictable pattern. Phasic arrhythmias may be respiratory, non-respiratory, or ventriculophasic.

Non-phasic sinus arrhythmia It refers to variability in the P-Pi/R-Ri without associated respiratory or predictable P-P interval variation. Occasionally, the dog or cat may have a non-phasic sinus arrhythmia where the rhythm/rate varies in an apparently random manner, though intermittent sinus tachycardia from intermittent sympathetic stimulation superimposed on a phasic sinus arrhythmia can mimic such a pattern.

Phasic sinus arrhythmia It is a predictable variation in sinus nodal discharge and is typically denoted as a respiratory sinus arrrhythmia (RSA) or normal sinus arrhythmia (NSA), which is characterized by a regularly irregular rhythm that increases in rate with inspiration and decreases in rate with expiration. This is often accompanied by predictable changes in the P wave morphology (wandering pacemaker), and the basic underlying respiratory rate is correlated with physical examination findings. A phasic but non-respiratory sinus arrhythmia is also common in the dog. This is often seen in canine patients where the EKG appears to show a gradual increase followed by a decrease in rate similar to that seen with respiratory/phasic sinus arrhythmia, but clearly unrelated to the respiratory cycle. The other type of phasic sinus arrhythmia is ventriculophasic, where the R-R variability depends on the preceding P-P interval.

Respiratory sinus arrhythmia This is physiologic/normal in the dog and associated with prevailing parasympathetic tone. Cats normally have sinus tachycardia in the veterinary office from elevated sympathetic tone, though sinus arrhythmia is common in cats in the home environment (documented on Holter monitors). A RSA in the cat tends to be pathologic in the veterinary office and often secondary to upper airway obstruction or vagotonia secondary to gastrointestinal disease. Brachycephalic dogs, likely due to some degree of pathological upper airway obstruction and associated enhanced vagal tone frequently, have an obnoxious phasic RSA and may have very long ventricular pauses occasionally terminated by escape beats. Respiratory sinus arrhythmia is the most common cause of a so-called regularly -irregular rhythm and no treatment is necessary.

Wandering pacemaker A "wandering" sinus or atrial pacemaker is said to be characterized by variable P wave amplitudes, which may even become isoelectric or negative.

> ***A Note:*** If the morphology of the P waves changes but the P wave axis remains the same, then the focus is considered to remain confined to the sinoatrial node (wandering *sinus* pacemaker). If the P wave axis changes as well, then the focus may be wandering outside of the sinus node (wandering *atrial* pacemaker).

Wandering pacemaker is associated with RSA, and the P waves tend to get taller (more positive in the inferiors) at higher heart rates during inspiration and progressively more negative at lower heart rates with expiration. The pacemaker complex is large in the dog, extending from the junction of the cranial vena cava and right atrium (the junction at the sulcus terminalis of which is sinoatrial node proper), extranodally and caudally to near the

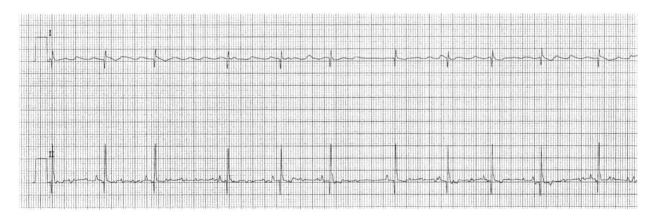

Figure 9.5 Paper speed 25 mm/s, 1 cm/mV, leads I and II, canine. **Non-phasic sinus arrhythmia**. Greater than 20% variability in P-P/R-Ri is present. Baseline artifact is undulating from respiratory artifact (panting, mimicking atrial flutter in lead I), and P waves are clearly preceding the QRS complexes in lead II consistent with a sinus origin. Here, the variability is random without apparent pattern. Phasic/respiratory sinus arrhythmia is ruled out by panting.

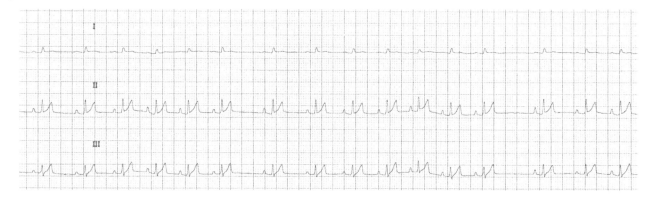

Figure 9.6 Paper speed 25 mm/s, 1 cm/mV, leads I, II, III, canine. **Phasic sinus arrhythmia** due to respiratory variation. The P-P/R-Ri shortens with inspiration and lengthens with expiration.

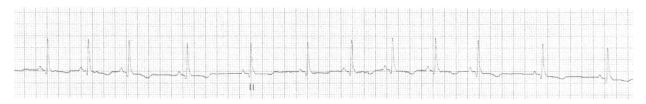

Figure 9.7 Paper speed 50 mm/s, 1 cm/mV, lead II, feline. **Respiratory sinus arrhythmia** secondary to upper airway obstruction. Note the long Q-T interval typical of bradycardia.

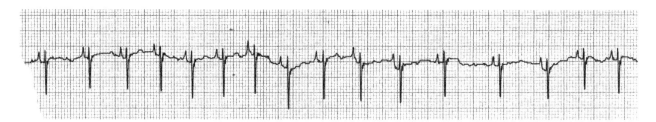

Figure 9.8 Paper speed 25 mm/s, 1 cm/mV, lead II, feline, **respiratory sinus arrhythmia** secondary to an upper airway obstruction. This cat also has very deep S waves.

coronary sinus and caudal vena cava. Cats are rarely noted to have a WPM. During respiration, inspiratory elevations in sympathetic tone shift the pacemaker within the sinus node to a superior/cranial focus, resulting in tall, normally oriented P waves. During expiration, parasympathetic tone dominates and shifts the pacemaker focus more caudally, altering the wavefront of atrial depolarization and its vector enough to make lower amplitude, isoelectric, and even negative P waves in the inferior leads on surface EKG. These late diastolic beats may confuse the examiner with junctional escape beats. The pacemaker complex in the sinus node has been described to be multicentric, with three to five separate conduction pathways in the dog, each capable of initiating atrial depolarization. Fusion of the wavefronts results in the propagated wave that depolarizes the atria. "Ectopic" atrial rhythms (i.e. "atrial escape" or "accelerated" atrial rhythms) may arise from one of the

caudal foci, and competition for pacing the atria may occur between one or more foci. Depending on which site spontaneously depolarizes first, variable degrees of atrial fusion can occur, leading to the changing P wave morphology on surface EKG. This makes the term "wandering pacemaker" misleading as the focus may be abruptly changing depending on prevailing sympathetic/parasympathetic tone and not "wandering" per se. Generally, no specific treatment is indicated for a WPM/RSA.

Phasic non-respiratory sinus arrhythmia It occurs with some frequency in the dog and is less commonly recognized in the cat. This is characterized on surface EKG with a gradual rate increase followed by a gradual rate decrease in SA nodal discharge that is apparently unrelated to respiratory phase. This may be secondary to regular changes in peripheral vascular resistance where the systemic capillary

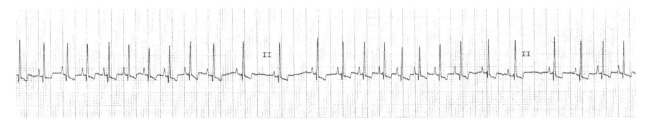

Figure 9.9 Paper speed 25 mm/s, 1 cm/mV, lead II, canine, **Respiratory sinus arrhythmia** with a **wandering pacemaker**. The P waves get taller in amplitude at higher HR.

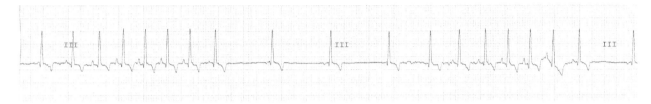

Figure 9.10 Paper speed 25 mm/s, 1 cm/mV, lead III, canine. Marked **respiratory sinus arrhythmia** with a **wandering pacemaker**. The P waves are tallest at high heart rates during inspiration, and progressively become isoelectric, then negative at slower HR associated with expiration. An argument could be made that the complexes with negative P waves could be junctional escapes; however, the P-Ri is consistent and the "interval of escape" is variable.

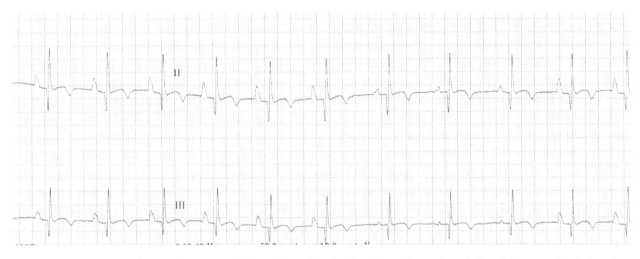

Figure 9.11 Paper speed 50 mm/s, 1 cm/mV, leads II and III, canine. A rather abrupt change in cycle length between the sixth and seventh complexes is associated with a different P wave morphology. This is consistent with a **sudden** shift from a pacemaker high in the SA node (the taller P waves) to a distinct pacemaker distal to that (complexes #8, #9, and #10). Strips like this support the notion of multiple atrial pacemakers, with some within or near the sinus node. Since the rate is slower than the sinus rate, this could be considered an **atrial escape rhythm,** though a focus within the SA node itself cannot be excluded.

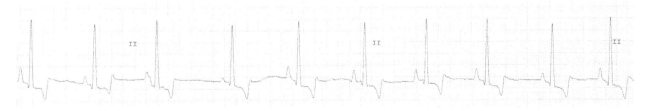

Figure 9.12 Paper speed 50 mm/s, 1 cm/mV, lead II, canine. **Wandering pacemaker** with mild sinus arrhythmia.

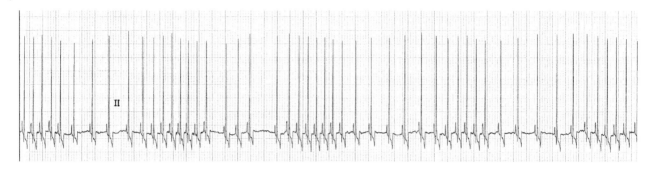

Figure 9.13 Paper speed 10 cm/s, 1 cm/mV, lead II, canine. **Phasic**, but **non-respiratory sinus arrhythmia**. This dog was not panting and had a resting respiratory rate of 24 per minute. Here, the phasic changes correspond to a rate of around 11 per minute and were not associated with obvious excitement or stimulation (excluding intermittent sinus tachycardia from transient increased sympathetic tone).

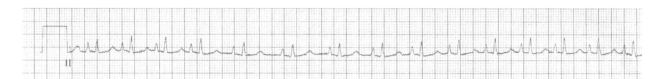

Figure 9.14 Paper speed 50 mm/s, 1 cm/mV, lead II, feline with renal failure. **Phasic**, but **non-respiratory sinus arrhythmia**. Here, the phasic changes in heart rate were not correlated with respiratory variation.

beds alternate periods of vasoconstriction with vasodilation, affecting the systemic blood pressure, which in turn stimulates a baroreceptor response and subsequent gradual change in HR. The most common example of this occurs in dogs that have an apparent phasic sinus arrhythmia while panting heavily during the recording. Intermittent sinus tachycardia superimposed on sinus rhythm is a rule out and is suggested by a concurrent increase in apparent anxiety in the patient. No treatment for this arrhythmia is warranted.

Ventriculophasic sinus arrhythmia It occurs when the ventricular rate is slow, commonly during incomplete (Type 1 second degree) or complete heart block (third degree AV block) and is characterized by P-P cycles that contain QRS complexes that are always shorter than P-P cycles without an intervening QRS. Similar lengthening can be present in the P-P cycle following a ventricular premature

complex with a compensatory pause. The changes in the P-P interval are likely due to the influence of the autonomic nervous system's response to changes in stroke volume (Bainbridge reflex – increased intra-atrial pressure results in vagal inhibition with acceleration of SAN discharge) or that the ventricular contraction produces increased coronary blood flow to the SAN, accelerating its discharge. Another theory is that the mechanical motion induced by ventricular contraction excites SA nodal cells, accelerating their discharge. Non-conducted bigeminal atrial premature complexes (APCs) may mimic VSA. *Paradoxical* VSA is marked by longer P-P intervals that encompass a QRS complex, has been described in humans, and is apparently rare (not documented) in dogs/cats. Treatment of this arrhythmia to consider includes sympathomimetics or pacemaker implantation if advanced AVB and symptomatic bradycardia are present.

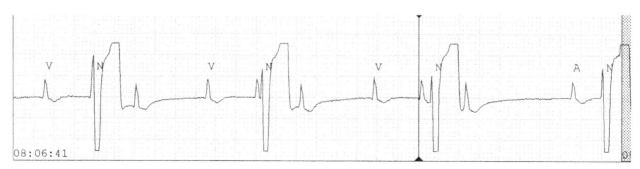

Figure 9.15 Paper speed 25 mm/s, 1 cm/mV, lead II, canine. Third degree AVB with **ventriculophasic sinus arrhythmia**. The monitoring system has misidentified the complexes (those labeled "V" and "A" are actually P waves followed by negative Ta waves, and the complexes labeled "N" are ventricular escape beats). The P waves containing QRS complexes have shorter intervals than those that do not. Ventricular escape rhythm is present.

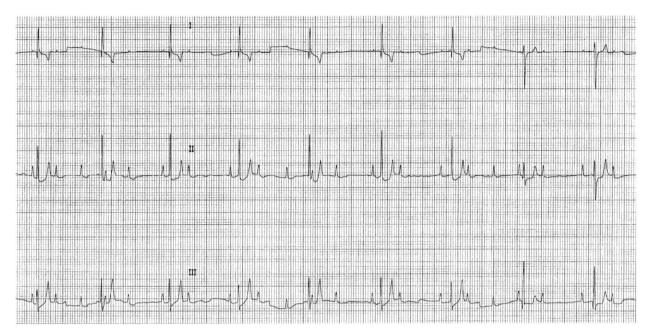

Figure 9.16 Paper speed 25 mm/s, 1 cm/mV, leads I, II, III, canine. **Ventriculophasic sinus arrhythmia** of the atria, junctional escape of the ventricles, complete AVD secondary to complete (third degree) AVB. The P-P intervals containing QRS complexes are shorter than those that do not, consistent with VSA. Intermittent LPFB results in periodic R axis deviation of the QRS. Competing escape foci is likely ruled out because the ventricular rhythm does not change with changes in QRS morphology.

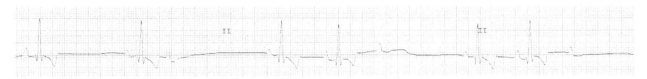

Figure 9.17 Paper speed 50 mm/s, 1 cm/mV, lead II, canine. Second degree AVB (Type I) with **ventriculophasic sinus arrhythmia**. The blocked P to P intervals are longer than the conducted P-blocked P intervals.

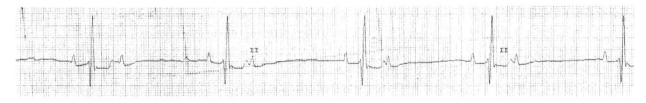

Figure 9.18 Paper speed 25 mm/s, 1 cm/mV, lead II, canine. **Ventriculophasic sinus arrhythmia**, this patient has second degree AVB (2:1 AV conduction), and the blocked P-P interval is longer than the P-blocked P interval.

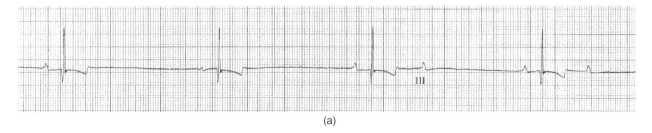

(a)

Figure 9.19a Paper speed, 50 mm/s, 1 cm/mV, lead III, canine with chronic bradycardia. The second beat has altered P wave morphology and may be late, suggestive of an **atrial escape complex**. The third beat is sinus, and 2:1 AVB with ventriculophasic conduction ensues. First degree AVB is present on conducted beats.

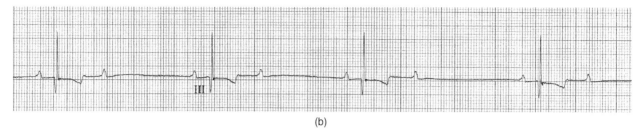

(b)

Figure 9.19b Paper speed 50 mm/s, 1 cm/mV, lead III, same dog. 2:1 AVB, **ventriculophasic sinus arrhythmia** with longer blocked P-conducted P intervals than conducted P-blocked P intervals.

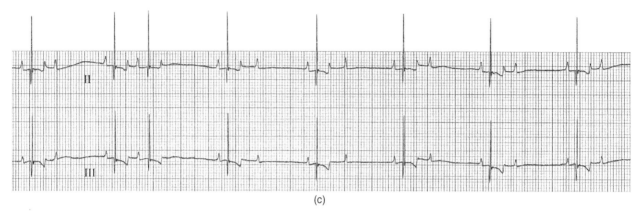

(c)

Figure 9.19c Paper speed 25 mm/s, 1 cm/mV, leads II and III, same dog. Occasionally, the early P waves are conducted, but ventriculophasic conduction and 2:1 AVB persists. The fourth P wave and non-conducted P waves have identical morphology with the sinus P waves, making non-conducted **atrial bigeminy** unlikely. The fourth P wave conducts to the ventricles with a longer P-R interval.

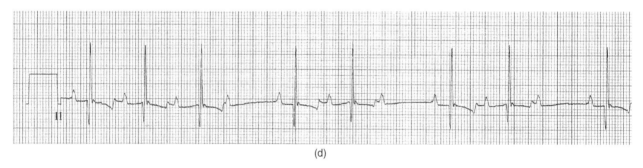

(d)

Figure 9.19d Paper speed 50 mm/s, 1 cm/mV, lead II, same dog immediately following **IV atropine** injection. The sinus node rhythm is now regular; however, second degree AVB persists with **Wenckebach phenomenon** (Type I). The P-R interval gradually prolongs before failure of conduction.

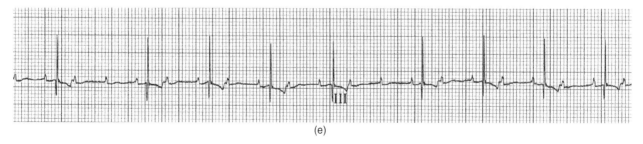

(e)

Figure 9.19e Paper speed 25 mm/s, 1 cm/mV, lead III, same dog, 30 second later. The sinus rate is faster yet and still regular. A **higher grade** of second degree AVB ensues, as two P waves fail to conduct following the first and fifth complexes. No two *consecutive* P waves are conducted, so Type I vs. Type II is indeterminate, though concurrent first degree AVB suggests *Type I* 2:1 and 3:1 AVB. Remember *transient* worsening of second degree AVB is common immediately following IV atropine.

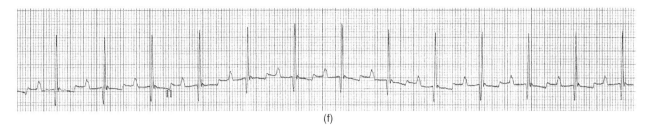

(f)

Figure 9.19f Paper speed 50 mm/s, 1 cm/mV, lead II, same dog two minutes post-IV atropine. **Normal sinus rhythm** with **1:1 AV conduction**. This patient's heart rate is still a bit low at under 100 bpm. Typically, dogs should attain a HR between 160 and 200 bpm following IV atropine, and this finding is suggestive of sinus nodal dysfunction.

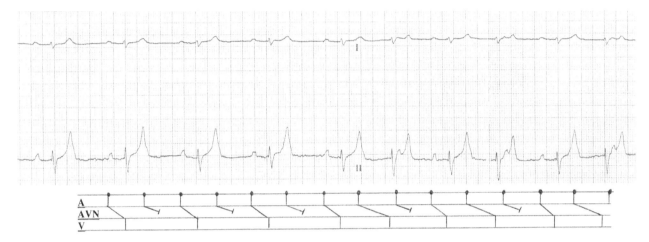

Figure 9.20 Paper speed 50 mm/s, 1 cm/mV, leads I and II, canine. At first glance, the rhythm appears to be simple sinus rhythm. However, the sixth complex is out of place, premature, and followed by a P wave in the S-T segment. This is an example of **ventriculophasic sinus arrhythmia with 2:1 Type I second degree AVB** that is revealed *after* 3:2 conduction occurs. The P-P intervals containing QRS complexes are just slightly shorter than the P-P intervals that do not. The non-conducted P waves are hiding in the T waves of the preceding beats.

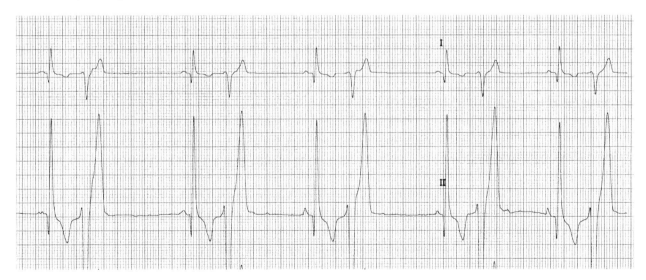

Figure 9.21 Paper speed 50 mm/s, 1 cm/mV, leads I and II, canine. **Ventriculophasic sinus arrhythmia, ventricular premature complexes in bigeminy** (1:1 extrasystole). The post-extrasystolic P wave is non-conducted and buried in the T waves of the VPCs, which are then followed by compensatory pauses. The P-P intervals encompassing QRS complexes (here two) are shorter than those that do not. Here, the VPCs temporarily accelerate SA nodal discharge and partial penetration of the AVN by the VPC leaves it refractory for the post-extrasystolic P wave creating the pauses and effective ventriculophasic sinus arrhythmia. Left ventricular enlargement is evident on the sinus QRS complexes and the VPCs have RBBB-like morphology, consistent with a LV origin.

Sinus bigeminy Occasionally, due to a fortuitous sinus arrhythmia (one breath for two heart beats), 3:2 sinoatrial block (sinus nodal escape-capture bigeminy) or 1:1 extrasystole from sinus nodal premature complexes, pairs of apparent sinus beats may occur separated by pauses. This is referred to as "sinus bigeminy." Fortuitous pairing with sinus arrhythmia is denoted by variable P-P intervals of paired beats with pauses correlated with respiratory phase. Sinus nodal premature complexes are favored if the P-Pi immediately prior to the onset bigeminy is obviously short (onset precipitated by a premature beat), and sinoatrial block with 3:2 conduction is favored if the P-Pi immediately prior to the onset is normal or minimally shortened (onset precipitated by the pause) (see Chapters 10 and 12). Since the HR and blood pressure generally remain within normal limits, this allorhythmia tends to be of little clinical importance if it occurs secondary to sinus arrhythmia and sinoatrial nodal premature beats other than being a rule out for bigeminal rhythms in general. However, if sinus bigeminy is secondary to sinoatrial block, then subclinical SSS may be a possibility. On rare occasion, more than one of these mechanisms may be at work to produce sinus bigeminy.

Sinoatrial escape-capture bigeminy If an impulse originating in the sinus node terminates a pause, it could be considered a sinus nodal "escape beat," which a questionably appropriate term if the original focus controlling the heart was also sinus. During ectopic rhythms, the sinus node may intervene and conduct to the ventricles, and the resulting premature beat is properly termed a "capture beat." Second degree sinoatrial block with 3:2 conduction produces a bigeminal rhythm with pauses terminated by sinoatrial escape/capture beats and can thus be referred to as sinoatrial escape-capture bigeminy.

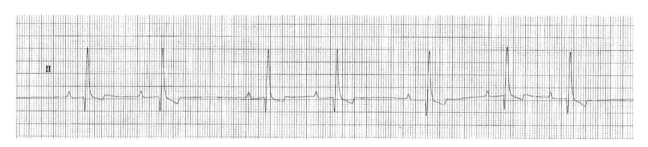

Figure 9.22 Paper speed 50 mm/s, 1 cm/mV, lead II, canine. **Sinus bigeminy**. Here, an underlying sinus arrhythmia is present and fortuitous timing allows for periods of sinus bigeminy. Note that no two P-P intervals are consistent. The last complex is the big giveaway here. If 3:2 sinoatrial block transitioning to 4:3 conduction was present, the P-P intervals between beats #1 and #2, #3 and #4, and the interval between beats #5 and #6 should be identical. First degree atrioventricular block with atypical Wenckebach periodicity is also present (prolonging P-R intervals without failure of conduction to the ventricles).

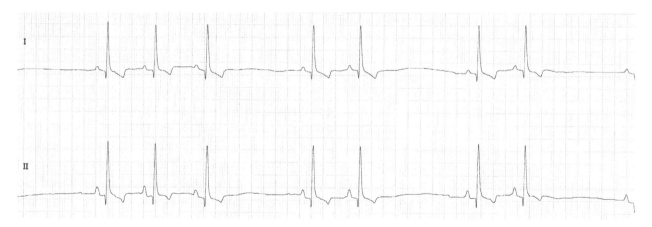

Figure 9.23 Paper speed 50 mm/s, 1 cm/mV, leads I and II, canine. Sinus arrhythmia with **sinus bigeminy** due to fortuitous timing of the respiratory rate. Sinoatrial block is excluded due to (albeit minor) P-P variability and the pauses were correlated on physical with respiratory phase.

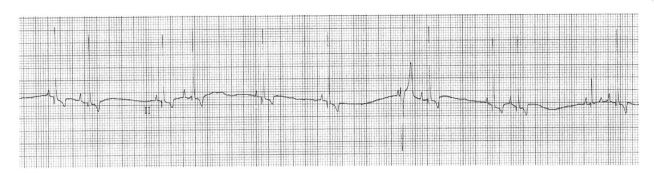

Figure 9.24 Paper speed 25 mm/s, 1 cm/mV, lead II, canine. **Sinus bigeminy**. At the beginning of the strip, a bigeminal rhythm is apparent. The second complex in each sequence has a slightly longer P-R interval and a slightly taller P wave. The seventh complex is a ventricular escape and the 11th complex represents a ventricular fusion complex. It is unclear on this strip whether the underlying cause of the bigeminy is secondary to SA nodal premature beats or if 3:2 sinoatrial block is to blame. Given that the pauses terminated by ventricular escapes/fusion are immediately followed by a "premature" complex (taller P wave, longer P'-Ri), sinus nodal premature beats seem most likely.

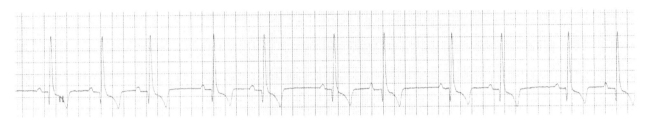

Figure 9.25 Paper speed 50 mm/s, 1 cm/mV, lead II, canine. **Sinoatrial escape-capture bigeminy**. A pause after the third beat is followed by an atrial escape (likely from within the sinus node itself since the P wave morphology is identical), then a sinus-capture, then bigeminy ensues. Again, this is likely secondary to sinoatrial block. Since the beats terminating pauses are sinus in origin, by definition, sinoatrial block with 3:2 conduction will result in sinoatrial escape-capture bigeminy.

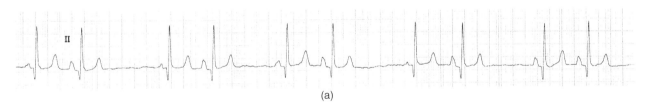

(a)

Figure 9.26a Paper speed 50 mm/s, 1 cm/mV, lead II, canine. **Sinus bigeminy**. Initially, this appears to be atrial or sinoatrial escape-capture bigeminy given that the P waves of the first beat in each pair is of altered morphology.

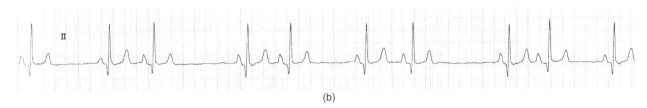

(b)

Figure 9.26b Paper speed 50 mm/s, 1 cm/mV, lead II, same dog immediately after. The P waves eventually become identical and the cycle length changes are variable suggestive of sinus bigeminy due to fortuitous pairing. Thus, sinus bigeminy in this individual appears to secondary to multiple mechanisms.

Sinus pause Sinus pauses occur when the P-P interval delimiting the pause does not equal an exact multiple of the normal P-P interval and is less than two normal P-P intervals. This is in contrast to sinoatrial block, which is suspected when the pauses are exact multiples of the underlying sinus cycle length (see Chapter 10). Sinus pauses are generally abrupt, independent of any underlying sinus arrhythmia, and are of short duration (less than two P-P intervals). Atrial premature complexes that are blocked in the AVN before reaching the ventricle may mimic sinus pause. Blocked APCs often cause deformed T wave – a P' without a QRS. Sinus pauses may also be confused with the post-extrasystolic pause associated with sinoatrial nodal premature complexes (which are denoted by a short P-P' interval prior to the pause). Sinus pauses may be a symptom of a sick sinus node.

Sinus arrest A disorder of impulse formation, sinus arrest occurs when the SA node apparently fails to fire for a longer period – typically described as a pause longer than two normal P-P/R-R intervals (but this may be seen with a severe sinus arrhythmia or high grade/paroxysmal sinoatrial block, so there is a gray zone). Sinus arrests in excess of 4–6 seconds may result in syncope. Profound sinus bradycardia and/or sinus arrest typically results in escape of a subsidiary pacemaker (junctional or ventricular escape rhythm). Sinus arrests with lazy escape foci are associated with SSS.

Asystole Asystole of the atria and ventricles is characterized by a lack of electrical as well as mechanical activity by the atria and ventricles for long periods of time

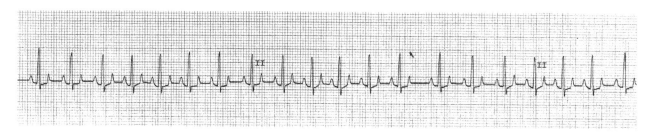

Figure 9.27 Paper speed 25 mm/s, 1 cm/mV, canine, **sinus pause**. The pause between the 13th and 14th beats is less than 2 P-P intervals, and not a multiple of the P-P interval. The underlying sinus rhythm is regular, making sinus pause more likely (vs. variation due to a sinus arrhythmia).

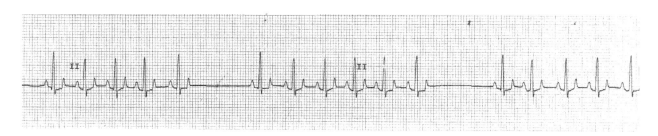

Figure 9.28 Paper speed 25 mm/s, 1 cm/mV, lead II, canine, **sinus arrest**. The pauses are greater than 2 P-P intervals, and not exact multiples of the P-P interval.

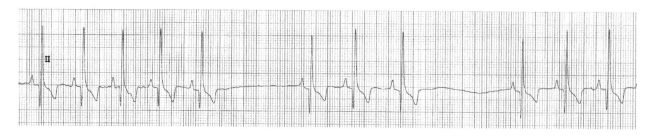

Figure 9.29 Paper speed 50 mm/s, 1 cm/mV, lead II, canine, **sinus arrest** simulating sinus arrhythmia. Unexpected pauses greater than 2 P-P intervals (inexact multiples) occur between sinus beats that are otherwise regular in rhythm. These pauses were not correlated with respiratory phase.

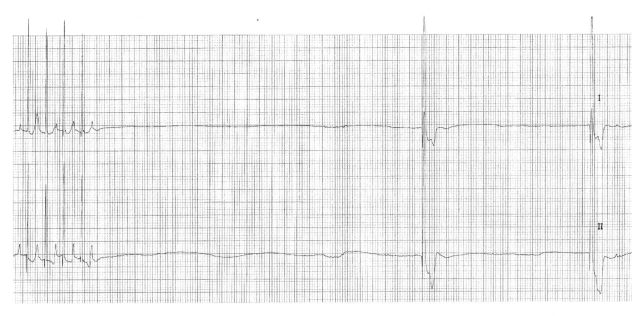

Figure 9.30 Paper speed 25 mm/s, 1 cm/mV, leads I and II, canine with sick sinus syndrome. Sinus tachycardia with QRS alternans terminates in a prolonged **sinus arrest** following a second degree atrioventricular block. A lazy ventricular escape focus rescues the dog from asystole.

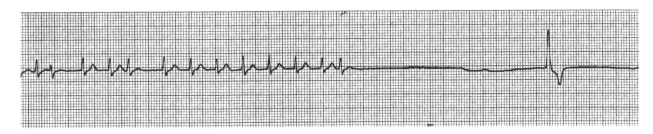

Figure 9.31 Paper speed 25 mm/s, 1 cm/mV, lead II, canine, sinus rhythm (low-amplitude P waves) with supraventricular premature complexes with dramatic **sinus arrest/asystole**, no indication of atrial activity (no P waves), followed by an escape beat likely originating in a Purkinje fiber in the R bundle (LBBB pattern). Note that the arrest is precipitated by a supraventricular premature beat.

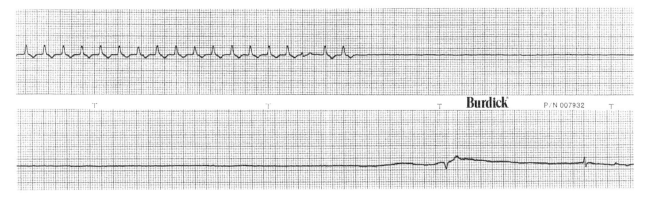

Figure 9.32 Paper speed 25 mm/s, 1 cm/mV, lead II, Holter recording from a syncopal cat. Prolonged **asystole** is terminated on the bottom strip by a ventricular escape beat.

(basically a prolonged sinus arrest without intervening escapes). No P waves and no QRS complexes are seen. The faster the HR prior to the onset of asystole, the longer the period of asystole tends to be. This is from so-called "overdrive suppression." Asystole may be precipitated by sinus arrest as seen with SSS and is associated with syncope. If no subsidiary pacemaker rescues the heart, death will ensue. It is important to remember that electrical defibrillation will not resolve asystole.

Further reading

Dubin, D. (2000). *Rapid Interpretation of EKG's*, 6e. Cover Inc.

Ilaria, S., Giuseppina, B.P., Paola, S. et al. (2013). ECG of the month. *JAVMA* 242 (9): 1222–1224.

Kalyanasundaram, A., Li, N., Hansen, B.J. et al. (2019). Canine and human sinoatrial node: differences and similarities in the structure, function, molecular profiles, and arrhythmia. *J. Vet. Cardiol.* 22: 2–19.

Kinoshita, S., Katoh, T., Tsujimura, Y. et al. (2000). Sinus escape-capture bigeminy and sinus extrasystolic bigeminy. *J. Electrocardiol.* 33 (1): 85–91.

Liu, T., Shehata, M., and Wang, X. (2011). Paradoxical ventriculophasic sinus arrhythmia during 2:1 atrioventricular block. *J. Cardiol. Cases* 3: e37–e39.

Murphy, L.A., Zuckerman, I.C., and Nakamura, R.K. (2015). ECG of the month. *JAVMA* 246 (7): 740–741.

Nakamura, R.K. and Yuhas, D.L. (2011). ECG of the month. *JAVMA* 239 (6): 751–753.

Skanes, A. and Tang, A. (1998). Ventriculophasic modulation of atrioventricular nodal conduction in humans. *Circulation* 97: 2245–2251.

Surawicz, B. and Knilans, T.K. (2001). *Chou's Electrocardiography in Clinical Practice: Adult and Pediatric*, 5e. Saunders.

Thorn, C.L. and Oyama, M.A. (2015). ECG of the month. *JAVMA* 247 (11): 1244–1246.

10

Sinoatrial Block

CHAPTER MENU

Sinoatrial block, 117
Type I second degree SA block, 117
Type II second degree SA block, 120

Sinoatrial block Sinoatrial block (SAB, SA block/SA exit block) occurs when the atrial tissue around the sinoatrial (SA) node fails to conduct a sinus beat because the wave of depolarization fails to exit the SA node. Thus, no P wave and subsequent QRS are seen when they are expected to otherwise. Most commonly, this is from so-called second degree SA block, where a pause is seen following a normal sinus beat and the interval between the last sinus beat and the next beat following a pause is *exactly* equal to a multiple of the normal P-P interval, and it is intermittent (like second-degree atrioventricular block/AVB).

Similar to AVB, sinoatrial block is categorized by degree. **First degree SAB** consists of a prolonged SA-P interval, which cannot be seen on surface EKG because SA nodal discharge is not recorded. Remember that P waves on surface EKG only show atrial depolarization, and if every sinus discharge eventually activates the atria, then the surface EKG is indistinguishable from that of sinus rhythm regardless of the duration of the SA-P interval. **Second degree SAB** may be inferred from surface EKG because the block is incomplete, resulting in missing P-QRS-T complexes when they are otherwise expected. Low-grade second degree SAB can thus be deduced from surface EKG by examining the intervals and pauses in the rhythm. High-grade second degree SAB often cannot be reliably differentiated from sinus arrest on surface EKG. Second degree SAB with 2:1 conduction may be suspected when the sinus rate abruptly halves in rate. **Third degree SA block** (complete SAB) can be manifested as complete absence of P waves, cannot be diagnosed without intracardiac EKG, or differentiated from protracted sinus arrest or atrial standstill on surface EKG. Since dogs commonly have exaggerated sinus arrhythmias, it is often difficult to diagnose SA block on surface EKG. Sinoatrial block may occur during excessive vagal stimulation, myocarditis, myocardial infarction, atrial fibrosis (thus associated with sick sinus syndrome, SSS), and intoxication with quinidine, procainamide, or digoxin/glycoside. Impostors of SA block include sinus or atrial bigeminy, blocked atrial premature complexes, sinus arrhythmia, ventriculophasic sinus arrhythmia, and sinus pause.

Type I second degree SA block (Wenckebach) occurs when the P-P interval progressively shortens prior to the pause, group beating occurs, and the duration of the pause is slightly less than two P-P intervals. The SA-P interval progressively prolongs, causing the acceleration of the P-P interval (typical Wenckebach periodicity) similar to the progressive R-R interval shortening seen with Type I second degree AV block, ultimately causing the group beating. We simply cannot see the SA-P interval on surface EKG. Typical and atypical Wenckebach periods may be seen, similar to what occurs during Type I second degree AVB. Type I second degree SAB can be difficult to justify in dogs due to sinus arrhythmia. A 3:2 SA conduction results in a bigeminal sinus rhythm ("sinus bigeminy") and 4:3 conduction results in a trigeminal rhythm (see Chapter 9).

Interpretation of the Electrocardiogram in Small Animals, First Edition. Nick A. Schroeder.
© 2021 John Wiley & Sons Inc. Published 2021 by John Wiley & Sons Inc.

Most of the time, Type I second degree SAB is a low grade of block, meaning no more than one consecutive sinus impulse is blocked. Rarely, a high grade of block may occur, and more than one consecutive sinus impulse may fail to conduct. Pauses created by sinoatrial block are not uncommonly thwarted/terminated by ectopic atrial escape beats and occasionally escape rhythm. The altered P′ wave morphology of these beats as well as apparent resetting of the sinus node are clues. Furthermore, sinoatrial block may be associated with a superimposed sinus arrhythmia and/or AVB. These phenomena make the diagnosis of SAB challenging at times.

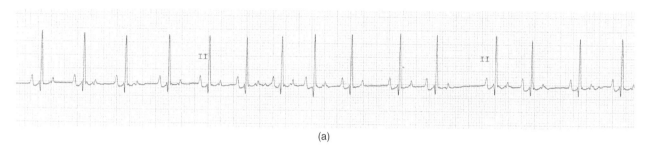

(a)

Figure 10.1a Paper speed 25 mm/s, 1 cm/mV, lead II, canine. **Type I second degree SA block**. Group beating is evident. The P-P intervals progressively shorten prior to the pauses seen between beats #9 and #10 and #11 and #12. The first four complexes are regular, and the group beating that occurs in the following beats was not correlated with inspiration. This, coupled with the conspicuous lack of a wandering pacemaker, favors a diagnosis of Type 1 second degree SAB over that of a sinus arrhythmia.

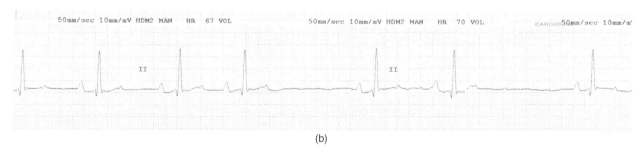

(b)

Figure 10.1b Paper speed 50 mm/s, 1 cm/mV, lead II, same dog. The progressive P-P shortening and group beating are evident in the first four complexes. The pause between the fourth and fifth beats is less than two P-P intervals, indicative of Wenckebach or Type I second degree SAB.

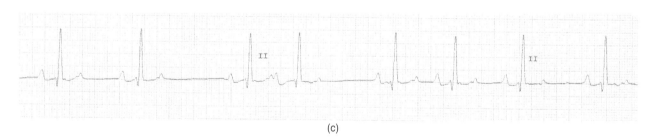

(c)

Figure 10.1c Paper speed 50 mm/s, 1 cm/mV, lead II, same dog. The fourth complex here may be an APC with a prolonged P′-R interval or a sinus beat with first degree AVB that occurred early enough to find the AVN partially refractory. The pause that follows this beat is less than two P-P intervals, and thus consistent with Type I second degree SAB. Resetting with a pause (if it is an APC) could explain it as well.

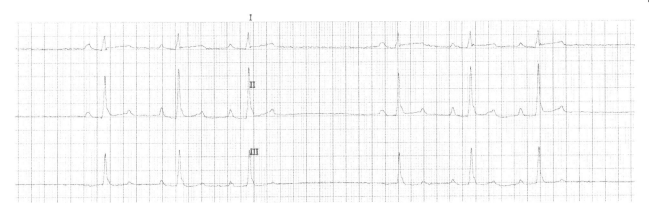

Figure 10.2 Paper speed 50 mm/s, 1 cm/mV, leads I, II, III, canine. **Sinoatrial block**, likely Type I second degree with 3:2 conduction with pauses interrupted by ectopic atrial escape beats, which reset the sinus node. This creates a repetitive trigeminal pattern. The first beat in each group is ectopic atrial. Note the altered P wave morphology, most notably in lead III.

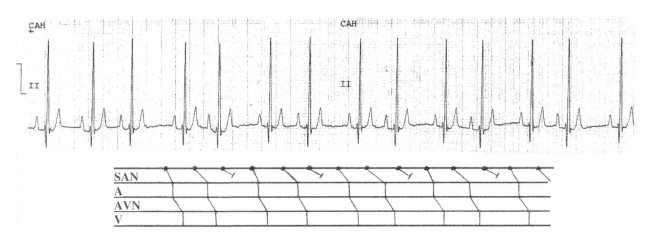

Figure 10.3 Paper speed 50 mm/s, 1 cm/mV, lead II, canine. **Type 1 second degree SA block** with 3:2 conduction. A ladder diagram illustrates the mechanism. Lengthening SA-P wave intervals result in an apparent shortening of the P-P interval before failure of conduction, manifested here as pauses that are less than twice the P-P interval and resulting in a *bigeminal* rhythm ("sinoatrial escape-capture bigeminy" or "sinus bigeminy").

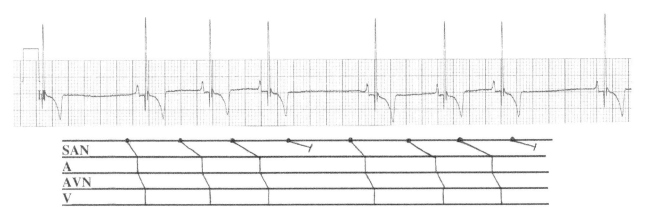

Figure 10.4 Paper speed 50 mm/s, 1 cm/mV, lead II, canine. **Type I second degree SA block** with 4:3 conduction. Lengthening SA-P wave intervals result in an apparent shortening of the P-P interval before failure of conduction. The pauses are less than twice the P-P interval immediately preceding the pause, resulting in a *trigeminal* rhythm.

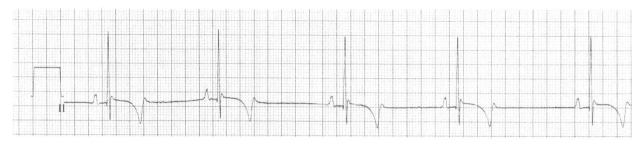

Figure 10.5 Paper speed 50 mm/s, 1 cm/mV, lead II, canine with *Bufo marinus* intoxication. Sinus bradycardia, possible 3:2 **Type I second degree SAB**, mild S-T segment elevation and long Q-T interval. Digitalis glycosides are present within the secretions of the parotid glands of the *Bufo* toad, and EKG changes and arrhythmias consistent with digitalis intoxication may result.

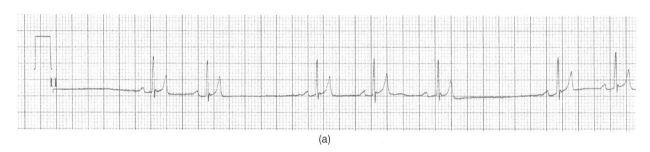

(a)

Figure 10.6a Paper speed 25 mm/s, 1 cm/mV, canine sedated with medetomidine. **Type I second degree SAB, atypical Wenckebach periodicity**. Here, there is P-P *lengthening* (between fourth and fifth complexes) before failure of SA nodal conduction and the resultant pause. This may actually be explained by a high grade of block (see below).

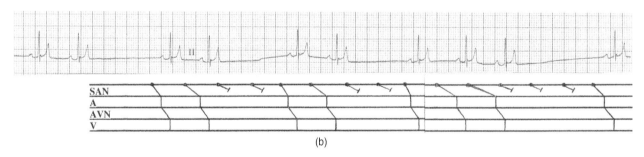

(b)

Figure 10.6b Paper speed 50 mm/s, 1 cm/mV, same dog. *Possible* **high-grade Type I second degree SAB**. The bigeminal sinus rhythm is suspicious for at least 3:2 Type I second degree SAB, and a typical Wenckebach period with 4:3 conduction may explain the triplet toward the end. However, when plotting the rhythm on a ladder, this pattern fits better with 4:2 conduction followed by 3:3 conduction, making this a potential example of high-grade Type I second degree SAB since more than one consecutive sinus impulse fails to conduct.

Type II second degree SA block

It has P-P intervals that are fixed and thus constant. The underlying sinus rhythm must be perfectly regular to diagnose Type II second degree SAB in dogs and is most commonly seen in association with SSS. Similar to Type II second degree AVB, Type II second degree SAB can be subdivided into low grade (no more than one consecutive non-conducted SA impulse) and high grade (2 or more consecutive non-conducted SA impulses). High-grade Type II SAB technically results in a sinus arrest if pauses last in excess of 2 P-P (or R-R) intervals (i.e. if 3+ sinus impulses are non-conducted). Abrupt and protracted ("paroxysmal") high-grade SAB results in sinus arrest (see Chapter 9).

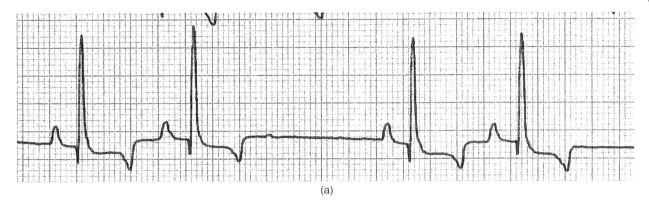

(a)

Figure 10.7a Paper speed 50 mm/s, 1 cm/mV, lead II, Miniature Schnauzer. Sinoatrial block, likely **low-grade Type II second degree SA block** as the P-R interval is fairly constant. The pause between the second and third beats is exactly 2 P-P intervals. This patient had sick sinus syndrome (**SSS**).

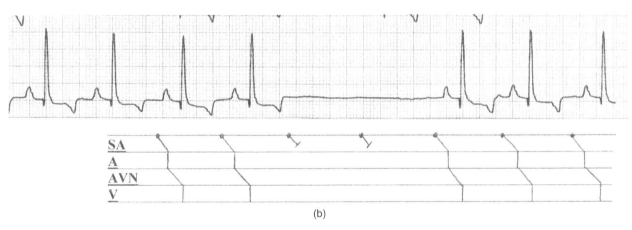

(b)

Figure 10.7b Paper speed 50 mm/s, 1 cm/mV, lead II, same dog, SA block, the pause shows exactly 2 P-P intervals before the next two beats, indicative of **high-grade Type II second degree SA block**. The ladder diagram illustrates the mechanism. The underlying sinus rhythm is perfectly regular between pauses.

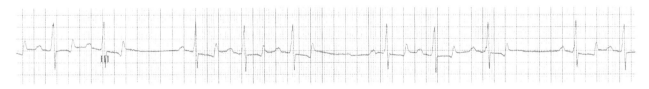

Figure 10.8 Paper speed 50 mm/s, 1 cm/mV, lead III, dog with renal failure and suspected digoxin toxicity. **Low-grade Type II second degree SA block**. The pauses occur secondary to 4:3 SA conduction, and are exactly 2 P-P intervals apart.

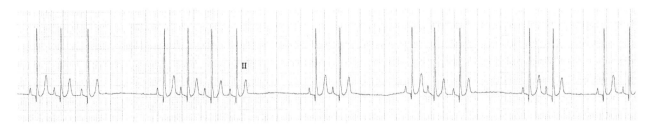

Figure 10.9 Paper speed 25 mm/s, 1 cm/mV, lead II, Miniature Schnauzer. **High-grade Type II second degree SA block masquerading as sinus arrhythmia.** Pauses in the rhythm are exact multiples of the underlying P-P interval (intermittent 3:1 SA conduction, 2:1 conduction at the end). Here, the pauses are coincident with expiration, but note that the P-P/R-R intervals are all *constant*. Simple sinus arrhythmia is generally denoted by a phasic and *gradual* increase and decrease in P-P/R-R intervals. Fixed intervals are consistent with exit block from the SA node and should alert the clinician to the likelihood of sinus nodal dysfunction/sick sinus syndrome.

Take Home Point: First and third degree SAB are not evident without intracardiac EKG – only second degree SAB may be diagnosed by examination of surface EKG. Distinguishing Type I second degree SAB from Type II is important. Type I is associated with elevated parasympathetic tone, physiologic, and unlikely to be a problem in of itself. Type II is more likely to be indicative of true conduction system disease (SSS), potentially becoming high grade and leading to symptomatic bradycardia eventually requiring intervention (i.e. potential pacemaker implantation).

Further reading

Marriot, H.J.L. and Conover, M.B. (1998). *Advanced Concepts in Arrhythmias*, 3e. Mosby.

Surawicz, B. and Knilans, T.K. (2001). *Chou's Electrocardiography in Clinical Practice: Adult and Pediatric*, 5e. Saunders.

11

Sick Sinus Syndrome

CHAPTER MENU

Sick sinus syndrome, 123
Overdrive suppression, 123
Sinus nodal dysfunction, 123
Bradycardia variant, 126
Tachycardia-bradycardia variant, 128

Sick sinus syndrome Sick sinus syndrome (SSS) is just that, a syndrome. It is not merely one arrhythmia, but rather a constellation of EKG findings that suggest there is abnormal sinus nodal activity associated with symptomatic bradycardia. Sick sinus syndrome is usually characterized by sinus bradycardia (intermittent or persistent, inappropriate to profound), sinus pause/arrest, sinoatrial block, transient atrial standstill, variable atrioventricular block (AVB), junctional bradyarrhythmias, and atrial flutter or atrial fibrillation with a slow ventricular rate response (see Chapters 9, 10, 13, and 17–20). Sick sinus syndrome is apparently rare in cats and not uncommon in female Miniature Schnauzers, Cocker Spaniels, and to a lesser extent West Highland White Terriers. Symptomatic patients are best treated with pacemaker implantation. Sick sinus syndrome may present as primarily bradycardia or manifest as a bradycardia-tachycardia syndrome, with bradyarrhythmias associated with intermittent supraventricular or ventricular tachycardia (VT), frequently irregular from exit block and post-tachycardia ventricular asystole. Common features include excessive overdrive suppression of the SA node following a relative tachycardia and lazy escape foci (atrial, junctional, and occasionally ventricular) following pauses resulting from block/arrests. Intact ventriculoatrial conduction is common.

Overdrive suppression Overdrive suppression is a feature of normal sinus nodal activity. Rapid depolarization of the sinus node by ectopic foci or atrial pacing will frequently cause some delay of a capture beat by the sinus node relative to the patient's underlying sinus cycle rate. This is what results in resetting with a pause that can occur following supraventricular premature complexes or sinus pauses/arrests following tachycardia. Excessive overdrive suppression of the SA node is a sign of a sick sinus node. As sinus nodal disease may progress to involve the atrioventricular junction and beyond (so-called "structural nodal disease"), junctional and ventricular escape foci may not appear when otherwise expected. This leads to very long sinus arrests with ventricular asystole. Pauses in the ventricular rhythm in excess of 6 seconds frequently produce clinical signs including weakness, lethargy, collapse, or overt syncope.

Sinus nodal dysfunction Patients with SSS may be subclinical or clinical, and subclinical individuals may be identified by the presence of sinus nodal dysfunction. Subclinical patients are often unmasked by general anesthesia and can often be managed on sympathomimetics such as theophylline or hyoscyamine. Blood pressure monitoring is recommended, as systemic hypertension may develop over time requiring medical intervention (i.e. amlodipine, angiotensin converting enzyme-inhibitors). Periodic echocardiography is also recommended to monitor for volume overload associated with bradycardia-induced cardiomyopathy. The intrinsic sinus rate may be induced by simultaneous muscarinic and beta-blockade with atropine/propranolol and may be abnormally low in subclinical SSS patients (<90–100 bpm in the dog). Intracardiac EKG can uncover abnormally prolonged SA nodal recovery time (overdrive pacing of the atria/SAN with a

Interpretation of the Electrocardiogram in Small Animals, First Edition. Nick A. Schroeder.
© 2021 John Wiley & Sons Inc. Published 2021 by John Wiley & Sons Inc.

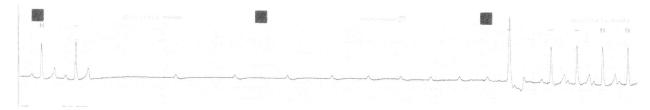

Figure 11.1 Paper speed 25 mm/s, 1 cm/mV, lead II, syncopal Cocker Spaniel. A long pause following the second beat is caused by a period of sinus arrest and paroxysmal AV block. Note the P wave rate gradually *increases* (P-P intervals decrease) until a ventricular escape beat rescues the heart. Sinus tachycardia ensues after the escape beat. The arrest following the second beat without P waves suggest **sinus nodal dysfunction** in addition to the AVB and late ventricular escape, all of which are consistent with SSS.

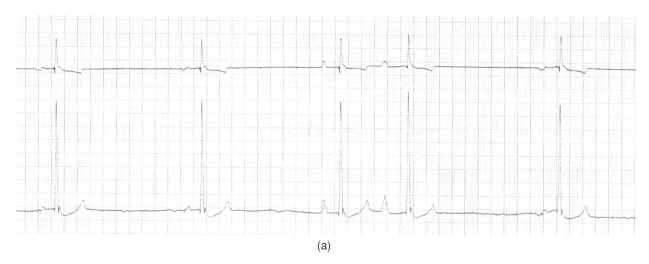

(a)

Figure 11.2a Paper speed 50 mm/s, 1 cm/mV, leads I (top) and II (bottom), F/S Miniature Schnauzer post-op lung lobectomy on a fentanyl constant rate infusion. A slow atrial escape rhythm has captured the ventricles secondary to sinus arrest. The third complex is a sinus capture, which is followed by another sinus beat with a prolonged P-R interval (functional first degree atrioventricular block secondary to short cycle length and elevated vagal tone from the fentanyl). The fourth beat is another atrial escape beat. This patient had an unremarkable EKG before anesthesia.

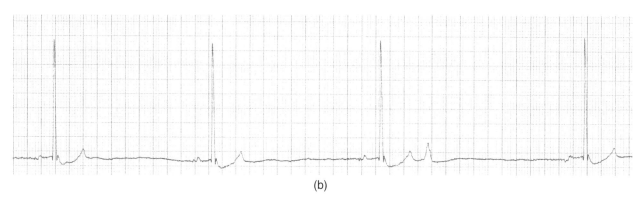

(b)

Figure 11.2b Paper speed 50 mm/s, 1 cm/mV, lead II, same dog. Atrial escape rhythm occurs for the first three beats, which is then followed by a sinus P wave that is AV blocked due to a short cycle length. The last complex is ectopic atrial induced by the sinus arrest. P mitrale is present with prolongation of the P waves (0.07 second). Interatrial block is not uncommon in patients with SSS and left atrial enlargement may or may not be present. The tall QRS complexes suggest left ventricular enlargement and increased amplitude of the sinus P waves suggests right atrial enlargement.

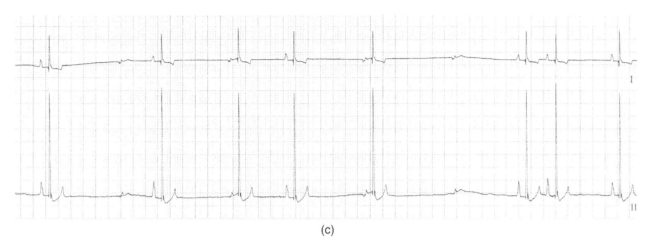

(c)

Figure 11.2c Paper speed 25 mm/s, 1 cm/mV, leads I and II, same dog. The first beat is sinus, which is then followed by an atrial ectopic escape beat which is AV blocked for no apparent reason. Then, atrial escape-capture bigeminy ensues for four beats, which is terminated by another blocked ectopic atrial beat. The sinus node then captures the rhythm again. These exaggerated vagal arrhythmias are evidence that this patient has **subclinical SSS**.

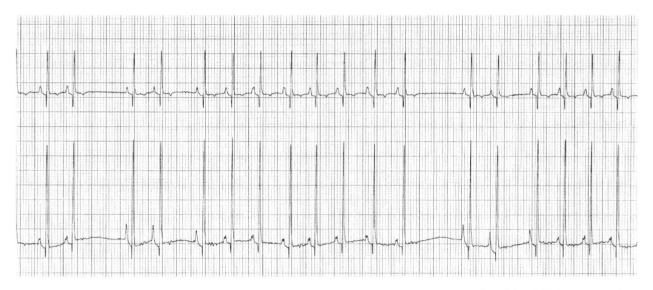

Figure 11.3 Paper speed 25 mm/S, 1 cm/mV, leads I (top) and II (bottom), F/S Miniature Schnauzer. **Subclinical SSS**. Sinus rhythm is interrupted by a sinus arrest, which is terminated by ectopic atrial (or higher SA nodal focus) for three beats, and sinus rhythm resumes with another arrest after beat #12. Sinus arrests here are relatively mild and less than 1 second in duration. This patient was asymptomatic. Anesthesia would likely provoke serious bradycardia.

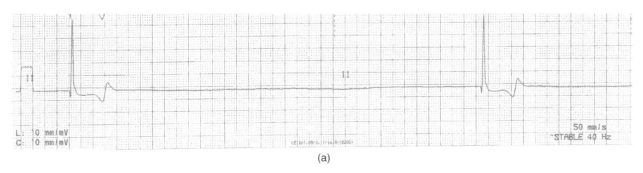

(a)

Figure 11.4a Paper speed 50 mm/s, 1 cm/mV, lead II. Cocker Spaniel under anesthesia. Sinus arrest with ventricular escape rhythm and a HR of approximately 17 bpm!

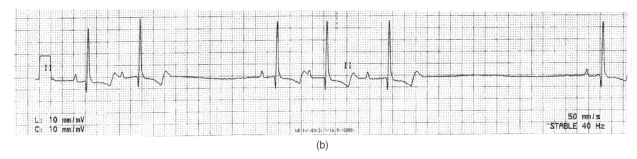

(b)

Figure 11.4b Paper speed 50 mm/s, 1 cm/mV, lead II. Same dog 24 hours after anesthesia. Sinus rhythm with **sinus arrests** and atypical Wenckebach periodicity (progressive P-Ri prolongation without failure of conduction). The heart rate of approximately 100 bpm allows for this dog to be asymptomatic.

longer than normal time until SAN capture) as well as evidence of interatrial block which may manifest as overdrive suppression and severe P mitrale on surface EKG, respectively (see Chapter 4).

Bradycardia variant Most often, patients with SSS have bradyarrhythmias. Profound sinus bradycardia, Type I or II second degree sinoatrial block, sinus pause/arrests/asystole are common. Sick sinus syndrome results from progressive idiopathic fibrosis in the SA node, which may progress to involve atrial tissue and the AV node and conduction system. Atrial standstill,

AVB, and junctional bradyarrhythmias may consequently develop with SSS. It should be noted that first and Type I second degree AVB, though considered "physiologic" and secondary to elevated parasympathetic tone, are quite commonly associated with SSS in at risk breeds. Even if the atria are rapidly depolarizing (i.e. if atrial fibrillation or atrial flutter is present), an excessively slow ventricular rate response in the absence of drug administration suggests a high grade of AVB and the possibility of SSS in susceptible breeds. Escape foci may be irregular from exit block or fail to appear when otherwise expected, resulting in prolonged asystole following sinus arrest and/or second degree AVB.

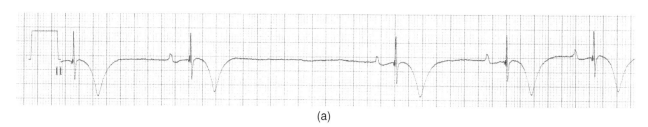

(a)

Figure 11.5a Paper speed 50 mm/s, 1 cm/mV, lead II, asymptomatic female Miniature Schnauzer. **Sinoatrial block** is likely creating sudden sinus **pauses/arrest** in this strip. No excessively long pauses are seen, and as such, treatment may not be indicated. **Long Q-T intervals** are present with deep, scoped-out T waves. Bradycardia in of itself typically results in some physiologic Q-Ti prolongation; however, this is excessive and suggests congenital long Q-Ti/repolarization abnormality. This patient should not only be monitored for syncope from bradycardia/sinus arrest, but this patient may also be predisposed to **torsades de pointes**, a potentially lethal polymorphic ventricular tachycardia, that may occur in this setting. Sinoatrial block/sinus arrest seen here may be the early manifestations of a **sick sinus node** in this patient. This patient unfortunately did die suddenly at home.

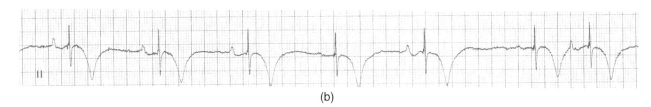

(b)

Figure 11.5b Paper speed 50 mm/s, 1 cm/mV, lead II, same patient. A pause after beat #3 is terminated by an atrial escape beat, which is followed by a sinus capture. A bigeminal rhythm ensues, and is termed **atrial escape-capture bigeminy**, secondary in this patient to sinoatrial block.

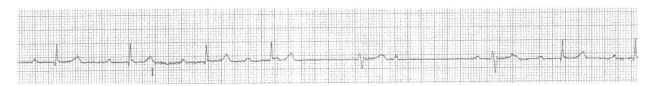

Figure 11.6 Paper speed 50 mm/s, 1 cm/mV, lead I, Cocker Spaniel with panting and episodic collapse. **First degree AVB** is present. A **sinus pause/arrest** ensues after the first four complexes. The P-P intervals gradually shorten prior to the pause, suggestive of **Type I second degree SAB**. A ventricular escape rhythm ensues for two beats, followed by sinus capture.

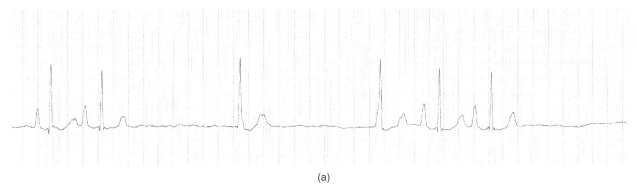

(a)

Figure 11.7a Paper speed 50 mm/s, 1 cm/mV, lead II, canine. **Sinus arrest** after the second beat is terminated by junctional escape. The escape complexes *thwart* attempts at sinus capture. Note the deformation of the QRS by the non-conducted P waves. P pulmonale is also present suggestive of right atrial enlargement.

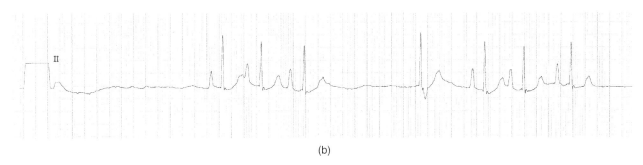

(b)

Figure 11.7b Paper speed 50 mm/s, 1 cm/mV, lead II, same dog. Sinus arrest is terminated by a capture beat. Another sinus arrest is then terminated by a junctional escape complex. Unimpeded by attempted sinus capture, this is immediately followed by a retrograde P′ wave just after the QRS within the S-T segment. Intact **VA conduction** is common in patients with **SSS**.

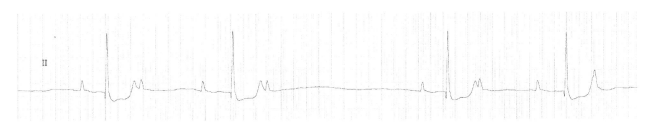

Figure 11.8 Paper speed 50 mm/s, 1 cm/mV, lead II. West Highland White Terrier with SSS. **Ventriculophasic sinus arrhythmia** is present, as is **first degree atrioventricular block**, **Type I second degree AVB**, and **sinus arrest** between the fourth and fifth P waves. Significant S-T segment depression is also present, suggestive of myocardial hypoxia.

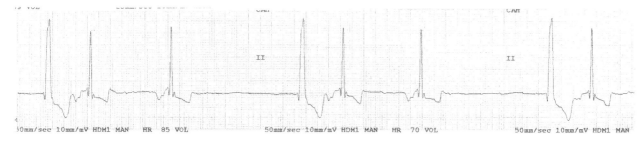

Figure 11.9 Paper speed 50 mm/s, 1 cm/mV, lead II, syncopal Cocker Spaniel, **SSS**. Here, the supraventricular beats have negative P waves. This is likely from a low RA focus at the periphery of the sinus node near the coronary sinus. A pause/arrest occurs after the third and sixth complexes and is followed by RV escape complexes.

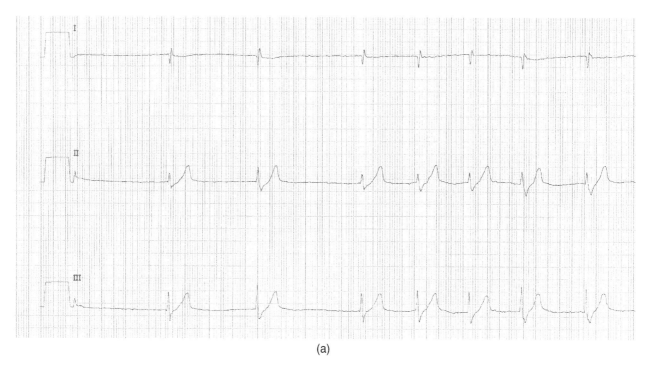

(a)

Figure 11.10a Paper speed 50 mm/s, 1 cm/mV, leads I, II, III, Dachshund on theophylline. At first glance, atrial activity is inapparent, the QRS complexes appear supraventricular, albeit prolonged in duration and with an irregular rhythm – all suggestive of atrial fibrillation with a relatively slow ventricular rate response and right bundle branch block of the QRS complexes.

Tachycardia-bradycardia variant Sick sinus syndrome can also present with periods of tachycardia. This may be sinus, non-sinus supraventricular tachycardia (SVT), or VT. These tachyarrhythmias may be irregular from exit block and secondary to progressive myocardial fibrosis. Pacing may eliminate syncope from bradyarrhythmias, but not that resulting from sustained tachycardia. Such patients may require pacemaker implantation and concurrent antiarrhythmic therapy to control

persistent tachyarrhythmias. Prolonged asystole following tachyarrhythmias from overdrive suppression is a feature.

Patients with clinical signs associated with SSS are candidates for implantation of a permanent artificial pacemaker. Most experience exercise intolerance, episodic weakness, collapse, or syncope and may present in congestive heart failure (often biventricular from bradycardia-associated cardiomyopathy ± superimposed chronic valvular degeneration). These symptoms are generally ameliorated

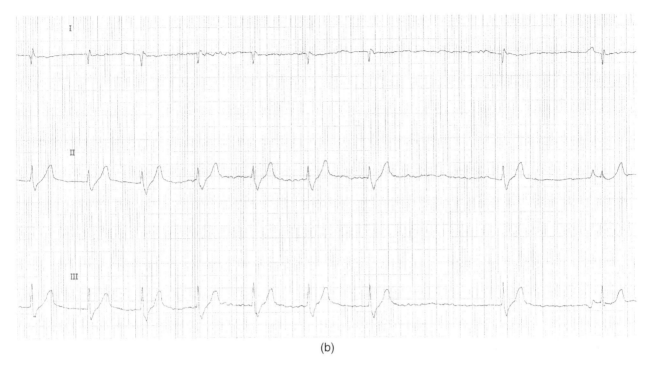

(b)

Figure 11.10b Paper speed 50 mm/s, 1 cm/mV, leads I, II, III, same dog. The last complex is the big reveal. The QRS complexes are indeed supraventricular, but junctional in origin. Retrograde P′ waves just follow the QRS complexes, distorting the S-T segment, so the junctional focus has **ventriculoatrial conduction**. The ninth complex appears to be a sinus capture with right axis deviation of the QRS. The junctional focus is accelerated and VA conduction is suppressing sinoatrial discharge; however, the SAN is not functioning properly as even long pauses between junctional beats (i.e. between beats #7 and #8) fail to always be terminated by sinus capture, which is random, rare, and thus consistent with a **sick sinus node**. Oddly, the prevailing **accelerated junctional arrhythmia** is *phasic* and *non-respiratory* (could not be correlated with respiratory phase on physical examination).

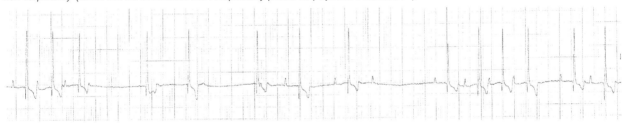

Figure 11.11 Paper speed 25 mm/s, 1 cm/mV, lead II, Cocker Spaniel with chronic mitral valvular disease. Sinus arrhythmia/sinus bradycardia, first degree atrioventricular block, low-grade (atypical) Type I second degree AVB, pauses terminated by junctional escapes. This dog was in left-sided congestive heart failure and sinus bradyarrhythmias are inappropriate. **Atrioventricular block** is not uncommonly associated with **SSS**.

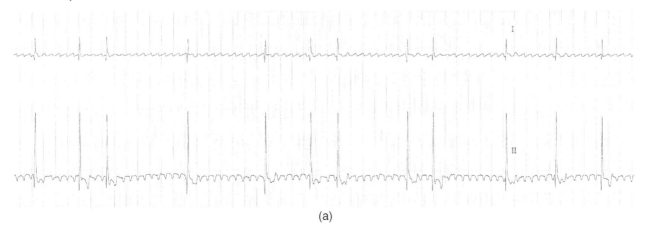

(a)

Figure 11.12a Paper speed 25 mm/s, 1 cm/mV, leads I and II, same dog. **Atrial flutter with high-grade atrioventricular block**. The ventricular rhythm is irregular and F-R intervals are variable, so which complexes are conducted and which ones represent junctional escapes is unclear (though QRS terminating longer pauses are more likely to be junctional escapes). This dog was not on antiarrhythmic or digoxin. Atrial flutter here with a **slow** ventricular rate response is a sign of **SSS**.

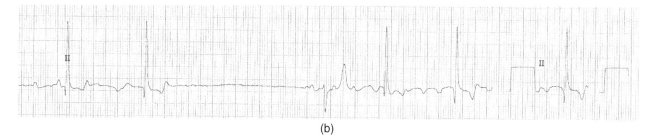

(b)

Figure 11.12b Paper speed 50 mm/s, 1 cm/mV, lead II, same dog. Variable AVB is followed by a junctional beat and sinus arrest terminated by an escape complex which in turn initiates paroxysmal atrial flutter.

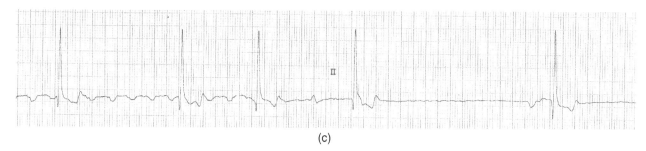

(c)

Figure 11.12c Paper speed, 50 mm/s, 1 cm/mV, lead II, same dog. The atrial flutter terminates with a sinus capture with marked first degree AVB. Sinus arrest ensues and is terminated by a junctional escape. Obvious overdrive suppression is another indicator of **SSS**.

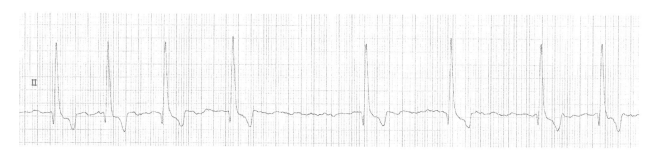

Figure 11.13 Paper speed 50 mm/s, 1 cm/mV, lead II, Miniature Schnauzer in left heart failure. **Atrial fibrillation with high-grade AVB** suggestive of **SSS**. The ventricular rate response (HR 120 bpm) is unusually slow in this small-breed dog with severe left atrial enlargement from underlying valvular disease. We would assume this patient should have a rapid ventricular rate response (malignant and secondary AF). This is especially the case given this patient was on no medications (i.e. no digoxin, diltiazem, or beta-blocker).

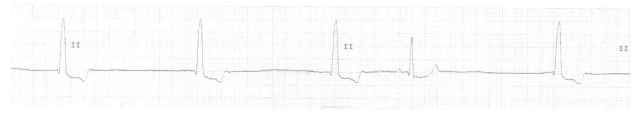

Figure 11.14 Paper speed 50 mm/s, 0.5 cm/mV, lead II, Miniature Schnauzer in right heart failure. Advanced sinus nodal disease left this patient with long periods of **atrial standstill** from prolonged sinus arrest and an escape rhythm of approximately 54 bpm. A single sinus capture beat occurs after the third escape beat here, demonstrating that this is not persistent atrial standstill, but advanced SA nodal dysfunction associated with **SSS**. The capture beat resets the escape focus, indicating the escape focus is junctional in origin by the **Rule of reset**. It is wide and bizarre due to LBBB aberration.

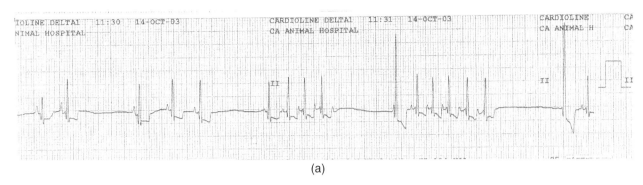

(a)

Figure 11.15a Paper speed 25 mm/s, 1 cm/mV, lead II, syncopal Miniature Schnauzer, **SSS**. Supraventricular tachycardia starts with the sixth complex and is followed by sinus arrest and RV escape complexes. The ninth complex is followed by a non-conducted P wave (second degree AVB).

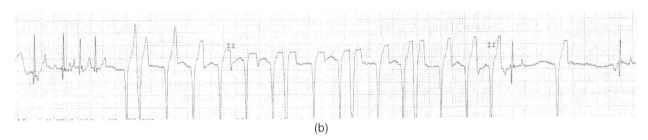

(b)

Figure 11.15b Paper speed 25 mm/s, 1 cm/mV, lead II, same dog. Occasionally **ventricular tachycardia** may be associated with **SSS**, demonstrating that the EKGs of dogs with SSS can show a variety of associated arrhythmias. The VT here is likely irregular from exit block and is terminated by a reciprocal complex.

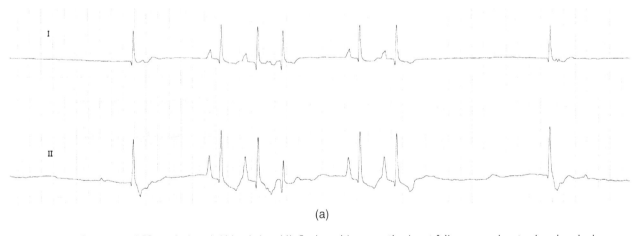

(a)

Figure 11.16a Paper speed 50 mm/s, 1 cm/mV, leads I and II. Canine with congestive heart failure secondary to chronic valvular disease. P-pseudobiatriale is present. The P waves were markedly increased in amplitude (p-pulmonale) and prolonged (p-mitrale), though only severe left atrial enlargement was documented via echocardiography. The first and last complexes are junctional escapes with ventriculoatrial conduction that terminate sinus arrests. The fourth complex is a junctional premature complex with mild aberrancy.

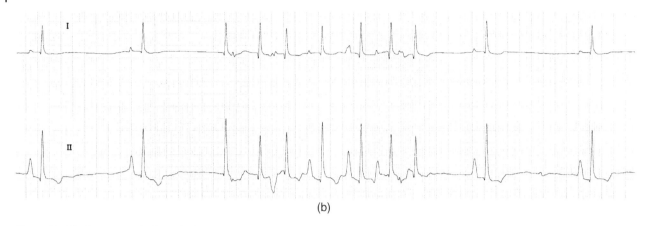

(b)

Figure 11.16b Paper speed 50 mm/s, 1 cm/mV, leads I and II, same dog. Sinus pauses are terminated by a junctional escape and non-sustained reentrant **SVT**. Sinus pauses with escapes and SVT are suggestive of **tachycardia-bradycardia** variant of **SSS**.

by pacing and those with heart failure may have some regression of cardiomegaly and be able to come off diuretics.

> *Take Home Point*: Sick sinus syndrome frequently produces bizarre EKGs with multiple arrhythmias, and it is very easy for the examiner to focus on minutia and miss the underlying cause. Sick sinus syndrome associated with bradycardia

usually is marked by bradyarrhythmias in general which are generally attributed to failure of impulse formation and propagation out of the SA node itself. Thus, profound sinus bradycardia, sinus pauses/arrests are features. The bradycardia-tachycardia variant is marked by intermittent SVT or VT. Pauses in the rhythm and episodes of tachycardia are often followed by long periods of asystole from overdrive suppression before sinus captures or rescue by escape foci.

Further reading

Kalyanasundaram, A., Li, N., Hansen, B.J. et al. (2019). Canine and human sinoatrial node: differences and similarities in the structure, function, molecular profiles, and arrhythmia. *J. Vet. Cardiol.* 22: 2–19.

Marriot, H.J.L. and Conover, M.B. (1998). *Advanced Concepts in Arrhythmias*, 3e. Mosby.

Santilli, R., Perego, M., Pariaut, R., and Sydney, M. (2018). *Electrocardiography of the Dog and Cat: Diagnosis of Arrhythmias*, 2e. Edna.

Surawicz, B. and Knilans, T.K. (2001). *Chou's Electrocardiography in Clinical Practice: Adult and Pediatric*, 5e. Saunders.

Treseder, J.R. and Jung, S. (2016). ECG of the month. *JAVMA* 248 (7): 762–764.

12

Sinoatrial Tachyarrhythmias

CHAPTER MENU

Sinus nodal premature systoles, 133
Sinoatrial reciprocal complexes, 133
Sinus nodal parasystole, 134
Sinus tachycardia, 136
Sinus nodal reentrant tachycardia, 137

Sinus nodal premature systoles Premature beats with a P′ morphology identical (or nearly identical) to that of the normal P waves of the sinus beats may actually be arising from a separate focus within the sinus node itself. These beats are early, reset the sinus node, and have a supraventricular QRS (unless pre-existing bundle branch block or rate-dependent aberrancy is present). The P′-P interval should be identical to the P-P interval (perfect resetting); however, it may be slightly longer from overdrive suppression (resetting with a pause). Sinus nodal premature beats may be indistinguishable from ectopic atrial premature complexes arising from a focus very near the sinus node and the reset may be mistaken for a sinus pause. If SANPCs have constant coupling intervals, then sinoatrial reentry may be suspected. If the coupling intervals are variable, increased automaticity and even a parasystolic focus is possible. Documentation requires intracardiac EKG. These are common in Cavalier King Charles Spaniels, have the same significance as atrial premature beats, and may occur with elevated sympathetic tone. Sinus nodal premature beats may be difficult to prove in the presence of an underlying sinus arrhythmia; however, truly premature beats have a cycle length that is markedly shortened by a greater percentage than that expected for the cyclic variability of the P-P intervals. P-R interval prolongation (first degree AV block) may be noted on conducted sinus nodal premature complexes. Rarely, sinus nodal premature beats may be non-conducted (blocked in the atrioventricular/AV node). This typically presents as a low-grade Type I second degree (Wenckebach) block, is physiologic and secondary to transient elevations in parasympathetic tone. Sinus nodal premature complexes may occur in 1 : 1 extrasystole presenting as a sinus bigeminy and second degree sinoatrial block with 3 : 2 conduction and sinus arrhythmia with fortuitous pairing should be excluded (see Chapters 9 and 10).

Sinoatrial reciprocal complexes A single microreentry involving the sinoatrial node may reexcite the atria and ventricles producing a sinoatrial reciprocal complex or echo beat. The sequence is A-SAN-A-V. This may appear as sinoatrial premature beats with constant coupling intervals or manifest as an apparently interpolated atrial premature complex (APC) or sinoatrial premature complex with the post-extrasystolic complex representing the sinoatrial echo (see Chapter 14). This may mimic a couplet of supraventricular premature complexes, especially if the P′ waves are buried in the previous S-T segment obscuring the morphology. If the post-extrasystolic P wave is slightly early, then a sinoatrial reciprocal (echo) beat is favored. If the post-extrasystolic sinus beat is right on time, then interpolation occurred. If it is slightly delayed, then incomplete interpolation occurred, but the dominant sinus focus still fails to be reset. Often the differentiation between a sinoatrial reentry and interpolation is confounded by underlying sinus arrhythmia.

Interpretation of the Electrocardiogram in Small Animals, First Edition. Nick A. Schroeder.
© 2021 John Wiley & Sons Inc. Published 2021 by John Wiley & Sons Inc.

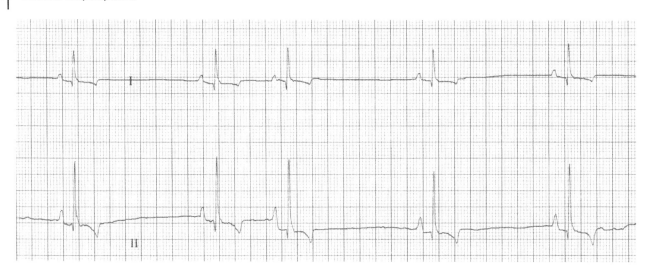

Figure 12.1 Paper speed 50 mm/s, 1 cm/mV, leads I and II, Cavalier King Charles Spaniel with premature beats. The third complex is premature, resets perfectly, and has a similar P wave morphology to the sinus P waves, consistent with a **sinus nodal premature beat**. Such supraventricular premature beats are common incidental findings in the breed.

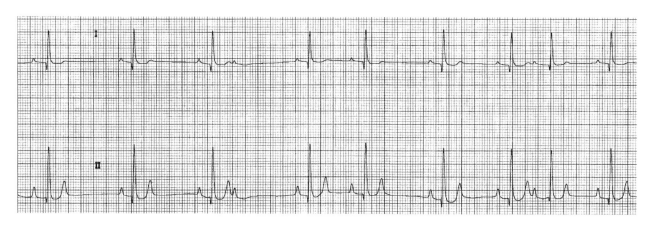

Figure 12.2 Paper speed 50 mm/s, 1 cm/mV, leads I and II, Cavalier King Charles Spaniel. **Sinoatrial nodal premature beats** with variable AV block. The fourth P wave is premature and **non-conducted** (AV blocked) due to physiologic refractoriness of the AVN (functional second degree AVB). The ninth P wave is premature but conducted with a long P-R interval due to partial refractoriness of the AVN (functional first degree AVB). Given that both these P waves have identical morphology to the sinus P waves, occur much earlier than expected (even considering the underlying sinus arrhythmia) with exact resetting of the rhythm, these are considered to be **sinus nodal premature complexes**. Note the degree of prematurity between the premature beats is not detectably different; therefore, the absolute refractory period of the AVN must become longer at relatively long cycle lengths. This means premature beats occurring during a relative bradycardia are less likely to be conducted than those occurring when the heart rate is faster.

Perpetuation of the reentry circuit results in sinoatrial reentrant tachycardia (see below). Documentation requires intracardiac EKG.

Sinus nodal parasystole

A parasystolic focus is one protected from the dominant pacemaker by entrance block, and subsequently fires independently of the underlying rhythm. Rarely, a separate focus within the sinoatrial node itself may produce sinoatrial premature beats independently of the dominant pacemaking cells. If the focus is parasystolic, the premature beats will have varied coupling intervals. Typically, reverse-coupling is present,

and the dominant SA nodal focus will be reset by the premature beats. The interectopic intervals have a common denominator, the ectopic P′ waves are nearly identical in morphology to the sinus P waves, and the QRS complexes of these beats are supraventricular. Fusion of the P and P′ waves is essentially indeterminate on surface EKG if both foci are within the SA node. Sinus nodal parasystole may also present as a sinus bigeminy but coupling interval variability may be difficult to document. Documentation requires intracardiac EKG, and sinus nodal parasystole may be indistinguishable from a right atrial parasystole if the ectopic focus is very close to the SA node.

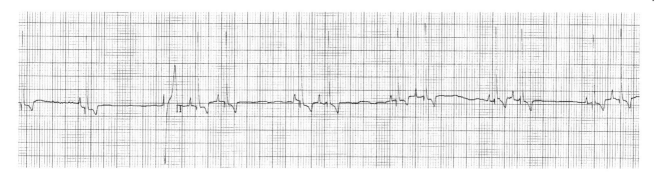

Figure 12.3 Paper speed 25 mm/s, 1 cm/mV, lead II, canine. Sinus rhythm, followed by a sinus pause terminated by ventricular escape, after which **sinus bigeminy** ensues. Note that the second complex in each pair has associated mild P-R interval prolongation (first degree atrioventricular block or atypical Wenckebach periodicity/second degree AVB without associated failure of conduction to the ventricles), suggesting elevated parasympathetic tone. Here, the P-Pi immediately prior to the onset of bigeminy is very short, suggesting that beat #4 is premature, and thus the sinus bigeminy that ensues is likely caused by sinus nodal premature complexes in **1 : 1 extrasystole** vs. second degree sinoatrial block with 3 : 2 conduction.

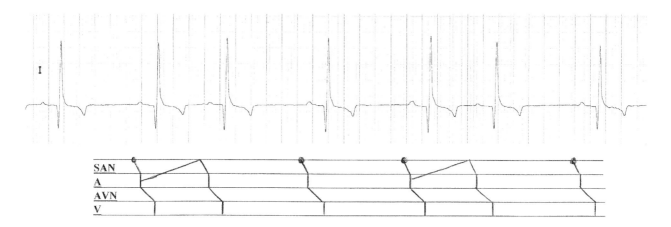

Figure 12.4 Paper speed 50 mm/s, 1 cm/mV, lead I, Cavalier King Charles Spaniel. Sinoatrial premature complexes/sinoatrial reciprocal beats. Here, supraventricular premature complexes with P′ nearly identical to the sinus P waves and perfect resetting consistent with sinoatrial premature complexes. The constant coupling intervals suggest reentry and thus these could be considered **sinoatrial reciprocal complexes**. The ladder diagram illustrates the mechanism of A-SAN-A-V conduction.

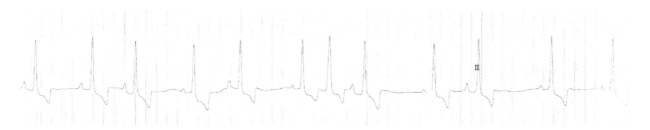

Figure 12.5 Paper speed 50 mm/s, 1 cm/mV, lead II, Cavalier King Charles Spaniel. The third beat is premature, resets the rhythm, and has a P′ nearly identical to the sinus P waves consistent with a **SANPC**, starting a run of sinus bigeminy. The seventh complex appears to be interpolated, making the eighth a possible sinoatrial reciprocal beat with post-extrasystolic P-Ri prolongation.

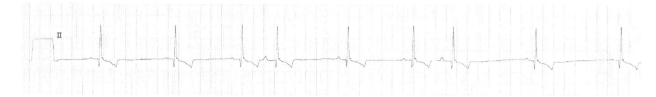

Figure 12.6 Paper speed 50 mm/s, 1 cm/mV, lead II, canine. The fourth and seventh complexes are sinoatrial premature complexes that reset or reset the rhythm with a pause. The *variable* coupling intervals suggests the possibility of **sinoatrial parasystole**. Long strips would be needed to establish a common denominator between interectopic intervals.

Sinus tachycardia This is really the most common supraventricular tachycardia (SVT) seen in small animals. Sinus tachycardia characteristically has a gradual warm-up and cool-down with changes in autonomic nervous tone. Typical sinus P waves (+ in II, III, aVF, usually slightly taller in amplitude) are seen preceding normal (supraventricular) QRS complexes occurring at a higher than normal rate (>180 bpm for dogs and >220 bpm for cats). There is a progressive shortening of P-R and R-R intervals with higher HR and the QRS amplitude may slightly increase. The Ta wave may become more apparent, resulting in P-R interval depression. Sinus tachycardia is expected to be present when prevailing sympathetic tone is high. Treatment of the underlying cause will be expected to resolve

sinus tachycardia. This is often a feature of congestive heart failure (CHF), can exacerbate CHF, and may warrant treatment (i.e. digoxin) if incessant. So-called "inappropriate sinus tachycardia" is a persistent sinus tachycardia in the absence of an obvious cause (i.e. no clear reason for elevated sympathetic tone). Congestive heart failure, exercise, fear/stress, hemorrhage, pain/acute injury, sympathomimetic/parasympatholytic drug administration, etc., must technically be excluded to diagnose truly inappropriate ST, which has not been reliably demonstrated in small animals thus far. Given the wide range of heart rates that are considered normal, sinus rhythm is not really ever considered to be "accelerated" in a specific distinction from sinus tachycardia.

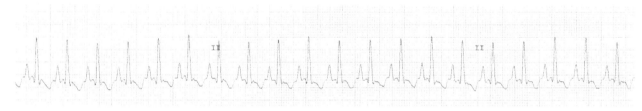

Figure 12.7 Paper speed 25 mm/s, 1 cm/mV, lead II, canine, **sinus tachycardia**. The HR is approximately 250 bpm. The T waves are negative, and the positive P waves come right after the T waves.

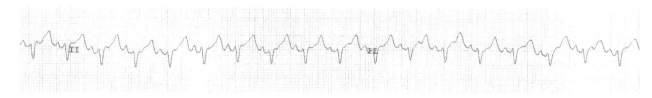

Figure 12.8 Paper speed 50 mm/s, 2 cm/mV, lead II, feline, **sinus tachycardia**. The HR is approximately 250 bpm. This patient has deep S waves characteristic of left anterior fascicular block or LAD.

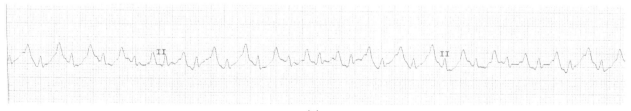

(a)

Figure 12.9a Paper speed 50 mm/s, 1 cm/mV, lead II, canine, **sinus tachycardia**, the P waves are buried in the T waves of the preceding beats.

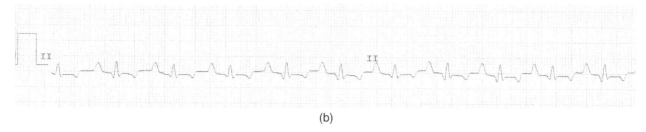

(b)

Figure 12.9b Paper speed 50 mm/s, 1 cm/mV, lead II, same dog. The HR has slowed exposing the T waves from the P waves, confirming ST in the previous strip. The P waves are mildly prolonged (0.05 second, p-mitrale), suggestive of left atrial enlargement.

Sinus nodal reentrant tachycardia

Sinus nodal reentrant tachycardia looks just like sinus tachycardia, only there is an abrupt onset and offset. The P waves are + in II, III, and AVF, are identical to (or possibly slightly higher in amplitude than) the sinus P waves, and the P′-Ri is identical to the P-Ri. Basically, this is a reentrant phenomenon, meaning a wave of depolarization circles back within the SA node repeatedly causing rapid depolarization, which ends up going through the atrioventricular node (AVN) causing ventricular depolarization. The R-P′ interval is characteristically long. This may be initiated and/or terminated by an APC (and SNRT should be inducible by atrial burst pacing during electrophysiologic studies). Vagal maneuvers tend to abruptly terminate SNRT, whereas they gradually decrease the heart rate with sinus tachycardia.

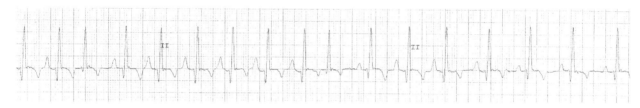

Figure 12.10 Paper speed 50 mm/s, 1 cm/mV, lead II, canine, the third complex is an APC that resets. The fourth–ninth complexes appear to be a supraventricular focus with just slightly different P wave morphology (slightly taller). The 10th complex is another APC, which initiates another short run of SVT. The last three complexes appear to be of sinus origin and are at a lower HR. This is suggestive of **SNRT**. APCs often cause temporary refractoriness of the SA node, allowing for a reentry circuit to start.

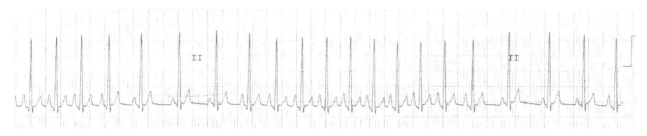

Figure 12.11 Paper speed 25 mm/s, 1 cm/mV, lead II, canine. Long R-P′ SVT, r/o **SNRT**. This SVT is relatively abrupt in onset and offset, and the P′ morphology is nearly identical to the sinus P waves, suggestive of SNRT.

Further reading

Childers, R.W., Amsdorf, M.F., de la Fuente, D.J. et al. (1973). Sinus Nodal Echoes. *Am. J. Cardiol.* 31 (2): 220–231.

Fisch, C. and Knoebel, S.B. (2000). *Electrocardiography of Clinical Arrhythmias.* Futurama Publishing Co.

Hafeez, Y. and Grossman, S.A. (2019). *Sinoatrial Nodal Reentrant Tachycardia (SANRT).* NCBI Bookshelf. StatPearls Publishing.

Narula, O.S. (1974). Sinus node re-entry: a mechanism for supraventricular tachycardia. *Circulation* 50: 1114–1128.

Rubenstein, J. and Abela, G.S. (2008). Sinoatrial Nodal Reentry Tachycardia: An Unusual Type of Sinus Tachyarrhythmia. HCP Live Network, MD Magazine.

Satullo, G. and Cavallaro, L. (1999). Intermittent sinus bigeminy as an expression of sinus parasystole: a case report. *J. Electrocardiol.* 32 (4).

Satullo, G. et al. (1991). Sinus parasystole. *Am. Heart J.* 121 (5): 1507–1512.

Wettersten, N. (2015). Not simply sinus tachycardia. *Am. J. Med.* 128 (9): e13–e14.

Atrial Arrhythmias

The atria are normally depolarized by the cells within the sinoatrial node. However, the atrial myocytes do have diastolic Phase 4 depolarization, which allows for escape complexes should the sinoatrial cells slow down enough. The internodal tracts are thought to allow for more rapid transmission of impulses from the sinoatrial node to the atrioventricular node. The atrial depolarization is denoted on surface EKG by the P wave. If the P wave axis is normal or high right atrial (i.e. approximately −20 to +100 degrees, "eccentric anterograde atrial activation") and the rate is within normal limits for sinoatrial discharge, then the sinus node is likely "in charge" of atrial depolarization. Ectopic lower right atrial foci outside the sinus node typically result in an "eccentric retrograde atrial activation" with a P' wave axis of −20 to −80 degrees and are positive in V1 and I. Higher ectopic left atrial foci typically have a P' wave axis of +90 to 180 degrees ("eccentric anterograde atrial activation"), lower ectopic left atrial foci have an axis of −100 −to 180 degrees ("eccentric retrograde atrial activation"), and both are negative in VI and I. Note that the actual polarity of an ectopic P' is not always reliable if the P' occurs within the S-T segment of the previous QRS-T complex. If an ectopic atrial focus is "in charge," then it will always precede the QRS complex, regardless of the QRS morphology and typically at least at a normal P-R interval for that patient. However, a P'-Ri that is longer than normal is not uncommon from physiologic first degree atrioventricular block or dual AV nodal pathway physiology. A short P'-Ri suggests a junctional origin in the absence of an accessory pathway. Exit block from an ectopic atrial focus is rare and probably associated with tachyarrhythmias. Atrial dissociation (double atrial rhythms) tends to be associated with tachycardia, and atrioventricular dissociation is not seen with atrial arrhythmias in the absence of atrioventricular block.

Atrial Bradyarrhythmias

Atrial escape complexes
    Atrial escape-capture bigeminy
Atrial escape rhythm
Atrial standstill
    Sinoventricular rhythm/hyperkalemia
    Atrial muscular dystrophy/persistent atrial standstill

Atrial Tachyarrhythmias

Atrial Premature Systoles

Left and right atrial premature complexes, resetting, resetting with a pause, interpolation
Atrial bigeminy and trigemy
Atrial premature complexes with aberrancy
    Supernormal excitation
Non-conducted atrial premature complexes
Atrial fusion complexes
Atrial reciprocal complexes
Atrial parasystole

Atrial Tachycardia

Accelerated atrial rhythm
    Transition of a pacemaker
Automatic atrial tachycardia
    Left atrial vs. right atrial tachycardia
    Multifocal atrial tachycardia
Intra-atrial reentrant tachycardia
Atrial dissociation

Bypass Tract Mediated Supraventricular Tachycardia/Ventricular Pre-excitation Syndromes

Ventricular pre-excitation and accessory pathways
Ventricular fusion
Atrial echo

Atrioventricular reentrant tachycardia
    Orthodromic atrioventricular reentrant tachycardia
    Antidromic atrioventricular reentrant tachycardia

Atrial Flutter
Type I (Isthmus-dependent)
    Counterclockwise (typical)
    Clockwise (reverse typical or atypical)
Type II (non-cavotricuspid isthmus-dependent)
Atrioventricular block
Artifacts

Atrial Fibrillation
Atrial fibrillation
Aberrancy
    Ashman's phenomenon
Ventricular ectopics
Atrioventricular dissociation
Concealed conduction

13

Atrial Bradyarrhythmias

CHAPTER MENU

Atrial escape beats, 141
   Atrial escape-capture bigeminy, 141
Atrial escape rhythm, 141
Atrial standstill, 141

Atrial escape beats Occasionally, a pause in a sinus rhythm will be terminated by an ectopic atrial beat. These beats have P′ morphologies dependent on the origin of the impulse and are thought to arise outside of the sinus node, though a separate focus (typically inferior to that of the prevailing sinus rhythm) within the sinus node itself may be a possibility. The QRS that follows is supraventricular in appearance unless pre-existing or transient bundle branch block (BBB) is present. Atrial escape beats are late by definition and follow sinus pauses, which may be the result of sinoatrial block or premature beats, the latter commonly misattributed to Chung's phenomenon (see Chapter 4). These beats often give rise to a misdiagnosis of wandering pacemaker; however, close scrutiny usually reveals abrupt albeit brief transitions of the atrial pacemaker. Atrial escape beats do not warrant specific therapy.

Atrial escape-capture bigeminy When a pause in the sinus rhythm elicits an atrial escape beat, which is then followed by a sinus capture, a bigeminal rhythm may ensue if the pattern repeats itself. This allorhythmia is termed atrial escape-capture bigeminy and is often confused with atrial bigeminy due to atrial premature beats.

Many EKGs that appear to show supraventricular (or atrial) bigeminy are actually examples of atrial escape-capture bigeminy due to sinoatrial block (see Chapter 10). The key to identifying the underlying mechanism lies in the onset of the arrhythmia. If the onset of a supraventricular bigeminal rhythm is initiated by a premature beat and continues as bigeminy, then true atrial bigeminy is likely. If the onset is initiated by a pause followed by late atrial escape beat, then atrial escape-capture bigeminy is likely.

Atrial escape rhythm If a pause in the rhythm occurs and is terminated by an atrial escape beat, the ectopic focus may capture the ventricles for a number of beats. If the ectopic atrial rhythm is slower than the prevailing sinus rhythm, it is properly termed an atrial escape rhythm. This is also termed transition of a pacemaker and is often mistaken for a "wandering pacemaker." Pauses in the sinus rhythm may be secondary to sinoatrial block which can elicit atrial escape rhythms. These typically persist for only a few beats. Escape rhythms in general should not be suppressed.

Atrial standstill This typically occurs when no P waves are visible on surface EKG and atrial fibrillation is not present. The heart rate will be normal to slow (if escape rhythm is present) and the rhythm will typically be regular in the absence of premature beats or atrial fibrillation. Make sure the P waves are not merely isoelectric, so check the other leads. Atrial standstill occurs when the atrial myocardia are unable to be depolarized. Two situations occur that allow for this to happen: atrial paralysis from hyperkalemia/sinoventricular rhythm and atrial muscular dystrophy causing persistent atrial standstill. While atrial fibrillation complicated by hyperkalemia may occur on occasion, patients with persistent atrial standstill by definition cannot have atrial fibrillation.

Interpretation of the Electrocardiogram in Small Animals, First Edition. Nick A. Schroeder.
© 2021 John Wiley & Sons Inc. Published 2021 by John Wiley & Sons Inc.

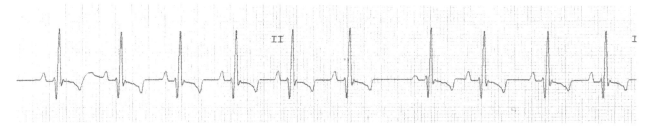

Figure 13.1 Paper speed 50 mm/s, 1 cm/mV, lead II, canine. The seventh complex is late, supraventricular, and has an altered P wave morphology suggestive of an **atrial escape complex**. The rest of the beats are fairly regular and all have the same P wave morphology suggesting a single focus in the SA node vs. a wandering pacemaker.

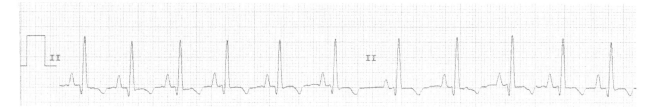

Figure 13.2 Paper speed 50 mm/s, 1 cm/mV, lead II, canine. The seventh complex is late, supraventricular, and has altered P wave morphology suggestive of an **atrial escape complex**.

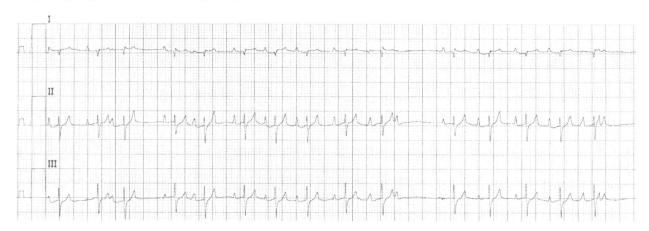

Figure 13.3 Paper speed 25 mm/s, 1 cm/mV, leads I, II, III, canine. Second degree AVB, atrial premature beats, possible sinoatrial block with pauses terminated by **atrial escape beats**. The first beat is sinus, which is followed by a pause, then an ectopic atrial escape beat, which is followed by an ectopic atrial premature beat from another focus. Note the two differing P′ morphologies. The 5th and 10th beats are also APCs, and the 10th beat causes *functional* block of the 11th sinus P wave. The pause that follows is terminated by an atrial escape, and another run of sinus beats is interrupted by another APC and blocked sinus P. This strip illustrates the difference between atrial *escape* beats and atrial *premature* beats. Escape beats are late, and premature beats are early.

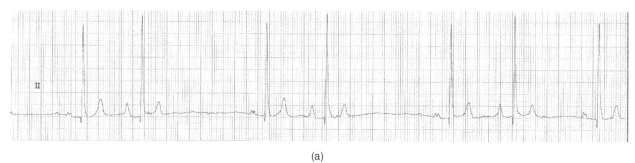

(a)

Figure 13.4a Paper speed 50 mm/s, 1 cm/mV, lead II, canine. At first glance, this appears to be **atrial bigeminy**, where every other beat is an APC. Careful examination, however, shows that the second complex has a slightly taller P wave, suggesting a high RA focus (likely within the sinus node) indicating that this may be a sinus capture. Sinoatrial block may be resulting in a pause which is terminated by an atrial escape beat, and thus this could be **atrial escape-capture bigeminy**.

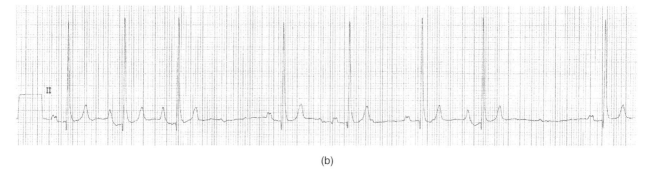

(b)

Figure 13.4b Paper speed 50 mm/s, 1 cm/mV, lead II, same dog. Two P wave morphologies are evident. The P waves with a lower amplitude appear on complexes following a pause. This suggests the bigeminal rhythm in the previous strip is really **atrial escape-capture bigeminy**. This is suggestive that the bigeminal rhythm that follows is really **atrial escape-capture bigeminy**.

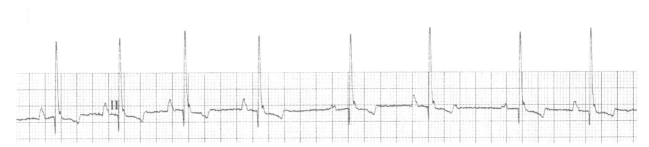

Figure 13.5 Paper speed 50 mm/s, 1 cm/mV, lead II, canine. **Atrial escape-capture bigeminy**. A pause following the fourth beat is terminated by an atrial escape beat. Bigeminy follows thereafter. The atrial escape beats have an obviously different P wave morphology than the sinus capture.

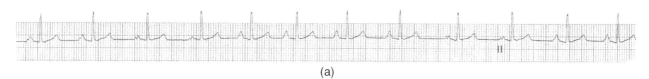

(a)

Figure 13.6a Paper speed 50 mm/s, 0.5 cm/mV, lead II, canine. The first four beats are ectopic atrial, followed by four sinus beats at a slightly faster rate. These are followed by two ectopic atrial beats (at a slower rate) following a pause. The ectopic atrial rate is slower than the sinus rate, consistent with **atrial escape rhythm**.

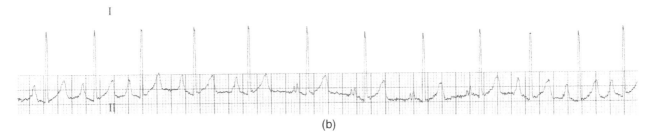

(b)

Figure 13.6b Paper speed 50 mm/s, 2 cm/mV, lead II, same dog. The sensitivity is higher here. A pause following the fifth sinus beat is terminated by an atrial escape beat with different P wave morphology. A slower **atrial escape rhythm** ensues for four beats, and then the sinus node takes over again.

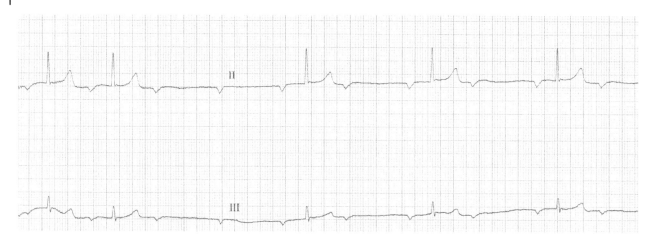

Figure 13.7 Paper speed 50 mm/s, 1 cm/mV, lead II and III, canine on fentanyl constant rate infusion. **Ectopic atrial (escape) rhythm**, high grade and 2:1 anterograde atrioventricular block. Fentanyl administration is commonly associated with vagal arrhythmias, which may be quite variable. In this case, the sinus focus has presumably slowed to the point of allowing a slower ectopic atrial focus to maintain control of the atrial rhythm. Atrioventricular block is also present. These arrhythmias typically subside following discontinuation of fentanyl.

Most commonly, hyperkalemia can result in the inability of the atrial myocardial to depolarize, resulting in an absence of P waves. Sinus node depolarization is conducted through three internodal tracts, which are bands of specialized conducting tissue, to the AV node. This has been documented in dogs. From there, the impulse is conducted through the normal His-Purkinje system to the ventricles, so the sinus node retains control of the ventricles though the atria are paralyzed. However, hyperkalemia also causes slowed SA nodal discharge, resulting in bradycardia, as well as slowed conduction through the ventricular myocardium, which results in prolongation/widening of the QRS complex. With severe hyperkalemia, the EKG is thus termed "sinoventricular rhythm." Cats typically have left axis deviation of the QRS, and dogs typically have a normal QRS axis with diphasic T waves (vs. peaked/tall T waves). Ectopic beats or accelerated rhythms may of course be seen with hyperkalemia, leading to irregular rhythms. Therapy is directed at resolving the hyperkalemia and any predisposing causes (insulin/dextrose, treatment for hypoadrenocorticism, correction of lower urinary tract obstruction, etc.).

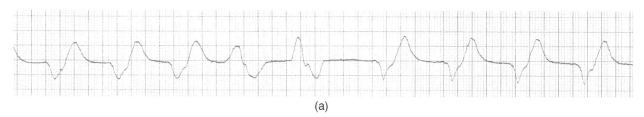

(a)

Figure 13.8a Paper speed 50 mm/s, lead II, feline with severe **hyperkalemia** (>9 mEq/l, pH 6.9) secondary to urethral obstruction. **Sinoventricular rhythm** with VPCs. No P waves are identifiable, and the QRS complexes are wide and bizarre with tall T waves. The fourth and fifth complexes are a couplet of VPCs.

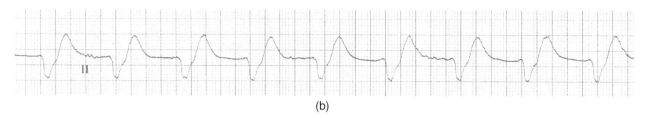

(b)

Figure 13.8b Paper speed 50 mm/s, lead II, same cat following treatment with IV insulin, dextrose, and calcium gluconate. The complexes are narrowing with decreasing serum potassium levels.

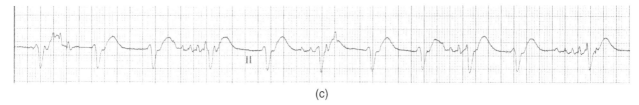

(c)

Figure 13.8c Paper speed 50 mm/s, lead II, same cat. The complexes are even narrower, and **purring artifact** is seen intermittently as an episodic sawtoothed baseline. Non-respiratory **sinus arrhythmia** (regularly irregular rhythm with gradual speeding up and slowing down of the rhythm) is present, as is **sinoventricular rhythm** (no P waves, sinus-controlled ventricular rhythm).

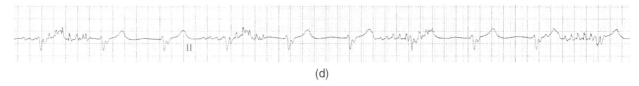

(d)

Figure 13.8d Paper speed 50 mm/s, lead II, same cat following sodium bicarbonate administration. The complexes are narrower yet, and the sinus arrhythmia has disappeared as evidenced by the *regular* rhythm (sinus rhythm). Purring artifact is still present, and P waves are still absent, so sinoventricular rhythm persists.

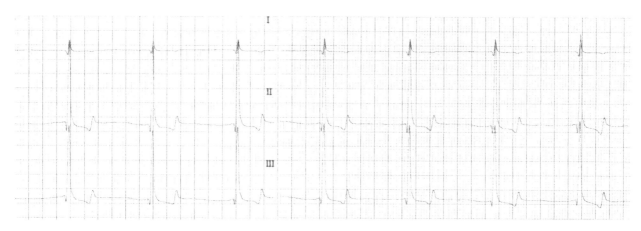

Figure 13.9 Paper speed 50 mm/s, 1 cm/mV, leads I, II, III, canine with chronic renal failure, serum potassium 6.8 mEq/l, sodium 120 mEq/l, suspect Addisonian crisis. **Sinoventricular rhythm**. No P waves are evident; however, the QRS complexes are regular at a rate of 60 bpm. The R waves are borderline tall at approximately 3 mV, possibly from LVH (and this patient had a history of systemic hypertension). The Q-Ti is long at approximately 0.22 second with diphasic T waves.

Sinoventricular rhythm may also be seen in the early stages of atrial muscular dystrophy and is diagnosed with typical EKG findings (absent P waves, regular and normal rate with supraventricular QRS complexes that are narrow unless conducted with BBB aberration) in association with biatrial enlargement and lack of mitral inflow A waves on echocardiography. Sinoventricular rhythm is distinguished from atrial standstill with permanent downward displacement of the pacemaker by a ventricular rate/rhythm within normal limits for that of sinus rhythm/sinus arrhythmia.

Atrial standstill also occurs when a particular form of cardiomyopathy or myocarditis affects the atria. Generally termed persistent atrial standstill, this may also result in "downward displacement of the pacemaker" as seen in third degree AV block. Transient atrial standstill may occur with significant sinus nodal disease (SSS) and is more properly termed sinus arrest (see Chapters 9 and 11). Persistent atrial standstill is most commonly seen in English Springer Spaniels, but other breeds have been reported. Advanced atrial muscular dystrophy causes the

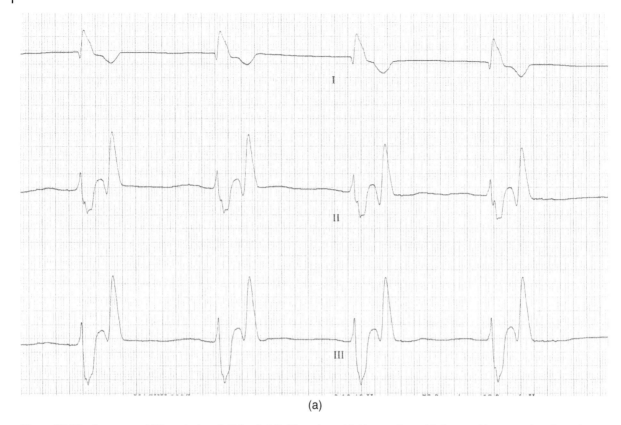

(a)

Figure 13.10a Paper speed 50 mm/s, 1 cm/mV, leads I, II, III, canine with history of renal failure and hypertension. Potassium 8.9 mEq/l. Sinoventricular rhythm. Note the absence of P waves, bradycardia, severe prolongation of the QRS complex, left axis deviation, prolonged QTi, and tall/diphasic T waves.

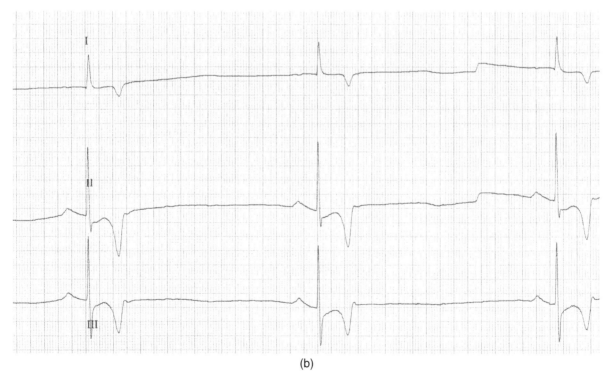

(b)

Figure 13.10b Paper speed 50 mm/s, 1 cm/mV, leads I, II, III, same dog following treatment with dextrose, insulin, calcium gluconate, sodium bicarbonate, and intravenous fluids. Serum potassium 7.8 mEq/l. P waves are now evident, the QRS duration has normalized, the T waves are now inverted, and the QTi is still prolonged.

Multifocal atrial premature complexes They have more than two P′ morphologies. These may have varying coupling intervals, variable P′-R intervals, and may reset the sinus rhythm or reset it with a pause. Persistent multifocal APCs may herald the onset of supraventricular tachycardia or atrial fibrillation. This may prompt the clinician to consider preemptive digitalization. Variable degrees of atrial fusion may simulate multifocal APCs and is suggested when a different morphology P′ wave occurs at a normal expected P-P′ interval. Differing coupling intervals are consistent with a multifocal origin.

One may usually determine whether premature beats are likely to be ventricular vs. supraventricular in origin based on what happens to the beats surrounding the premature beats. This is why it is important to know the different types of pauses. Resetting and resetting with a pause are two phenomena that are strongly associated with SVPCs.

The ectopic beats causing these create "non-compensatory pauses" ("less than fully compensatory pauses"). The SA node is depolarized by the premature beats, so the sinus rhythm resets or resets with a pause from overdrive suppression.

Resetting It occurs when a premature stimulus perfectly resets the underlying rhythm. No overdrive suppression of the SA node occurs, and the interval from the ectopic P′ wave/R wave to the following sinus P/R wave is exactly equal to one normal P-P/R-R interval.

Resetting with a pause It occurs when a premature stimulus resets the underlying rhythm and the interval from the ectopic P′/R′ wave to the following sinus P/R wave is longer than one normal P-P/R-R interval. This

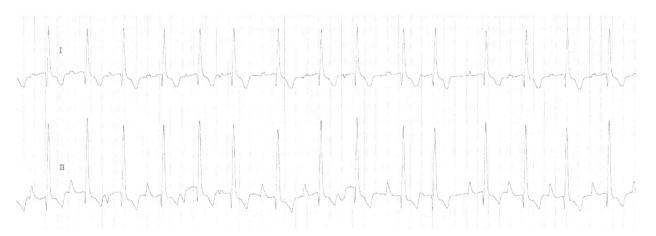

Figure 14.4 Paper speed 50 mm/s, 1 cm/mV, leads I and II, canine. **Multifocal APCS.** Sinus rhythm with p-biatriale is present. At least three ectopic P′ wave morphologies are evident with differing coupling intervals consistent with multifocal APCs. This patient would be expected to be at an increased risk for sudden development of atrial fibrillation given underlying atrial enlargement and an electrically unstable atrial myocardium. Digoxin could be considered.

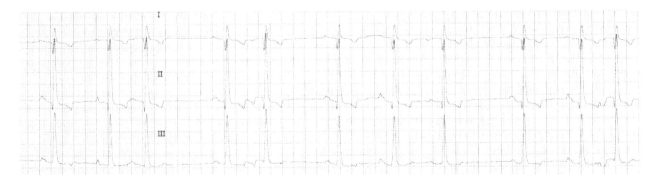

Figure 14.5 Paper speed 50 mm/s, 1 cm/mV, leads I, II, III, canine. **Multifocal APCs and ectopic atrial escapes**. The 1st, 4th, 6th, and 9th beats are ectopic atrial escapes, as they follow pauses and have P′ morphology different from that of the sinus beats (#2, #7, and #10). The third complex is an APC that resets with a pause long enough to elicit an atrial escape. The fifth complex is another SVPC with a retrograde P′ that resets with a pause long enough to again elicit an atrial escape. The eighth complex is another APC that has a different coupling interval and P′ morphology, again causing a pause terminated by an escape. The last beat is likely from the same focus as beat #5. Some of the variable P′ morphologies may be explained by atrial fusion.

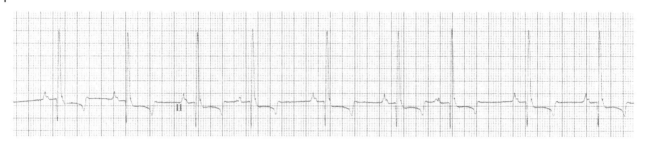

Figure 14.6 Paper speed 50 mm/s, 1 cm/mV, lead II, canine, the fourth and seventh complexes are premature and **reset** the rhythm. The R'-R interval is approximately the same as the R-R interval. This is likely an **APC**. The P' wave is very small, but positive.

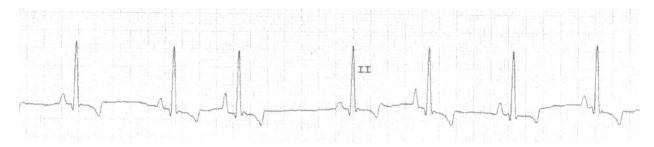

Figure 14.7 Paper speed 50 mm/s, 1 cm/mV, lead II, canine. The third complex is an APC with a tall P' wave that **resets with a pause** (the P'-post-extrasystolic P interval is longer than the preceding P-P cycle length). The fifth complex is another APC (note the same tall P') and resets the sinus rhythm without a pause. This strip illustrates that the earlier the APC, the more likely SAN overdrive suppression occurs, leading to resetting with a pause. The fifth complex is relatively less premature and simply resets.

phenomenon is due to overdrive suppression of the SA node. If the pause is long enough, it may mimic a fully compensatory pause (the preceding R to post-extrasystolic R interval fortuitously equals two R-R intervals) that is otherwise typically associated with ventricular premature complexes (VPCs). Excessive overdrive suppression is evident if the pause exceeds a fully compensatory pause ("overcompensatory" pause). The earlier the APC occurs, the more likely it will reset with a pause. Very early APCs may conduct to the ventricles with a long P'-R interval (functional first degree atrioventricular block/AVB) or may find the AVN completely refractory and be blocked (functional second degree AVB).

Interpolation A premature beat may be sandwiched in between two normal sinus beats (true extrasystole). Only rarely are APCs interpolated. Typically, ectopic atrial foci will depolarize the SAN along with the atrial myocardium, resetting the sinus node and subsequent rhythm. If an APC fails to penetrate the sinus node due to entrance block, it may capture the ventricles and be followed by another sinus beat that occurs on time and undisturbed. The post-extrasystolic P wave may be slightly delayed (incomplete interpolation) from concealed conduction of the ectopic atrial beat creating a functional first degree sinoatrial block, prolonging the conduction time for the impulse exiting the sinus node. This is analogous to the

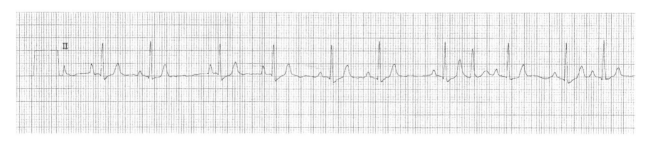

Figure 14.8 Paper speed 50 mm/s, 1 cm/mV, lead II, canine. The eighth complex appears to be an **interpolated atrial premature complex** (APC) which is mildly aberrant and followed by a *possible* **sinoatrial reciprocal complex** with post-extrasystolic P-Ri prolongation. The 2nd and 11th complexes are clearly ectopic atrial. Underlying sinus arrhythmia confounds whether this is simple interpolation of an APC vs. an APC followed by sinoatrial reentry.

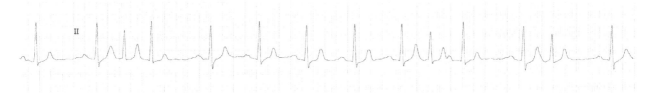

Figure 14.9 Paper speed 50 mm/s, 1 cm/mV, lead II, canine with a large heart-based mass. The 3rd and 10th complexes are interpolated APCs with **post-extrasystolic P-Ri prolongation**. The 13th complex is an APC that resets the rhythm.

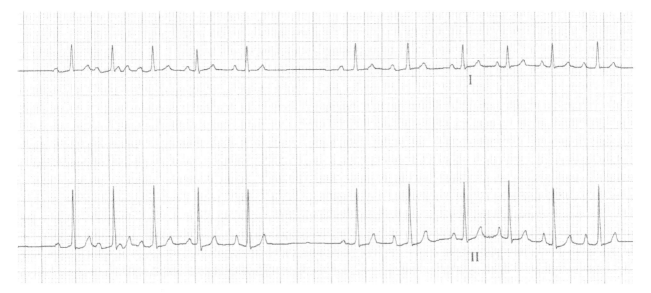

Figure 14.10 Paper speed 50 mm/s, 1 cm/mV, leads I and II, canine. The second complex is followed by an **interpolated APC** that is **non-conducted**. Physiologic refractoriness of the AVN prevented conduction to the ventricles. Entrance block to the sinus node prevented resetting of the sinus node. Respiratory sinus arrhythmia is present, and the P-R intervals vary secondary to changes in autonomic tone.

functional first degree AVB seen on post-extrasystolic beats following interpolated ventricular premature beats, which may also occur following interpolated APCs. Rarely, SVPCs may be interpolated and non-conducted, resulting in a P′ wave sandwiched between two conducted P waves, but not immediately followed by its own QRS. Underlying baseline artifact is a rule out.

Rarely, a postponed compensatory pause may follow interpolated APCs with post-extrasystolic P-R prolongation (and reciprocal R-P shortening) and AV block of the second post-extrasystolic P wave. Even less common is a doubly postponed compensatory pause with progressive post-extrasystolic P-R interval prolongation culminating with AV block of the third post-extrasystolic P wave (basically a Wenckebach sequence initiated by an interpolated premature beat). Impostors of interpolated APCs include ectopic atrial couplets, sinoatrial reentry, one-is-to-two conduction over dual AV nodal pathways, and interpolated

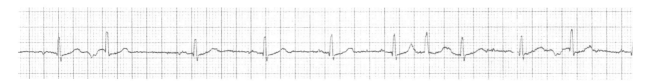

Figure 14.11 Paper speed 50 mm/s, 1 cm/mV, lead II, canine. The seventh complex is an **interpolated APC**. It does not reset the rhythm or create a pause due to entrance block of the APC to the SAN. The ninth complex has marked P-R interval prolongation, but ultimately conducts, and the immediately following P wave is AV blocked (**doubly postponed compensatory pause**). The 2nd and 10th complexes are supraventricular premature beats (junctional or low ectopic atrial) with retrograde P′ waves preceding the QRS that reset the rhythm with a pause.

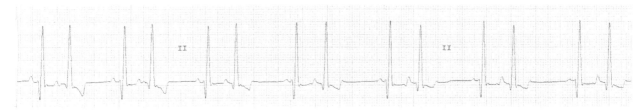

Figure 14.12 Paper speed 50 mm/s, 1 cm/mV, lead II, canine. **Atrial bigeminy** is present. Every other beat is an APC that resets.

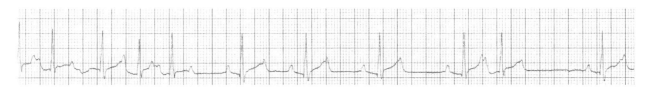

Figure 14.13 Paper speed 50 mm/s, 1 cm/mV, lead II, canine. **Non-conducted atrial bigeminy**. The fourth complex is followed by a non-conducted P′ that terminates a run of atrial tachycardia. Atrial bigeminy ensues, however, the APCs are not conducted until the ninth complex. This mimics 2 : 1 ventriculophasic sinus arrhythmia.

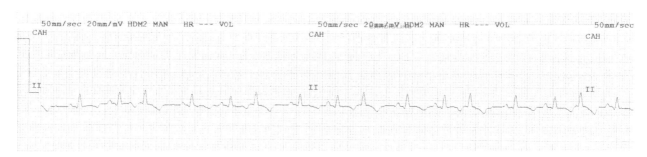

Figure 14.14 Paper speed 50 mm/s, 2 cm/mV, lead II, feline. **Atrial trigeminy (2 : 1 extrasystole)** is present. Every third complex is a supraventricular premature beat that resets the rhythm.

fascicular premature complexes. If the P′ wave associated with the "post-extrasystolic beat" differs from the P waves associated with sinus beats in morphology and/or the P′-P interval differs from the underlying P-P interval, this suggests a couplet of APCs. Sinoatrial reentry is suspected if the post-extrasystolic P wave is slightly early, though concurrent sinus arrhythmia frequently makes the distinction difficult, if not impossible (see Chapter 12). Dual AV nodal physiology is suspected if two discreet P-R intervals can be demonstrated. Ventricular premature complexes arising from the His bundle or one of the left fascicles may not be reliably differentiated from interpolated APCs if axis deviation of the QRS or a preceding P′ cannot be positively identified on surface EKG.

Atrial bigeminy Atrial premature complexes may follow every sinus beat, resetting the rhythm and occur in a bigeminal pattern. Each sinus beat is followed by an APC in a repetitive pattern and constitutes 1 : 1 extrasystole. Atrial bigeminy is often confused with sinoatrial block or atrial escape–capture bigeminy and may result from an atrial parasystolic focus. Non-conducted atrial bigeminy may mimic sinus bradycardia if the P′ waves are hiding in the T waves of preceding beats or ventriculophasic sinus arrhythmia if the P′ waves happen to be positive in the inferior leads.

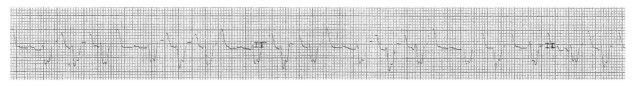

Figure 14.15 Paper speed 50 mm/s, 1 cm/mV, lead II, feline. **Atrial trigeminy (1 : 2 extrasystole)** is present. Each sinus beat is followed by a couplet of APCs in a repetitive pattern. Complete RBBB has resulted in wide sinus and ectopic atrial QRS complexes.

Atrial trigeminy   Atrial premature complexes may occur singly following two sinus beats in a repetitive pattern. This is from 2 : 1 extrasystole. Atrial trigeminy may also occur with 1 : 2 extrasystole and can be the result of atrial parasystole.

APCs with aberrancy   Atrial premature complexes may be conducted to the ventricles aberrantly. This results in a wide and bizarre QRS complex due to bundle branch block (BBB). If the APC occurs early enough in Phase 3 of the action potential, acceleration-dependent LBBB may result.

If the APC occurs following a suddenly prolonged cycle, Ashman's phenomenon may result in RBBB. Occasionally, SVPCs may be associated with QRS complexes that are slightly taller than that of the sinus QRS complexes, and this is thought to be from a left medial fascicular block (and more common with junctional premature complexes). Atrial premature complexes are by definition preceded by atrial activity at a normal or prolonged P′-Ri. An important rule out is simultaneous APCs and VPCs with or without ventricular fusion, which would be expected to have a short P′-R′i (see Chapter 24).

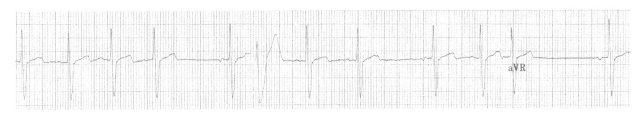

Figure 14.16 Paper speed 50 mm/s, 0.5 cm/mV, lead aVR, canine with CMVDz. A pause in the sinus rhythm after the fourth complex is followed by another sinus beat, then an aberrant supraventricular premature beat with RBBB morphology from **Ashman's phenomenon**. The **aberrant APC** resets the sinus rhythm. The 11th complex is another APC but is of normal morphology as it follows a short cycle.

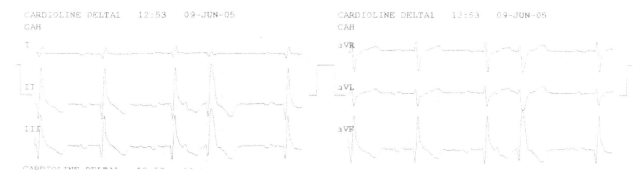

Figure 14.17 Paper speed 25 mm/s, 1 cm/mV, canine, the fourth complex is premature and conducted with aberrancy (**LBBB**) and *resets* the rhythm consistent with an **APC**. The P′ of the APC is in the S-T segment of the previous complex. The long P′-R interval is also suggestive that this beat is actually an APC. This is an example of Phase 3 block. This patient was a Boxer, and RVPCs are quite common in this breed. These premature beats are unlikely to be ventricular in origin in this case, however, because the rhythm is reset by the premature beat.

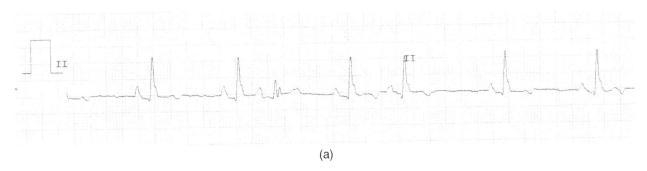

(a)

Figure 14.18a Paper speed 50 mm/s, 1 cm/mV, lead II, canine. The third complex is an **aberrantly conducted APC**. A positive P′ is seen on the T wave of the preceding beat, and the APC resets the rhythm. If an APC occurs when the ventricles have not finished repolarizing, aberrant conduction may occur. The fifth complex is an APC that also resets the rhythm. The notch on the downstroke of the R wave may indicate microscopic intramural myocardial infarction (MIMI) in this patient with severe CMVDz.

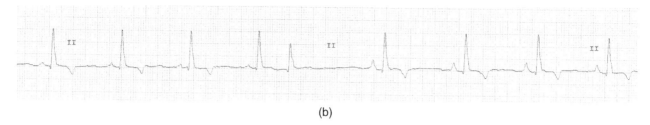

(b)

Figure 14.18b Paper speed 50 mm/s, 1 cm/mV, lead II, same dog. **Transition of a pacemaker**. The first four complexes have a different P wave morphology than the last four complexes of sinus origin. This suggests that a slow ectopic atrial focus (accelerated atrial rhythm) originally had captured the rhythm (displaced pacemaker secondary to concealed conduction?). The fifth complex is an **aberrantly conducted APC** that resets the rhythm and allows the normal sinus pacemaker to take back over control of the heart.

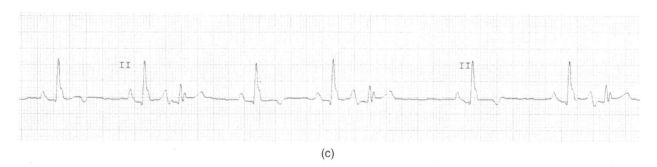

(c)

Figure 14.18c Paper speed 50 mm/s, 1 cm/mV, lead II, same dog, **atrial trigeminy with aberrancy**. Every third beat is premature, aberrantly conducted, and resets the rhythm consistent with APCs.

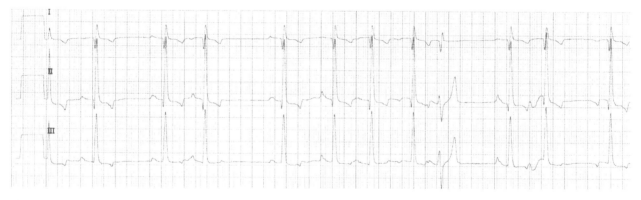

Figure 14.19 Paper speed 50 mm/s, 1 cm/mV, leads I, II, III, canine. **Multifocal SVPCs**. The third and fifth beats are ectopic atrial escapes. The seventh and eighth beats are APCs, and the ninth beat is **aberrantly conducted** (RBBB) secondary to *Ashman's phenomenon* (long-short sequence). This beat also has a different P′ and coupling interval. The 11th beat is another ectopic premature (possibly junctional, but different focus than beats #7 and #8. The last beat is ectopic junctional (or low left atrial) escape.

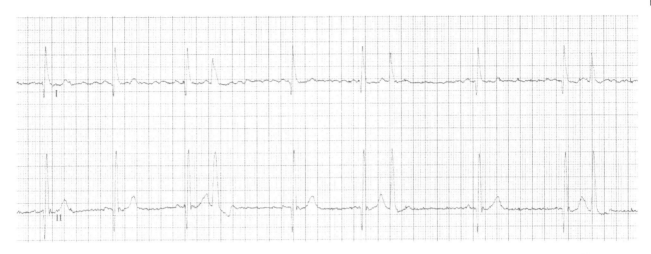

Figure 14.20 Paper speed 50 mm/s, 1 cm/mV, leads I and II, canine. **Atrial trigeminy with aberrancy**. Note here that the APCs have a wide-and-bizarre appearance secondary to LBBB aberration. From left to right, the coupling intervals get slightly longer, resulting in better intraventricular conduction and less aberrancy of the last APC. Note that the APCs reset the sinus rhythm. The baseline is undulating from muscle tremor artifact – potentially confusing the examiner with atrial fibrillation. Variable coupling intervals seen here is also suggestive of an **atrial parasystolic** focus.

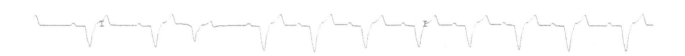

Figure 14.21 Paper speed 50 mm/s, 1 cm/mV, lead I, canine. **Supernormal excitation**. This patient had a persistent RBBB in sinus rhythm. The third complex is premature, slightly narrower than the rest of the beats, and resets the rhythm suggestive of an APC. The P′ may be buried in the preceding T wave. Supernormal excitation occurs during the "vulnerable period" or Phase 3 of the action potential (AP), but in contrast to vulnerability (in which an increased susceptibility to VF is found), supernormality is a lowered threshold in which stimuli smaller than those needed to reach normal threshold levels may propagate an AP.

Supernormal excitation It occurs when conduction is better than expected, but usually not as good as "normal." A classic example is a patient with permanent or rate-dependent BBB in sinus rhythm has an APC that is narrower than expected. The P-R interval should remain unchanged or shortened, which rules out equal prolongation of the bundle branches. If conduction time in both bundles is more synchronized, then cancelation of forces results in a narrow complex. While demonstrated *in vitro*, convincing examples *in vivo* are lacking and are yet to be proven. Supernormality may be mimicked by the so-called "gap phenomenon," peeling back refractoriness, shortening of refractoriness via changing preceding cycle length, Wenckebach phenomenon in the bundle branches, bradycardia-dependent BBB, summation, or dual AV nodal pathways. Abrupt normalization of aberration by a VPC proves retrograde concealment as the mechanism of perpetuation of the aberration. The gap phenomenon is the most common cause of so-called pseudo-supernormality

and basically is a period of time following a native sinus beat in which conduction of an APC can occur before or after (the "gap"), but never during. Multiple types of gap phenomena have been described and are beyond the scope of this text.

Non-conducted ("blocked") APCs Atrial premature complexes may fail to conduct to the ventricles if they occur early enough to encounter the absolute refractory period (ARP) of the AV nodal tissue. Blocked APCs typically will, however, penetrate and reset the sinus node, resetting the rhythm. This affords our clue to the presence of a blocked APC – leading to unexpected pauses and a disturbed sinus rhythm. If atrial bigeminy occurs and all of the APCs are blocked, it mimics ventriculophasic sinus arrhythmia (2 : 1 second degree AVB) or sinus bradycardia if the P′ waves are not obvious. Given that the failure of propagation is

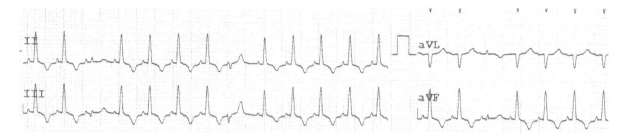

Figure 14.22 Paper speed 25 mm/s, 1 cm/mV, leads II and III, aVL and aVF, feline. **Supernormal excitation**. This patient had rate-dependent LBBB. The third complex is slightly early, conducted with a more normal QRS duration, and resets the rhythm (an APC). The eighth complex is a VPC that creates a compensatory pause.

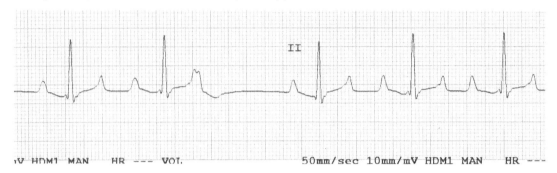

Figure 14.23 Paper speed 50 mm/s, 1 cm/mV, lead II, canine. The second complex has a distorted T wave and is followed by a pause that resets the rhythm. This is an example of a **blocked APC**. The P′ wave of the ectopic beat distorts the T wave, and while the SA node is depolarized (as evidenced by the reset rhythm), the impulse occurs too early (the AVN is still refractory), so the impulse fails to conduct to the ventricles. Blocked APCs are imposters of SA block/sinus pause.

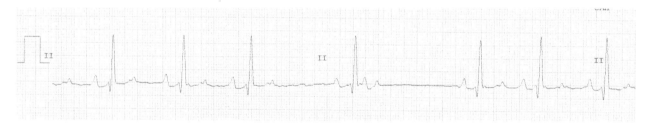

Figure 14.24 Paper speed 50 mm/s, 1 cm/mV, lead II canine. **Blocked APC** and SA block. The fourth complex has a P′ within the S-T segment, possibly causing the pause following this beat. The pause prior to this beat was secondary to sinoatrial block.

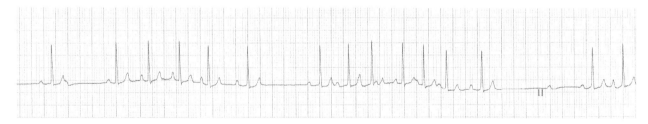

Figure 14.25 Paper speed 25 mm/s, 1 cm/mV, lead II, canine. The first complex is followed by a **non-conducted APC**. An underlying respiratory sinus arrhythmia is present. The ninth ventricular complex is followed by another non-conducted APC. The ninth and 11th complexes are APCs that are conducted to the ventricles. The 16th P wave is non-conducted due to Wenckebach periodicity.

attributed to the normal physiological refractoriness of the AV node, some authors prefer the term "non-conducted" vs. "AV-blocked" (which implies a pathological condition). Depending on the degree of prematurity, the APC may encounter the relative refractory period (RRP) of the AVN, resulting in functional first degree AV block

of the APC and a long P′-R interval. If the APC occurs earlier yet, a functional second degree AV block and/or blocked/non-conducted/non-propagated APC will occur (P′ without a following QRS) as it runs into the ARP. Non-conducted APCs may be mimicked by baseline artifact.

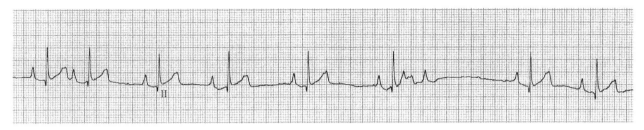

Figure 14.26 Paper speed 50 mm/s, 1 cm/mV, lead II, canine. The first complex here is followed by a conducted APC which resets the rhythm. The sixth complex is followed by a couplet of APCs that are *both* AV blocked (non-conducted) because they occurred early enough to conduct to the atria, but the AV node was refractory enough to prevent conduction to the ventricles from concealed conduction. This is followed by a long pause caused by overdrive suppression of the SA node. If the "second non-conducted APC" were actually sinus (possible given P′ morphology nearly identical to that of sinus P wave), it would still be too early though a sinoatrial reentry is always a possibility.

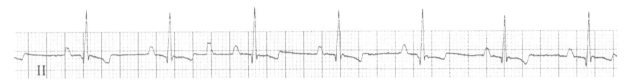

Figure 14.27 Paper speed 50 mm/s, 1 cm/mV, lead II, canine. An apparently non-conducted APC occurs between the second and third complexes; however, this is more likely an **artifact**. The "APC" fails to reset the SA node and underlying rhythm. If this were truly a non-conducted APC, it would have to be interpolated with entrance block to the SA node, an unlikely sequence of events. The presence of conducted APCs with P′ waves of similar morphology would support the notion that this is actually a non-conducted interpolated APC.

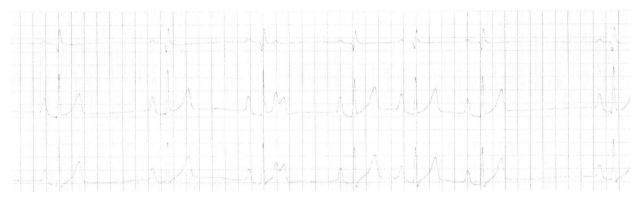

Figure 14.28 Paper speed 50 mm/s, 1 cm/mV, leads I (top), II (middle), and III (bottom), canine. P-biatriale, sinus arrhythmia, and **blocked APC**. The third complex has a retrograde P′ wave in the T wave, and resets the rhythm, consistent with an APC that is AV blocked. This has the appearance of being interpolated, as the interval from the preceding P wave to the post-extrasystolic P wave matches that of the preceding P-P interval. However, the P′-P interval is the same as the interval from the post-extrasystolic P to the following P wave, making it more likely that the sinus node was reset. Sinus arrhythmia accounts for the varied P-P intervals.

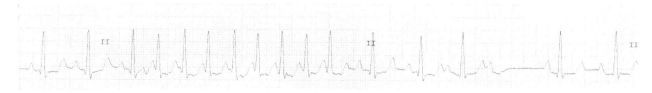

Figure 14.29 Paper speed 50 mm/s, 1 cm/mV, lead II, canine. The fourth complex starts a run of SVT. The 14th beat is sinus conducted with a long P-R interval and is apparently followed by a blocked APC that resets the sinus node. Alternatively, the 13th, 14th, and blocked P may simply be a **Wenckebach period** (Type I second degree AVB), which are not uncommon during the offset of SVT. The P′ waves "skip" the immediately following QRS and conduct the second, making this a "long R-P′" SVT.

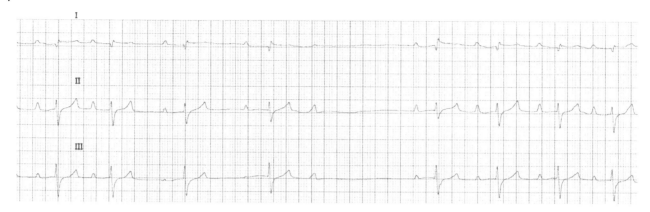

Figure 14.30 Paper speed 50 mm/s, 1 cm/mV, leads I, II, III, canine. The first two beats are sinus, which are followed by a short pause terminated by an **ectopic atrial (escape)** focus, which persists for two beats. The non-conducted P′ that follows is a **non-conducted APC**, with SAN overdrive suppression causing a long pause. Note the two different P′ morphologies vs. the normal sinus P wave morphology.

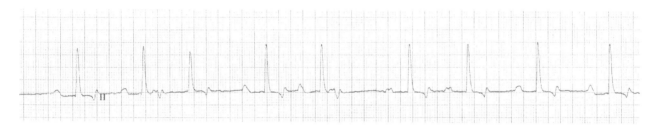

Figure 14.31 Paper speed 50 mm/s, 1 cm/mV, lead II, canine. The third complex is an **APC** with a **long P′-R interval** that resets the rhythm. The fifth complex is followed by a pause created by a **non-conducted APC** (within the S-T segment of the fifth complex). The pause is terminated by a short, two-beat run of ectopic atrial rhythm, demonstrating a **transition of the pacemaker** from the sinus node to an ectopic atrial site. The sinus node then takes back over the rhythm.

Atrial fusion complexes

They are signified by complexes with P waves that are intermediate in morphology between sinus P waves and ectopic P′ waves, but the QRS complexes are normal in morphology and are not premature. This is because the ectopic focus fires approximately at the same time as the SA node, and in the case of a supraventricular premature beat, depolarization of the ventricles occurs at about the same time as the sinus beat would have otherwise. Atrial fusion is most obvious with sinus and ectopic supraventricular foci; however, atrial fusion can occur following a ventricular beat if intact ventriculoatrial conduction (VA conduction, that is, retrograde conduction over the AV node) is present. Basically, each focus depolarizes a portion of the atria.

Atrial reciprocal complexes

Conduction delay within the AV node may result in reentry and reactivation of the atria. The resultant P′ wave is typically retrograde in the inferiors and is termed an atrial reciprocal beat/complex, "echo," or return extrasystole. The sequence is A-V-A. Atrial echoes may be precipitated by APCs, are often indistinguishable from ectopic atrial or junctional foci, and are suggested when P-R interval prolongation occurs prior to the P′ (as in Wenckebach periods) or when premature retrograde P′ waves interrupt the sinus rhythm during complete AVB. They may be dependent on intraventricular conduction delay and to some extent on supernormal conduction. The atrial echo is usually non-conducted to the ventricles and resets the supraventricular (usually sinus) rhythm. If the atrial echo happens to be conducted, it will be followed by a supraventricular QRS complex. Retrograde P′ waves following conducted QRS complexes that are not associated with at least second or third degree AV block suggest retrograde activation of the atria over an accessory pathway, thus indicating the potential for atrioventricular reentrant tachycardia (AVRT, see Chapter 16). The apparent polarity of a P′ wave occurring within the S-T segment of a QRS cannot always be a reliable indicator of the atrial vector (so positive P′ waves may actually be the result of retrograde activation of atrial tissue and vice versa).

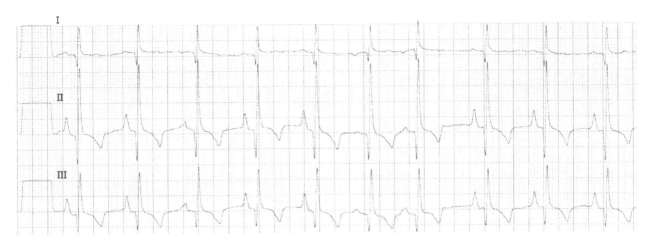

Figure 14.32 Paper speed 50 mm/s, 1 cm/mV, leads I, II, III, canine. The third complex is an **atrial fusion complex**. This beat comes on time, is neither early nor late, and has a P′ morphology intermediate between that of the premature beats. The sixth and seventh complexes are a couplet of APCs (likely left atrial due to the negative P′ in I). Atrial fusion complexes may also occur with junctional premature beats and ventricular premature beats with intact VA conduction.

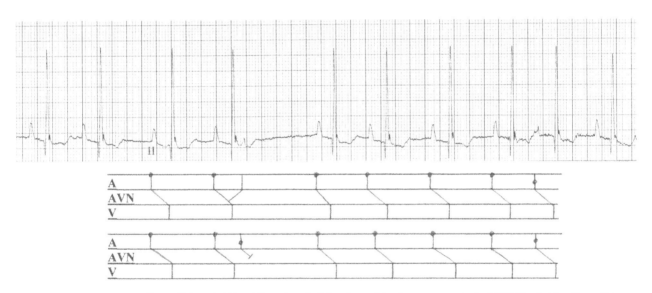

Figure 14.33 Paper speed 50 mm/S, 1 cm/mV, lead II, canine. **Atrial reciprocal beat** vs. **non-conducted APC**. The ladder diagrams illustrate the mechanisms. The small positive deflection (P′) within the S-T segment of the fourth complex is either the result of a reversed echo (atrial echo) beat or is simply ectopic supraventricular (atrial) that failed to conduct due to refractoriness of the AVN. Either situation creates the resetting of the sinus node. Since P-R interval prolongation (i.e. from a Wenckebach period) is not evident prior to the P′, which would favor an atrial echo, either mechanism may be at work. The ninth complex is ectopic atrial and obviously resets the rhythm, which makes the previous P′ wave more likely to be a non-conducted APC.

Atrial parasystole Ectopic atrial foci may be protected from depolarization by the sinus node due to entrance block. This results in a regular, independent ectopic atrial impulse that does reset the SA node, resulting in reverse-coupling (so the post-extrasystolic beat is coupled to the premature beat as opposed to the premature beat being coupled to the preceding sinus beat). The interectopic intervals will have a common denominator, fusion beats may occur, and the ectopic focus will fail to propagate if the sinus impulse is earlier than the ectopic impulse. Many cases of atrial bigeminy and trigeminy are actually secondary to atrial parasystolic foci.

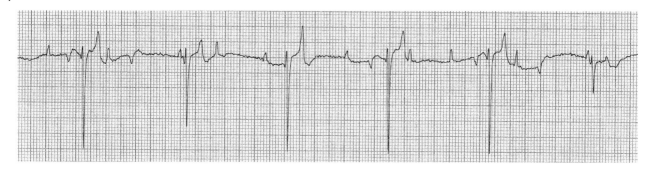

Figure 14.34 Paper speed 25 mm/s, 1 cm/mV, lead II, canine. **Atrial reciprocal complexes**. The basic rhythm is sinus with apparent third degree AV block. The first, second, sixth, eighth, and ninth sinus P waves are followed by reciprocal (atrial echo) complexes. These reset the sinus rhythm and fail to conduct to the atria (proven by the fact none of the P-R intervals are constant). An idioventricular rhythm with variable morphologies is in control of the ventricles.

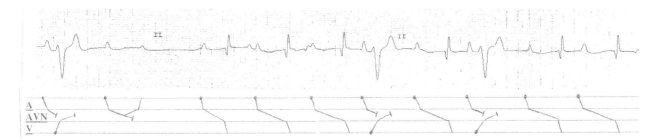

Figure 14.35 Paper speed 50 mm/s, 1 cm/mV, lead II, canine. Wenckebach periods interrupted by VPCs. The first sinus P wave is AV blocked by a VPC. The second sinus impulse finds the anterograde path refractory, but is able to re-enter the atria retrogradely, producing an **atrial reciprocal beat**. This resets the sinus rhythm at a new interval, and the Wenckebach period restarts. The mechanism is illustrated in the ladder diagram. Alternatively, the "atrial echo" here may really be an ectopic atrial premature complex that resets the sinus rhythm, especially given that the P′ has an ambiguous morphology (i.e. not clearly retrograde). Intracardiac EKG would be needed for documentation.

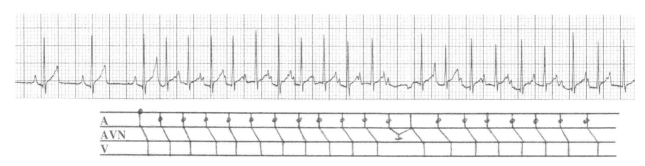

Figure 14.36 Paper speed 25 mm/s, 1 cm/mV, lead II, canine. Atrial tachycardia occurs following the third beat. Midway through, a non-conducted beat occurs following P′-R interval prolongation (a typical Wenckebach period terminating atrial tachycardia). This is followed by a retrograde P′ wave, which may well be an **atrial reciprocal beat** which then returns to excite the ventricles. Atrial tachycardia then follows. Since this retrograde P′ wave follows a non-conducted supraventricular beat in association with P′-R interval prolongation, an atrial echo is favored.

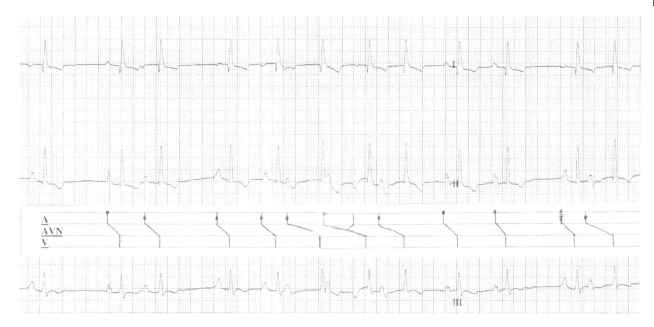

Figure 14.37 Paper speed 50 mm/s, 1 cm/mV, leads I, II, III, canine. Multifocal APCs with variable P′-R intervals illustrating PR/RP reciprocity, and **atrial echo**. The earlier a premature beat is (i.e. the shorter the R-P′ interval), the longer the P′-R interval will be. The first complex is ectopic atrial (note the negative P′ in I). This is followed by a sinus complex as illustrated on the ladder diagram. The third beat is ectopic atrial with a normal P′-R interval. The sixth beat is ectopic atrial, occurs relatively earlier, and is conducted with a longer P′-R interval, which causes the following sinus beat to reenter the atria as an echo (atrial reciprocal beat) prior to conducting to the ventricles. The 12th complex appears to be an atrial fusion.

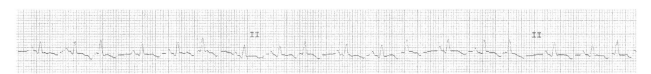

Figure 14.38 Paper speed 50 mm/s, 2 cm/mV, lead II, feline. **Atrial trigeminy, R/O atrial parasystole**. The APCs have slightly variable coupling intervals, and the interectopic intervals are consistent. Due to *reverse coupling*, the SA node is reset after each APC.

Further reading

Achen, S.E. and Miller, M.W. (2008). ECG of the month. *JAVMA* 233 (4) 15: 561–562.

Fisch, C. and Knoebel, S.B. (2000). *Electrocardiography of Clinical Arrhythmias*. Futurama Publishing Co.

Goldreyer, B.N. and Damato, A.N. (1971). Sinoatrial-node entrance block. *Circulation* XLIV: 789–802.

Guimond, C., Leblanc, A., Pelletier, B. et al. (1981). Supernormal conduction and atrial echo beats in the dog. *Eur. Heart J.* 2 (6): 499–507.

Marriot, H.J.L. and Conover, M.B. (1998). *Advanced Concepts in Arrhythmias*, 3e. Mosby.

Marriott, H.J. (1998). *Pearls & Pitfalls in Electrocardiography, Pithy, Practical Pointers*, 2e. Williams & Wilkins.

Santilli, R, Moise NS, Pariaut R, Perego M. *Electro-cardiography of the Dog and Cat: Diagnosis of Arrhythmias*, 2e, Edna. 2018.

Scheinman, M. (2016). *Cardiac Electrophysiology Clinics. Interpretation of Complex Arrhythmias: A Case-Based Approach*, vol. 8. Elsevier.

Schuilenburg, R.M. and Durrer, D. (1968). Atrial Echo beats in the human heart elicited by induced atrial premature beats. *Circulation.* 37: 680.

Surawicz, B. and Knilans, T.K. (2001). *Chou's Electrocardiography in Clinical Practice: Adult and Pediatric*, 5e. Saunders.

Varghese, J.P., Damato, A.N., Caracta, A.R. et al. (1974). Intraventricular conduction delay as a determinant of atrial Echo beats. *Circulation* 49: 805.

15

Atrial Tachycardia

CHAPTER MENU

Accelerated atrial rhythm, 166
Automatic atrial tachycardia, 166
Intra-atrial reentrant tachycardia, 171
Atrial dissociation, 171

Accelerated atrial rhythm Ectopic atrial rhythms may occasionally capture the ventricles and compete with the sinus node for control. If these are faster than the prevailing sinus rhythm and atrial escape rhythm, but slower than atrial tachycardia (i.e. less than 180–200 bpm), then the ectopic rhythm is referred to as an accelerated atrial rhythm. Whether it is referred to as accelerated or escape depends on the underlying sinus rate. If the sinus rate is faster, then the ectopic atrial rhythm is considered to be atrial escape rhythm (see Chapter 13). If the ectopic atrial rhythm is faster than the prevailing sinus rhythm, then it is referred to as accelerated atrial rhythm. Accelerated atrial rhythm typically requires no specific therapy.

> *A Note*: Fortunately, the term non-paroxysmal idioatrial tachycardia (analogous to non-paroxysmal idiojunctional or idioventricular tachycardia) never caught on (see Chapters 22 and 25). During an accelerated rhythm, the heart rate is usually similar to that of the sinus node (i.e. not a tachycardia per se), the onset and offset tend to be inapparent (thus non-paroxysmal), and the term idioatrial rhythm implies atrial dissociation (which is generally not the case with an accelerated atrial rhythm).

Automatic atrial tachycardia Think of this one as a rapid run of APCs. (Just like ventricular tachycardia/VT is a rapid run of ventricular premature complexes/VPCs). The P′ configuration (duration and polarity) depends on the site of the atrial focus, and AAT generally has a gradual onset and offset with prolongation of the P′ to P′ interval right before it stops. Usually, the P′ is positive in II, III, and aVF in dogs, but this may vary. Often a long R-P′ interval is present, but it varies with the SVT rate. If the P′ is negative in II, III, and aVF, it is an inferior focus, and if it is positive, a superior focus. If the P′ is + or biphasic in aVL, it is likely a right atrial focus (right atrial tachycardia or **RAT**), and if it is + in V1, then it is likely a left atrial focus (left atrial tachycardia or **LAT**). Automatic atrial tachycardia typically produces a regular narrow-QRS tachycardia but may present as a wide-complex tachycardia if pre-existent/rate-dependent bundle branch block (BBB) or ventricular enlargement is present. **Atrial tachycardia with atrioventricular block** is not uncommon and may lead to an irregular rhythm. The atrioventricular block may be physiologic or a manifestation of digoxin toxicity, and if atrial tachycardia is rapid enough, it may be confused with atrial flutter. **Multifocal (chaotic) atrial tachycardias (MAT)** have also been described. A normal or prolonged P′-R interval is present, and subsequent P′ waves should have the same morphology if it is a single focus. Most supraventricular tachycardia (SVTs) in dogs are really atrial tachycardias, and these generally have a low likelihood of benefiting from a radioablation procedure. Treatment with calcium channel blockers, beta-blockers, or digoxin may be considered.

Interpretation of the Electrocardiogram in Small Animals, First Edition. Nick A. Schroeder.
© 2021 John Wiley & Sons Inc. Published 2021 by John Wiley & Sons Inc.

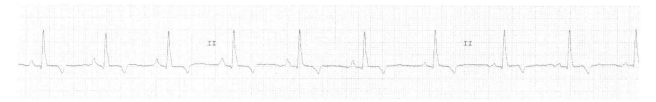

Figure 15.1 Paper speed 50 mm/s, 1 cm/mV, lead II, canine. An **accelerated atrial rhythm** ensues after a slight pause after the sixth complex. The P waves are slightly different than the sinus P waves, suggesting an *ectopic* atrial focus. The seventh complex is an atrial escape complex. The initial HR is approximately 109 bpm and the ectopic atrial rate is approximately 111 bpm. This is an example of **transition of a pacemaker**.

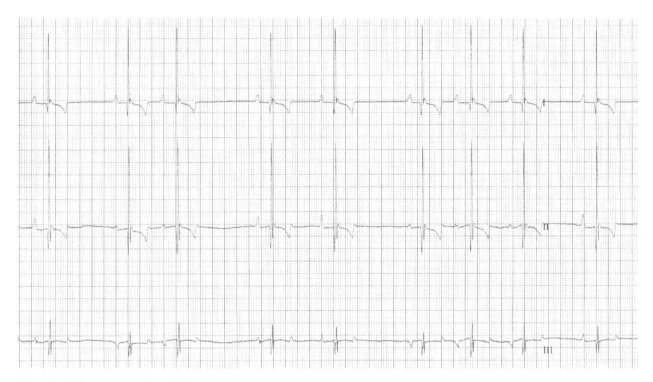

Figure 15.2 Paper speed 50 mm/s, 1 cm/mV, leads I, II, III, canine. **Accelerated atrial rhythm.** The first complex is sinus, which is followed by a two-beat salvo of ectopic atrial rhythm at a slightly faster rate than the prevailing sinus rhythm. This focus is likely an inferior right atrial focus, as the P′ is still positive in I, but negative in III. This is followed by two sinus beats, then a three-beat ectopic atrial salvo. Here, control of the heart is alternating between the competing foci of the sinus node and ectopic atrial tissue.

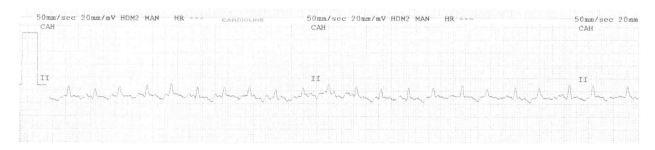

Figure 15.3 Paper speed 50 mm/s, 2 cm/mV, feline. **Atrial tachycardia** is present. The 15th complex is sinus, and atrial bigeminy occurs after.

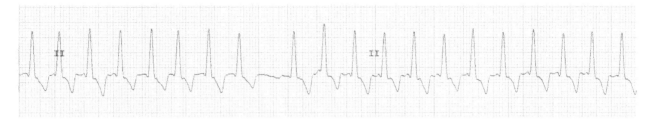

Figure 15.4 Paper speed 50 mm/s, 1 cm/mV, lead II, canine, the SVT terminates midway through the strip. The pause uncovers a negative P′ wave preceding the next QRS (beat #9), making this a long R-P′ SVT. If this is AAT, the negative P′ waves suggest an inferior focus, and negative P′ in V1 (not shown) suggest a RA focus. The 10th beat is somewhat aberrant in morphology and is so because it of the **second-in-the-row anomaly** (short cycle follows long cycle, Ashman's type aberration), a not uncommon occurrence during SVT. The QRS complexes are mildly **prolonged** at 0.06 second due to underlying left ventricular enlargement.

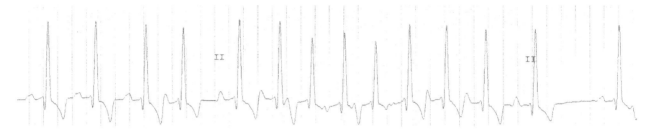

Figure 15.5 Paper speed 50 mm/s, 1 cm/mV, lead II, canine, the fourth complex is an APC that resets, the sixth complex starts a run of **multifocal atrial tachycardia** (the P′ waves are multiforme, and the R-R′ intervals vary).

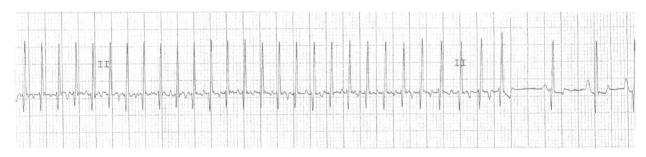

Figure 15.6 Paper speed 25 mm/s, 1 cm/mV, lead II, canine, rapid SVT which terminates. The last three complexes are sinus in origin. The R-P′ prolongs just before conversion into sinus rhythm, suggestive of **AAT**.

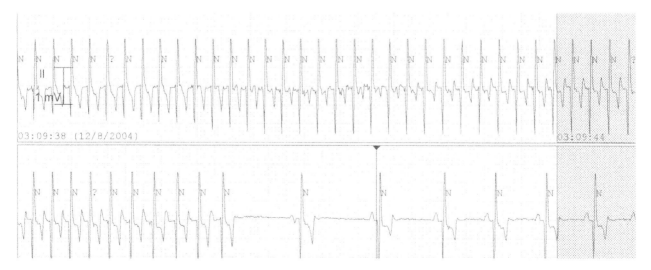

Figure 15.7 Paper speed 25 mm/s, 1 cm/mV, lead II, canine. Another example of **AAT**. The P′-R interval prolongs before conversion.

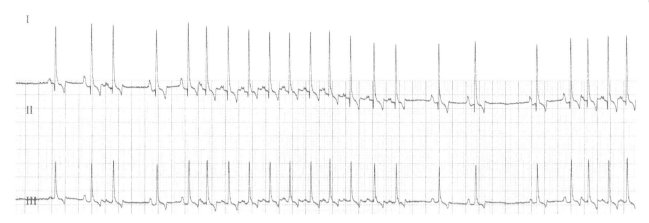

Figure 15.8 Paper speed 25 mm/s, 1 cm/mV, leads II and III, canine. **Automatic atrial tachycardia**. An APC follows the second beat and resets the sinus rhythm with a pause. The fourth beat terminates a short cycle preceded by a relatively long cycle and induces a run of AAT. The ventricular rate gradually speeds up and slows down just before termination. Another run of AAT is induced after a long-short sequence at the end of the strip. Presumably, the AAT is initiated by *reentry* (because of the long-short sequences) and is maintained by *abnormal automaticity* (evident by the gradual warm-up and cool-down of the tachycardia). The P′-R interval prolongs just before termination of the tachycardia.

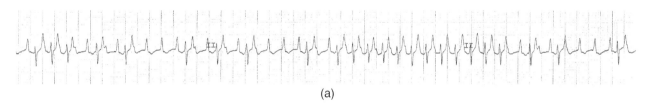

(a)

Figure 15.9a Paper speed 25 mm/s, 1 cm/mV, lead II, canine. **Atrial tachycardia with atrioventricular block**. The P′ waves are tall and buried in the T waves of the preceding beats until nonconduction occurs.

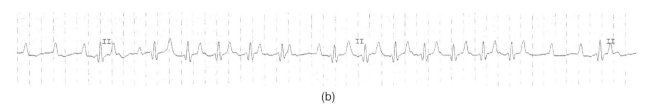

(b)

Figure 15.9b Paper speed 50 mm/s, 1 cm/mV, lead II, same dog. The fifth P wave (second P-QRS-T complex) is a sinus capture. Atrial tachycardia resumes. The atrioventricular block here appears physiologic as the P′-R intervals gradually prolong prior to failure of conduction to the ventricles.

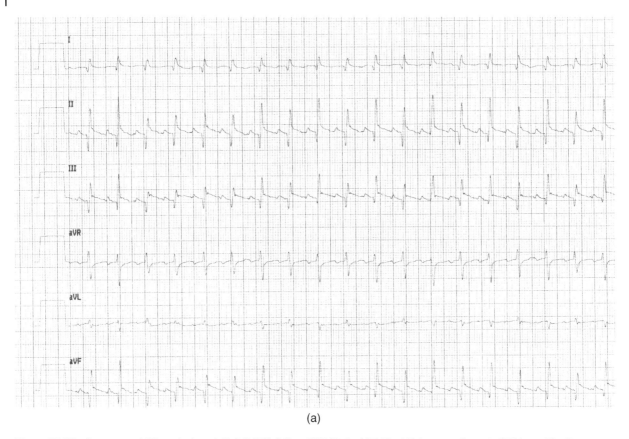

(a)

Figure 15.10a Paper speed 50 mm/s, 1 cm/mV, full EKG, feline, SVT, likely **AAT**. The HR is approximately 275 bpm. The P waves are superimposed on the T waves. Note the QRS alternans, typical of tachycardia.

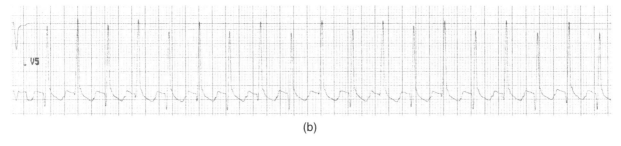

(b)

Figure 15.10b Paper speed 50 mm/s, 1 cm/mV, lead V5, same cat. SVT with electrical alternans.

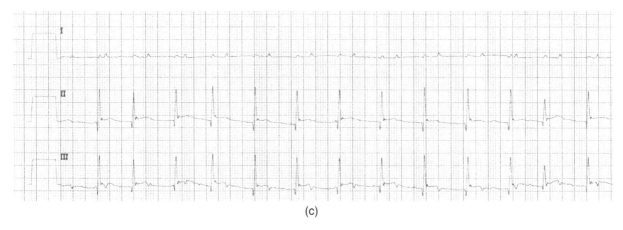

(c)

Figure 15.10c Paper speed 50 mm/s, 1 cm/mV, leads I, II, III, same cat following conversion. Sinus rhythm with severe first degree AVB, P-Ri 0.2 second. Note that the P waves are actually in the S-T segment just after the QRS complex. These are most evident in lead I following the APCs (beats #2, 4, and 12). The P waves in this lead happen to be taller than the isoelectric QRS complexes.

Intra-atrial reentrant tachycardia This is characterized by variable P′ waves that differ from the sinus P, an often long R-P′ interval (but varies with the SVT rate) with an abrupt onset and offset. Intra-atrial microreentry may develop around atrial scars and is distinguished from the macroreentrant circuit associated with atrial flutter (see Chapter 17). Treatment with digoxin and/or diltiazem could be considered.

Atrial dissociation Rarely, one of the atria (or a portion of one of the atria) may be dissociated from the rest of the atrial tissue. The ventricles may be controlled by the sinus node or by ectopic atrial rhythm. The usual manifestation of this is the development of a separate set of P′ waves that are seen marching through the normal sinus P-QRS-T complexes at an independent rate/rhythm. These ectopic P′ waves are usually small in amplitude, and the focus is protected by simultaneous entrance and exit block. In human infants, this arrhythmia may be benign, though atrial dissociation may be a harbinger of death in the elderly and may be seen post-cardiac transplantation as an incidental manifestation of native sinus nodal tissue and transplanted sinus nodal tissue both producing independent P waves. Most of the time, atrial dissociation is supposedly benign and incidental in the dog; however, in this author's experience, it tends to be associated with significant underlying structural heart

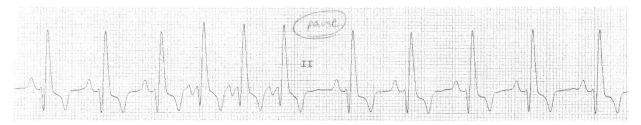

Figure 15.11 Paper speed 50 mm/s, 1 cm/mV, lead II, canine, the fourth beat is premature and preceded by a negative P′ wave and is followed by a short run of SVT. This may be AAT or **interatrial reentrant tachycardia** (IART).

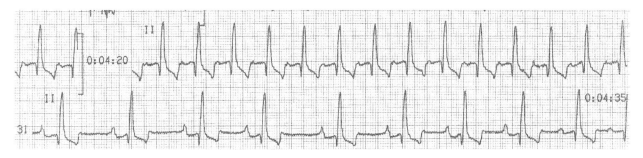

Figure 15.12 Paper speed 25 mm/s, 1 cm/mV, lead II, canine, the bottom strip shows sinus rhythm and the top strip shows SVT, possibly **IART**, since the R-P′ interval is long, and the onset and offset is apparently abrupt.

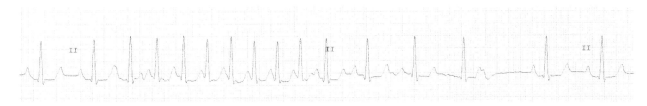

Figure 15.13 Paper speed 50 mm/s, 1 cm/mV, lead II, canine with acute rupture of the left atrium. Suspected **IART**. The third complex starts a run of SVT. Note that the QRS complexes are "skipped" with the P′ actually conducting the second QRS complex following it. The 13th complex has an atrial fusion complex, which is followed by a blocked APC that resets the sinus node.

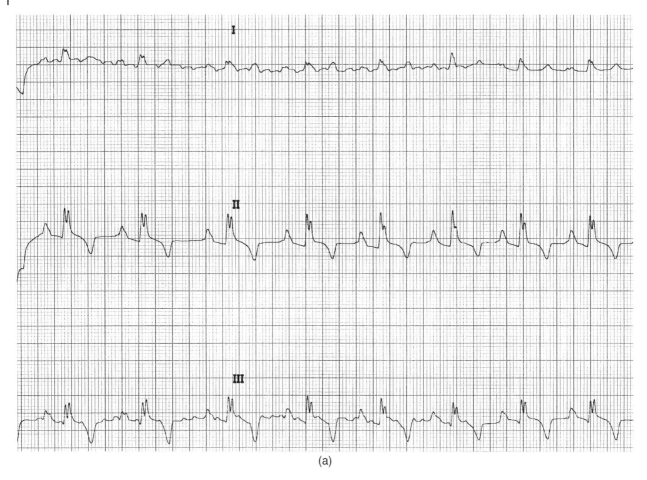

(a)

Figure 15.14a Paper speed 50 mm/s, 1 cm/mV, leads I, II, III, canine with severe chronic mitral and tricuspid valvular disease, pulmonary hypertension, biventricular failure, and multifocal supraventricular premature complexes. *Paroxsymal* **atrial dissociation**. A sinus rhythm is present with a regular HR of 120 bpm. At the beginning of the strip, the baseline in I and III apparently show independent microfibrillatory or microflutter waves that spontaneously terminate after the sixth QRS complex. The underlying sinus rhythm is undisturbed, indicating concurrent entrance and exit block. P-mitrale and a nonspecific intraventricular conduction defect with mild prolongation and splintering of the QRS are present and secondary to concurrent left heart chamber enlargement. This dog was not trembling or having labored inspiration during the recording, so baseline artifact and pseudo-atrial dissociation seems less likely.

disease. If the dissociated atrial rhythm is slow, it tends to be incidental; however, if it is a tachycardia, it may be more significant. Atrial dissociation may be sustained or less commonly paroxysmal. One atrium may be fibrillating, and the other may be in sinus rhythm or atrial flutter (in which case differentiation from Type II atrial flutter may not be possible on surface EKG). Many combinations are possible, and documentation of atrial dissociation is done with intracardiac EKG. Digoxin toxicity is a potential cause. Baseline artifact and atrial parasystole should be excluded. Pseudo-P′ waves associated with laborious inspiration has been termed as Dietz-Marques phenomenon. Treatment with digoxin and/or diltiazem could be considered.

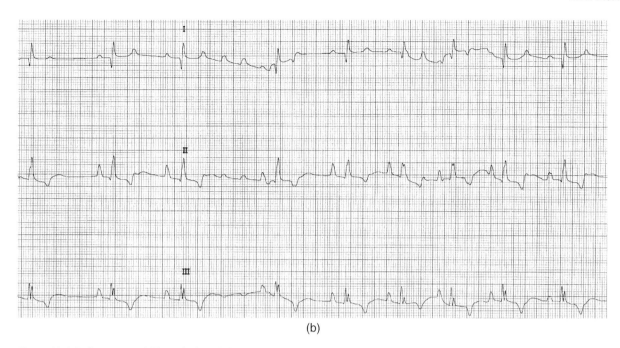

(b)

Figure 15.14b Paper speed 50 mm/s, 1 cm/mV, leads I, II, III, same dog. Another episode of paroxysmal atrial dissociation occurs following the third complex. Here, an atrial tachycardia is briefly dissociated from the prevailing underlying sinus rhythm. Note that the sinus P waves are not reset and the ectopic atrial focus is also not conducted to the ventricles.

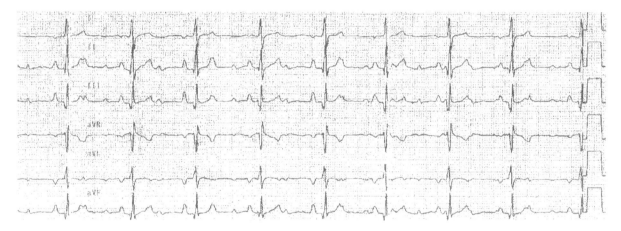

Figure 15.15 Paper speed 50 mm/s, 1 cm/mV, full EKG, canine. **Atrial dissociation,** sinus rhythm in control of the ventricles and dissociated atrial tachycardia. The sinus rate is approximately 111 bpm, and a separate and lower amplitude set of P′ waves are seen marching through the underlying sinus rhythm at an independent rate of approximately 300 bpm. The ectopic P′ waves do not reset or interfere with the sinus rhythm in any way and are blocked from propagating to the ventricles. Furthermore, this ectopic rhythm does not overtly appear to be influenced by the sinus rhythm. This is indicative of a functionally independent significant area of atrial tissue that is dissociated from the rest of the atria, which are under control of the sinus node. *Tracing courtesy of Lynnette D'Urso-Tsugawa.*

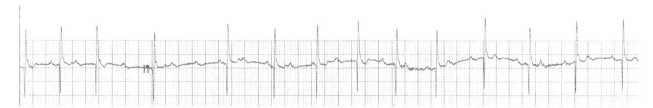

Figure 15.16 Paper speed 25 mm/s, 1 cm/mV, lead II, canine with an intracardiac mass within the interatrial septum. **Unilateral atrial fibrillation** is present, and the atrium that is fibrillating has control of the ventricles, as evidenced by the irregularly irregular supraventricular rhythm and undulating baseline. *P waves* are also seen dissociated from the ventricular rhythm (marching through the QRS complexes) and occur at an independent rate of approximately 150 bpm. This is suggestive of **atrial dissociation** with one atrium fibrillating and controlling the ventricular rate response, and the other atrium in sinus or ectopic atrial rhythm. Perhaps the invasive atrial tumor has electrically isolated the atria in this patient.

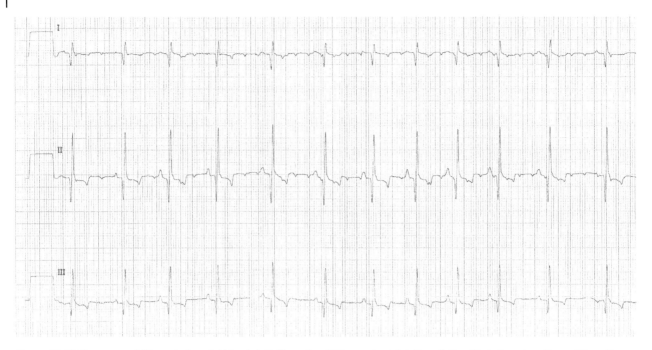

Figure 15.17 Paper speed 50 mm/s, 1 cm/mV, leads I, II, III, canine. R/O ***pseudo*-atrial dissociation** likely from baseline artifact. Sinus arrhythmia is present. Small-amplitude negative possible P′ waves are visualized in leads I and II marching through the P-QRS-T complexes. The rate for the P′ waves appears to be around 500 bpm, which is unphysiologically rapid for an atrial tachycardia, flutter or even fibrillation (which would be irregular and likely indeterminate from surface EKG if dissociated from a sinus rhythm). Lead III has no obvious P′ waves at all (this implies the L forelimb is the culprit). This dog had no structural heart disease evident on echocardiography and was trembling during the recording, making baseline artifact seem to be a more plausible explanation.

Further reading

Achen, S.E., Saunders, A.B., and Miller, M.W. (2008). ECG of the month. *JAVMA* 233 (1): 44–46.

Cheriex, E.C., Brugada, P., and Wellens, H.J.J. (1986). Pseudo-atrial dissociation: a respiratory artifact. *Eur. Heart J.* 7 (4): 357–359.

Deitz, G., Marriott, H.J.L., Fletcher, E. et al. (1657). Atrial dissociation and uniatrial fibrillation. *Circulation* 15: 883–888.

Goldkamp, C. and Estrada, A.H. (2007). ECG of the month. *JAVMA* 230 (5): 668–670.

Hajsadeghi, S., Oraii, S., Riahi, H. et al. (2014). Atrial dissociation in a middle aged patient: a case report. *Cata Medica Iranica* 52 (8): 641–643.

Harmon, M.W. and Fine, D.M. (2012). ECG of the month. *JAVMA* 240 (6): 668–669.

Khan, A.H. (1972). Atrial dissociation. *Br. Heart J.* 34: 1308–1310.

Kimiaki, N. and Osamu, T. (1976). False atrial dissociation (The Deitz-Marques Phenomenon), and its dependence on Dyspnea. *Jpn. Circ. J.* 39 (12): 1329–1334.

Sanghvi, L.M. (1962). Atrial dissociation and double atrial arrhythmias. *Br. Heart J.* 24 (2): 249–252.

Surawicz, B. and Knilans, T.K. (2001). *Chou's Electrocardiography in Clinical Practice: Adult and Pediatric*, 5e. Saunders.

Tanner, J.C.M., Lake-Bakaar, G.A., and Kittleson, M.D. (2013). ECG of the month. *JAVMA* 243 (5): 637–639.

16

Bypass Tract–Mediated Macroreentrant Tachycardias/Ventricular Pre-excitation Syndromes

CHAPTER MENU

Ventricular pre-excitation and accessory pathways, 175
  RV accessory pathway, 176
  LV accessory pathways, 176
Ventricular fusion, 178
Atrial echo, 179
Atrioventricular reciprocating tachycardia/circus movement tachycardia, 179

Ventricular pre-excitation and accessory pathways

Tachycardias may be the result of bypass tracts (accessory pathway or AP), which are embryonic muscular remnants of conductive tissue that connect the atria and the ventricles outside the AV node along the atrioventricular groove. Most commonly, these are associated with narrow-QRS (supraventricular) tachycardia and given that atrial myocardial tissue is a prerequisite part of the circuit, bypass tract–mediated macroreentry is usually included under supraventricular/atrial tachyarrhythmias. When the rhythm is sinus in origin, ventricular pre-excitation (VPE, short P-R interval, and delta waves, which are a notch or slurring of the upstroke of the R wave) may be present on surface EKG if anterograde conduction over the AP is possible. This indicates that the impulse produced by the sinus node actually bypasses the AV node, traveling down the bypass tract to depolarize the ventricles early. The result is a special type of ventricular fusion complex, with depolarization of the ventricles occurring via the AP and via the normal AV node and His-Purkinje system. The more the ventricles are activated by the AP, the shorter the P-Ri, and the wider and more bizarre the QRS is. The more the ventricles are activated over the AV node and normal His-Purkinje system, the longer the P-Ri is and the more normal and narrow the QRS complex is. Thus, various degrees of pre-excitation can be present – from none, to minimal, to maximal pre-excitation. Cats commonly display VPE if they have an AP. Unless pre-excitation is present on the EKG ("manifest"), you do not know that the heart has these bypass tracts (no pre-excitation on surface EKG or "concealed," with only retrograde conduction). Latent accessory pathways may conduct in either direction. A recent small study in dogs suggested that most dogs have concealed bypass tracts, most commonly in the posteroseptal region of the tricuspid annulus. As a result, VPE is uncommon to rare in the dog. The presence of a special type of atrial echo – a retrograde P′ wave that follows the QRS on sinus beats – may be the only clue that a canine patient has an AP that conducts only in the retrograde direction (concealed AP). Three bypass tract types have been historically described as below:

Kent bundles are AV connections completely bypassing the AVN, is characterized by VPE on surface EKG, and if associated with atrioventricular reentrant tachycardia and clinical signs, constitutes *"Wolff-Parkinson-White"* (WPW) syndrome in people. Rarely seen in dogs and in cats with hypertrophic cardiomyopathy (HCM).

James bundles are atrio-His, intranodal or paranodal connections that bypass the AVN, causing a short P-R interval without a widened QRS (no delta wave), that when associated with SVT (usually atrioventricular nodal reentrant tachycardia) results in so-called *"Lown-Ganong-Levine"* (LGL) syndrome in people. Occasionally seen in dogs with congestive heart failure (CHF). "Short P-R/normal QRS syndrome" *without* associated SVT in people is thought to be the result of retention of a juvenile-associated rapid AV

Interpretation of the Electrocardiogram in Small Animals, First Edition. Nick A. Schroeder.
© 2021 John Wiley & Sons Inc. Published 2021 by John Wiley & Sons Inc.

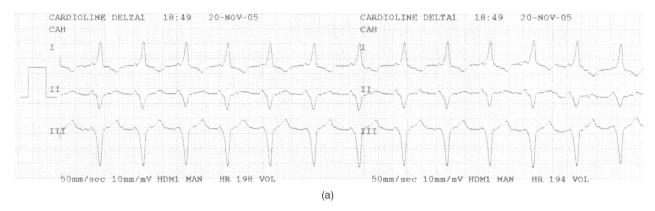

(a)

Figure 16.1a Paper speed 25 mm/s, 1 cm/mV, feline, **ventricular pre-excitation** is evident in this asymptomatic cat. This could be a posteroseptal AP of the LV since this patient had a positive delta wave and QRS in V1. This patient also has a LAFB. The P-R interval is short at approximately 0.04 second. The delta wave indicates the atrial impulse is traveling across an atrioventricular connection (**Kent bundle**) to prematurely activate the ventricles.

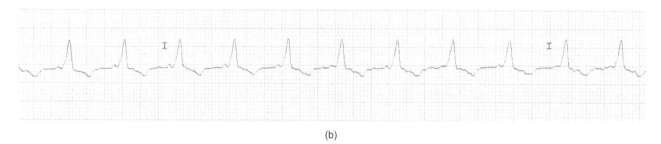

(b)

Figure 16.1b Paper speed 50 mm/s, 1 cm/mV, lead I, same cat. Ventricular pre-excitation is evident: the delta waves are seen as a notch on the upstroke of the R wave, and the P-R interval is short. If this cat were syncopal, this would constitute **Wolff-Parkinson-White (WPW) syndrome**. This cat actually became syncopal (see below).

nodal conduction, and intranodal connections can result in LGL syndrome.

Mahaim fibers: AV nodal ventricular connections bypassing the His bundle, causing a normal P-R interval with a wider QRS than that seen in Kent bundle aberration. Not yet described in small animals.

This simple classification system has failed to address the full spectrum of pre-excitation syndromes seen in humans. Many different types have been described and include atrioventricular connections, as well as nodoventricular, atriofascicular, intranodal, and fasciculoventricular connections, etc.

The location of an AP can be suggested by surface EKG if the AP is manifest:

RV accessory pathway If there is a negative delta wave and QRS in V1, then it is a right ventricular AP.

Posteroseptal pathways have a negative delta wave and QRS in II, III, and aVF, positive in I and aVL.

Right ventricular free wall APs have a left axis orientation (negative in III, aVR and positive in I, II).

Anteroseptal RV APs have an inferior axis (positive in I, II and negative in V1, V2).

Midseptal APs have delta waves similar to anteroseptal APs, except the delta waves are negative in II, III, and aVF.

LV accessory pathways If there is a positive delta wave and QRS in V1, then the AP is left ventricular.

Posteroseptal APs have a negative delta wave and QRS in II, III, and aVF.

Lateral (left ventricular free wall) APs have an isoelectric or negative delta wave in I, aVL, V5, and V6.

Thus, the transition zone of the delta wave in the V leads (where the rS becomes an Rs pattern, or where the most isoelectric V lead is with an RS pattern) is important. Early transitions are transition zones shifted to the right (counterclockwise), and delayed transitions are shifted to the left (clockwise). Identification of the transition zone helps delineate where the AP is. The AP will be perpendicular to the zone of transition. The leads with the negative delta waves "point" to the location of the AP. Precise localization of the AP required intracardiac EKG/mapping.

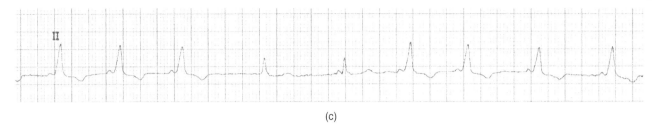

(c)

Figure 16.1c Paper speed 50 mm/s, 1 cm/mV, lead II, same cat. Sinus arrhythmia produces a pause in the rhythm after the third complex long enough to elicit a **junctional escape beat** (beat #4). Note the absence of an obvious P wave (retrograde or sinus), and the *narrow* QRS consistent with conduction down the normal His-Purkinje system. Junctional beats would be expected to produce a normal duration QRS complex in patients with accessory pathways given the absence of underlying BBB. The fifth complex may be another junctional escape with a sinus P wave that happens to precede the QRS, then the sinus node takes over ventricular activation via the accessory pathway as evidenced by the widened QRS, short P-Ri typical of pre-excited sinus rhythm.

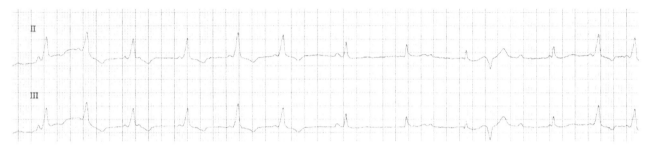

Figure 16.1d Paper speed 50 mm/s, 1 cm/mV, leads II and III, same cat. Sinus arrhythmia reveals some degree of rate-dependent ventricular pre-excitation. The seventh beat is only mildly prolonged, and the P-Ri is longer, indicating more activation of the myocardium over the normal His-Purkinje system vs. activation via the accessory pathway with *minimal* **ventricular pre-excitation**. The eighth and ninth beats appear to be junctional escapes with normal QRS duration, and the 10th beat is a VPC that blocks the following P wave. The 11th beat appears to be junctional escape with a superimposed sinus P wave on the QRS complex, and this is followed by a sinus beat with *maximal* **ventricular pre-excitation**.

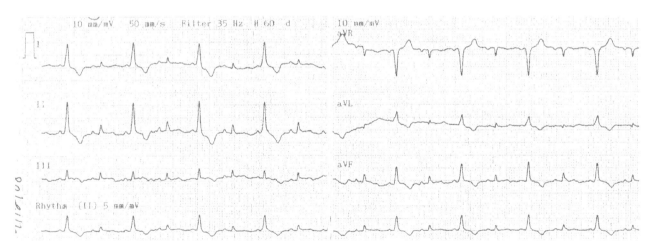

Figure 16.2 Paper speed 50 mm/s, 1 cm/mV, full EKG, feline with history of episodic open-mouthed breathing. **2:1 ventricular pre-excitation**. Anterograde conduction over the accessory pathway occurs on every-other-beat. This mimics right ventricular bigeminy. The clues here are that the P-R′ intervals are consistent despite a mild variation in the P-P intervals from sinus arrhythmia, and the QRS axis does not change whether or not the beat is pre-excited. *Tracing courtesy of Scott Forney*.

The gradual onset of VPE over a series of beats is termed the "concertina effect." Normal conduction over the AVN is present at first, then minimal progressing to maximal VPE occurs over a number of complexes as more and more of the ventricular myocardium is activated over the AP vs. the normal His-Purkinje system. The P-R intervals progressively shorten associated with the appearance of delta waves, resulting in progressive QRS prolongation and repolarization abnormality (T wave opposite in deflection of the main QRS vector). The concertina effect suggests

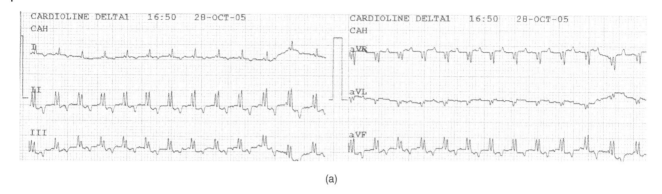

(a)

Figure 16.3a Paper speed 25 mm/s, 2 cm/mV, full EKG, asymptomatic feline. If this cat had been syncopal, this would constitute **Lown-Ganong-Levine (LGL) syndrome**. The P-R interval is very short, but the QRS complex is of normal duration. This is suggestive that there is ventricular pre-excitation; however, there is no obvious delta wave. This could mean there is an abnormal atrio-His bundle connection (**James fiber**) or juvenile-type rapid AVN conduction, allowing the atrial impulse to prematurely activate the ventricles.

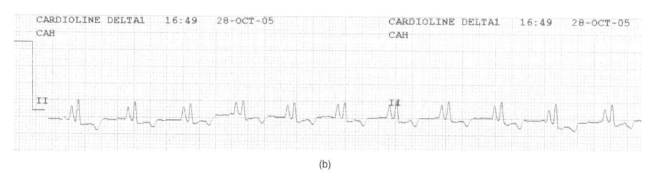

(b)

Figure 16.3b Paper speed 50 mm/s, 2 cm/mV, lead II, same cat. The P-R interval is approximately 0.04 second (normal is 0.05–0.09 second).

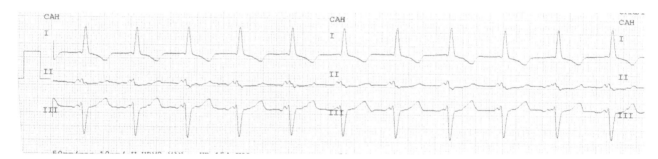

Figure 16.4 Paper speed 50 mm/s, 1 cm/mV, leads I, II, III, feline. Ventricular pre-excitation (**LGL** or James fiber type) in a cat with bifascicular block (RBBB + LAFB or LAD), which prolongs the QRS duration without the presence of a delta wave.

the AP has a long refractory period and should be differentiated from the gradual onset of bundle branch block (which has static or prolonging P-R intervals with the onset of ventricular aberration) and the gradual onset of ventricular fusion with an accelerated idioventricular rhythm (which has shortening P-R intervals with no delta waves). Wenckebach and Mobitz conduction over the AP is presumably difficult to recognize on surface EKG, but Wenckebach would be expected to be progressive and Mobitz to be random. 2:1 conduction over the AP results in every-other-beat displaying VPE.

Ventricular fusion Rarely, supraventricular premature beats during pre-excited sinus rhythm can occur with narrowed QRS complex and are the result of a ventricular fusion between the sinus and ectopic atrial or junctional origin foci. This is the exception to the rule that ventricular fusion indicates a ventricular arrhythmia. That rule holds true if the AVN is the only electrical connection between the atria and the ventricles. In the presence of an AP, supraventricular foci may conduct to the ventricles via the AVN or the AP, allowing for ventricular fusion complexes. The presence of supraventricular premature

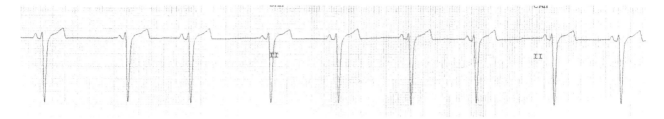

Figure 16.5 Paper speed 50 mm/s, 1 cm/mV, lead II, canine with asymptomatic VSD. Ventricular pre-excitation (LGL) and RBBB. Note the short P-R interval (0.05 second) and lack of obvious delta wave.

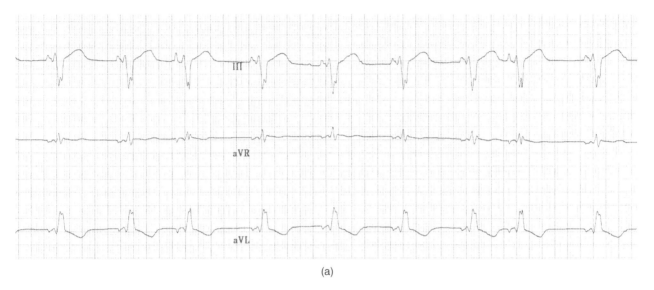

(a)

Figure 16.6a Paper speed 50 mm/s, 1 cm/mV, leads III, aVR, aVL, feline. Ventricular **pre-excited sinus rhythm** with **APCs**. The 3rd and 8th beats are premature, reset the sinus rhythm, and have ectopic P′ morphology consistent with ectopic atrial supraventricular premature beats.

beats and a short P′-Ri on a narrower QRS supports the diagnosis of ventricular fusion. However, pre-excitation can be intermittent, so if the P-Ri is normal, conduction over the AP is minimal on that particular beat and normal intraventricular conduction is expected.

Atrial echo

Often in dogs with retrogradely conducting APs will have retrograde P′ waves seen following sinus beats. This indicates the sinus impulse depolarized the atria, went through the AVN, depolarized the ventricles, and then traveled retrogradely across the AP to reactivate the atria -producing a special type of atrial echo (AP-mediated vs. those generated from reentry within the AVN itself). If the impulse finds the AVN excitable, then orthodromic atrioventricular reentrant/reciprocating tachycardia (OAVRT) ensues. If the AVN is refractory, the impulse is AV blocked and OAVRT is averted.

An APC or VPC can initiate (or terminate) SVT involving the bypass tract and cause atrioventricular reciprocating tachycardia or circus movement tachycardia (described

below). These SVTs may only be able to be induced during electrophysiologic studies and are best treated with radiofrequency catheter ablation. An inciting VPC is differentiated from the so-called "second-in-the-row" anomaly (BBB on the second complex of an SVT) by failure to identify preceding atrial activity with a normal to long P-R interval.

Atrioventricular reciprocating tachycardia/circus movement tachycardia

When an APC travels down the AV node then up a bypass tract, back down the AV node, a circuit can be created, depolarizing the atria and the ventricles nearly simultaneously. This is termed orthodromic AVRT (**OAVRT**). The P′ waves follow the QRS complexes. This is characterized on EKG by negative P′ waves in II, III, and aVF, visible in the ST-T segment, a short R-P′ interval, and is abrupt in onset and offset. Vagal maneuvers usually terminate OAVRT. If the P′ is negative in lead I, then it is a left-sided AP. There is always 1:1 AV conduction. This arrhythmia has been associated with tricuspid valve dysplasia/Ebstein's anomaly in Labrador

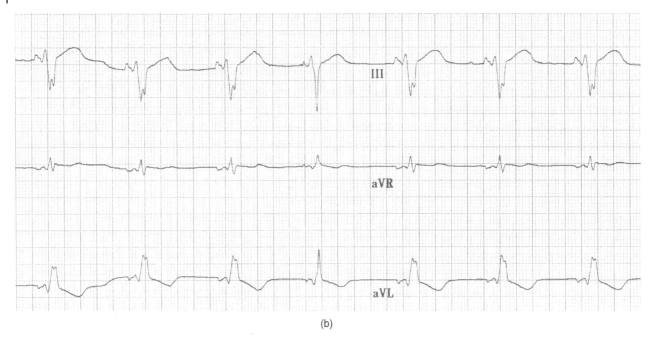

(b)

Figure 16.6b Paper speed 50 mm/s, 1 cm/mV, leads III, aVR, aVL, same cat. **Ventricular fusion with an APC**. The fourth complex is on time but has an altered P′ morphology with a short P′-Ri, and the QRS that follows is narrower than those of pure sinus origin with full pre-excitation. This is a rare example of a ventricular fusion beat that results from the fusion of two supraventricular foci with conduction over the AP and the AVN with a resultant narrowing of the QRS from better intraventricular conduction. Typically, ventricular fusion is an indication of a ventricular arrhythmia; however, in the presence of an accessory pathway, ventricular fusion can occur with a supraventricular arrhythmia. The presence of APCs in the above strip confirms the diagnosis.

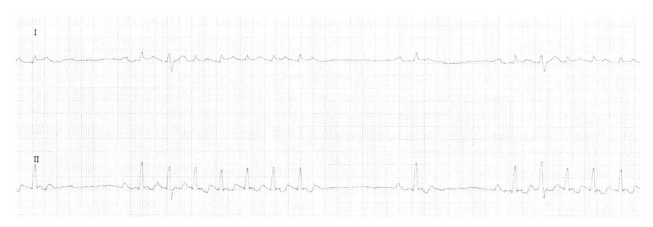

Figure 16.7 Paper speed 50 mm/s, 1 cm/mV, leads I and II, canine. The second beat is sinus followed by **atrial echo/retrograde P′** in the S-T segment, initiating a run of **OAVRT**. The third complex is aberrant with RBBB due to the long-short sequence (Ashman's type phenomenon, "second-in-the-row anomaly" given preceding atrial activity). Note the ninth beat has a retrograde P′ in the S-T segment that is AV blocked. OAVRT resumes following the 10th beat.

Retrievers. Orthodromic AVRT may also be initiated by a VPC traveling up the AP then down the AVN, or by sinus tachycardia, and often displays electrical alternans during the tachycardia. While cats may commonly have manifest VPE (indicating antegrade conduction over the AP), dogs rarely do. Dogs, however, may have atrial echoes following the QRS complexes in sinus rhythm if only unidirectional retrograde conduction over the AP is present.

If an APC travels down the bypass tract and retrogradely up the AV node (VA or ventriculoatrial conduction), traveling back down the tract to create a circuit, then antidromic AVRT (**AAVRT**) is created. Alternatively, a VPC may travel retrogradely up the AV node, activating the atria, then down the bypass tract, initiating the same arrhythmia. This often results in a wide-complex SVT that mimics VT. This is from the delta waves widening the QRS complexes and

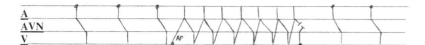

Figure 16.8 Ladder diagram illustrating the mechanism of **OAVRT**. Sinus rhythm for three beats occurs, then a VPC activates the accessory pathway (labeled AP) retrogradely, activating the atria, which then returns anterogradely across the AVN to activate the ventricles. A VPC then terminates the tachycardia.

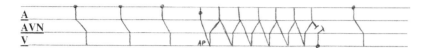

Figure 16.9 Ladder diagram illustrating the mechanism of **AAVRT**. Sinus rhythm occurs for three beats, then an APC finds the AVN refractory, but proceeds antegrade across the AP to activate the ventricles, then retrograde across the AVN to reactivate the atria. A VPC terminates the tachycardia.

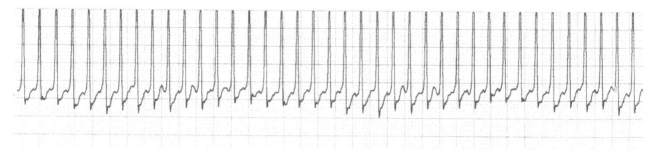

Figure 16.10 Paper speed 25 mm/s, 1 cm/mV, lead II, canine, this Rottweiler puppy had tricuspid valve dysplasia, suspected Ebstein's anomaly, and an incessant SVT that was unresponsive to medications and eventually led to the puppy's sudden death. Suspect **OAVRT**. The ventricular rate is over 300 bpm.

a P′ following the QRS and is terribly rare in veterinary patients. Other SVTs that cause wide-complex tachycardias include CMT using nodoventricular or fasiculoventricular fibers, CMT with two APs, and CMT with BBB aberration. Atrial fibrillation with conduction over an AP results in a very rapid, irregular, wide-complex tachycardia that mimics ventricular tachycardia, and may predispose to sudden cardiac death from ventricular fibrillation. When in doubt, the human literature says to use procainamide. Digoxin and verapamil are contraindicated in AVRT because it may accelerate conduction over the AP, leading to dangerously fast ventricular rate responses.

Electrical alternans (QRS), where the QRS complexes alternate in amplitude on a beat-to-beat basis, is relatively common during AVRT, especially if there is a concealed AP. This is probably secondary to alternating prolongation of the refractory phase of the heart. QRS alternans is a helpful clue to circus movement tachycardia but may happen during tachycardia of any origin.

Frequent or sustained SVT can lead to syncope and/or worsening of CHF, and prolonged tachycardias of any origin can result in a form of cardiomyopathy known as "tachycardia-induced cardiomyopathy." Pacing studies in animals are used to create models for dilated cardiomyopathy (DCM). Whether these models are really representative of naturally acquired DCM is the big question. If a normal dog is paced at 180–240 bpm for 2–4 weeks, it will be in CHF and have a dilated, weakly contracting heart. Treatment of SVT is aimed at interrupting the abnormal circuit or slowing conduction through the AV node if it is involved in the circuit. Diltiazem and beta-blockers can be considered. Medical therapy can be unrewarding, and radiofrequency ablation offers a reasonable chance at a cure.

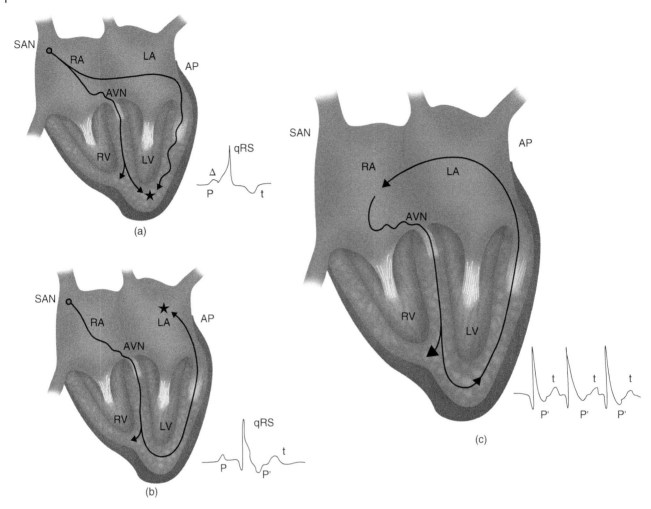

Figure 16.11 Diagrams illustrating bypass tract–mediated arrhythmia. (a) **Ventricular pre-excitation**. A sinus impulse simultaneously activates the ventricular myocardium over the AVN and the accessory pathway resulting in a short P-Ri and prolonged QRS from the presence of a delta wave. (b) **Atrial echo**. A sinus impulse activates the ventricular myocardium normally over the AVN and the atria are depolarized again over the accessory pathway resulting in a retrograde P′ following the QRS. (c) **Circus movement tachycardia/ atrioventricular reentrant tachycardia**. Sustained supraventricular tachycardia results from macroreentry over the AVN and the accessory pathway. Orthodromic physiology is illustrated here. **SAN**: sinoatrial node, **AVN**: atrioventricular node, **RA**: right atrium, **LA**: left atrium, **RV**: right ventricle, **LV**: left ventricle, **AP**: accessory pathway, **P**: p wave, **qRs**: QRS complex, **t**: t wave, δ: delta wave, **P′**: atrial echo.

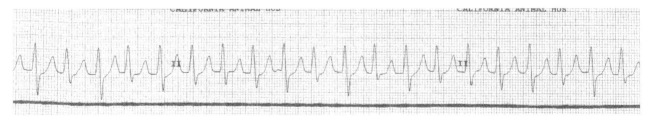

Figure 16.12 Paper speed 50 mm/s, 1 cm/mV, lead II, canine with hyperthyroidism secondary to thyroid adenocarcinoma and SVT. **QRS alternans** is apparent, and suggestive of CMT.

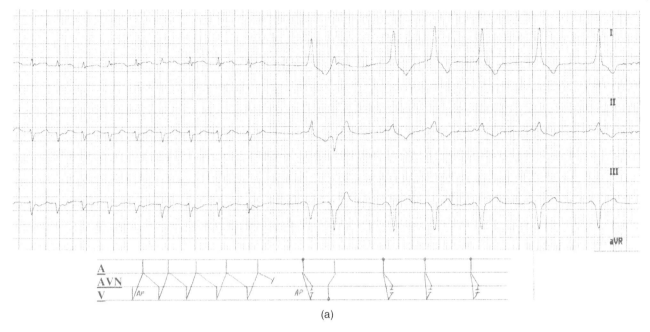

(a)

Figure 16.13a Paper speed 50 mm/s, 1 cm/mV, leads I, II, III, feline given IV diltiazem to interrupt CMT. **OAVRT** with a HR of approximately 300 bpm is present at the beginning of the strip until the impulse is finally blocked in the AVN. A single pre-excited beat occurs followed by a VPC, which thankfully does not initiate another run of OAVRT. The VPC may be conducting retrogradely across the AVN or the AP (note the retrograde P′ in the S-T segment, most obvious in lead I). Sinus rhythm with **ventricular pre-excitation** (HR approximately 150–200 bpm) follows. The QRS complexes are narrow (0.04 section) in duration, indicative of orthodromic physiology. The ladder diagram illustrates the mechanism. The pre-excited beats are a special type of fusion complex, with the ventricles being simultaneously excited by the AP as well as across the AVN. This cat was lethargic and weak during tachycardia, and thus has **Wolf-Parkinson-White syndrome**.

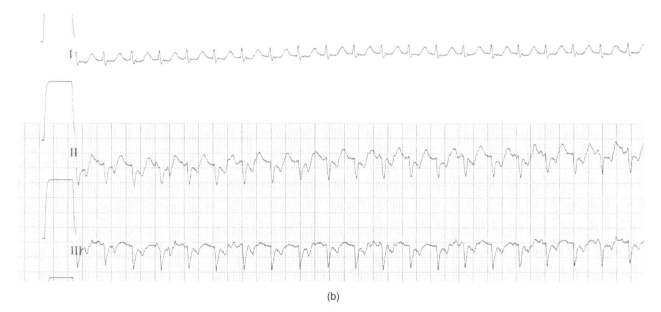

(b)

Figure 16.13b Paper speed 50 mm/s, 2 cm/mV, leads I, II, III, same cat. **OAVRT**. HR approximately 300 bpm. The sensitivity is set higher here, and the retrograde P′ waves are more obvious here immediately following the QRS complexes within the S-T segment. It took multiple boluses of diltiazem followed by procainamide to terminate this tachycardia.

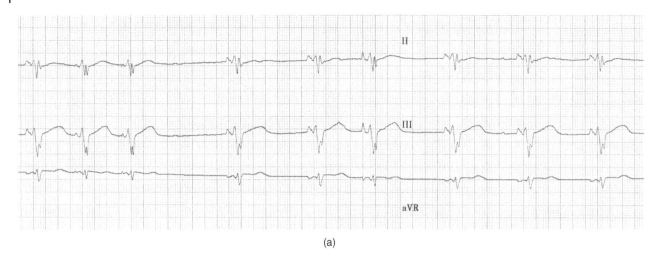

(a)

Figure 16.14a Paper speed 50 mm/s, 1 cm/mV, feline with severe unclassified cardiomyopathy and history of SVT. Sinus rhythm, ventricular pre-excitation, *multifocal* **atrial premature beats**. The second and third complexes are a couplet of APCs that reset the sinus rhythm with a long pause. The sixth complex is another APC with a different P′ morphology that resets the rhythm. These beats are not junctional in origin, as JPCs that occur in patients with manifest ventricular pre-excitation would be expected to be conducted with a narrow QRS. Premature beats can easily initiate circus movement as seen below.

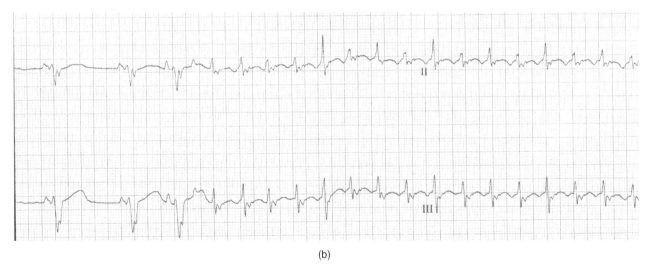

(b)

Figure 16.14b Paper speed 50 mm/s, 1 cm/mV, leads II and III, same cat. Onset of **OAVRT**. The third and fourth beats are a couplet of APCs that initiate circus movement tachycardia. Note the transition from wide, pre-excited QRS complexes to the narrow QRS complexes (with electrical alternans midway through the strip) typical of orthodromic SVT.

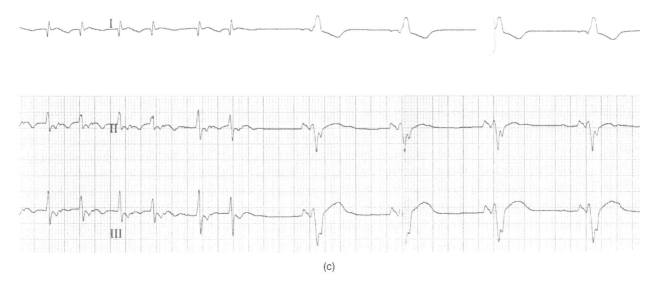

(c)

Figure 16.14c Paper speed 50 mm/s, 1 cm/mV, leads I, II, III, same cat. Offset of OAVRT with resumption of sinus rhythm with ventricular pre-excitation.

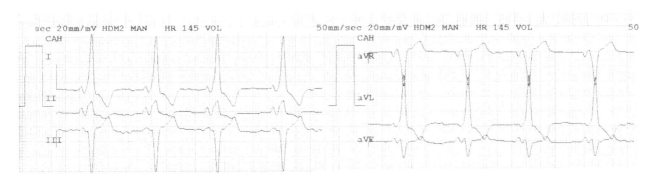

Figure 16.15 Paper speed 50 mm/s, 2 cm/mV, full EKG, feline with VPE in sinus rhythm with LAD. Delta waves are present with a shortened P-R interval, indicative of an accessory pathway. This patient was being administered propranolol orally to control SVT.

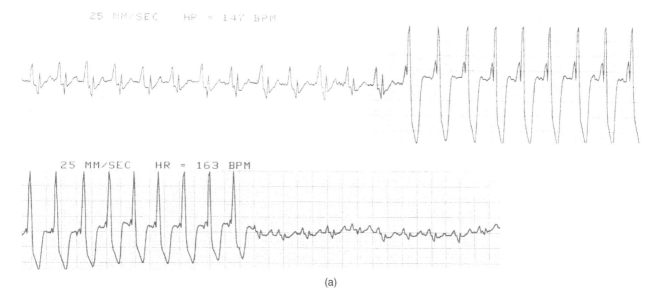

(a)

Figure 16.16a Paper speed 25 mm/s, 2 cm/mV on top and 1 cm/mV on bottom lead II, feline. The top strip shows sinus rhythm with an abrupt transition to NSR and VPE and the HR goes from 150 to 167 bpm. The P waves are tall in sinus rhythm. The bottom strip shows NSR/VPE and transition to NSR without pre-excitation. The HR is approximately 188 bpm throughout, so this patient's pre-excitation does not appear to be rate-dependent.

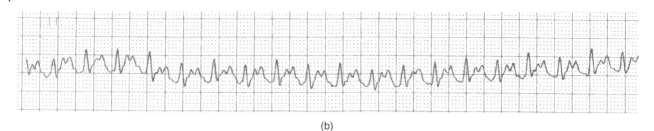

(b)

Figure 16.16b Paper speed 50 mm/s, 1 cm/mV, lead II, same cat. **OAVRT.** The HR is approximately 300 bpm, and negative P′ waves follow the QRS complexes and appear within the S-T segments, indicating *orthodromic* physiology. The circuit is directed anterogradely over the AVN and retrogradely over the AP. *Antidromic* physiology (AAVRT) would show retrograde P′ waves followed by widened QRS complexes since the AP is used in an anterograde direction and the AVN is used in a retrograde direction. Since this patient has manifest pre-excitation, AVRT, and clinical signs of syncope, **Wolff-Parkinson-White** (WPW) syndrome is present.

Further reading

Fogoros, R.N. (1999). *Electrophysiologic Testing*, 3e. Blackwell Publishing.

Hart, T.M. and Stauthammer, C.D. (2010). ECG of the month. *JAVMA* 237 (6): 641–643.

Johnson, M., Martin, M., and Smith, P. (2006). Cardioversion of supraventricular Tachycardia using Lidocaine in five dogs. *J. Vet. Intern. Med.* 20: 272–276.

Ometto, R., Thiene, G., Corrado, D. et al. (1992). Enhanced A-V nodal conduction (Lown-Ganong-Levine Syndrome) by congenitally hypoplastic A-V node. *Eur. Heart J.* 13 (11): 1579–1584.

Mandel, W.J., Danzig, R., and Hayakawa, H. (1971). Lown-Ganong-Levine Syndrome: a study using his bundle electrograms. *Circulation* 44: 696–708.

Santilli, R.A., Spadacini, G., Moretti, P. et al. (2007). Anatomic distribution and electrophysiologic properties of accessory atrioventricular pathways in dogs. *JAVMA*. 231 (3).

Santilli, R.A., Critelli, M., and Toaldo, M.B. (2010). ECG of the month. *JAVMA* 237 (10): 1142–1144.

Singla, V., Singh, B., Sing, Y. et al. (2013). Concertina effect: a subtle but specific marker. *BMJ Case Reports* https://doi .org/10.1136/bcr-2013-009328.

Sternick, E.B. and Wellens, H.J.J. (2006). *Variants of Ventricular Preexcitation: Recognition and Treatment*. Blackwell Futura.

Surawicz, B. and Knilans, T.K. (2001). *Chou's Electrocardiography in Clinical Practice: Adult and Pediatric*, 5e. Saunders.

17

Atrial Flutter

CHAPTER MENU

Atrial flutter, 187
  Type I AFL, 187
  Type II AFL, 188
Atrioventricular block, 193
Artifacts, 194

Atrial flutter Atrial flutter is characterized on surface EKG by often irregular but rapid supraventricular QRS complexes with a "sawtooth" baseline that represent flutter waves. Flutter waves are rapid atrial depolarization waves that are one after another without rest usually at an atrial rate of over 300 bpm. The cause and treatment is similar to that of atrial fibrillation (AF), and atrial flutter may degenerate into coarse AF. It caused by a macro-reentrant, self-perpetuating circuit usually located within the right atrium. Rapid atrial rates generally induce physiologic atrioventricular block (AVB). The Bix Rule states that if the T waves are evenly spaced between QRS complexes, then additional P waves may be hiding within the QRS complexes, and atrial flutter (or ectopic atrial tachycardia) is suspected, though this is not always a feature. If what initially appears to be a sinus tachycardia remains at an elevated/locked rate for long periods, then supraventricular tachycardia such as AFL (with a fixed conduction ratio) should be suspected. While the atrial rhythm is regular, the ventricular rhythm in AFL may or may not be. The P′ waves ("F" waves, flutter or AFL waves) are usually negative in the inferior leads with positive T waves with 2:1 or 4:1 AV conduction. This means that there are either 2 or 4 flutter waves seen before a QRS complex. Atrial flutter with alternating 2:1 and 4:1 conduction and aberration of the QRS complexes ending shorter cycles (Ashman's phenomenon) famously mimics ventricular bigeminy. Atrial flutter may be difficult to distinguish from rapid focal atrial tachycardia with AVB and is much more common in dogs than in cats. Treatment with digoxin and diltiazem can be considered. Beta-blockers may be used in refractory cases. There are two types of atrial flutter based on the atrial rate.

Type I AFL The atrial rate is 240–340 bpm (in humans, no established values in dogs in cats; however, spontaneous flutter rates in dogs generally exceed those rates established in the human literature), aka "Isthmus-Dependent."

"Typical" (Counterclockwise): It is the common form, with negative atrial flutter waves in II, III, and aVF. Positive flutter waves in V1 with transition to negative by V6. The flutter path proceeds caudocranially along the RA septum and craniocaudally along the RA free wall. A zone of slow conduction may exist bounded by the tricuspid annulus, the caudal vena cava, and the coronary sinus.

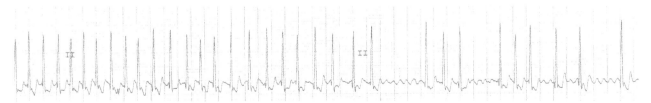

Figure 17.1 Paper speed 25 mm/s, 1 cm/mV, lead II, canine, **atrial flutter**, the flutter waves are evident during the pauses (at a flutter rate of 375 bpm).

Interpretation of the Electrocardiogram in Small Animals, First Edition. Nick A. Schroeder.
© 2021 John Wiley & Sons Inc. Published 2021 by John Wiley & Sons Inc.

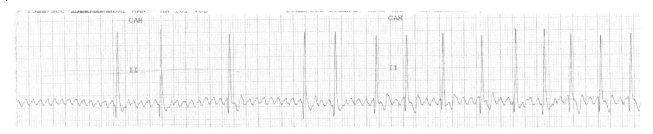

Figure 17.2 Paper speed 25 mm/s, 1cm/mV, lead II, canine, **atrial flutter**. Longer pauses are present between the conducted beats at the beginning of the strip, highlighting the sawtoothed baseline from rapid atrial depolarization. The flutter rate is approximately 375 bpm.

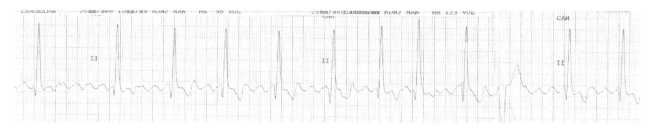

Figure 17.3 Paper speed 50 mm/s, 1 cm/mV, lead II, same dog. Atrial flutter rate 428 bpm. The 10th complex *may* demonstrate *Ashman's phenomenon*, as it ends a relatively short cycle preceding a relatively long cycle and is of RBBB morphology. Alternatively, it may just be a VPC. With variable AV conduction present, it is difficult to call the pause following this beat a compensatory-like pause, since the R-R intervals vary. This is similar to the phenomenon of concealed conduction during atrial fibrillation.

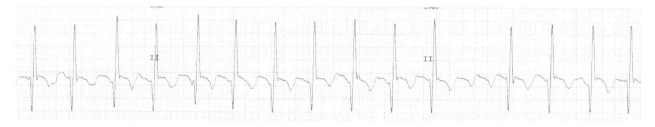

Figure 17.4 Paper speed 50 mm/s, 1 cm/mV, lead II, canine with severe CMVDz, **Type I (typical Isthus-dependent) AFL**. At the beginning of the strip, there is **2:1 conduction**. The flutter rate is 333 bpm, and the ventricular rate is approximately 166 bpm. Flutter waves are evenly spaced between R waves and summate with the T waves. According to the **Bix Rule**, additional flutter waves are suspected hiding within QRS complexes, which can be seen on the initial slurred downstroke of the Q waves. A **vagal maneuver** was performed in this patient, resulting in a higher level of AVB, resulting in **4:1 conduction** toward the end of the strip, uncovering the sawtoothed baseline characteristic of AFL. Here, the flutter waves are negative in II, suggestive of Type I AFL.

"Reverse Typical" or "Atypical" (Clockwise): It is the rare form, with + atrial flutter waves in II, III, and aVF. It is almost always abolished by overdrive (atrial) pacing, and more amenable to catheter ablation. The flutter path proceeds cranially up the RA free wall and caudally down the interatrial septum.

Type II AFL The atrial rate is 340–433 bpm in humans (no established values for dogs and cats, again likely faster than in humans, notably faster than in Type I AFL). AKA "Non-Cavotricuspid Isthmus-Dependent." Also known as "fibrillo-flutter," it mimics AF, is almost never abolished by overdrive pacing, is poorly characterized, and less amenable to catheter ablation. The flutter waves do not conform to typical patterns associated with Type I AFL and are often irregular. The ventricular rate response is thus irregularly irregular in rhythm. Due to the less organized atrial activity, some consider this more closely related or a transition to AF. This is generally impossible to differentiate on surface EKG from atrial dissociation where one atrium (typically the right atrium) is in flutter and the other (usually left) atrium is in fibrillation (see Chapter 15).

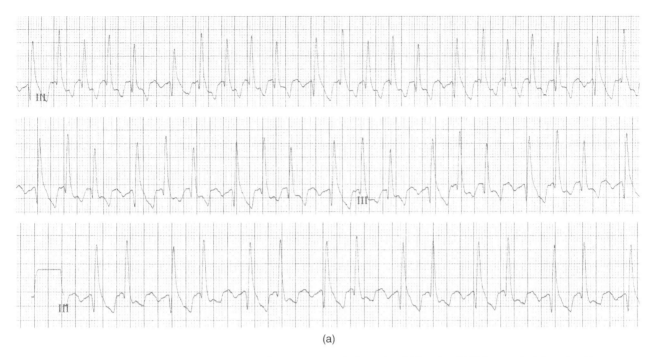

(a)

Figure 17.5a Paper speed 50 mm/s, 1 cm/mV, lead III, Bernese Mountain Dog with SVT, during IV diltiazem administration. From top to bottom, **6:5**, **4:3**, and **3:2** conduction leading to group beating. **Electrical alternans** is present as well, and likely a function of HR.

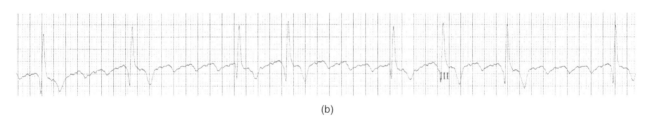

(b)

Figure 17.5b Paper speed 50 mm/s, 1 cm/mV, lead III, same dog. Higher grade AVB ensues, revealing the regular undulating baseline of AFL. The negative flutter waves in III indicate **Type 1 Typical (counterclockwise) AFL**.

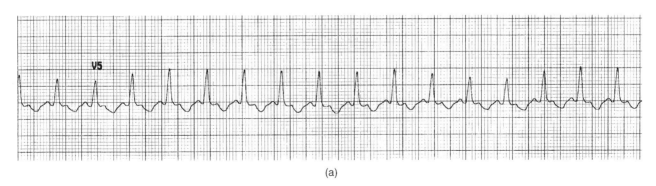

(a)

Figure 17.6a Paper speed 50 mm/s, 1 cm/mV, lead V5, canine with heart-based mass and tachycardia-induced cardiomyopathy. Sustained SVT. Atrial activity uncertain. Note that the T waves are spaced halfway between QRS complexes and the S-T segment seems irregular. This is suggestive of **AFL** via the **Bix Rule**.

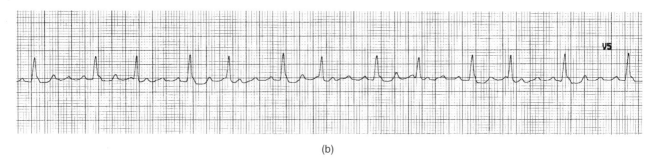

(b)

Figure 17.6b Paper speed 50 mm/s, 1 cm/mV, lead V5, same dog. A few minutes later following a bolus of diltiazem IV, AVB increases to 3:1 alternating with 2:1 AVB revealing the flutter waves.

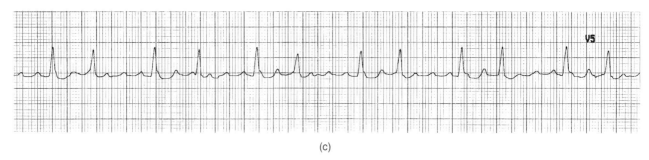

(c)

Figure 17.6c Paper speed 50 mm/s, 1 cm/mV, lead V5, same dog. A few minutes later yet, the degree of AVB increases to 4:1 conduction.

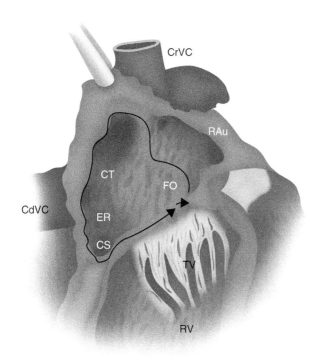

Figure 17.7 Illustration of the mechanism of Type I counterclockwise AFL. View of the heart from the right, with the right atrium and right ventricle opened. **CrVC**: cranial vena cava, **CdVC**: caudal vena cava, **RAu**: right auricle, **CT**: crista terminalis, **FO**: fossa ovalis, **ER**: Eustachian ridge, **CS**: coronary sinus, **TV**: tricuspid valve (septal leaflet), **RV**: right ventricle. The macroreentrant pathway of atrial flutter is shown by the line, the direction of the wavefront by the arrow, and the zone of slow conduction is indicated by waviness of the line.

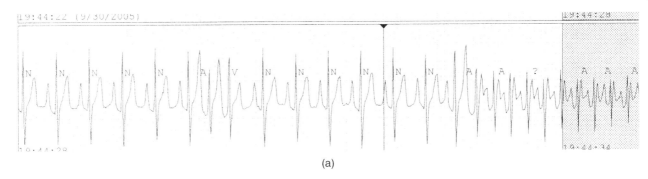

(a)

Figure 17.8a Paper speed 25 mm/s, 1 cm/mV, lead II, a Husky with rapid **atrial flutter** at approximately 280–300 bpm. The T waves are nearly spaced evenly between QRS complexes. This dog was quite syncopal during these episodes of tachycardia, and the only cardiac abnormality noted was **annuloaortic ectasia** (an idiopathic dilation of the ascending aorta similar to that seen in humans with *Marfan's syndrome*).

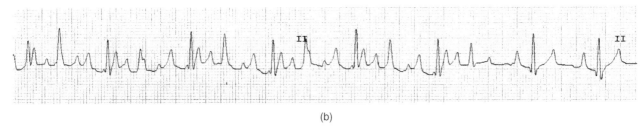

(b)

Figure 17.8b Paper speed 50 mm/s, 1 cm/mV, lead II, same dog, atrial flutter, the beginning of the strip shows AFL with variable degrees of AVB.

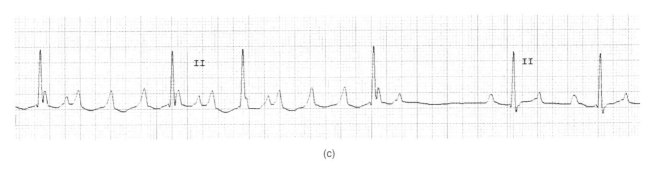

(c)

Figure 17.8c Paper speed 50 mm/s, 1 cm/mV, lead II, same dog, atrial flutter following IV diltiazem administration. The flutter waves are obvious and there is 4:1 conduction, then 2:1, then 4:1 conduction before the break into NSR.

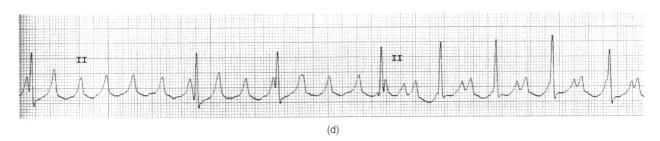

(d)

Figure 17.8d Paper speed 50 mm/s, 1 cm/mV, lead II, same canine, showing variable degrees of AVB during atrial flutter. The positive flutter waves in lead II suggest **reverse typical Isthmus-dependent atrial flutter**.

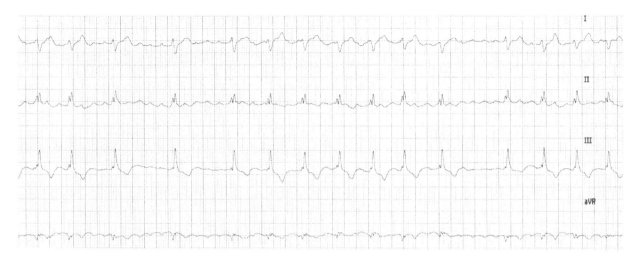

Figure 17.9 Paper speed 50 mm/s, 2 cm/mV, leads I, II, III, avR, feline with severe tricuspid dysplasia and right atrial enlargement. **Atrial flutter**, likely Type I clockwise. Note the regular baseline undulations (positive in the inferiors) at an approximate rate of 600 bpm, indicative of organized atrial activity. Variable degrees of AVB results in an irregular ventricular rate response. In the middle of the strip, 4:1 conduction results in a regular ventricular rate response. The QRS complexes are widened from pre-existing **RBBB**.

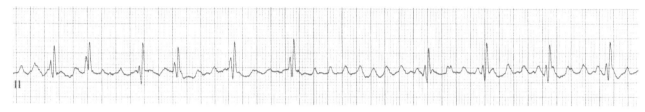

Figure 17.10 Paper speed 50 mm/s, 1 cm/mV, lead II, canine with TVDysplasia/Ebstein's-type anomaly. **Type II AFL**. The ventricular rate response in this patient was grossly irregular and during pauses, irregular flutter waves are seen (i.e. between the sixth and seventh complexes) at a rate of approximately 600 bpm. The QRS complexes are splintered (rsR') typical of that associated with TVD.

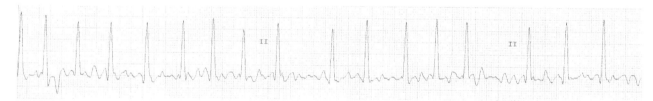

Figure 17.11 Paper speed 50 mm/s, 1 cm/mV, lead II, canine. **Atrial flutter/fibrillation**. This may be non-cavotricuspid isthmus-dependent AFL (Type II, flutter rate nearly 750 bpm) or simply coarse atrial fibrillation. This patient had hepatic neoplasia and annuloaortic ectasia.

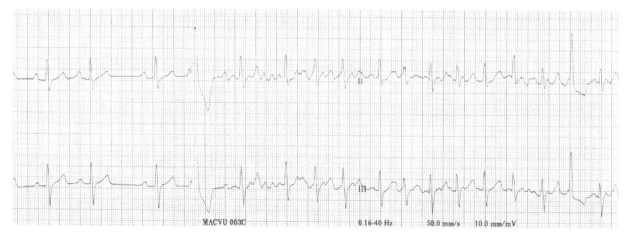

Figure 17.12 Paper speed 50 mm/s, 1 cm/mV, leads II and III, canine undergoing pericardiocentesis. A VPC initiates transient **atrial flutter/fibrillation**. Note that the first P wave following the VPC is immediately followed by an ectopic P' that occurs during the Ta wave – this so-called "**P on Ta**" is a common trigger for atrial fibrillation.

Atrioventricular block Due to the rapid atrial rate during AFL, functional/physiologic AVB is the rule and may result in a regular or irregular ventricular rhythm. AVB can change from a low to a higher grade (progressive AVB) or from a high to a lower grade of block (regressive AVB). Progressive AVB is typified by Wenckebach periodicity where the F-R intervals of conducted beats gradually increase until a greater degree of block ensues. Regressive AVB has two forms. Most commonly, an initially consistent number of non-conducted F waves suddenly changes to a lower grade of block, and an increase in the ratio of conducted to non-conducted F waves is seen. The F wave responsible for the regression has a longer F-R interval than the previous F-R intervals. Rarely, no constant F-R intervals are seen, and this is termed "reverse alternating Wenckebach mode." In these situations, regression from low- to high-grade block is associated with gradually decreasing F-R intervals and R-R intervals that are not constant. The lower grade of block is characterized by a conducted F-R interval that is longer than the previously gradually decreasing F-R intervals.

Furthermore, more than one level of AVB within the AVN may occur. The AVN is functionally divided into three levels: an upper (atrionodal or AN) level, a middle (nodal or N) level, and a lower (nodal-His or NH) level. Integral conduction block (non-Wenckebach) in an upper level can even coexist with a non-integral conduction block (Wenckebach) at a more distal level. The ventricular rate response pattern may occasionally only be explained by such phenomena during AFL. Rate-related aberrancy may frequently produce right bundle branch block on complexes terminating short cycle lengths. Such alterations in cycle length frequently occur during AFL, especially with alternation of 2:1 and 4:1 conduction. This is from Ashman's phenomenon and should not be confused with ventricular ectopy (see Chapter 6).

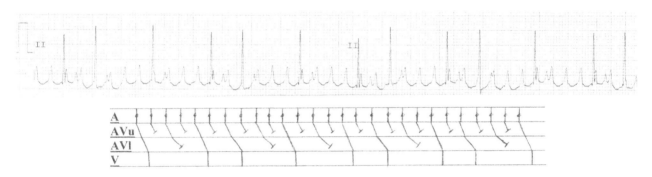

Figure 17.13 Paper speed 25 mm/s, 1 cm/mV, lead II, canine. **AFL** is present with two levels of block within the AVN. This arrhythmia can be explained by 2:1 block in the upper AVN region and 3:2 alternating with 2:1 block in the lower AVN region with Wenckebach phenomenon.

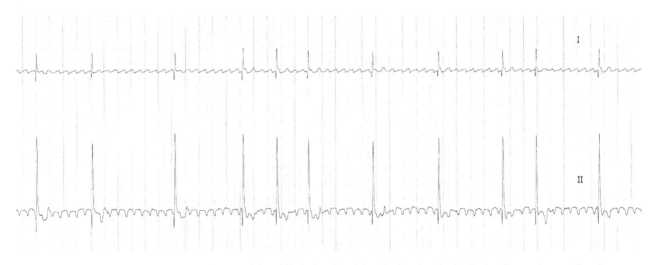

Figure 17.14 Paper speed 25 mm/s, 1 cm/mV, leads I and II. Cocker Spaniel with chronic mitral valvular disease (not on digoxin or antiarrhythmics). **Type I typical AFL**. *High-grade atrioventricular block* is present with a slow and irregular ventricular rate response. Which complexes may represent junctional escape beats is unclear given the irregular ventricular rhythm and variable F-R intervals. The relatively slow ventricular rate response is actually a good thing for the dog, at least for the time being. Progression to third degree AVB could lead to symptomatic bradycardia, however, necessitating pacemaker implantation.

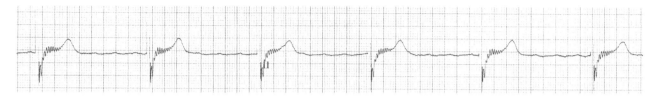

Figure 17.15 Paper speed 50 mm/s, 1 cm/mV, lead II, *feline* with history of third degree AVB and epicardial pacemaker. Fine, regular, positive undulations of the baseline here are indicative of reverse-typical Isthmus-dependent **atrial flutter** *or* focal atrial tachycardia. The atrial rate is approximately 300 bpm. Lack of associated supraventricular complexes indicates third degree AVB. The ventricular pacemaker is capturing the ventricles at a rate of approximately 63 bpm. Atrial flutter is extremely rare in the cat. A 60-Hertz interference ("ringing") artifact is present in the S-T segment.

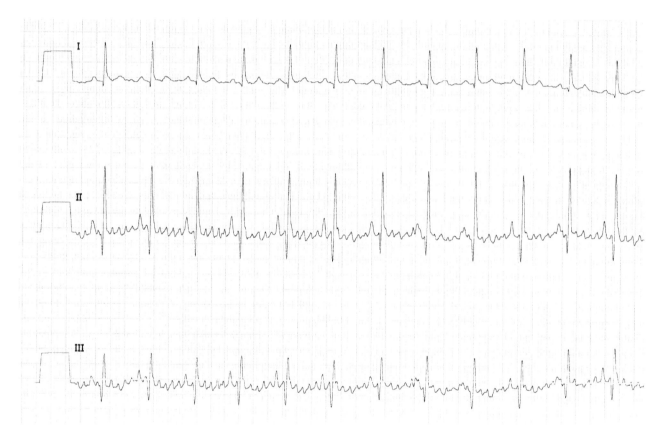

Figure 17.16 Paper speed 50 mm/s, 1 cm/mV, leads I, II, III, canine. A quick glance at lead II shows seemingly regular baseline deflections occur suggestive of atrial flutter; however, these most likely represent **artifact.** They do not disturb the underlying rhythm, which marches through the deflections unchanged. Lead I appears fairly normal as the flutter-like deflections as seen in the other leads here are isoelectric. This suggests movement in LL electrode as the culprit.

While functional AVB is the norm during AFL, pathologic AVB is characterized by an inappropriately low ventricular rate response and may be associated with sick sinus syndrome (see Chapter 11). If the second degree AVB is high grade, the ventricular rate response may be irregular and which QRS complexes represent junctional escapes may be unclear if the F-R intervals are variable. A regular, slow supraventricular rhythm during AFL suggests third degree AVB with junctional escape rhythm (if the rate is consistent with junctional escape). A regular, slow rhythm with prolongation of the QRS complexes suggests third degree AVB with ventricular escape rhythm (if the rate is consistent with ventricular escape). The combination of AF or atrial flutter and third degree AVB has been termed as Frederick syndrome.

Artifacts Atrial flutter may be mimicked by a variety of EKG artifacts. Baseline artifact from muscle tremors or panting may give the appearance of atrial flutter. Purring baseline artifact in cats is not uncommon and produces a phasic respiratory flutter on EKG at an unphysiologically high flutter rate.

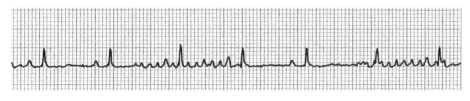

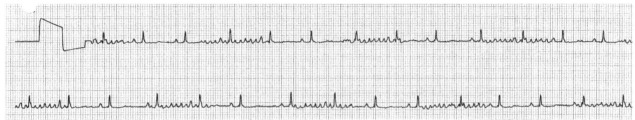

Figure 17.17 Paper speed 50 mm/s, 1 cm/mV, lead II, feline. The top strip appears to have baseline undulations that may be mistaken for atrial flutter. A longer continuous strip reveals the undulations are phasic with respiration, and independent of the underlying sinus rhythm. This cat was **purring**. Note that the atrial rate for the "flutter" is at least 1500 bpm, which is not physiologic.

Further reading

Adams, A.K. and Keene, B.W. (2007). ECG of the month. *JAVMA* 231 (2): 209–211.

Armenano, R.A., Schmidt, M.K., and Maisenbacher, H.W. III, (2010). ECG of the month. *JAVMA* 236 (1): 51–53.

Cocchiaro, M.F. and Kittleson, M.D. (2010). ECG of the month. *JAVMA* 236 (8): 836–838.

Fisch, C. and Knoebel, S.B. (2000). *Electrocardiography of Clinical Arrhythmias*. Futurama Publishing Co.

Good, L., Cote, E., and Wright, K. (2002). ECG of the month. *JAVMA* 221 (8).

Machen, M.C., Estrada, A.H., and Prosék, R. (2008). ECG of the month. *JAVMA* 233 (11): 1694–1696.

Marriott, H.J. (1998). *Pearls & Pitfalls in Electrocardiography, Pithy Practical Pointers*, 2e. Williams & Wilkins.

Marriot, H.J.L. and Conover, M.B. (1998). *Advanced Concepts in Arrhythmias*, 3e. Mosby.

Nelson, W.P., Marriott, H.J.L., and Schocken, D.D. (2007). *Concepts & Cautions in Electrocardiography*. MedInfo Inc.

Wiley, L.E. and Trafny, D.J. ECG of the month. *JAVMA* 248 (11): 1245–1247.

18

Atrial Fibrillation

CHAPTER MENU

Atrial fibrillation, 196
Aberrancy, 201
   Ashman's phenomenon, 201
Ventricular ectopics, 203
Atrioventricular dissociation, 204
Concealed conduction, 207

Atrial fibrillation Though atrial fibrillation may manifest with a rapid, normal, or slow ventricular rate response, it is included under atrial tachyarrhythmias as the atrial myocardium is rapidly depolarizing in a chaotic manner. You should be able to not only suspect atrial fibrillation from physical, but also be able to identify it on surface EKG from across the room. Generally, the examiner is unable to discern AF on physical examination from an animal in sinus rhythm with very frequent (often multifocal) premature beats. That said, AF sounds like "tennis shoes in a dryer" or bongo drums on auscultation of the heart. Usually, the ventricular rate is rapid (>170–180 bpm), pulse deficits are present, and the rhythm is classically "irregularly irregular." Atrial tissue needs a certain surface area to generate and sustain AF. This means larger animals such as horses, humans, and giant breed dogs possess enough atrial tissue with atria of normal dimensions to generate and sustain AF. Giant breed dogs with so-called "lone AF" (Primary AF) with otherwise normal hearts and a relatively slow ventricular rate response are a particular treatment dilemma for us (do we cardiovert or manage ventricular rate response with drugs?).

Atrial fibrillation is said to beget AF, meaning the electrical instability of AF is shown to create permanent changes in atrial tissue that further predisposes it to AF. Animals with rapid and sustained AF frequently go on to develop myocardial disease (tachycardia-induced cardiomyopathy), and humans are known to be at significant risk of stroke (not seen in dogs, but certainly the case in cats). Slow AF can also be trickier to discern by auscultation, whereas fast or malignant AF (Secondary AF) is usually obvious. One or more "mother rotor" waves, usually originating in or around the pulmonary venous ostia of the left atrium, may be the root cause of atrial fibrillation, which is why the surgical "maze" procedures and radiofrequency ablation with electrical isolation of the pulmonary venous ostia are therapeutic options in humans suffering from chronic or paroxysmal AF. Grossly, the atria in fibrillation have the so-called appearance of a "bag of worms," with irregular and uncoordinated mechanical activity.

During AF, multiple "microreentrant" wavelets of depolarization (atrial rate often 700–900 bpm) course across the atrial tissue, which cause complete lack of organized contraction. This lack of coordinated atrial contraction is what contributes to the decrease in cardiac output (up to 25% decrease). The atrioventricular (AV) node acts as the electrical gatekeeper, allowing impulses to be transmitted only when it is no longer refractory. The chaotic atrial electrical wavelets bombard the AV node randomly, and concealed conduction results in the irregularly irregular ventricular rate and so-called "absolute ventricular arrhythmia." Criteria for malignant AF include:

1) **High ventricular rate: 180 + bpm** (usually, however the rate may be normal if controlled on medication, or low if significant AVB is present).
2) **Supraventricular/narrow QRS complexes** (usually, but commonly may be prolonged from ventricular enlargement or rarely wide/bizarre from underlying bundle branch block/interventricular conduction defect

Interpretation of the Electrocardiogram in Small Animals, First Edition. Nick A. Schroeder.
© 2021 John Wiley & Sons Inc. Published 2021 by John Wiley & Sons Inc.

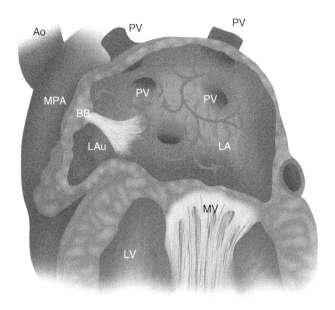

Figure 18.1 Illustration of the left atrium and mechanism of atrial fibrillation. **Ao**: aorta, **MPA**: main pulmonary artery, **PV**: pulmonary vein, **LA**: left atrium, **LAu**: left auricle, **BB**: Bachman's bundle, **MV**: mitral valve, **LV**: left ventricle.

or escape rhythm during complete atrioventricular block/AVB).

3) **Irregularly irregular rhythm** (usually, but may be pseudonormal from very fast or very slow rates; may be regular if complete AVB and escape rhythm present or if atrioventricular dissociation/AVD is present secondary to usurpation from an accelerated idiojunctional/idioventricular rhythm or junctional/ventricular tachycardia). If fibrillating atria are in control of the ventricles, the rhythm will always be irregularly irregular.

4) **Complete absence of P waves in all leads** (the baseline may be apparently flat or undulating).

If the R-R interval is not consistent whatsoever and P waves are not present, you are likely looking at AF. Normal sinus P waves are replaced by "f" waves representing fibrillatory activity of the atria. These f waves may be most evident in V1. Fine AF has a very minimally undulating baseline, and the baseline in coarse AF is all over the place. Absolute ventricular arrhythmia is the hallmark of AF and usually most obvious when the heart rate is between 100 and 200 bpm. The only time AF is confusing is when it is occurring at such a rapid rate and the QRS complexes come so close together (or when the ventricular rate response is so slow and the QRS complexes far apart) that the R-R interval artifactually may appear regular. Fortuitous pairing during AF may result in a bigeminal

rhythm. Run your strips at 50 mm/s if the heart rate is over 200 bpm and 25 mm/s if the heart rate is under 100 bpm and get your calipers out. You can detect R-R variability much easier this way. Examine the other leads, as P waves may be yet present and simply not obvious in lead II. On occasion, AF can mimic ventricular tachycardia (VT). This occurs most often when AF is conducted with a bundle branch block, giving wide, negative QRS complexes (if right bundle branch block, RBBB), that if occurring at a rapid rate may really look like VT. Left ventricular enlargement, frequently concomitant with the prerequisite left atrial enlargement associated with AF, will similarly prolong the QRS complexes, potentially confusing the clinician with VT. If AF is present, there should be no P waves otherwise indicative of coordinated atrial depolarization. Remember, P waves should be seen during VT, they are just typically dissociated, so they march in and out of the ventricular complexes or are retrograde and follow the QRS complexes if ventriculoatrial/VA conduction is present. If P waves are buried within QRS complexes or T waves, they are generally inapparent.

Atrial fibrillation is one of the most common arrhythmias in small animals. It takes significant atrial enlargement in small breed animals with heart disease (usually chronic mitral valvular disease/CMVDz in dogs and cardiomyopathy in cats) to allow for the development of AF. Sudden onset of AF in an otherwise compensated dog with valvular disease often results in decompensation (sudden pulmonary edema), syncope, etc. Atrial fibrillation may be triggered by very early supraventricular premature complexes (SVPCs) that occur during the vulnerable period of atrial repolarization (so-called "P on Ta", analagous to R on T phenomenon for the triggering of ventricular fibrillation). Killip's rule has stated that if the P-P' interval is less than ½ of the preceding P-P interval, then ectopic beat can possibly land on the Ta wave, initiating AF. Interratrial block (profound P mitrale), frequent and often multifocal SVPCs, persistent sinus tachycardia, and other supraventricular tachycardias (paroxysmal automatic atrial tachycardia, multifocal atrial tachycardia, atrial flutter) are considered to be risk factors for the eventual development of AF, especially if associated with severe atrial enlargement. Atrial fibrillation can be paroxysmal and has been reportedly associated with hypothermia. Generally, AF is usually sustained. Thus, treatment of AF is directed at controlling the ventricular rate response (i.e. slowing conduction through the AV node with digoxin and calcium-channel blockers if active CHF/secondary AF or using beta-blockers if primary AF). Due to the risk of stroke in humans, AF is usually attempted to be converted medically or with catheter ablation or surgery. However, studies have shown that rate control is as effective as conversion to sinus rhythm. The longer the R-R interval, the more time for ventricular filling, the better the cardiac output, and the stronger the pulse. Cardioversion in dogs/cats typically requires general anesthesia, which presents risks in those with severe underlying heart disease. Dogs in AF are not generally considered to be at risk for arterial thromboembolism, though cats (and possibly Cavalier King Charles Spaniels with macrothrombocytopenia?) in AF almost always are. Atrial fibrillation that (usually temporarily) happens to convert to sinus rhythm in small animals with severe cardiac disease and left atrial enlargement can be associated with a paradoxical decrease in blood pressure and transient worsening of the clinical signs of congestive heart failure. This is from post-tachycardia "stunning" of the myocardium. This is why gradual reduction of the ventricular rate response with drug therapy is often preferable to cardioversion to sinus rhythm. Remember that the response to CHF is usually tachycardia in an effort to maintain perfusion in the face of decreased cardiac output. Drastic and rapid reduction of the heart rate in this situation may be a bad thing for the patient.

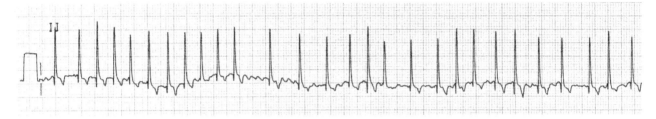

Figure 18.2 Paper speed 25 mm/s, 1 cm/mV, lead II, canine, **AF**. The HR varies between 150 and 300 bpm.

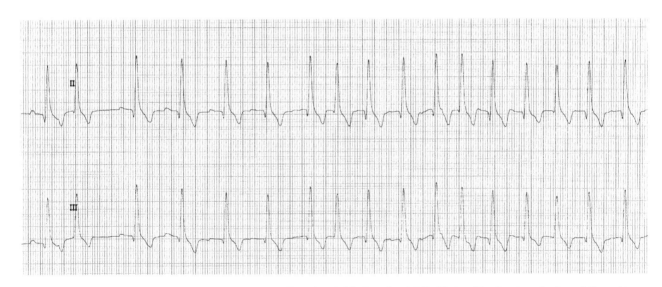

Figure 18.3 Paper speed 50 mm/s, 1 cm/mV, leads II and III, canine. **Initiation of atrial fibrillation**. The first beat is sinus, followed by an APC. Atrial fibrillation ensues at beat #5 with an onset of an irregularly irregular ventricular rhythm with absent P waves on baseline. Presumably, an APC occurred on Ta wave, initiating AF ("P on Ta"). The P'-Pi of the first APC is shorter than half the P-Pi cycle length in keeping with *Killip's rule*.

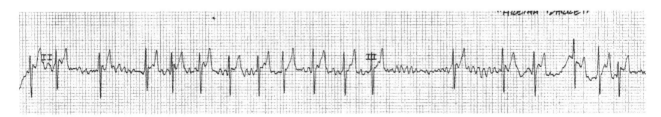

Figure 18.4 Paper speed 25 mm/s, 1 cm/mV, lead II, canine, coarse **AF** with **right axis deviation** (deep S waves).

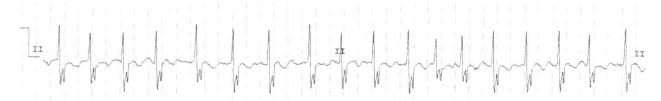

Figure 18.5 Paper speed 25 mm/s, 1 cm/mV, lead II, feline, coarse **AF** with **RAD** and QRS prolongation from an **interventricular conduction disturbance**.

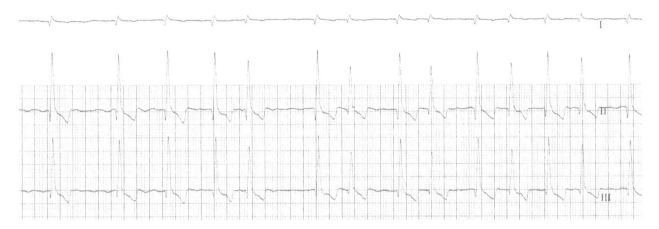

Figure 18.6 Paper speed 50 mm/s, 1 cm/mV, leads I, II, III, canine. **Atrial fibrillation** and **electrical alternans with fortuitous pairing**. After the fifth complex, the QRS-T amplitudes alternate, which is most evident in leads II and III. This is likely a function of the HR as the shorter amplitudes occur after short cycle lengths. Fortuitous pairing during AF is a cause of a bigeminal rhythm. Close examination of the R-R intervals reveals enough variation to be consistent with atrial fibrillation with intact anterograde conduction.

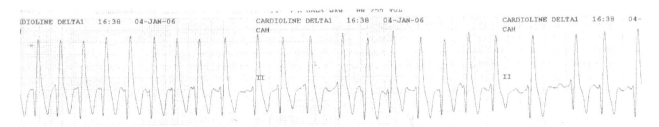

Figure 18.7 Paper speed 50 mm/s, 1 cm/mV, lead II, canine with generalized cardiomegaly, **fast AF**. Biventricular enlargement is evident as the QRS complexes are prolonged from ventricular enlargement, and deep Q waves are present. The ventricular rate is approximately 200–300 bpm.

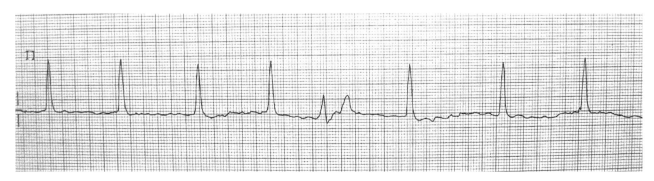

Figure 18.8 Paper speed 50 mm/s, 1 cm/mV, lead II, canine, **slow atrial fibrillation**, the fifth complex may be a VPC or an aberrantly conducted supraventricular complex. Slow AF can be difficult to discern as the R-R intervals may not be obviously variable (pseudo-regularized ventricular rhythm). The HR is approximately 120 bpm.

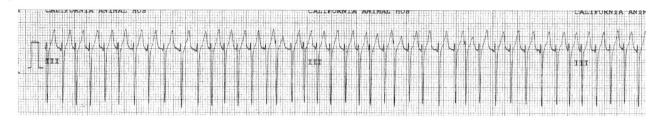

Figure 18.9 Paper speed 25 mm/s, 1 cm/mV, lead III, feline, fast AF. **Left axis deviation** resulted in negative R waves in this patient. The R-R interval variability also becomes more difficult to ascertain at such rapid heart rates, resulting in **pseudo-regularization** of the ventricular rhythm.

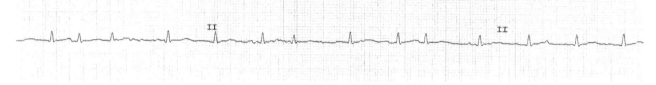

Figure 18.10 Paper speed 50 mm/s, 1 cm/mV, lead II, feline, AF with slow ventricular response rate due to propranolol administration.

Atrial fibrillation may be characterized by how undulating the baseline is. The so-called f waves of AF may not be obvious in a single lead depending on projection. Thus, it is often better to look for the characteristically "irregularly irregular" ventricular rate response. This leads to a so-called "absolute arrhythmia" in which the R-R intervals constantly change and is an indication of atrioventricular association during AF (i.e. the fibrillating atria are "in-charge" of the ventricles). Atrial fibrillation may be termed fine, medium, or coarse. Coarse AF may be more common in patients with extremely severe left atrial enlargement, especially if it is new in onset.

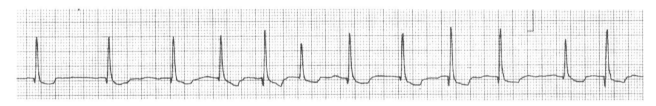

Figure 18.11 Paper speed 50 mm/s, 1 cm/mV, lead II, canine. **Fine AF**. The baseline is only minimally undulating. Thus, "f" waves may not always be obvious.

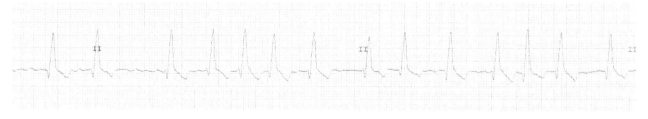

Figure 18.12 Paper speed 50 mm/s, 1 cm/mV, lead II, canine. **Medium AF**. The baseline is more undulatory.

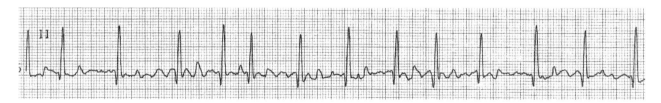

Figure 18.13 Paper speed 50 mm/s, 1 cm/mV, lead II, canine. **Coarse AF**. The baseline undulates markedly, nearly mimicking atrial flutter. Alternatively, this may represent fibrillo-flutter (or **Type II AFL**), which may also be the result of the left atrium being in fibrillation, while the right atrium is in atrial flutter (**atrial dissociation**).

Aberrancy While it is not uncommon to see mild prolongation of the QRS complex in patients with atrial fibrillation from underlying left ventricular enlargement, aberrancy of the QRS will prolong the complexes from bundle branch block or occasionally from nonspecific interventricular conduction disturbances (see Chapter 8). Atrial fibrillation and RBBB classically mimics left ventricular tachycardia. The clue to atrioventricular association is the irregularly irregular rhythm, which is rare with monomorphic ventricular tachycardia and a hallmark of atrial fibrillation.

Ashman's phenomenon It is thought to be relatively common during AF due to the variable R-R intervals and is frequently confused with ventricular premature complexes/VPCs. During AF, if a relatively long cycle length occurs, the short one that follows may be aberrant in conduction. RBBB of a supraventricular impulse is favored (since the relative refractory period of the right bundle branch is shorter than that of the left bundle branch). Two reasons why this may just be wrong have been postulated. First, by Rule of bigeminy, a lengthened cycle tends to precipitate a VPC. Second, because of concealed conduction, it is never known when a bundle branch is activated from surface EKG. If an aberrant beat does end a long-short cycle during AF, it may be due to refractoriness of a bundle branch secondary to concealed conduction into it rather than due to changes in the length of the ventricular cycle. Left ventricular originating VPCs (with a RBBB-like morphology) are also common in patients with left ventricular enlargement associated with chronic mitral valvular disease or dilated cardiomyopathy regardless of whether or not the patient is in AF. Aberrancy is favored if the preceding R-R interval is disproportionately long (considering underlying R-R variability) and the post-extrasystolic beat is relatively closely coupled. If the post-extrasystolic beat is very closely coupled, then reentry from a V-A-V echo

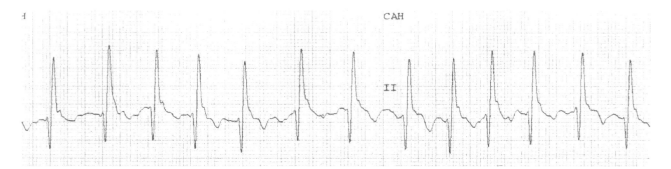

Figure 18.14 Paper speed 50 mm/s, 1 cm/mV, lead II, Doberman with cardiomyopathy. **Atrial fibrillation** is present. The notch on the downward stroke of the R waves is suggestive of **microscopic intramural myocardial infarction** (MIMI) representing a nonspecific intraventricular conduction defect occasionally seen in advanced cardiac disease.

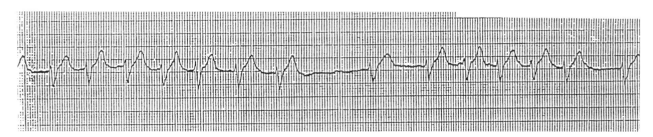

Figure 18.15 Paper speed 50 mm/s, 1 cm/mV, lead II, canine. **Atrial fibrillation** with **RBBB**. This arrhythmia is a classic impostor of VT. There are no visible P waves and the R-R interval is irregularly irregular, indicative of AF. The deep and wide S waves are consistent with RBBB.

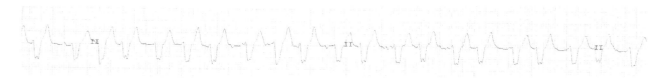

Figure 18.16 Paper speed 50 mm/s, 1 cm/mV, lead II, feline. **Atrial fibrillation** with **RBBB**. AF was paroxysmal in this patient and the second complex is a sinus capture.

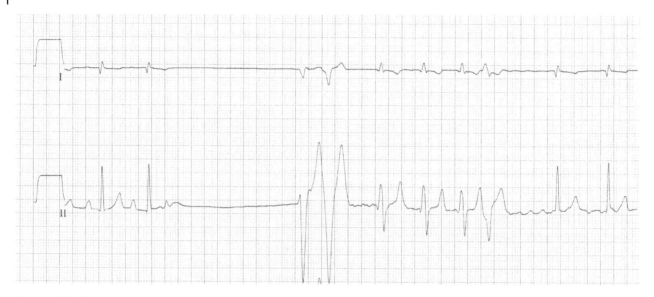

Figure 18.17 Paper speed 50 mm/s, 1 cm/mV, leads I and II, canine undergoing pericardiocentesis. **Initiation of atrial fibrillation.** The first two beats are sinus. A non-conducted APC occurs on the T wave of beat #2. This is followed by a sinus arrest terminated by a pair of ventricular ectopics, which initiate atrial fibrillation. Note the retrograde P′ following the first ventricular beat indicating VA conduction. The fifth–eighth beats appear to be supraventricular with RBBB aberration, and the irregularly irregular rhythm and undulating baseline indicates atrial fibrillation. Normal intraventricular conduction resumes after a pause in the rhythm, indicating a rate-dependent BBB.

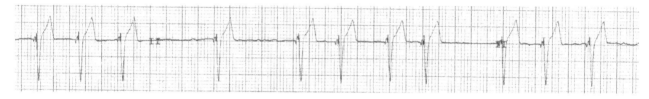

Figure 18.18 Paper speed 25 mm/s, 1 cm/mV, lead II, canine. **Atrial fibrillation** with **RBBB** and a slower ventricular response rate (HR approximately 75–100 bpm).

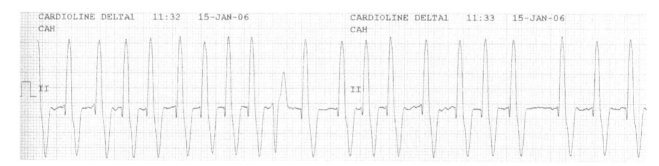

Figure 18.19 Paper speed 25 mm/s, 0.5 cm/mV, lead II, canine. **Atrial fibrillation** with **LBBB**. This is another example of AF mimicking VT. No visible P waves are present, and the R-R interval is irregularly irregular, indicating AF. The ninth complex is a VPC.

(reciprocal beat following a VPC from concealed reentry) is possible. This concept is important clinically, as the presence of VPCs during AF suggests active congestive heart failure, fibrosis associated with cardiomyopathy, myocardial ischemia, or even digoxin toxicity. This should signal the clinician to treat accordingly (i.e. give more diuretic, start positive inotropic administration, discontinue or reduce digoxin). If aberrancy secondary to Ashman's phenomenon is evident, then it is largely incidental, should be ignored, and treatment of the underlying AF is the focus.

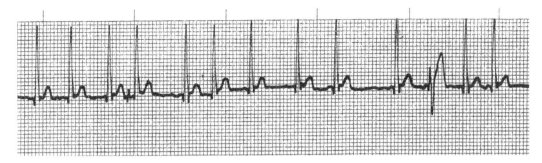

Figure 18.20 Paper speed 25 mm/s, 1 cm/mV, lead II, canine. AF. The 11th complex may demonstrate *Ashman's phenomenon*. A long interval between R waves makes it more likely that an early stimulus will result in RBBB aberration since the refractory period of the R bundle branch is longer than that of the left bundle branch. The interval between the 9th and 10th complexes is approximately 640 milliseconds. The 11th complex comes approximately 400 milliseconds after the 10th complex and is conducted with RBBB morphology. The lack of a "compensatory-like pause" following this beat is suggestive of aberrancy vs. ventricular ectopy. Alternatively, if the 11th complex is actually a VPC, then the 12th could arguably be a reciprocal complex (as opposed to a supraventricular beat).

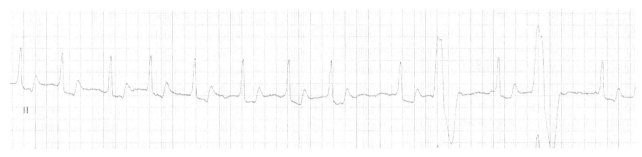

Figure 18.21 Paper speed 50 mm/s, 1 cm/mV, lead II, Great Dane. **Atrial fibrillation and ventricular bigeminy**. The relatively long R-R interval between the eighth and ninth beats elicits a VPC, which in turn creates a "compensatory-like" pause. This creates another long-short sequence that favors the formation of another VPC and perpetuation of ventricular bigeminy by the Rule of bigeminy.

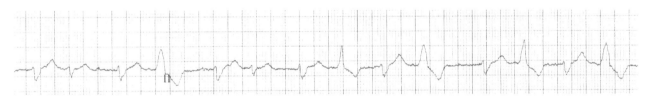

Figure 18.22 Paper speed 50 mm/s, 1 cm/mV, lead II, feline with UCM. Atrial fibrillation and **ventricular bigeminy**. The supraventricular complexes display RBBB, and the underlying rhythm is irregularly irregular without identifiable P waves, indicative of atrial fibrillation. The ventricular rate is approximately 150–200 bpm since this cat was digitalized. VPCs appear following beats that end relatively long cycles following short cycles. The VPCs here are wide and bizarre (LBBB-like pattern, inferior axis). The VPCs tend to create "compensatory-like pauses," which in turn create another long cycle, which initiates another VPC, perpetuating a bigeminal rhythm according to the *Rule of bigeminy*. The sudden appearance of ventricular bigeminy in this patient may be an indication of digoxin toxicity, and a serum digoxin level is warranted.

Ventricular ectopics

Ventricular ectopy during atrial fibrillation posits a conundrum for interpreters of the EKG for many reasons. Ventricular premature complexes during AF can only be defined by vague terms under the best of circumstances. During the irregularly irregular ventricular rhythm associated with atrial fibrillation and intact AV nodal conduction, what exactly constitutes a "premature beat" is quite dubious. If a wide-complex premature beat occurs during AF, is it the result of Ashman's phenomenon/functional RBBB or is it a left ventricular extrasystole (see below and Chapter 24)? What constitutes interpolation vs. a "compensatory like pause" (see Chapter 24)? If a wide-complex beat occurs following a pause in the rhythm during AF, at what point can it be considered to be a junctional escape with deceleration-dependent aberrancy, a ventricular escape, or an accelerated ventricular escape (see Chapters 6, 19, and 23)? Ventricular fusions support ventricular ectopy. The lack of a compensatory-like pause

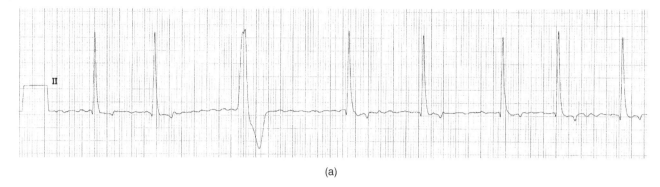

(a)

Figure 18.23a Paper speed 50 mm/S, 1 cm/mV, lead II, canine. **Atrial fibrillation**. The third complex had a prolonged QRS and is of unknown origin. Critical rate deceleration bundle branch block or junctional escape with aberrancy seems unlikely due to a LBBB-like morphology and the fact that the post-extrasystolic R-Ri is longer than the R-R' interval.

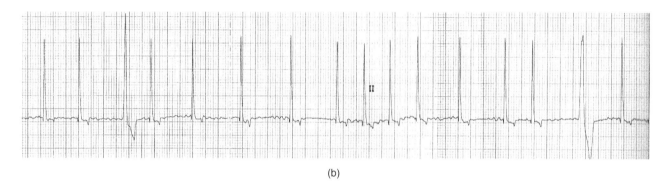

(b)

Figure 18.23b Paper speed 25 mm/S, 1 cm/mV, lead II, same dog. Atrial fibrillation with **ventricular ectopics**. The third QRS is a ventricular fusion evidenced by the slightly narrower QRS duration – making the ectopic beats almost certainly ventricular in origin. Though pauses precede the prolonged QRS complexes, the R-R' interval is variable – making left ventricular escapes a little less likely.

and bigeminal rhythms also support ventricular ectopy. If a pause is terminated by an escape with a wide QRS complex within the expected range of interval of escape and is of RBBB morphology, then a junctional escape with deceleration-dependent aberrancy is favored. If a pause during AF is terminated with a wide QRS complex with a consistent and longer interval of escape, then a ventricular escape focus is favored. Practically, it may be nearly impossible to determine if intermittent wide QRS complexes during atrial fibrillation represent ventricular premature beats, escape complexes, accelerated escapes, or aberrantly conducted supraventricular beats from surface EKG.

> *A Note:* Obviously, SVPCs (ectopic sinoatrial or atrial extrasystoles) are not possible during AF with intact AV nodal conduction. Junctional premature complexes are indeterminate from those impulses generated from fibrillatory conduction from the atria. Junctional escapes may occur during AF with a slow ventricular rate response or high-grade AV block by default and acceleration of a junctional focus may result in a regular rhythm with supraventricular QRS during AF, indicative of AV dissociation secondary to usurpation (see below).

Atrioventricular dissociation A regular ventricular rhythm usually disputes AF or suggests AV block or supports usurpation in the presence of intact AV nodal or accessory pathway anterograde conduction. Pseudo-regularization of the ventricular rhythm during AF with intact anterograde AV nodal conduction may occur with an excessively slow or fast ventricular rate response during AF. Atrial fibrillation and AVD by default from high-grade second degree AVB may have a slow, irregular ventricular rate response. If isolated junctional escapes are present, they are likely indistinguishable from supraventricular captures, but they are expected following long pauses and suspected if the rhythm is periodically supraventricular, regular, slow, and consistent in rate with junctional escape for short periods of time. Wide QRS complexes following long pauses are consistent with ventricular escapes. A slow ventricular rate response during untreated atrial fibrillation suggests the possibility of sick sinus syndrome in susceptible breeds (i.e. Miniature Schnauzers, Cocker Spaniels). If third degree AVB develops, the ventricular rhythm is regular, slow, and the QRS complexes are supraventricular at a rate consistent with junctional escape rhythm. If bundle branch block of the escape focus is concomitant, junctional escape rhythm is indistinguishable from an accelerated idioventricular rhythm. If the QRS complexes are prolonged and the rate is consistent with a ventricular escape focus, then ventricular escape is likely and the term Fredrick's syndrome has been coined. Pacemaker implantation may be considered for clinical bradycardia if the ventricular rate response and/or escape rate is excessively slow. Atrioventricular dissociation secondary to usurpation may occur during AF if an accelerated idiojunctional rhythm or accelerated idiofascicular/idioventricular

rhythm captures the ventricles. The heart rate will be between 80 and 180 bpm and the rhythm will be regular. The sudden appearance of such accelerated rhythms during otherwise controlled AF suggests the possibility of digoxin toxicity or occult neoplasia (i.e. splenic/hepatic masses). Atrioventricular dissociation from overt junctional or ventricular tachycardia during otherwise controlled AF may produce a rapid, regular ventricular rhythm as well, and appropriate therapy (i.e. discontinuation of digoxin if toxicity is suspected, use of diltiazem, sotalol, or mexiletine) should be instituted.

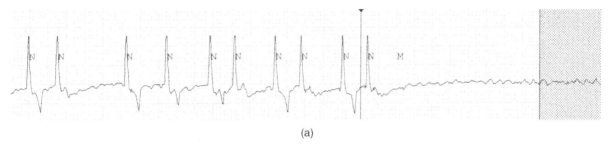

(a)

Figure 18.24a Paper speed 25 mm/s, 1 cm/mV, lead II, canine, **AF** with **AVB**. This patient was normally in rapid AF but had bouts of syncope related to intermittent ventricular asystole from paroxysmal AVB.

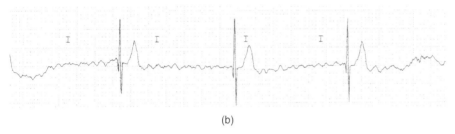

(b)

Figure 18.24b Paper speed 25 mm/s, 1 cm/mV, lead II, same dog, **AF** with **AVB** and a **junctional escape rhythm** of 45 bpm. AF is diagnosed by the absence of P waves and the undulation of the baseline between QRS complexes. If the QRS complexes appear at a fixed, regular rate, this suggests a subsidiary pacemaker below the AVN has captured the ventricles. Usually if this occurs, a wide and bizarre ventricular escape rhythm is present. The relatively narrow QRS complexes seen here suggest a His bundle focus and possibly supernormal conduction. The upright T waves are also different than the negative T waves during typical AF in the above strip.

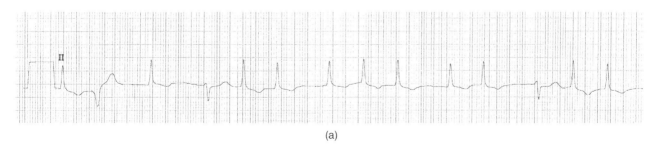

(a)

Figure 18.25a Paper speed 50 mm/s, 1 cm/mV, lead II, feline. **Atrial fibrillation** with **AVB** and **junctional escape complexes**. The first complex is conducted and is followed by a VPC. The 3rd and 11th complexes are followed by pauses terminated by an escape complex with an aberrant QRS. The rest of the complexes are upright and the rhythm irregularly irregular with no discernable P waves consistent with AF. This cat was on no antiarrhythmic medication at the time. The relatively slow ventricular rate response with escape beats suggests significant AV block.

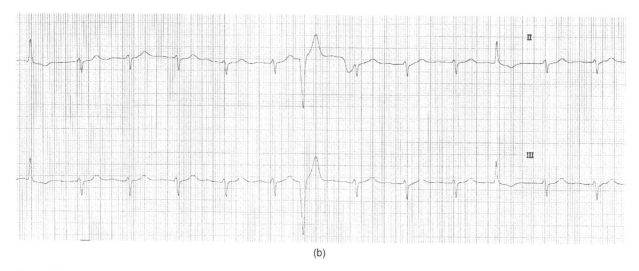

(b)

Figure 18.25b Paper speed 50 mm/s, 1 cm/mV, leads II and III, same cat. Longer periods of regular **escape rhythm** with one VPC appear consistent with AVD by *default* secondary to AVB. The escape rhythm at approximately 140 bpm is most consistent with a junctional escape rhythm (with iRBBB aberrancy). A less likely rule out would be an accelerated idiofascicular rhythm.

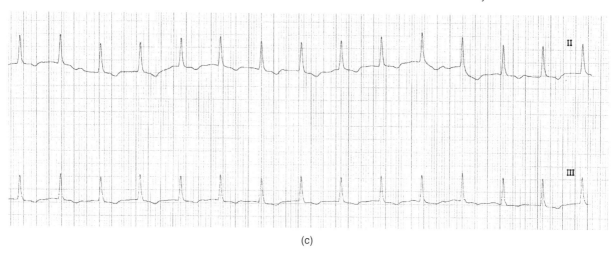

(c)

Figure 18.25c Paper speed 50 mm/s, 1 cm/mV, leads II and III, same cat. Atrial fibrillation, apparently complete AVD secondary to *usurpation* now from an **accelerated idiojunctional rhythm/junctional tachycardia** (HR 188 bpm). No aberrancy is seen and the rhythm is supraventricular and perfectly regular. This cat was on no antiarrhythmic medication, including digoxin. Serum potassium was 3.1 mE/dl, excluding sinoventricular rhythm.

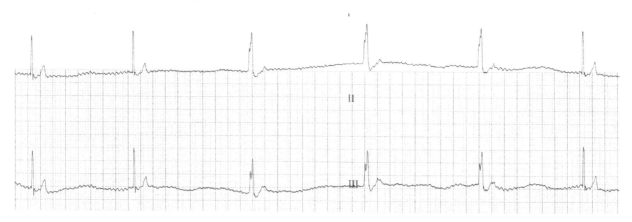

Figure 18.26 Paper speed 25 mm/s, 1 cm/mV, leads II and III, canine. **Atrial fibrillation** with **high-grade AVB** and **ventricular escape rhythm**. The baseline is undulating, and no P waves are evident, indicative of AF. The first two QRS complexes are supraventricular, then a long pause elicits a three-beat run of ventricular escape rhythm. Note the LBBB-like morphology and very slow but regular rhythm. The last beat is a supraventricular capture. The excessively *slow* ventricular rate response in this patient indicates a high-grade (though incomplete) AVB.

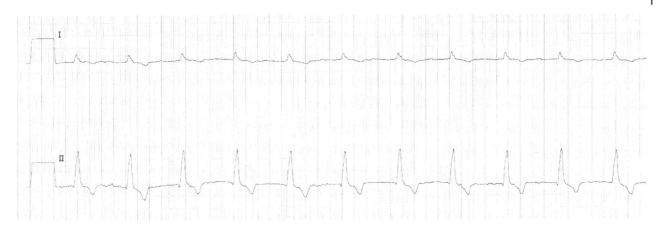

Figure 18.27 Paper speed 50 mm/s, 1 cm/mV, leads I and II. Canine treated with digoxin and diltiazem for chronic atrial fibrillation. Fibrillation of the atria, apparently complete **atrioventricular dissociation** secondary to usurpation by **accelerated idiojunctional rhythm**. The QRS complexes are mildly prolonged from L ventricular enlargement. The rhythm is completely regular and at a rate of 140 bpm. No visible P waves are present and the baseline finely undulating from AF. This finding should alert the clinician to the possibility of digoxin toxicity.

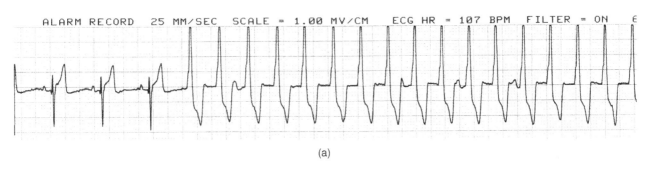

(a)

Figure 18.28a Paper speed 25 mm/s, 1 cm/mV, canine, post-op gastric-dilatation volvulus. This patient had a wide variety of arrhythmias. The first three beats show sinus rhythm with incomplete RBBB. This is followed by a right-ventricular originating tachycardia. The VT has intermittent P waves visible between ventricular beats indicating AV dissociation.

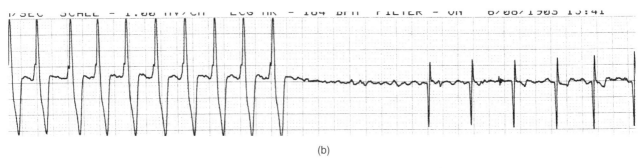

(b)

Figure 18.28b Paper speed 25 mm/s, 1 cm/mV, lead II, same dog. **Atrial fibrillation** and **ventricular tachycardia**. The ventricular tachycardia terminates and reveals AF with incomplete RBBB. Double tachycardia is often associated with digoxin intoxication, and usually consists of atrial tachycardia and VT (or fascicular tachycardia). Note the long pause following termination of VT. This is consistent with overdrive suppression from concealed retrograde conduction into the AVN by the ventricular focus.

Concealed conduction Electrical activity that is not seen on surface EKG accounts for the varied R-R interval of AF. Incomplete penetration of the AVN by rapid atrial activity occurs so that not all impulses can propagate to the ventricles. These non-conducted impulses leave the AV nodal tissue with varying degrees of refractoriness, resulting in irregular R-R intervals between conducted beats. The AVN is anterogradely depolarized to different levels. If this did not occur, AF would be totally regular, as the ventricular rate would depend on the time it took for the AVN to return to a resting state following the refractory period, and the subsequent impulses would conduct to the

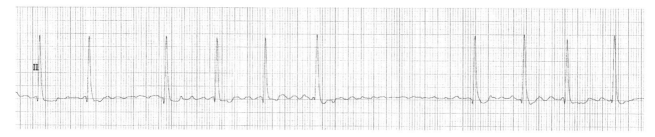

Figure 18.29 Paper speed 50 mm/s, 1 cm/mV, lead II, canine. Atrial fibrillation with an initially rapid ventricular rate response is suddenly interrupted by a long pause. This is consistent with repetitive **concealed conduction** vs. a high-grade AV block.

ventricles at apparently regular intervals. Dual AV nodal physiology has been implicated as a contributing cause of the irregularly irregular ventricular rate response of AF, as the pathways have differing refractory periods. Ablation of the slow pathway (that has the shortest refractory period and is responsible for antegrade conduction with the shortest R-R intervals during AF) reduces the heart rate. Concealed conduction also results in a slower ventricular rate response during AF than dur-

ing atrial flutter within the same patient. Repetitive concealed conduction may result in unexpectedly long pauses during otherwise rapid AF. Exit block of junctional or ventricular escapes may contribute to the pauses if they exceed expected intervals of escape. Concealed reentry may manifest as ventricular echoes following interpolated VPCs during AF with shorter than expected coupling intervals (lack of a "compensatory-like pause").

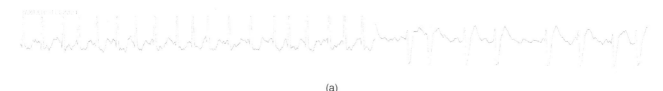

(a)

Figure 18.30a Paper speed 25 mm/s, 1 cm/mV, lead II, canine with a history of atrial fibrillation and congestive heart failure, strips are sequential, but not continuous, during euthanasia. **Atrial fibrillation** is present at the beginning of the strip with a typical upright QRS and an irregularly irregular rhythm. The second half of the strip shows a slower ventricular rate response, and BBB aberration (RBBB) of the QRS, and a persistent irregular rhythm.

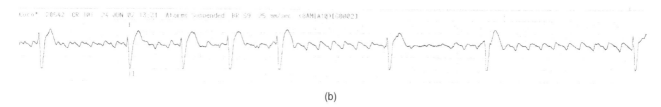

(b)

Figure 18.30b Paper speed 25 mm/s, 1 cm/mV, lead II, same dog, shortly after the above strip. The atrial fibrillation has converted to an **atrial flutter** with high-grade AVB and an irregular ventricular rate response. Between the sixth and seventh complexes, the atria transiently fibrillate again before converting into an atrial flutter.

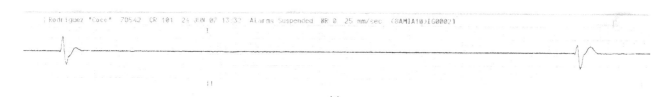

(c)

Figure 18.30c Paper speed 25 mm/s, 1 cm/mV, lead II, same dog, shortly after the above strip. **Asystole** of the atria with ventricular escape beats. The patient subsequently expired.

Further reading

Damato, A.N. and Lau, S.H. (1971). Concealed and supernormal atrioventricular conduction. *Circulation* XLIII: 967–970.

Fisch, C. and Knoebel, S.B. (2000). *Electrocardiography of Clinical Arrhythmias*. Futurama Publishing Co.

Marriot, H.J.L. (1998). *Pearls & Pitfalls in Electrocardiography*, 2e. Williams & Wilkins.

Marriot, H.J.L. and Conover, M.B. (1998). *Advanced Concepts in Arrhythmias*, 3e. Mosby.

Nelson, W.P., Marriott, H.J.L., and Schocken, D.D. (2007). *Concepts & Cautions in Electrocardiography*. MedInfo Inc.

Peckens, N.K. and Lefbom, B.K. (2008). ECG of the month. *JAVMA* 232 (11): 1642–1644.

SeungWoo, J. and Griffiths, L.G. (2011). ECG of the month. *JAVMA* 238 (10): 1258–1260.

Singletary, G.E., Kent, M., and Calvert, C.A. (2007). ECG of the month. *JAVMA* 231 (1): 44–46.

Surawicz, B. and Knilans, T.K. (2001). *Chou's Electrocardiography in Clinical Practice*, 5e. Saunders.

Junctional Arrhythmias

The atrioventricular node (AVN) is the electrical "gate-keeper" between normally electrically isolated atrial and ventricular myocytes in a region also known as the junction. There are two approaches composed of transitional cells that lead from atrial myocardium to the AVN itself. The anterosuperior (craniodorsal, "fast path") tract is located in the anterior interatrial septum near the apex of Koch's Triangle (bordered by the Tendon of Todaro, the annulus of the tricuspid valve, and the coronary sinus) and the posterioinferior (caudoventral, "slow path") tract extends from the coronary sinus. The AVN itself is situated at the base of the interatrial septum at the apex of Koch's Triangle. The cells within the AVN are densely packed, identical to the P cells in the sinoatrial node, and have interspersed transitional cells, Purkinje, and myocardial cells. The proximal portion (upper AVN) is marked by automaticity. The middle region (N region) is transitional, and the NH region is transitional from the AVN to the His bundle, which also has features of automaticity.

The P′ wave originating from a junctional focus normally has a superior axis of −80 to −100 degrees from so-called "concentric retrograde atrial activation" and the P′ wave may precede, occur during or follow the associated supraventricular QRS complex. The term "coronary sinus rhythm" (negative P′ in inferiors, P′-Ri WNL) has caused some degree of confusion, and such rhythms should actually be classified as ectopic atrial (given that atrial pacing at other sites will produce the same P′ morphology) or junctional (since the P′-R interval may be the same as the P-R interval due to fortuitous anterograde and retrograde conduction delay). The term "block" is associated with reduced conduction. Extreme conduction delay (vs. an actual physical obstruction) can result in block, which if antegrade, is associated with bradyarrhythmias (atrioventricular block with Type I/Wenckebach and Type II/Mobitz varieties). If block is retrograde (ventriculoatrial block), then it is typically associated with tachyarrhythmias, and ventriculoatrial/VA block or exit block from an ectopic focus can also be of Wenckebach or Mobitz varieties. Atrioventricular dissociation is common during atrioventricular block or

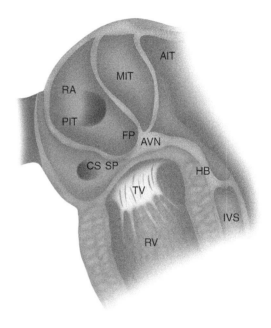

Figure JAI.1 Illustration of the atrioventricular node. **RA**: right atrium, **RV**: right ventricle, **IVS**: interventricular septum, **AVN**: atrioventricular node, **FP**: fast pathway, **SP**: slow pathway, **HB**: His bundle, **TV**: tricuspid valve, **PIT**: posterior internodal tract, **MIT**: middle internodal tract, **AIT**: anterior internodal tract, **CS**: coronary sinus.

junctional tachyarrhythmias; however, junctional dissociation (double junctional rhythms) tends to occur in the setting of bradycardia.

Junctional Bradyarrhythmias
Junctional escape complexes
    Junctional escape-capture bigeminy
Junctional escape rhythm
    Isorhythmic dissociation
    Rule of Reset
Reciprocation
Junctional dissociation (double junctional rhythms)
    Ventriculophasic junctional arrhythmia

Interpretation of the Electrocardiogram in Small Animals, First Edition. Nick A. Schroeder.
© 2021 John Wiley & Sons Inc. Published 2021 by John Wiley & Sons Inc.

Atrioventricular Block
First degree atrioventricular block (prolonged P-Ri)
Second degree atrioventricular block
    Type I (Wenckebach)
    Type II (Mobitz)
    Block-acceleration dissociation
    Paroxysmal atrioventricular block
Third degree AVB
    Junctional escape
    Ventricular escape
    Atrioventricular dissociation
        Atrioventricular dissociation with usurpation
Ventriculoatrial block
Exit block

Junctional Tachyarrhythmias

Junctional Premature Systoles
Resetting, resetting with a pause and interpolation
Junctional bigeminy and trigeminy

Further Reading

Marriot, H.J.L. and Conover, M.B. (1998). *Advanced Concepts in Arrhythmias*, 3e. Mosby.

Santilli, R., Moïse, S., Pariaut, R., and Perego, M. (2018). *Electrocardiography of the Dog and Cat: Diagnosis of Arrhythmias*, 2e. Edna.

Junctional premature complexes with aberrancy
Non-conducted junctional premature complexes
Concealed conduction
Atrial fusion
Junctional reciprocal complexes
Junctional parasystole

Junctional Tachycardia
Accelerated junctional/idiojunctional rhythm
    Isorhythmic dissociation
Automatic junctional tachycardia
Atrioventricular nodal reentrant tachycardia
    Orthodromic atrioventricular nodal reentrant tachycardia
    Antidromic atrioventricular nodal reentrant tachycardia

19

Junctional Bradyarrhythmias

CHAPTER MENU

Junctional escape beats, 213
   Junctional escape-capture bigeminy, 213
Junctional escape rhythm, 216
   Rule of reset, 219
Reciprocation, 219
Junctional dissociation, 223
Ventriculophasic junctional arrhythmia, 226

Junctional escape beats A pause in the sinus rhythm, whether due to sinus bradycardia, exaggerated sinus arrhythmia, sinus pause/arrest, sinoatrial block, or atrioventricular block, may allow the subsidiary pacemakers in the junctional tissue to escape. Junctional escape beats commonly have negative P′ waves that may precede or follow the QRS (or may be lost within the QRS and thus not apparent). If retrograde conduction is blocked, no P′ wave is generated. Rarely, junctional foci may be associated with positive P′ waves if retrograde conduction from the junction proceeds up to Bachman's bundle, activating the atria from "top-down" producing P waves similar to those seen with sinus nodal origin. These are suggested when the positive P′ wave occurs at an unphysiologically short P′-Ri, within the S-T segment or following the QRS and would be expected to reset sinus nodal discharge (as sinus nodal entrance block tends to be rare). Positive P waves preceding QRS complexes at normal P-R intervals generally indicate sinus capture or fortuitous discharge of the SA node and the AV junction when the sinus node by chance happens to fire prior to the dissociated junctional focus. Positive P waves with unphysiologically short P-R intervals (or R-P intervals) are more likely to be sinus nodal in origin and thus dissociated from the junctional discharge that actually conducts to the ventricles, producing the QRS complex.

The interval of escape should be consistent with the inherent junctional discharge rate for the species (i.e. 40–80 bpm in dogs, and 80–140 bpm in cats). This is calculated by measuring the R-R interval from the last

sinus/supraventricular capture to the escape beat and determining the instantaneous HR. This can certainly be variable, however, as overdrive suppression may delay the escape focus. Furthermore, patients with sick sinus syndrome commonly have "lazy escape foci" that do not appear when otherwise expected. The actual escape rate is thus best determined by calculating the instantaneous HR (R'-R'i) after stable and sustained junctional escape rhythm ensues (see below). The QRS of the junctional escape beat is expected to be supraventricular in appearance, matching that associated with conducted sinus complexes. Occasionally, junctional escape beats may have slight QRS aberration from left medial fascicular block (producing a taller than normal QRS in lead II with normal duration). This phenomenon may, however, be explained by increased filling of the left ventricle from the pause (Brody effect). Less commonly, junctional escapes may have right or left bundle branch block (BBB) aberration. This may be bradycardia-dependent or from pre-existent BBB. The interval of escape can help sort these cases out.

Junctional escape-capture bigeminy When a pause in the rhythm elicits a junctional escape beat followed by a sinus capture in a repetitive pattern (allorhythmia), junctional escape-capture bigeminy ensues. This may be secondary to sinus pause/arrest, sinoatrial block, or atrioventricular block. With this situation, the first QRS in each pair is junctional escape in origin and the second

Interpretation of the Electrocardiogram in Small Animals, First Edition. Nick A. Schroeder.

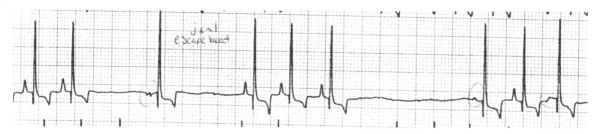

Figure 19.1 Paper speed 25 mm/s, 1 cm/mV, lead II, canine, the third and seventh complexes are late and supraventricular with P′ waves that are different from the sinus P waves consistent with **junctional escape beats**. The last complex is a junctional premature beat. Note the interval of escape is variable.

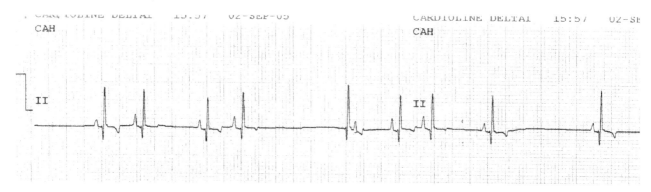

Figure 19.2 Paper speed 25 mm/s, 1 cm/mV, lead II, canine. Atrial bigeminy followed by a sinus pause and **junctional escape beat** (fifth complex). A positive P′ wave follows the escape beat, possibly indicating retrograde activation of the atria (with the impulse traveling up to the interatrial septum via the cranial internodal tract to the area of Bachmann's bundle, then activating the atria from a dorsocranial location, resulting in the positive P′ waves). Alternatively, this may simply represent a sinus P wave that happened to occur just *after* the escape complex conducted to the ventricles; however, the sinus node appears to be reset by this focus. P waves that occur during the S-T segment may have altered morphology that belies the site of origin. The QRS complex is taller, suggestive of left medial fascicular block or the Brody effect.

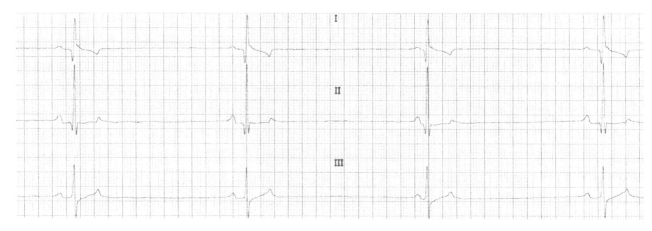

Figure 19.3 Paper speed 50 mm/s, 1 cm/mV, leads I, II, III, canine. Sinus bradycardia elicits a **junctional escape beat** (beat #3). Note the supraventricular QRS. A sinus P wave happens to occur just preceding the escape beat, but at too short of a P-R interval to have conducted to the ventricles. The junctional escape *thwarts* the attempt at a sinus capture.

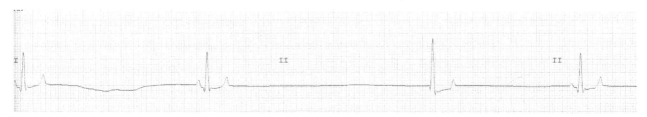

Figure 19.4 Paper speed 50 mm/s, 1 cm/mV, lead II, canine with marijuana toxicity. Severe sinus bradycardia is present. The longer pause following the second beat is a **junctional escape beat**. The QRS complex is taller, again suggestive of left medial fascicular block or Brody effect.

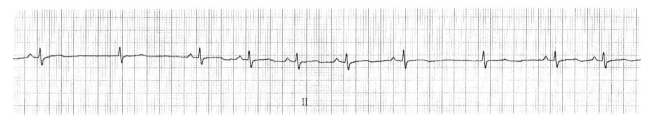

Figure 19.5 Paper speed 50 mm/s, 1 cm/mV, lead II, feline on atenolol. A sinus arrhythmia is present and long cycle lengths are terminated by **junctional escape complexes** (second and eighth complexes). No P waves are associated with these beats and the QRS is of normal/supraventricular appearance with an escape interval of approximately 90 bpm.

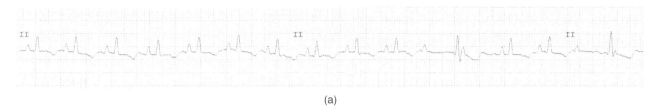

(a)

Figure 19.6a Paper speed 50 mm/s, 2 cm/mV, lead II, feline. Transition from sinus rhythm to periods of Type II second degree AVB.

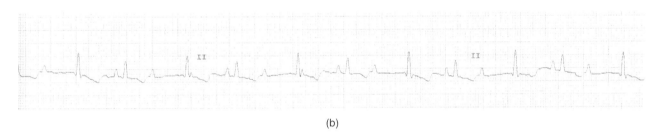

(b)

Figure 19.6b Paper speed 50 mm/s, 2 cm/mV, lead II, same cat. A higher grade of block occurs shortly thereafter (3 : 1 AV conduction). Junctional escape beats follow the first non-conducted P wave in each repeating sequence (sinus conducted, blocked P, escape, blocked P, sinus conducted). This particular sequence is also known as *junctional* **escape-capture bigeminy**. The bigeminal rhythm is produced by the sinus and (here, junctional) escape complexes. The escape complexes themselves induce a functional block of the third P wave in each sequence.

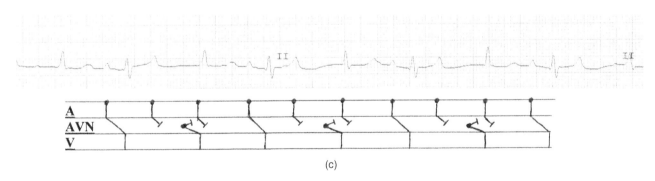

(c)

Figure 19.6c Paper speed 50 mm/s, 1 cm/mV, lead II, same cat. A ladder diagram illustrates the functional block; the junctional escape complexes induce, creating the bigeminal pattern with conducted beats. Importantly, an alternative explanation for this EKG could be dual AV nodal pathways with alternating conduction over the fast path ("capture beats") and the slow path ("escape beats") could be sinus conducted. 1 : 2 block over the fast path could potentially explain this. The slight variation in the slow P-Ri favors a diagnosis of escape-capture bigeminy over dual AV nodal physiology.

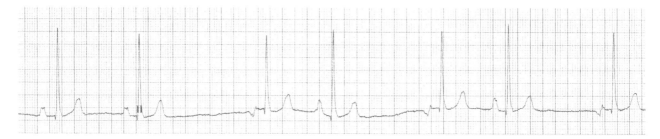

Figure 19.7 Paper speed 50 mm/s, 1 cm/mV, lead II, canine. *Junctional* **escape-capture bigeminy** secondary to sinoatrial block.

QRS complex represents a sinoatrial capture. A rule out for junctional escape-capture bigeminy from second degree atrioventricular block is dual atrioventricular nodal pathway physiology with 1 : 2 block in the fast pathway and conduction over the slow path on every-other-beat.

Junctional escape rhythm

If the SA node or atria fail to pace the ventricles (i.e. during severe sinus bradycardia, sinus arrest, atrial standstill, high-grade second degree or third degree atrioventricular block), a junctional escape rhythm may rescue the heart from stopping altogether. Junctional escape rhythms in the dog range from 40 to 80 bpm (80–140 bpm in cats), usually respond to atropine administration if from upper nodal regions (typified by faster escape rates), and may display bradycardia-dependent or pre-existent BBB or axis deviation (especially from lower nodal regions or associated with diffuse conduction system disease). Junctional escape

rhythm occurs if the rhythm persists for three or more QRS complexes in a row without intervening supraventricular (usually sinus) capture. If junctional escape rhythm is sufficiently slow or fails altogether, a ventricular escape rhythm may take over. Atrioventricular dissociation (AVD) may occur by default. Ventriculoatrial (VA) conduction may occur resulting in retrograde capture of the atria. This may happen before, during, or after the QRS complexes and typically will interrupt or suppress the prevailing sinus rhythm if still present.

Uninterrupted by captures, premature beats, or competing escape foci, junctional escape rhythms are usually metronomically regular, but may be somewhat responsive to changes in sympathetic tone. Rarely, "respiratory or non-respiratory junctional arrhythmia" may occur when junctional escape rhythm has markedly variable R-R intervals that may progressively lengthen and shorten in a cyclic manner with respiratory phase like phasic/respiratory sinus arrhythmia or vary randomly

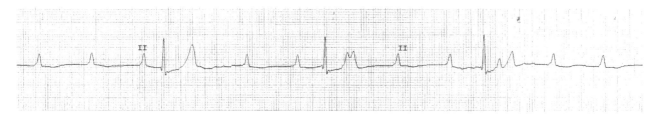

Figure 19.8 Paper speed 50 mm/s, 1 cm/mV, lead II, canine. Third degree AVB has resulted in AV dissociation and a **junctional escape rhythm**. The ventricular complexes are narrow, suggestive of a junctional focus. In this case, the junctional focus is *slow*, with a ventricular rate of approximately 46 bpm. The atrial rate is approximately 136 bpm.

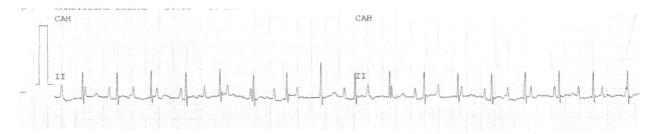

Figure 19.9 Paper speed 25 mm/s, 2 cm/mV, lead II, feline. Third degree AVB has resulted in AVD and a **junctional escape rhythm** of approximately 125 bpm. Atrioventricular block in cats is commonly well tolerated, as the ventricular rate is generally acceptable enough to keep them clinically asymptomatic.

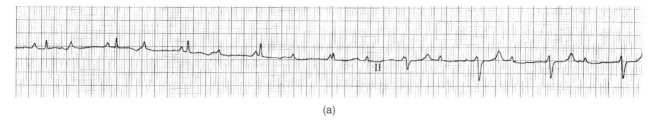

(a)

Figure 19.10a Paper speed 50 mm/s, 1 cm/mV, lead II, feline. Third degree AV block with **junctional escape**. The ventricular rate is 107 bpm and the QRS complexes initially appear supraventricular, but halfway through the strip gradually become negative and prolonged without a change in rate. P waves march through the QRS complexes with an atrial rate of 220 bpm indicating AVD by default from third degree AVB. Why the junctional focus gradually develops a possible **RBBB** is unclear. Interestingly, when the P waves happen to precede the QRS complexes at a normal P-R interval, the complexes are normal in appearance, suggesting the aberrancy could somehow be related to AV dyssynchrony.

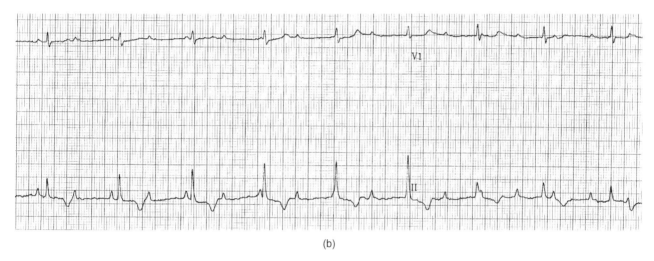

(b)

Figure 19.10b Paper speed 50 mm/s, 2 cm/mV, lead II, same cat. Here, the QRS complexes start fairly normal in morphology, then gradually become more positive, and no obvious prolongation occurs. The axis shift would suggest a LBBB aberration, and again this occurs when the P waves are farthest from the QRS complexes. Lead V1, however, looks fairly consistent throughout and does not change, making a gradual onset of BBB unlikely altogether.

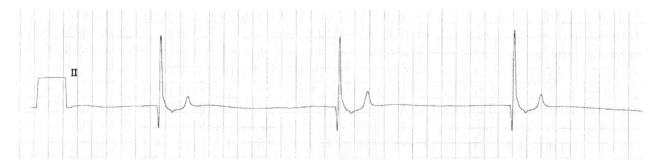

Figure 19.11 Paper speed 50 mm/s, 1 cm/mV, lead II, canine. Profound sinus bradycardia or sinus arrest, **junctional escape rhythm** with **ventriculoatrial conduction**. Retrograde (negative) P′ waves are visualized following the QRS complexes within the S-T segment.

similar to that seen with non-phasic sinus arrhythmias. Occasionally, exit block from the junctional focus will also produce an irregular junctional escape rhythm. Sinus captures interrupting junctional escape rhythm should have a premature supraventricular QRS and associated

with a believable and repeatable P-Ri. Junctional escape beats may be coupled to premature beats. These are usually ventricular premature complexes, although reciprocal beats may also occur. Escape rhythms should never be suppressed.

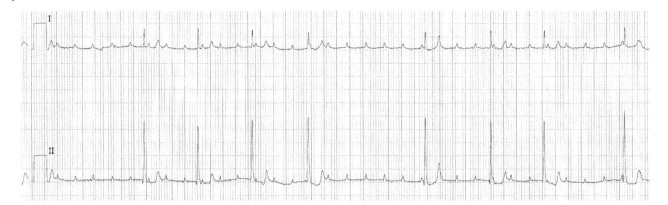

Figure 19.12 Paper speed 25 mm/s, 1 cm/mV, leads I and II, canine. Sinus tachycardia of the atria, *possibly phasic respiratory junctional (escape) arrhythmia* of the ventricles, complete atrioventricular dissociation secondary to complete atrioventricular (third degree) atrioventricular block. The escape rhythm is regularly irregular at a cyclic variation consistent with a plausible respiratory rate (20 breaths/min). Alternatively, this could be a high-grade Type II second degree atrioventricular block interrupted by junctional escape complexes (QRS #5 and #8). Variable P-R intervals argue against this interpretation.

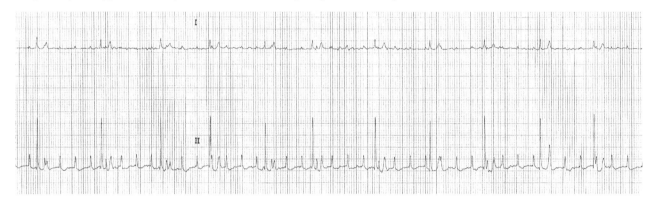

Figure 19.13 Paper speed 25 mm/s, 1 cm/mV, leads I and II, canine. Sinus tachycardia of the atria, *non-phasic junctional escape arrhythmia* of the ventricles, complete AV dissociation secondary to complete AV block (third degree). Variable P-R intervals again argue against supraventricular capture. R-R interval variation did not correlate with respiratory phase in this individual.

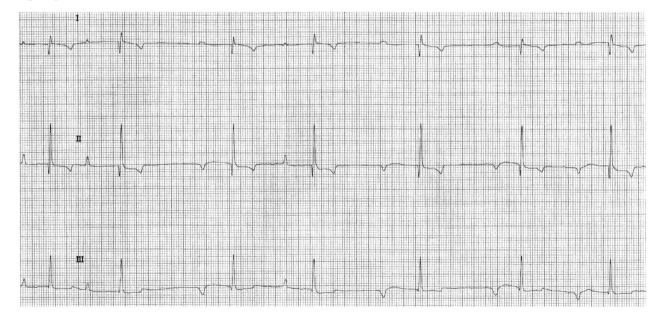

Figure 19.14 Paper speed 50 mm/s, 1 cm/mV, leads I, II, III, canine. Sinus rhythm, first degree AVB, aborted Wenckebach sequences (atypical Type II second degree AVB) with sinus pause terminated by junctional escape rhythm. The third beat is a single junctional escape complex, and junctional escape rhythm with *variable* P'-R intervals and some degree of variation in rhythm (**non-phasic junctional arrhythmia**) ensues after the sinus capture (complex #4).

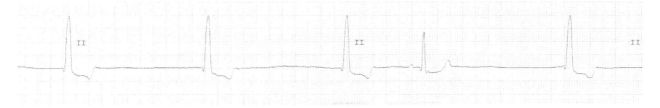

Figure 19.15 Paper speed 50 mm/s, 0.5 cm/mV, lead II, Miniature Schnauzer with right heart failure. Advanced sinus nodal disease left this patient with long periods of atrial standstill and an escape rhythm of approximately 54 bpm. A single sinus capture beat occurs after the third escape beat here, demonstrating that this is not persistent atrial standstill, but advanced SA nodal dysfunction associated with **SSS**. The capture beat resets the escape focus, suggesting the escape focus is junctional in origin by the **Rule of reset**. It is wide and bizarre due to LBBB aberration. The escape rate is more consistent with a junctional focus (vs. a ventricular escape focus) as well.

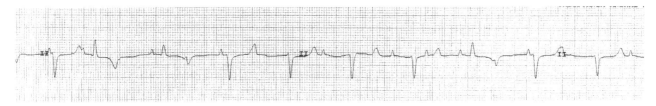

Figure 19.16 Paper speed 50 mm/s, 1 cm/mV, lead II, feline. High-grade Type II second degree AVB has left this cat with periods of what *appears* to be ventricular escape rhythm. AV dissociation is incomplete in this patient, as the 2nd, 4th, and 13th P waves are conducted normally. The atrial rate is approximately 214 bpm, and the escape rhythm is approximately 115 bpm. The rate of the escape rhythm is inconsistent with a ventricular focus, and the escape focus is reset by the capture beats, which suggests that the escape focus is actually junctional in origin by the **Rule of reset**. The junctional focus is conducted with a RBBB, resulting in the wide QRS complexes that are negative in lead II. Intracardiac EKG would be required to rule out an accelerated idioventricular rhythm (so-called block/acceleration dissociation).

Rule of reset Occasionally, a junctional escape focus will be conducted with aberrancy resulting in a wide and bizarre QRS that appears to be idioventricular. Similarly, a ventricular escape focus may be fascicular in origin resulting in a relatively narrow QRS that appears to be supraventricular (junctional). Noting how the escape focus is affected (or not affected by capture (or other clearly supraventricular) beats can help elucidate the site of origin of the escape focus. The Rule of reset states that if the escape focus is reset by capture beats, then the focus is more likely to be junctional regardless of the morphology of the QRS. Thus, if the escape to escape interval is longer than the capture to escape interval (even by a few milliseconds), the escape focus was reset by the impulse traveling through the AVN (junctional area) within the P-R interval of the preceding capture, indicating the escape focus was most likely junctional in origin. This also implies that escape foci that are ventricular in origin may more often be parasystolic. As usual, rules are meant to be broken, so there are exceptions of course. Ventricular foci near or in the His bundle region may also be reset by supraventricular captures. Junctional escape foci can similarly be reset by ventricular ectopic foci with retrograde conduction into the AV node. Concealed reentry within the AV node may

also reset a junctional escape rhythm with a pause. The escape interval is typically consistent with that expected from a junctional escape focus.

Reciprocation Junctional escape beats may occasionally be followed by a reciprocal (reentrant) complex. Basically, what happens is a supraventricular QRS is followed by a negative P′ wave from VA conduction, which in turn is followed by another supraventricular QRS that interrupts the underlying junctional escape focus creating a pause in the rhythm. The sequence here is thus V-A-V, and the reciprocal beats are relatively premature and followed by a pause (perfect resetting or resetting with a pause if overdrive suppression occurs). So-called "R-P′ reciprocity" may be obvious. The shorter the R-P′ interval, the more likely the following P′-R interval will be long, and the longer the R-P′ interval, the more likely the P′-R interval will be short. This is analogous to the P-R/R-P reciprocity seen with Type I second degree atrioventricular block. Prolonged retrograde conduction through the AV node (first degree VA block, a long R-P′ interval) favors reentry. Bigeminal rhythms may occur if there is 1:1 extrasystole from reciprocation (every-other-beat is a reciprocal complex

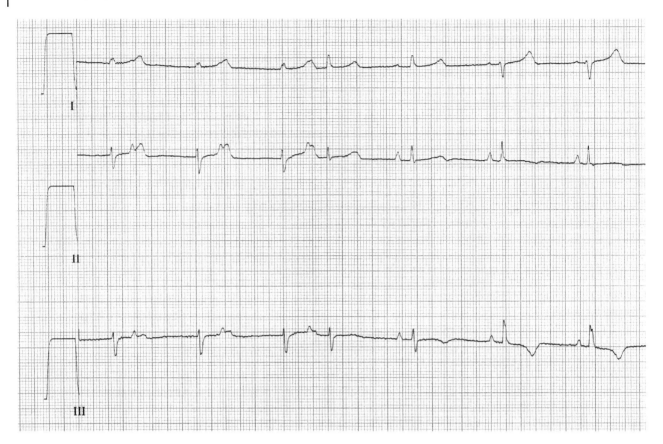

Figure 19.17 Paper speed 50 mm/s, 2 cm/mV, leads I, II, III, feline. R/O **block/acceleration dissociation**. Sinus bradycardia of the atria and escape rhythm of the ventricles, origin uncertain. The atrial and ventricular rates are similar at about 105 bpm, resulting in periods of isorhythmic dissociation with accrochage. The P waves gradually march through the T waves of the first three beats, resulting in a sinus capture (beat #4). This resets the escape focus and AV dissociation immediately ensues with a change in morphology of the QRS complex. The QRS complexes are mildly prolonged at 0.05 second. Given that the escape rate remains steady, the escape focus is likely unifocal, but is either a slow junctional escape focus with changing aberrancy or it is an accelerated ventricular focus near the His bundle with progressive ventricular fusion.

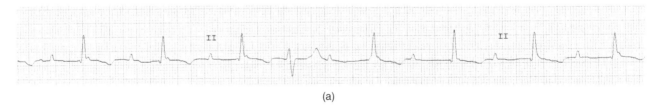

(a)

Figure 19.18a Paper speed 50 mm/s, 1 cm/mV, lead II feline presented for thromboembolism. This arrhythmia *mimics* **isorhythmic dissociation**. This is actually **third degree AVB with junctional escape with synchronization** and an atrial rate (200 bpm) exactly *double* that of the ventricular rate (100 bpm). P waves actually occur independent of all ventricular complexes, indicating AVD. At first glance, the P waves appear to precede the ventricular complexes at relatively regular (albeit prolonged) intervals until a JPC occurs (complex # 4, conducted with LAFB aberration) which resets the junctional escape focus to create an apparently longer P-R interval, exposing the rhythm as AVD. However, additional P waves are hiding *within* the QRS complexes and are seen just peeking out from the QRS complexes during the first three beats. The atrial rate is approximately 200 bpm and the junctional escape rhythm is approximately 100 bpm. If the atrial rate is *exactly* twice that of the ventricular rate during AVD, P waves may occur between ventricular complexes, as well as hiding within them, and can thus give the illusion that the atrial rate is *half* of what it really is, therefore mimicking isorhythmic dissociation. The fourth complex may alternatively be ventricular in origin, *retrogradely* depolarizing the junctional escape focus and resetting it.

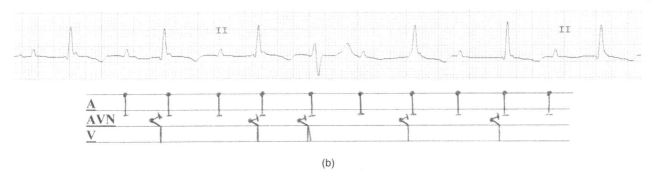

(b)

Figure 19.18b Paper speed 50 mm/s, 1 cm/mV, lead II, same cat. Ladder diagram illustrating a possible mechanism of the above strip.

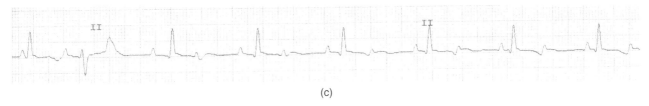

(c)

Figure 19.18c Paper speed 50 mm/s, 1 cm/mV, lead II, same cat. **Third degree AVB with junctional escape rhythm and synchronization.** The fifth complex is narrow, conducted with aberrancy, likely LAFB, and resets the underlying escape focus, suggesting the escape focus is junctional in origin by the Rule of reset. However, a VPC is a possibility as well, since VPCs can retrogradely depolarize junctional foci, resetting them. There is complete atrioventricular dissociation (AVD) as the P waves march through the ventricular rhythm completely unaffected by it. It is tempting to call the fifth complex a sinus capture, but careful examination shows that the P waves are coming immediately before the QRS complexes and right after the T waves in the first four complexes, then happen to precede the QRS complexes and come right before the T waves in the latter four complexes. The atria and ventricles are synchronized with a 2 : 1 response (two atrial beats for every one ventricular beat).

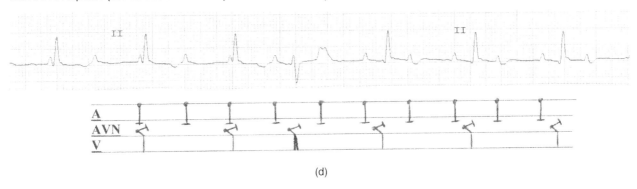

(d)

Figure 19.18d Paper speed 50 mm/s, 1 cm/mV, lead II, same cat. Ladder diagram illustrating the mechanism of the above strip.

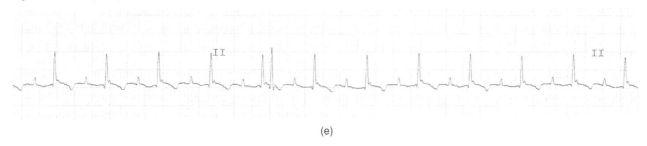

(e)

Figure 19.18e Paper speed 50 mm/s, 1 cm/mV, lead II, same cat. Here, the P waves appear to precede each QRS by an apparently regular, albeit prolonged P-R interval. Careful examination reveals additional P waves just peeking out from the QRS complexes, so the atrial rate is exactly twice that of the ventricular rate, again mimicking isorhythmic dissociation, even though the underlying abnormality is third degree AVB with junctional escape. The sixth complex appears to be premature, narrow and upright, and interpolated between QRS complexes, disturbing neither the atrial rhythm nor the junctional escape. This is suggestive that the sixth complex is actually a ventricular premature ectopic complex. However, careful examination shows that this "beat" occurs during phase 2 of the action potential of the fifth complex (at time when the ventricles ought to be refractory to another depolarization wave). Additionally, the T wave of the fifth complex occurs at the normal Q-T interval, right on time as well. In all likelihood, this deflection, creating a **double QRS complex,** must be an artifact. The monitor lead may occasionally freeze with no associated markings (i.e. no recalibration marks) duplicating a portion of the recording leading to artifactual simulation of sinus nodal reentry (double P waves), shortened or prolonged P-R intervals, intermittent bundle branch block or double QRS complexes, depending on the timing.

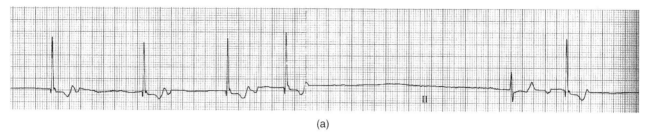

(a)

Figure 19.19a Paper speed 50 mm/s, 1 cm/mV, lead II, canine. Sinus arrest or profound sinus bradycardia. A **junctional escape** focus with VA conduction has captured the ventricles and the atria. The third complex is followed by a short R-P′ interval (0.22 second). The fourth complex occurs prematurely, consistent with a **reciprocal (reentrant) beat** with a long P′-R interval (0.32 second). The stimulus turned around in the AV node and reactivated the ventricles. This elicits a pause (as the junctional focus resets with a long pause from overdrive suppression) that is terminated by a ventricular escape, which in turn is followed by a reciprocal beat with a long R-P′ (0.30 second) and a much shorter P′-R interval (0.16 second).

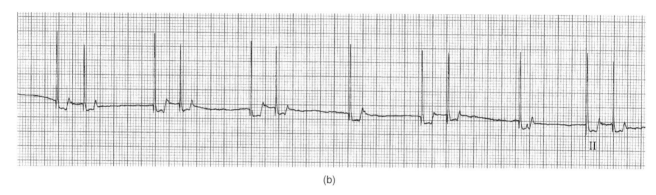

(b)

Figure 19.19b Paper speed 25 mm/s, 1 cm/mV, lead II, same dog. Junctional escape with reciprocal bigeminy ("**escape-echo bigeminy**"). Here, each junctional escape beat is followed by a reciprocal complex creating a bigeminal rhythm. This is interrupted at the seventh complex during which the P′ that follows the QRS fails to reenter the ventricles. This occurs due to progressive shortening of the R-P′ interval where the absolute refractory period of the AVN encroaches on the P′ wave until failure of conduction occurs. The reciprocal beats here display perfect resetting of the junctional escape focus since the interval from the reciprocal beat to the next junctional "capture" is equal to the junctional escape interval.

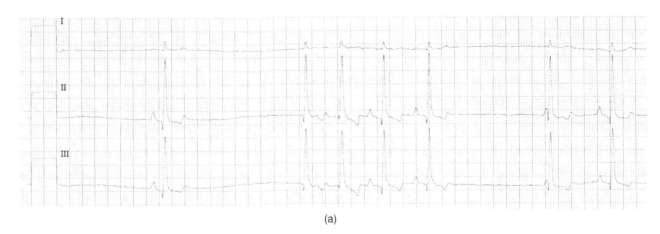

(a)

Figure 19.20a Paper speed 50 mm/s, 1 cm/mV, leads I, II, III, canine. Sinoatrial block is likely creating the long pauses. The pause after the first complex (sinus origin) is terminated by a junctional escape beat, which is then followed by a **reciprocal complex**. The fourth and fifth beats are sinus, which is then followed by another pause eliciting another junctional escape beat (sixth complex). A sinus P wave occurs just before this junctional escape, causing retrograde block, preventing another reciprocal cycle.

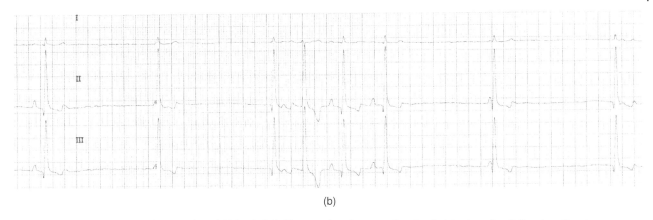

(b)

Figure 19.20b Paper speed 50 mm/s, 1 cm/mV, leads I, II, III, same dog. A pause after the first beat again elicits a junctional escape beat, which is prevented from conducting retrogradely to the atria by a preceding sinus impulse. The third complex is another junctional escape and is followed by a reciprocal beat that finds the left bundle branch partially refractory (acceleration-dependent, phase 3 block), leading to incomplete LBBB aberration. The seventh and eighth beats are junctional escapes, the seventh has VA block again from a preceding sinus impulse, and the eighth is followed by a retrograde P′ just following the QRS complex.

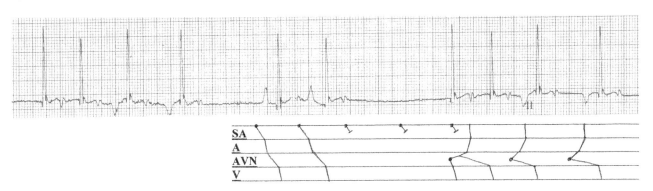

Figure 19.21 Paper speed 50 mm/s, 1 cm/mV, lead II, canine. **Junctional escape beats with reciprocal beats**. The first complex terminated a sinus arrest and is followed by a negative P′ in the T wave, which reenters to form a reciprocal beat (beat #2). Ectopic junctional beats then occur. Two intervening sinus beats occur, and sinus arrest ensues. The allorhythmic sequence then repeats itself (junctional escape, reciprocal complex, ectopic junctional rhythm for two beats), and is illustrated by the ladder diagram. The second beat in each allorhythmic sequence *resets* the junctional focus, implying not only that the last two beats were junctional in origin by the rule of reset, but also that the second beat must be supraventricular in origin. Since the first beat in each sequence is supraventricular (junctional) escape, and the ectopic junctional focus is reset by the interval from the negative P′ following the first QRS, the second beat is most likely a reciprocal (reentrant) beat.

followed by pauses, so-called "escape-echo bigeminy"). Prerequisites for reentry/reciprocation include dual pathways, slowing or asynchrony of conduction, unidirectional block, and recovery of excitability.

Junctional dissociation

Very rarely, two independent foci within the junction may actually dominate both the atrial and the ventricular rhythms. This usually manifests as apparent third degree atrioventricular block with retrograde P′ waves dissociated from a slower supraventricular (junctional) escape focus. Often, a severe sinus bradycardia or sinus arrest develops, allowing a junctional escape rhythm to occur. The atria are controlled by an upper AV nodal rhythm, and the ventricles are controlled by a lower nodal escape rhythm; these are dissociated from each other

via bidirectional entrance/exit block. This can result in AV dissociation secondary to usurpation or default, depending on the heart rate. If the atrial rhythm is rapid and ventricular rhythm is slow (i.e. within heart rate range of a typical junctional escape 40–80 bpm in the dog, 80–140 bpm in the cat), then the AV dissociation is secondary to default (third degree atrioventricular block). If the atrial rhythm and ventricular rhythm are in the accelerated range (i.e. 80–200 bpm in the dog, 140–200 bpm in the cat), then the AV dissociation is secondary to usurpation. Digoxin toxicity has been implicated in double nodal rhythms associated with QRS alternans. Typically, the upper nodal rhythm will exceed the lower nodal rhythm in rate and is usually regular in rhythm. Rarely, the rhythm may be irregular or ventriculophasic conduction may be seen. If the different

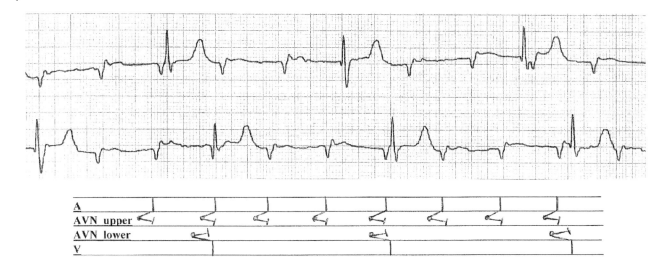

Figure 19.22 Paper speed 50 mm/s, 1 cm/mV, lead II, continuous strip. **Junctional dissociation**. Accelerated idiojunctional rhythm of the atria, junctional escape rhythm of the ventricles, apparently complete atrioventricular dissociation by default secondary to apparently complete (third degree) atrioventricular block. The ladder diagram illustrates the mechanism. Because the upper nodal rhythm is accelerated, it may be suppressing sinoatrial discharge, usurping control of the atria.

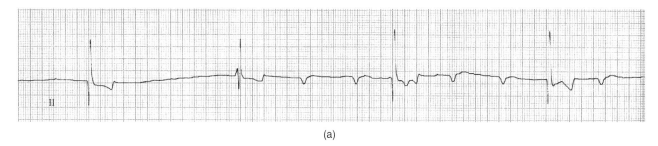

(a)

Figure 19.23a Paper speed 50 mm/s, 1 cm/mV, lead II, canine. Junctional dissociation. Sinus arrest (or profound sinus bradycardia) with a regular supraventricular rhythm at 48 bpm consistent with a junctional escape focus. Midway through the strip a series of dissociated and inverted P waves appear consistent with a junctional focus with a spontaneous rate of 133 bpm without apparent capture of the ventricles. This indicates a "**double nodal rhythm**" with an upper nodal focus in charge of atrial depolarization that is dissociated from a lower nodal focus in charge of ventricular depolarization.

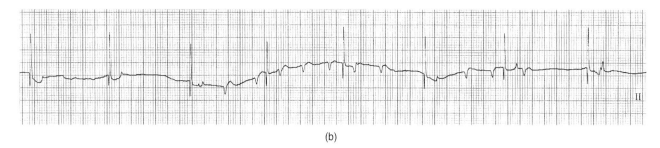

(b)

Figure 19.23b Paper speed 25 mm/s, 1 cm/mV, lead II, same dog. **Junctional dissociation**. The upper nodal rhythm is fast and irregular, while the lower nodal escape focus is regular.

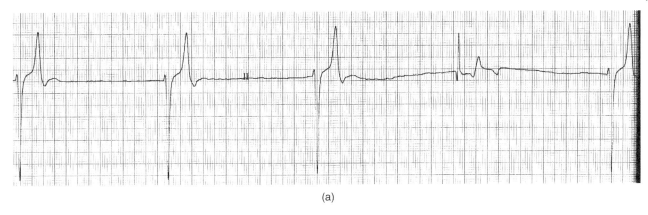

(a)

Figure 19.24a Paper speed 50 mm/s, 1 cm/mV, lead II, canine. Sinus arrest with a regular, apparently ventricular escape rhythm (spontaneous rate of 46 bpm). That rate is a bit fast for ventricular escape in the canine. Each of the ventricular beats is followed by negative P waves suggestive of VA conduction. A more supraventricular appearing QRS follows at a slightly shorter cycle length and again is followed by a negative P wave.

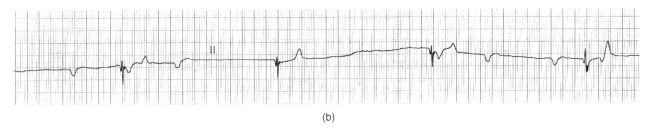

(b)

Figure 19.24b Paper speed 50 mm/s, 1 cm/mV, lead II, same dog. The QRS complexes are much narrower suggestive of a supraventricular (likely junctional focus) and the rate is identical at 46 bpm. This suggests the previous rhythm was probably the same focus, albeit conducted with a RBBB. Negative P waves are visualized marching through the QRS complexes at more rapid rate with an irregular rhythm consistent with **junctional dissociation**.

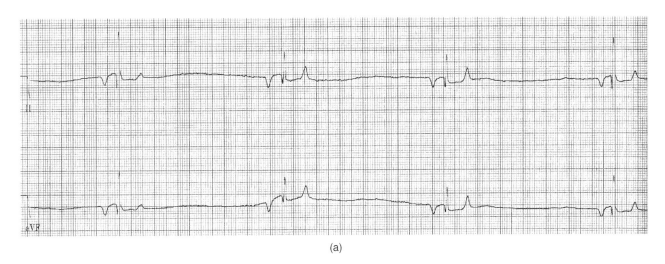

(a)

Figure 19.25a Paper speed 50 mm/s, 1 cm/mV, leads II and aVF, canine. Sinus arrest or profound sinus bradycardia. A regular set of negative P wave precede supraventricular QRS complexes (with some degree of **alternans**) at a rate of 44 bpm. This is suggestive of a junctional escape focus with retrograde P′ waves preceding the QRS complexes with synchrony. However, close scrutiny of the P′-R intervals shows they are not exactly constant.

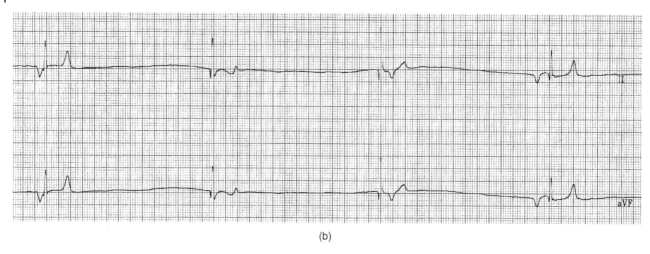

(b)

Figure 19.25b Paper speed 50 mm/s, 1 cm/mV, leads II, aVF, same dog. The QRS complexes appear supraventricular and at a rate of 44 bpm consistent with a junctional escape focus. The atria are apparently beating nearly at the same rate, but the negative P waves march in and out of the QRS complexes indicating AV dissociation. Here, the rates are similar, but the rhythms dissociated, making this an example of "**isorhythmic junctional dissociation**" or double nodal rhythms with accrochage. QRS-T alternans is also evident.

nodal foci have similar rates, then the term isorhythmic junctional dissociation/double junctional rhythm may be used. Similar to that seen with accrochage/synchrony with simple AV dissociation, whether these foci are actually somehow "tethered together" begs the question how dissociated they really are. If the atrial rhythm appears to be irregular with progressive lengthening retrograde conduction, the P′-P′ intervals will vary, and a single junctional rhythm with reciprocal beating should be considered. Junctional dissociation appears to be associated with sick sinus syndrome (see Chapter 11) and if symptomatic bradycardia is encountered, sympathomimetics or permanent pacing may be considered.

Ventriculophasic junctional arrhythmia

Rarely, during junctional dissociation or junctional rhythm with 2 : 1 anterograde AV block, the P′-P′ intervals that encompass the QRS complexes will be shorter than the ones that do not. The ventricular contraction somehow stimulates a more rapid firing of the subsequent junctional impulse, which in turn results in refractoriness of the ventricles with failure of antegrade conduction. If the P′-Ri is regular, then intact anterograde conduction from a single junctional focus with 2 : 1 anterograde AV block is likely. If the P′-Ri interval varies, then junctional dissociation is more likely.

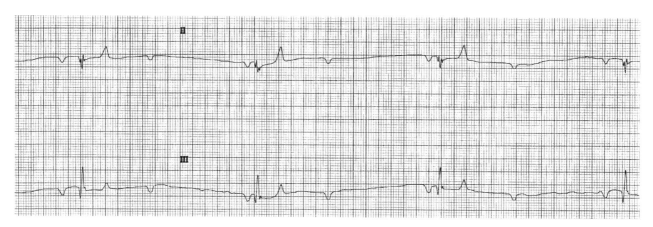

Figure 19.26 Paper speed 50 mm/s, 1 cm/mV, leads II and III, canine. Double nodal rhythms in a dog with a history of sick sinus syndrome. Sinus arrest or profound sinus bradycardia. **Ventriculophasic junctional arrhythmia of the atria.** The P′-P′ intervals including a QRS are shorter than the P′-P′ intervals than those that do not include a QRS. **Junctional escape rhythm** of the ventricles. The lower junction has control of the ventricles and has a pre-existing LPFB accounting for the R axis deviation. The rhythms are dissociated from each other evidenced by variable P′-R intervals. The upper nodal (atrial) rate is approximately 80 bpm and the lower nodal (ventricular) rate is 42 bpm.

Further reading

Barold, S.S. and Herweg, B. (2012). Escape-echo bigeminy. *J. Electrocardiol.* 45 (2): 167–169.

Bernard, R., Vainsel, H., and Schamroth, L. (1972). Atrioventricular dissociation between two atrioventricular nodal rhythms. *Br. Heart J.* 34: 1078–1080.

Chung, E.K. (1968). Digitalis-induced double atrioventricular nodal rhythm associated with electrical Alternans. *Jpn. Heart J.* 9 (5): 504–508.

Dubin, D. (2000). *Rapid Interpretation of EKG's*, 6e. Cover Inc.

Fisch, C.F. and Knoebel, S.B. (2000). *Electrocardiography of Clinical Arrhythmias*. Futura Publishing Co.

Fletcher, E., Morton, P., Murtagh, J.G. et al. (1971). Atrioventricular dissociation with accrochage. *Br. Heart J.* 33: 572–577.

Johnson, C.D. (1978). Intermittent double junctional rhythm with complete atrioventricular block. Electrocardiogram of the month. *Chest* 74: 2.

Knoebel, S.B. (1974). Accelerated junctional escape: a clinical and electrocardiographic study. *Circulation* 50: 151–158.

Marriott, H.J. (1998). *Pearls & Pitfalls in Electrocardiography, Pithy Practical Pointers*, 2e. Williams & Wilkins.

Pick, A. (1956). Aberrant ventricular conduction of escaped beats: preferential and accessory pathways in the A-V junction. *Circulation* 13: 702–711.

Pick, A. and Langendorf, R. (1979). *Interpretation of Complex Arrhythmias*. Lea & Febiger.

Rosen, K.M. (1973). Junctional tachycardia: mechanisms, diagnosis, differential diagnosis, and management. *Circulation* XLVII: 654–664.

Scheinman, M. (2016). *Cardiac Electrophysiology Clinics. Interpretation of Complex Arrhythmias: A Case-Based Approach*, vol. 8. No.1. Elsevier.

Surawicz, B. and Knilans, T.K. (2001). *Chou's Electrocardiography in Clinical Practice: Adult and Pediatric*, 5e. Saunders.

20

Atrioventricular Block

CHAPTER MENU

Atrioventricular block, 228
First degree AVB, 229
Second degree AVB, 231
   Mobitz Type I second degree AVB, 231
      Low-Grade Type I second degree AVB, 231
      2 : 1 Wenckebach, 234
      High-Grade Type I second degree AVB, 235
   Mobitz Type II second degree AVB, 240
      Low-Grade Type II second degree AVB, 240
      2 : 1 Mobitz, 240
      High-Grade Type II second degree AVB, 241
   Block/acceleration dissociation, 242
   Paroxysmal atrioventricular block, 247
Third degree AVB, 248
   Atrioventricular dissociation, 253
Ventriculoatrial block, 256
Exit block, 257

Atrioventricular block This can be confusing but is really not all that difficult to get a grasp on. Basically, antegrade atrioventricular block (AVB) is conduction delay or block interrupting propagation of the supraventricular rhythm (usually sinus) to the ventricles at the level of the AVN or His bundle and is classically subdivided into three "degrees." These include first, second, and third degree AVB. Isolated first degree AVB simply represents AV nodal conduction delay manifesting as a longer than normal P-R interval; however, all supraventricular beats are eventually conducted (1 : 1 conduction). Second degree AVB is incomplete with some supraventricular conduction and intermittent failure to conduct to the ventricles ("dropped beats"). Second degree AVB is further subdivided into Type I and Type II. In third degree AVB, the block is complete and occurs when no supraventricular beats conduct to the ventricles, resulting in atrioventricular dissociation by default. An escape focus must be present to rescue the heart in these patients (permanent downward displacement of the pacemaker) and is either junctional or ventricular in origin.

These subdivisions are simplistic, however, so keep this in mind. The term "block" itself is also misleading. Extreme delay of conduction can result in apparent block on surface EKG. Furthermore, the word "block" implies an anatomic and/or fixed obstruction, which is rarely the case in patients with AVB. Generally speaking, first degree AVB and Type I second degree AVB are considered physiologic, though may be seen in states of "pathologically" elevated parasympathetic tone (vagotonia) or in patients with sick sinus syndrome. Type II second degree AVB and third degree AVB are considered pathologic and secondary to AV nodal disease/fibrosis (Lev's/Legenere's dz). The prevailing autonomic tone is generally sympathetic and often manifested by sinus tachycardia that is associated with progressive ventricular bradycardia. Subsidiary junctional escape rhythms may somewhat be responsive to elevations in sympathetic tone or parasympatholysis, whereas ventricular escape foci are typically unresponsive.

Certain phenomena associated with AVB do not fit neatly into traditional classification schemes. These include 2 : 1 AVB, multiple levels of AVB, block/acceleration

Interpretation of the Electrocardiogram in Small Animals, First Edition. Nick A. Schroeder.
© 2021 John Wiley & Sons Inc. Published 2021 by John Wiley & Sons Inc.

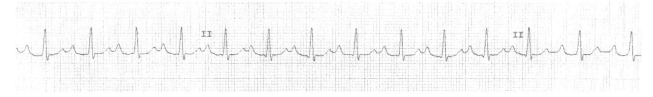

Figure 20.1 Paper speed 50 mm/s, 1 cm/mV, lead II, canine, **first degree AVB**. The P-R interval is 0.14 second.

dissociation, and transient ventricular asystole from paroxysmal AVB. Retrograde AVB may occur when ventricular or lower junctional foci penetrate the AVN from the bottom-up and has analogous degrees/Types. Exit block may manifest as irregular rhythms from ectopic foci and likewise has similar degrees/Types. While retrograde (ventriculoatrial) block and exit block are not generally associated with antegrade AVB, they are briefly discussed here as they pertain to second degree blocks in general and examples are provided in other chapters (see Chapters 10, 16, 19, 24, and 25) based on the primary underlying rhythm disturbance.

First degree AVB This is characterized on surface EKG by prolongation of the P-R interval (beginning of P to the beginning of the q wave if present or to the R wave if no q wave). In dogs, this is greater than 0.13 second, and greater than 0.09 second in cats. First degree AVB represents delay in conduction through the AV node is associated with high vagal tone. Every supraventricular (typically sinus) impulse eventually results in ventricular activation, so this is an instance where the term "block" is technically a misnomer. First degree AVB may also be transient, physiologic, and is commonly seen on atrial premature complexes, post-extrasystolic beats (i.e. the beats following interpolated premature complexes) as well as on beats terminating relatively short cycles that follow longer ones. Treatment of isolated first degree AVB is unnecessary.

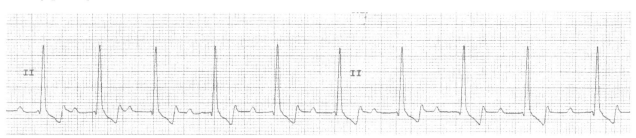

Figure 20.2 Paper speed, 50 mm/s, 1 cm/mV, lead II, canine, the P-R interval is 0.16 second.

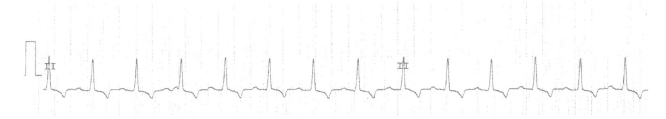

Figure 20.3 Paper speed 50 mm/s, 1 cm/mV, hyperkalemic cat, **first degree AVB** and sinus bradycardia. The P-R interval is 0.10 second.

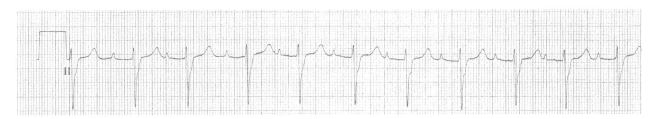

Figure 20.4 Paper speed 50 mm/s, 1 cm/mV, lead II, feline. Severe **first degree AVB** is present (P-Ri of 0.16 second), with sinus rhythm and RBBB.

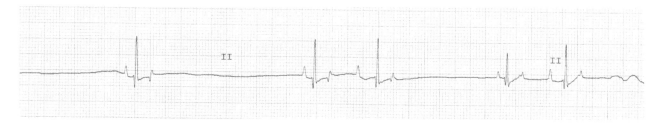

Figure 20.5 Paper speed 25 mm/s, 1 cm/mV, lead II, canine sedated with medetomidine. **Alternating P-R interval prolongation** causes first degree AVB on beats ending short cycles in this bradycardic and normotensive patient. This is likely secondary to changes in autonomic tone caused by alpha antagonism. The third and fifth beats show marked P-R interval prolongation as the AVN is still partially (and variably – arguing against dual AV nodal pathway physiology) refractory from the preceding beats. Electrical alternans also occurred in the patient independent of respiratory excursion, and the second and especially the fourth beats are smaller than the rest of the complexes.

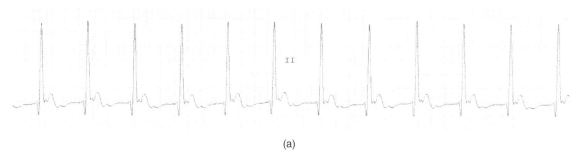

(a)

Figure 20.6a Paper speed 50 m/s, 1 cm/mV, lead II, canine with digoxin toxicity. **Sinus tachycardia with** *severe* **first degree AVB** with P waves just following the QRS complexes within the S-T segment of the previous beats. The P-R interval is apparently 0.3 second.

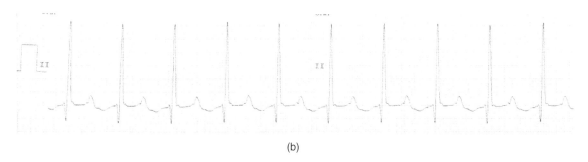

(b)

Figure 20.6b Paper speed 50 m/s, 1 cm/mV, lead II, same dog. The ventricular rate is the slightly slower, and the P waves have moved to nearly midway between complexes. They are right on top of the T waves and are followed by negative Ta waves. First degree AVB is present with a very long P-R interval at 0.22 second (clearly different than above, which suggests worsened AV nodal conduction time with relative tachycardia).

Obnoxious first degree (and Type I second degree) AVB (often associated with an exaggerated sinus arrhythmia ± sinus pauses/arrests) may be associated with elevated parasympathetic tone that is considered pathologic. High vagal tone (vagotonia) is associated with four disease states:

1) **Respiratory disease**: chronic obstructive pulmonary disease, heartworm infestation, fungal pneumonitis, pneumonia, bronchitis, airway collapse/upper airway obstruction, diffuse infiltrative neoplastic disease, etc., are all associated with a pathologic increase in vagal tone.

2) **Neurologic disease**: granulomatous meningoencephalitis, lymphosarcoma, etc., may be associated with elevations in vagal tone.

3) **Gastrointestinal disease**: too many to list, but, hemorrhagic gastroenteritis, inflammatory bowel disease, severe malnutrition, etc., are often associated with vagal tone increases.

4) **Intoxication**: i.e. digitalis glycosides, being sympatholytic, is associated with pathologic vagal tone increase. Remember, digoxin can cause any arrhythmia including AVB – not just accelerated rhythms and ventricular premature beats.

(5) **Normal variant:** athletic dogs may normally have high vagal tone, brachycephalics typically have high vagal tone (secondary to their chronic effective upper airway obstruction, so this really falls under respiratory disease though it is considered normal for the breed).

Second degree AVB

Also known as "Incomplete" Heart Block: this is characterized on surface EKG by the presence of intermittent failure of conduction through the AVN ("dropped QRS" or a P wave without a corresponding QRS complex). Mechanically, this means the atria contract, but since the impulse fails to conduct through the AVN, the ventricles periodically fail to contract. There are two Types of second degree AVB. Type I block is associated with high vagal tone and may be seen incidentally in puppies and brachycephalics. Transient (Type I) second degree AVB is commonly seen immediately following IV injection with atropine and goes away in a few minutes. This is because atropine affects the SA node before the AV node. Type II block is pathologic and more likely to progress to third degree AVB. Second degree AVB is the rule when the atria are beating rapidly (i.e. during atrial fibrillation [AF] or flutter [AFL]), a situation in which the AVN acts as an electrical "gatekeeper," preventing the ventricles from beating too quickly, which otherwise could result in ventricular tachycardia and/or fibrillation. Second degree AVB also includes so-called "block-acceleration dissociation" and paroxysmal AV block.

Mobitz Type I second degree AVB

Also known as "Wenckebach phenomenon," in which there is critical progressive prolongation of the P-R interval prior to a failure of conduction. This is incidentally the most common physiologic arrhythmia in the horse. The block is in the AVN usually and results from prolongation of the relative refractory period. The term "group beating" refers to the phenomenon seen when the sinus rate (P-P interval) remains constant while the decreasing increments in the P-R interval cause a slight acceleration of ventricular rate

during the period of increasing P-R prolongation until a blocked cycle occurs. R-P/P-R reciprocity is typical. The shorter the R-P interval, the longer the P-R interval of the following cycle, and vice versa. Typically, Wenckebach is a low grade of AVB, with no more than one consecutive P wave failing to conduct (so-called "dropped" QRS). First degree AVB on the conducted complexes is expected, and if the P-Ri is sufficiently prolonged combined with a high enough atrial rate, QRS complexes may be "skipped" and P waves appear just before the previously conducted QRS complex.

> ***Quick and Dirty***: Comparing the P-R interval of the beats on either side of a non-conducted beat can help you quickly determine if a second degree AVB is likely to be from Wenckebach periodicity or not. If the P-R interval of the beat following the non-conducted beat is shorter than the P-R interval of the beat preceding the non-conducted beat, then it is probably Wenckebach. This can be unreliable, however. Pauses can elicit junctional escape beats, and a dissociated sinus P wave may fortuitously precede the escape complex and thus mimic a capture with a short P-R interval. These may be unmasked by an unphysiologically short P-R' interval.

Wenckebach periodicity is thought to occur for two potential reasons. First, increasing depression of the AVN can be from the series of impulses inactivating an increasing fraction of the calcium or sodium channels. Second is the fact that the R-P interval progressively shortens. This means the impulses conducted from the atria begin to reach the AV junction earlier during the relative refractory period left behind after the preceding beat until an atrial impulse reaches the AVN (or bundle) before it is able to generate a propagated action potential during the absolute refractory period. Type I second degree AVB generally warrants no specific therapy.

Low-Grade Type I second degree AVB

This occurs when no more than one consecutive P wave that fails to conduct to the ventricles.

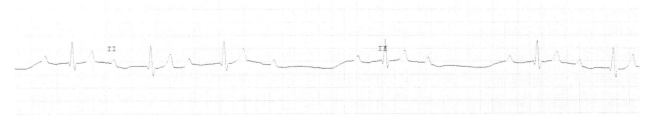

Figure 20.7 Paper speed 50 mm/s, 1 cm/mV, lead II, canine, classic **Wenckebach** with gradual P-R interval prolongation prior to failure of conduction. The first P-R interval is 0.22 second, then 0.28 second, then 0.3 second. The atrial rate is higher than the ventricular rate, which tells you there is at least second degree AVB.

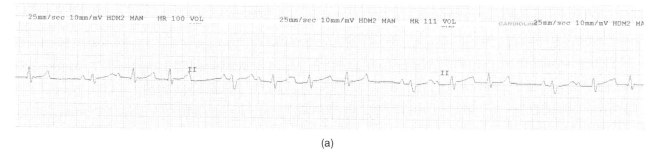

(a)

Figure 20.8a Paper speed 50 mm/s, 1 cm/mV, lead II, feline, classic **Wenckebach** with obvious group beating. The P-R interval gradually prolongs until a P wave is not conducted (these are buried in the T waves of the 3rd, 7th, and 10th complexes). Typical of Wenckebach, the second P-R interval in each group displays the most prolongation vs. the previous complex. There is 4 : 3, 4 : 3, then 5 : 4 conduction.

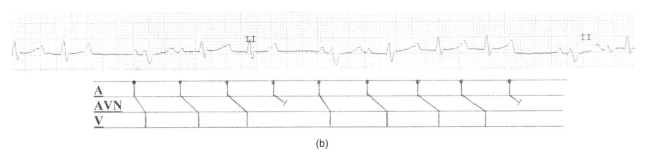

(b)

Figure 20.8b Paper speed 50 mm/s, 1 cm/mV, lead II, same cat. Ladder diagram of the above EKG. One can quickly see that 4 : 3 and then 5 : 4 conduction occurs.

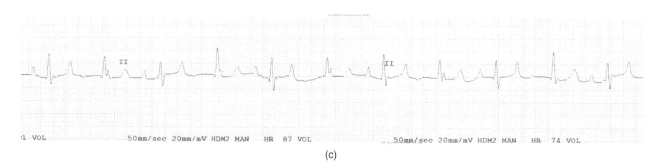

(c)

Figure 20.8c Paper speed 50 mm/s, 2 cm/mV, lead II, same cat, Type I second degree AVB with 3 : 2 conduction. This can be tricky to sort out from Type II second degree AVB, as successive conducted impulses are not clearly evident. The giveaway here is that the second conducted P wave in each group prior to failure of conduction is buried in the T wave of the preceding complexes.

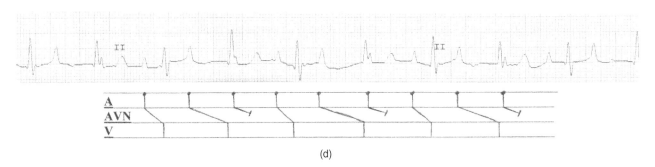

(d)

Figure 20.8d Paper speed 50 mm/s, 1 cm/mV, lead II, same cat. Ladder diagram of the above EKG. 3 : 2 conduction is evident. The second conducted complex in each group displays marked prolongation of the P-R interval, indicating Wenckebach periodicity. Alternatively, the "second conducted complex" in each group could be interpreted as a junctional escape, which prevents the sinus impulse immediately following it from being conducted (junctional escape-capture bigeminy). Typical Wenckebach periodicity in the preceding strips confirms the above interpretation.

Low-grade Type I second degree AVB is often transiently induced by ventricular premature complexes (VPCs). Partial retrograde penetration into the AVN causes a "compensatory pause" if the post-extrasystolic P wave is non-conducted (functional second degree AVB). An interpolated VPC causes a functional first degree AVB on the post-extrasystolic beat. This is from concealed conduction into the AVN by the VPC. Dual AV nodal physiology has been used to explain this post-extrasystolic P-Ri prolongation. Retrograde conduction into the AVN by the VPC renders the fast path refractory and allows conduction to proceed over the slow pathway. Rarely, the compensatory pause may be "postponed" and the VPC is interpolated, the post-extrasystolic beat has P-Ri prolongation, and the next sinus beat is AV blocked. The VPC basically induces a Wenckebach period.

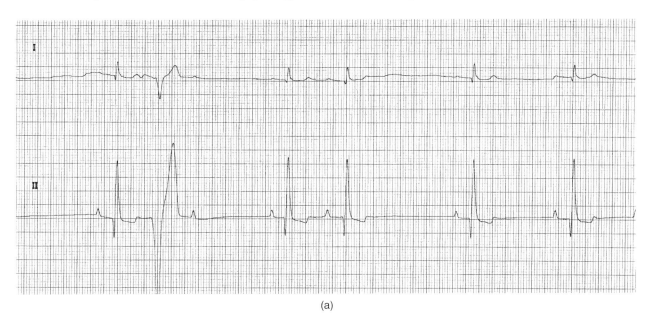

(a)

Figure 20.9a Paper speed 50 mm/s, 1 cm/mV, leads I and II, canine. The second complex is a VPC that causes a compensatory pause. The post-extrasystolic P wave is non-conducted. The following QRS complexes display progressive P-Ri prolongation without failure of conduction (Variant III atypical Wenckebach periodicity).

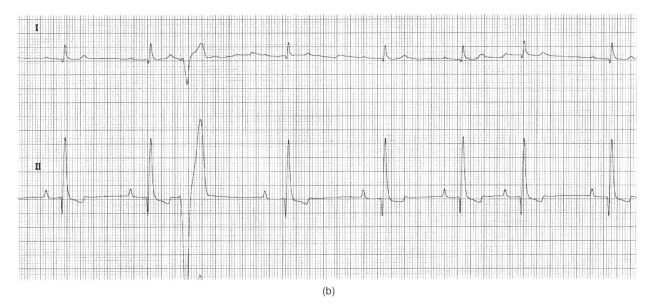

(b)

Figure 20.9b Paper speed 50 mm/s, 1 cm/mV, leads I and II, same dog. This time, the VPC is interpolated, and causes post-extrasystolic P-Ri prolongation without failure of conduction. The P-Ri prolongation persists for a few beats. This is indicative of concealed conduction. The VPC partially penetrated the AVN retrogradely, causing the conduction delay of subsequent sinus complexes. This dog had apparently elevated parasympathetic tone with sinus arrhythmia, first degree AVB, and Wenckebach periodicity, albeit atypical.

Atypical Wenckebach periods Not all Type I AV blocks will result in classical Wenckebach periodicity with a gradually prolonging P-R interval and shortening R-R interval prior to failure of conduction. In fact, atypical Wenckebach periodicity can be seen in 50% or more cases of Type I second degree AVB, making the term "atypical" somewhat of a misnomer. Concealed reentry within the AVN with abortive attempts at atrial echoes may cause sudden, otherwise unexplained P-R interval prolongation, as can dual AV nodal physiology. Abrupt and unexpected P-R interval shortening (i.e. following a relatively short R-P interval) may also be explained by the gap phenomenon, which may mimic supernormal conduction. Conduction ratios of 5:1 or 6:1 or higher have atypical Wenckebach periodicity most of the time. Many variants have been described:

Variant I: The last R-R interval may prolong as well as the P-R interval right before failure of conduction.

Variant II: Sudden, marked (vs. gradual) prolongation of the P-R interval may occur, usually followed by a blocked P wave.

Variant III: The P-R interval may gradually prolong, then shorten without failure of conduction (no "dropped QRS").

2:1 Wenckebach The classification of Type I vs. Type II second degree AVB becomes problematic when there is 2:1 AV conduction. If RP/PR reciprocity is present, then 2:1 block is Type I. If the PR is independent of the RP, then 2:1 block is Type II (Mobitz). These are features obvious only when consecutive conducted beats are analyzed. 2:1 Wenckebach is suggested when the

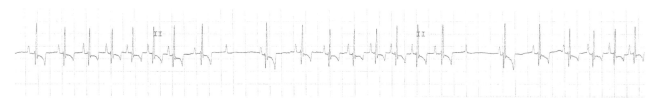

Figure 20.10 Paper speed 25 mm/s, 1 cm/mV, lead II, canine. **Type I second degree** AVB (Wenckebach) with obvious group beating. The P-R interval gradually prolongs before failure of conduction to the ventricles. The ventricular rate gradually accelerates (shortening the R-R intervals) in each group up until the very last conducted complex in each period, which follows a *long R-R interval*. Note that the conduction ratios are high (8:1).

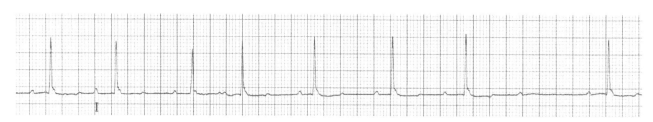

Figure 20.11 Paper speed 50 mm/s, 1 cm/mV, lead I, canine. **Atypical Wenckebach periodicity**. Long P-R intervals persist for the first four complexes, then shorten on the fifth and sixth beats. The seventh beat shows *sudden P-R interval prolongation* and is followed by a blocked P wave.

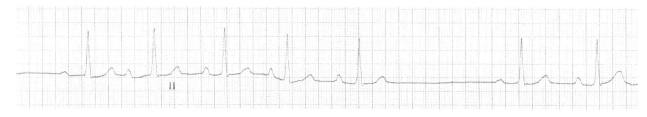

Figure 20.12 Paper speed 50 mm/s, 1 cm/mV, lead II, canine. **Atypical Wenckebach periodicity** with sudden increase in P-Ri without failure of conduction to the ventricles. The second complex shows a marked and abrupt prolongation of the P-Ri, the third complex has a shorter P-Ri, and the fourth and fifth complexes have mild progressive P-Ri prolongation without a blocked P wave following the sequence. Underlying sinus arrhythmia is present, as well as a wandering pacemaker.

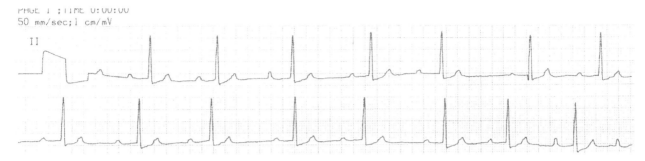

Figure 20.13 Paper speed 50 mm/s, 1 cm/mV, lead II, canine. **Atypical Wenckebach** with gradually increasing P-R intervals *without* failure of conduction to the ventricles.

P-R interval is prolonged, but the QRS is of normal duration. Ventriculophasic sinus arrhythmia is also more commonly associated with Wenckebach periodicity. 2 : 1 Mobitz is suggested when the P-R interval is normal and often has a widened QRS due to concurrent bundle branch block. Classically, vagal maneuvers increase parasympathetic inhibition of the AVN, increasing the number of cycles/series to produce 3 : 2 or 4 : 3 Wenckebach. Vagal maneuvers either eliminate 2 : 1 Mobitz, producing 1 : 1 conduction, or have no effect at all.

Take Home Point: When evaluating AVB, rate is more important than ratio. Type I second degree AVB can be "high" grade and Type II second degree AVB may be "low" grade. The classical divisions of AVB here should not be overemphasized. The emphasis should rather be placed on the prevailing rate as well as differentiating pathologic from physiologic refractoriness of the AV junction and bundle branches.

High-Grade Type I second degree AVB This occurs when more than one consecutive P wave fail to conduct to the ventricles. It is unusual to see more than one consecutive

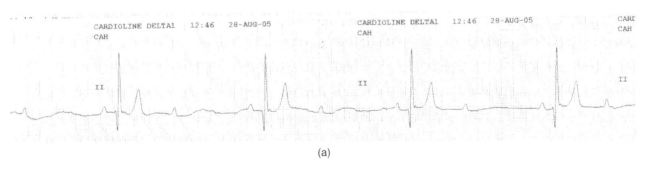

(a)

Figure 20.14a Paper speed 50 mm/s, 1 cm/mV, lead II, canine. **2 : 1 AVB**. The P-R interval is slightly prolonged (0.13 second) and normal duration QRS complexes (as well as ventriculophasic sinus arrhythmia) suggest this is Wenckebach.

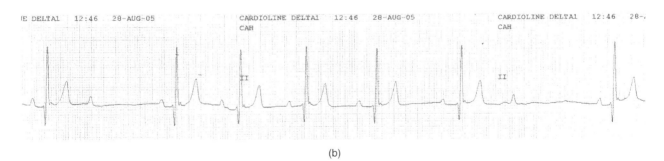

(b)

Figure 20.14b Paper speed 50 mm/s, 1 cm/mV, lead II, same dog. Type I second degree AVB is obvious. The P-R interval gradually prolongs prior to failure of conduction, demonstrating that the above strip was **2 : 1 Type I AVB (Wenckebach)**.

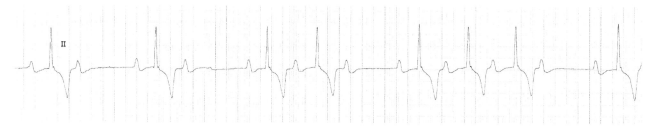

Figure 20.15 Paper speed 50 mm/s, 1 cm/mV, lead II, canine. Type 1 second degree AVB with **2 : 1 conduction** at the beginning of the strip transitions to 3 : 2, then 4 : 3 conduction with obvious P-Ri prolongation prior to failure of conduction. The P-Ri is prolonged on all conducted complexes (*first degree AVB*), *ventriculophasic sinus arrhythmia* is present, and R-P/P-R reciprocity is evident on consecutively conducted complexes – all supportive of Type I AVB/Wenckebach periodicity. Negative Ta waves are most obvious on non-conducted beats, and the T waves are incidentally deep. This patient had a laryngeal mass with invasion into the trachea, effective upper airway obstruction, and was mentally inappropriate. Pathologically elevated parasympathetic tone was suspected, as well as possible intracranial disease.

P wave fail to conduct following Wenckebach periods. However, this can occur with excessively high vagal tone, and there are usually more conducted complexes than those that are blocked overall. This happens when the first non-conducted impulse penetrates relatively deeply into the AVN, prolonging the refractory period long enough for multiple impulses to be blocked. The cycle lengths/P-P intervals of the consecutively blocked complexes are almost invariably longer than those that are conducted, so worsened block occurs with the slowing of the SA nodal discharge during a sinus arrhythmia. Rarely, pauses from the high grade of block may be terminated by escape beats from subsidiary pacemakers. This is because vagotonia also depresses normal automaticity of the normal (especially junctional) escape centers. High-grade Type I second degree AVB is the rule when the atria are undergoing rapid and coordinated depolarization, as seen in atrial tachycardia and atrial flutter (AFL). Treatment of high-grade Type I second degree AVB is directed at alleviating pathologically elevated parasympathetic tone, removing parasympathomimetics or considering antiarrhythmic medication for atrial tachycardia or flutter.

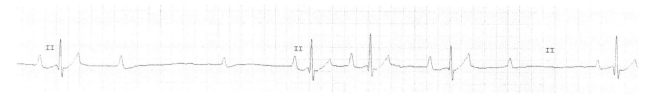

Figure 20.16 Paper speed 50 mm/s, 1 cm/mV, lead II, canine. ***High-grade** Type I second degree AVB*. Two consecutive P waves fail to conduct following the first complex, which is considered a "high grade" of block, no matter where the block is. An atypical Wenckebach period follows with the next group (with a longer R-R interval seen prior to failure of conduction). First degree AVB is also present, as is a marked respiratory and ventriculophasic sinus arrhythmia.

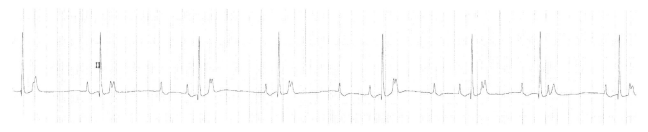

Figure 20.17 Paper speed 50 mm/s, 1 cm/mV, lead I, canine. **Ventriculophasic sinus arrhythmia, high-grade Type I second degree AVB** with up to 3 : 1 conduction. First degree AVB with variable P-R intervals is present, and by the end of the strip, 2 : 1 conduction ensues. Fortuitous junctional escape is unlikely, as P-R/R-P reciprocity is evident, P waves always precede supraventricular QRS complexes at plausible P-R intervals and irregular junctional escape rhythms are uncommon in general. Ta waves are evident and P waves are superimposed on T waves.

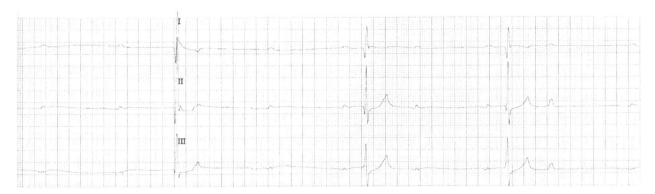

Figure 20.18 Paper speed 50 mm/s, 1 cm/mV, leads I, II, III, canine. **Ectopic atrial rhythm** with *high-grade* **Type I second degree AVB**. Two consecutive atrial impulses are AV blocked, eliciting a junctional escape beat (first complex) with retrograde conduction block. Note the ectopic atrial focus is not reset. The third and fourth beats are ectopic atrial conducted. The last beat is followed by a sinus P wave. The impulse is also AV blocked, and is followed by another ectopic atrial beat. The captures are conducted with a long P′-R interval, and this patient had typical Wenckebach periodicity in sinus rhythm.

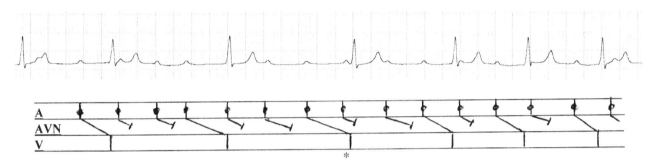

Figure 20.19 Paper speed 50 mm/s, 1 cm/mV, lead V4, canine treated with metoprolol and digoxin for chronic SVT (atrial tachycardia). High-grade Type I second degree AVB with *"skipped" QRS complexes*. The eighth P′ wave shown on the ladder diagram skips the immediately following QRS (*), which was in fact conducted by the previous P′ wave. The P′-Ri is too short to be consistent with AV conduction. Given more than one P′ wave is intermittently AV blocked, this constitutes a high grade of block. The first degree AVB on conducted complexes combined with a relatively rapid atrial rate (260 bpm) allows for "skipping" of the QRS complexes on occasion.

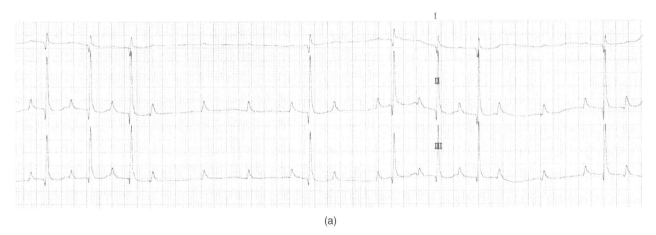

(a)

Figure 20.20a Paper speed 50 mm/s, 0.5 cm/mV, leads I, II, III, canine with severe atrioventricular valvular disease, biatrial enlargement, and history of congestive heart failure. **P-biatriale, first degree AVB, High-grade Type I second degree AVB, sinus arrhythmia with 4 : 1 and 3 : 1 conduction during expiration**. The first three complexes represent a typical Wenckebach period with first degree AVB (P-Ri of 0.14 second on the first cycle), and progressive P-Ri prolongation before failure of conduction. Interestingly, up to three consecutive sinus impulses fail to conduct, making this a *very* high grade of AV block, and this is coincident with expiration and slowing of the sinus node. This is followed by a brief period of 2 : 1 conduction, another Wenckebach period, then 3 : 1 conduction on the second expiration/slowing of the sinus rate. More than 1 non-conducted complex following a Wenckebach period is unusual, and 3 non-conducted complexes are even rarer. Even with a high grade of AVB, typically no more than two sinus impulses fail to conduct. Perhaps, the marked slowing of the sinus node encouraged a transient Phase 4 block of the following complexes.

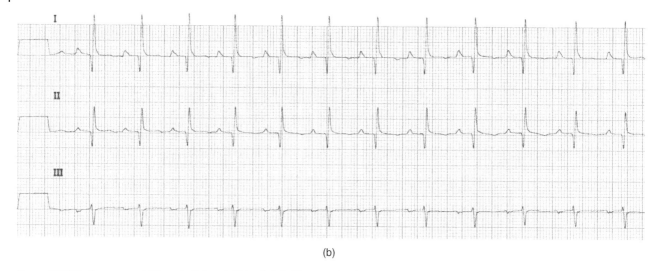

(b)

Figure 20.20b Paper speed 50 mm/s, 0.5 cm/mV, leads I, II, III, same dog following administration of atropine. Sinus rhythm is present with 1 : 1 conduction. This demonstrates that although the above strip shows a high grade of AVB, it was vagal in origin, and the block was likely AV nodal.

"Pseudo Mobitz Type II second degree AVB": Wenckebach periodicity may occasionally simulate Type II second degree AVB. Most often, these involve atypical Wenckebach periods. Long Wenckebach cycles in which at least the last 3 cycles show relatively constant P-R intervals before the block, but the P-R interval following the blocked P wave will still be shorter than that of the P-R before the block. Look for other clues to Wenckebach periodicity or elevated vagal tone: sinus arrhythmia, first degree AVB,

etc. Other causes of a pseudo Mobitz Type II second degree AVB include concealed junctional premature beats (causing unexpected conduction blockade), blocked atrial ectopics and artifacts, of course.

Muscarinic blockade with an atropine trial is in order if a second degree or higher grade of block is diagnosed and can help distinguish physiologic block secondary to elevated parasympathetic tone from pathologic block if it is unclear based on surface EKG. Atropine is administered

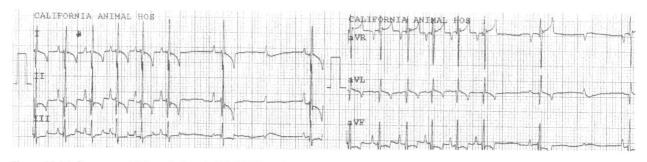

Figure 20.21 Paper speed 25 mm/s, 1 cm/mV, full EKG, canine. Atypical Wenckebach periodicity, **pseudo Mobitz Type II second degree AVB**. The P-R intervals are pretty consistent for the first six complexes. A long cycle is terminated with a P-Ri that is longer and is followed by a blocked P wave, and the following complex has a shorter P-R interval.

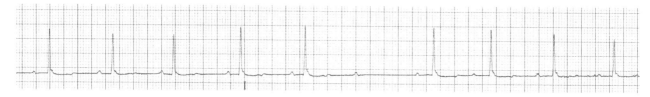

Figure 20.22 Paper speed 50 mm/s, 1 cm/mV, lead I, canine. Atypical Wenckebach periodicity, **pseudo Mobitz Type II second degree AVB**. The first beat has a P-R interval (0.12 second), and the second through fourth complexes have a shorter and *relatively constant* P-R interval (0.10 second). An AV block occurs, and the last four beats which show longer P-R intervals (0.12 second). The presence of two discreet P-R intervals suggests **dual AV nodal physiology**.

at a high dose (0.04 mg/kg SQ/IM), and the patient's EKG is re-evaluated. It is critical to remember there is a differential effect on the SAN vs. the AVN and this is dose-dependent. The SAN usually has more vagal innervation and is expected to respond before the AVN. Sinus nodal discharge accelerates before the AVN has time to respond, initially worsening conduction, resulting in a higher grade of AV block. This effect is transient, more pronounced following IV injection and given enough time (usually 15–20 minutes), the AVN will become responsive and conduction should improve resulting in sinus tachycardia with 1 : 1 conduction *if* the AV block was physiologic and secondary to vagotonia. Importantly, low-dose atropine (0.006 mg/kg, < 0.5 mg per human) can cause a paradoxical slowing of SA nodal discharge with resultant sinus bradycardia and is thought to be secondary to a central vagotonic effect. The AVN usually has improved conduction following low-dose atropine, though differential vagal innervation has been suggested in humans with persistent first degree AV block and low-dose atropine administration resulting in paradoxical worsening of AVB. This means the AV node may abnormally have more vagal innervation than the SA node in rare cases leading to abnormal responses to atropine administration.

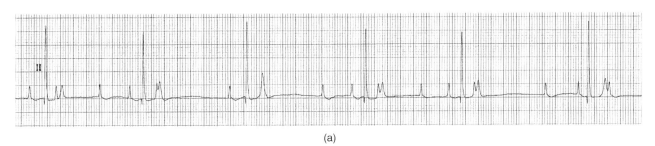

(a)

Figure 20.23a Paper speed 25 mm/s, 1 cm/mV, lead II, canine. **High-grade second degree AVB**. Ventriculophasic sinus arrhythmia of the atria is present with an atrial rate of around 100 bpm. The ventricular rate is slower at approximately 80 bpm. R-P/P-R reciprocity is present with better conduction at higher atrial rates suggestive of Type I second degree AVB despite the P-Ri variability. First degree AVB is present on all conducted beats.

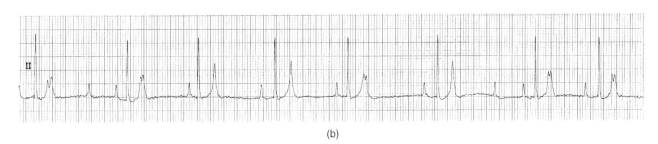

(b)

Figure 20.23b Paper speed 25 mm/s, 1 cm/mV, lead II, same dog. Five minutes post-injection of atropine (0.04 mg/kg). The sinus rate has paradoxically *slowed* to 90 bpm and 2 : 1 conduction (ventriculophasic sinus arrhythmia) ensues for most of the time. Non-conducted P waves are hiding in the T waves. Slowing of the sinus nodal discharge despite a high dose of atropine suggests an exaggerated central vagal effect. Persistent first degree AVB with less variability appears to be present.

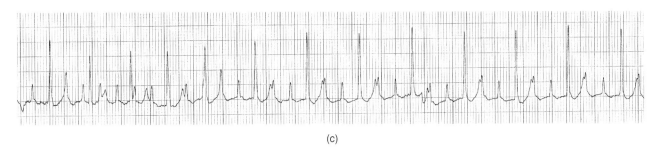

(c)

Figure 20.23c Paper speed 25 mm/s, 1 cm/mV, lead II, same dog. Fifteen minutes post-injection, the sinus rate has finally increased to 250 bpm and the ventricular rate up to 85 bpm, albeit with a 3 : 1 conduction ratio. P waves are superimposed over the T waves and the QRS complexes. The P-Ri becomes more fixed at 0.24 second. The second QRS is likely conducted from the P wave hiding in the T wave of the first QRS, *skipping* the fourth P wave here. Paradoxical worsening of the AVB here may suggest differential vagal innervation of the AVN vs. the SAN. We would expect 1 : 1 AV conduction by now.

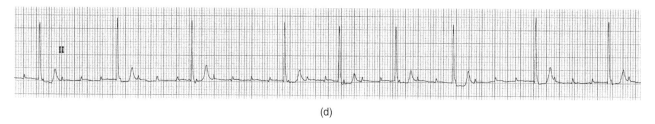

(d)

Figure 20.23d Paper speed 25 mm/s, 1 cm/mV, lead II, same dog. Twenty minutes post-injection. The sinus rate has slowed to 200 bpm. The P-Ri remains constant and prolonged at 0.24 second. Conduction ratios worsen (up to 5 : 1 conduction) despite slowing of the atrial rate as the atropine starts to wear off. The P wave morphology has changed but may be due to slightly altered limb lead placement (or displacement of the pacemaker to a lower sinus or R atrial ectopic focus).

Mobitz Type II second degree AVB AKA "Mobitz" or "Hay" in which there is no relation between the P-R interval and when P waves fail to conduct. The P-R interval is generally fixed, and the P-R interval tends to be independent of the R-P interval. The conduction tends to follow an "all or none" response, and failure of conduction occurs unexpectedly and in a random fashion. This means conduction occurs normally (i.e. with a normal P-Ri) or not at all. Concomitant conduction disturbances, such as bundle branch block are frequent. Type II second degree AVB may be of low or high grade. The block is usually in the AV bundle, bundle branches, and fascicles or distal His-Purkinje system and results from pathologic prolongation of the absolute refractory period.

Low-Grade Type II second degree AVB No more than one consecutive non-conducted beat occurs. Low-grade Type II second degree AVB tends to be less commonly seen vs. high-grade Type II second degree AVB. Low-grade Type II second degree AVB warrants watchful waiting.

2 : 1 Mobitz When conduction proceeds on every-other-beat and the block is of Type II variety, then 2 : 1 Mobitz is present. Clues to this include constant P-R intervals and often prolongation of the QRS from underlying bundle branch block. When the P-R interval is normal and the QRS is of normal duration, then the differentiation of Type I vs. Type II 2 : 1 AVB may not be possible on surface EKG. This is more likely secondary to distal conduction

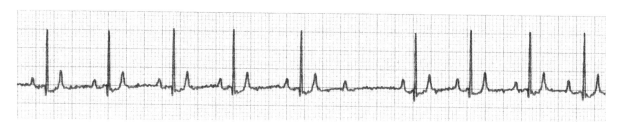

Figure 20.24 Paper speed 25 mm/s, 1 cm/mV, lead II, canine, *low-grade* **Type II second degree AVB**. The P-R interval is constant at 0.12 second.

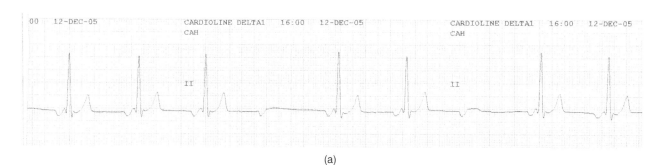

(a)

Figure 20.25a Paper speed 50 mm/s, 1 cm/mV, lead II, canine. An **accelerated junctional rhythm** (faster than junctional escape, slower than junctional tachycardia) is present, evident by the negatively oriented P waves. **Low-grade Type II second degree AVB** is present. The fourth and seventh P' waves fail to conduct to the ventricles. The P'-R interval is constant.

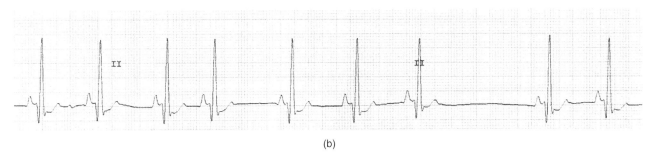

(b)

Figure 20.25b Paper speed 50 mm/s, 1 cm/mV, lead II, same dog, different day. The previous junctional rhythm has disappeared and been replaced by a sinus rhythm with occasional unexpected sinus pauses. These may be due to sinoatrial block.

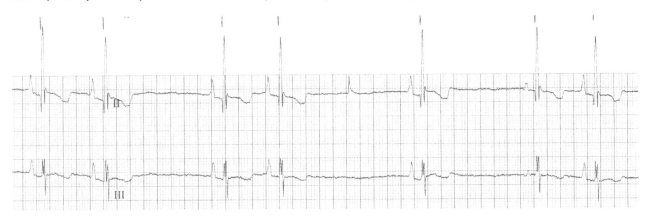

Figure 20.26 Paper speed 50 mm/s, 1 cm/mV, leads II and III, canine with hepatic encephalopathy. *Pseudo* **Mobitz Type II second degree AVB**. There appears to be a non-conducted P wave in lead II following the fourth complex. However, careful examinations show that this deflection is absent in lead III, making it unlikely to be a real atrial depolarization (certainly not sinus as the sinus P's in III are clearly positive). This "non-conducted P wave" is most likely an **artifact**. The pauses in the rhythm are secondary to sinoatrial block. The sixth complex is an ectopic atrial escape beat.

disease/bilateral bundle branch block and likely to progress to high-grade AVB.

High-Grade Type II second degree AVB There are more non-conducted beats than conducted beats (more than one consecutive non-conducted beats). Escape complexes/rhythms may be seen and of course capture beats as well since the block is still incomplete. Technically, if two or more consecutive P waves are blocked, it constitutes a high grade or advanced AVB, which can also

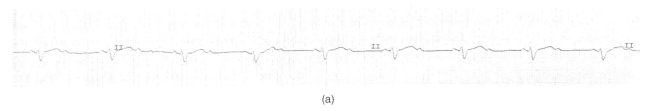

(a)

Figure 20.27a Paper speed 50 mm/s, 1 cm/mV, lead II, feline, 2:1 AVB. Whether this is **2:1 Type II (Mobitz)** is indeterminate from this strip; however, the P-R interval is normal and the QRS complexes are slightly widened (RBBB), suggesting Mobitz. Since pre-existing RBBB is present, intermittent block in the LBB may be causing failure of conduction, making this a *bilateral BBB*.

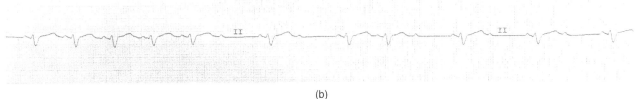

(b)

Figure 20.27b Paper speed 50 mm/s, 1 cm/mV, lead II, same cat. **Type II second degree AVB**. The P-R interval is constant.

occur with Type I AVB. The P-R intervals on captures are generally of normal duration and constant. The QRS complexes of captures may be prolonged from concurrent bundle branch block. High-grade Type II second degree AVB is more closely related to third degree AVB, often misdiagnosed as third degree AVB (especially if extended periods of escape rhythm are present) and is more likely to progress to third degree AVB. Therapy with sympathomimetics can be considered; however, permanent pacing is indicated for individuals with symptomatic bradycardia.

The differentiation between Type I and Type II second degree AVB can become even more problematic when two or more levels of AVB exist within the AVN. If the atrial rate is variable, a Type I block can change to a Type II. Patients with Type II block may convert into a Type I block if the atrial rate increases. Patients with AFL frequently have functional AVB due to high atrial depolarization rates, occasionally with two or more levels of block within the AVN. Furthermore, concealed premature depolarizations of the His bundle (from JPCs or VPCs) may create patterns that simulate Type I or Type II AVB.

Block/acceleration dissociation This is a term that has been coined by Marriot to describe a situation in which a relatively slow sinus rhythm, combined with a mild or undetermined (but incomplete) degree of AVB *and*

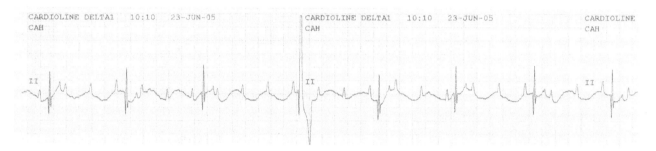

Figure 20.28 Paper speed 25 mm/s, 1 cm/mV, lead II, canine with **second degree AVB** that *worsened* after IV atropine injection. The P-R interval is 0.2 second and relatively constant. Initially, there is 3 : 1 AV conduction. A RV escape complex occurs after four P waves fail to conduct. Baseline undulation is present from panting artifact.

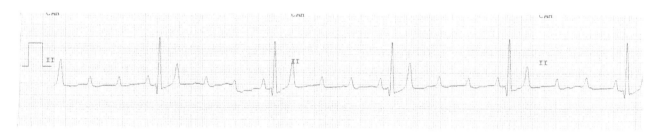

Figure 20.29 Paper speed 50 mm/s, 1 cm/mV, lead II, canine, **high-grade Type II second degree AVB** with 4 : 1 AV conduction. P waves are hiding in the T waves of the conducted QRS complexes.

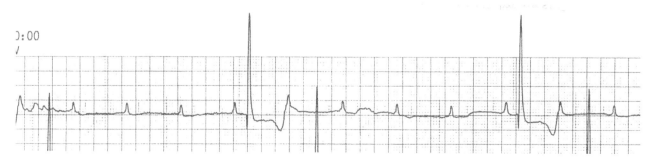

Figure 20.30 Paper speed 25 mm/s, 1 cm/mV, lead II, canine, **high-grade Type II second degree AVB** with 5 : 1 AV conduction.

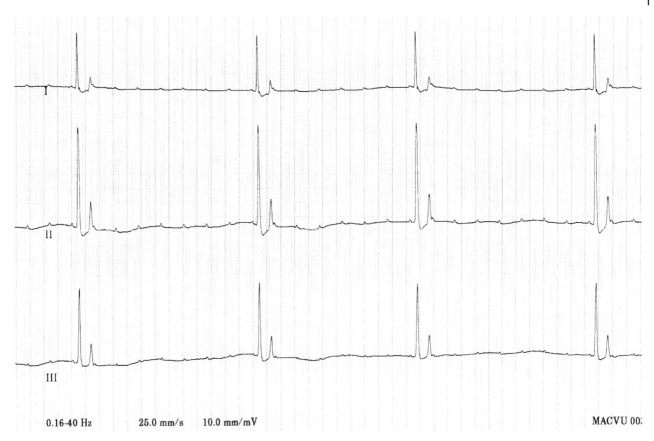

0.16-40 Hz   25.0 mm/s   10.0 mm/mV   MACVU 00:

Figure 20.31 Paper speed 25 mm/s, 1 cm/mV, leads I, II, III, canine. This six-month-old GSD puppy that presented for collapse. **Congenital high-grade Type II second degree AVB** with 8:1, 7:1, 8:1 conduction. The QRS complexes are tall, mildly prolonged with a long QTi, and have S-T segment depression likely from heart enlargement, bradycardia, and myocardial hypoxia, respectively.

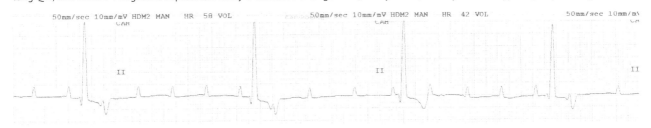

Figure 20.32 Paper speed 50 mm/s, 1 cm/mV, lead II, canine. During periods of extended AVB and ventricular escape rhythm, this dog's atrial rate would vary with respiration (sinus arrhythmia), causing the P waves gradually speed up then slow down, as seen here.

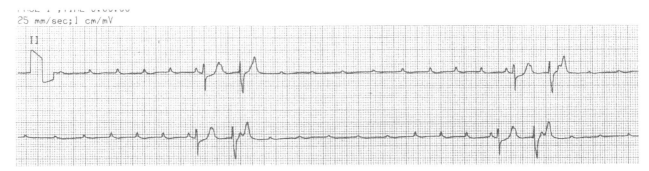

Figure 20.33 Paper speed 25 mm/s, 1 cm/mV, lead II, canine. **High-grade type II second degree AVB with ventricular bigeminy**. The narrow QRS first beat in each couplet is sinus conducted, and they each have a regular P-R interval. The wide-and-bizarre second beat in each couplet is a VPC. There is 9:1 AV conduction. There is some functional block of the P waves following the VPCs. These occur during the S-T segment of the VPCs. Because of the long-short sequence induced by prolonged periods of AVB, VPCs frequently appear due to re-entry (by **Rule of bigeminy**). Note the regular coupling intervals. Note the gradually increasing sinus *rate* and *amplitude* of the P waves prior to conduction. This is from progressively increasing sympathetic tone that occurs during the ventricular pause.

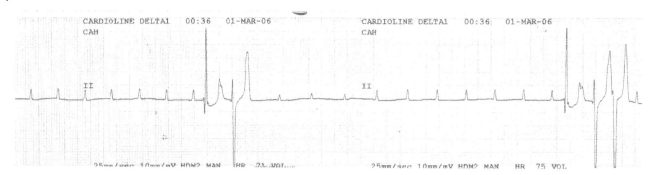

Figure 20.34 Paper speed 25 mm/s, 1 cm/mV, lead II, canine. High-grade Type II second degree AVB vs. third degree AVB. The beats following the apparently conducted beats may be aberrantly conducted sinus beats (RBBB). This *may* be a manifestation of ***Ashman's phenomenon***, as these beats (#2 and #4) end a short cycle preceded by a relatively long cycle (here, very long cycles due to advanced AVB). The P waves occur in the T wave of the preceding conducted sinus beats (#1 and #3). The fifth complex is clearly early and ventricular (VPC). The P-R intervals *appear* constant, suggesting aberrancy of the following beats and ***supernormal conduction***. Alternatively, the narrow complexes may simply be junctional escapes (with P waves that *happen* to precede them by a seemingly constant interval) and are followed by LVPCs by Rule of bigeminy and occur due to re-entry. This explanation is simpler, and thus more likely.

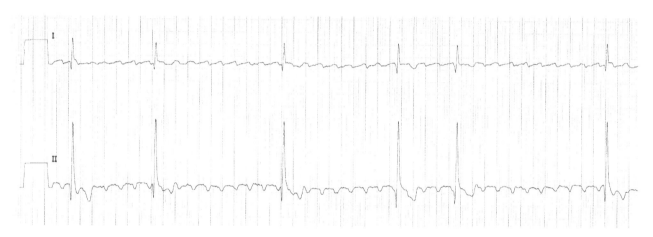

Figure 20.35 Paper speed 50 mm/s, 1 cm/mV, leads I and II, canine. ***Atrial flutter*** with ***high-grade second degree AVB***. The atrial rate is approximately 500 bpm, and the ventricular rate much slower at around 80 bpm. The ventricular rhythm is irregular and which QRS complexes may represent junctional escape beats is unclear given variable F-R intervals. This dog was on no antiarrhythmic medication or digoxin.

an accelerated idiojunctional or idioventricular rhythm produces AV dissociation. This frequently leads to a misdiagnosis of high-grade AV block, potentially prompting unnecessary pacemaker implantation. The clue to deciphering these EKGs is to note the faster than normal escape rate of the QRS complexes and at least intermittent failure of supraventricular conduction over the AVN when conduction would otherwise be expected (i.e. seeing P waves occurring without a corresponding supraventricular QRS within a "reasonable" amount of time). Examining the capture beats closely can help elucidate what the patient requires for 1 : 1 conduction. Close scrutiny of the R-P/P-R intervals is necessary. The faster the atrial or ventricular rate, the worse AV conduction tends to be, and in patients with incomplete AV block, a critical R-Pi is present that determines the capacity for anterograde AV nodal conduction. If the R-Pi is too short, conduction fails. If the R-Pi exceeds this critical length, conduction proceeds unless it is interrupted by an impulse from an accelerated focus from the junction itself or from the ventricles. The block may be physiologic and rather mild vs. truly high grade and pathologic.

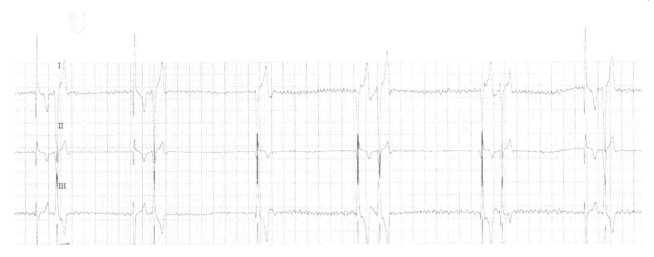

Figure 20.36 Paper speed 50 mm/s, 0.5 cm/mV, leads I, II, III, canine. **High-grade second degree AVB, fibrillation of the atria, ventricular bigeminy, ventricular escape rhythm with ventricular bigeminy**. The first and third beats are supraventricular and are followed by VPCs in a bigeminal rhythm. The fifth complex is ventricular escape, as are the sixth and eighth beats, which in turn are followed by VPCs in a bigeminal rhythm. The 10th complex is another supraventricular capture. The baseline is undulating and no P waves are identifiable, and the supraventricular captures occur at irregular intervals, indicative of atrial fibrillation. This patient had a high grade of AVB leading to excessively low ventricular rate response, frequent periods of ventricular bigeminy, and occasional periods of ventricular escape rhythm. Ventricular bigeminy and escape rhythm with ventricular bigeminy may be seen in patients with high-grade second degree (incomplete) AVB. The VPCs here are coupled to the preceding beats at a regular coupling interval, suggesting a reentrant mechanism.

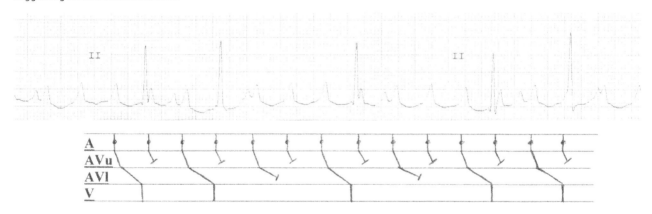

Figure 20.37 Paper speed 50 mm/s, 1 cm/mV, canine with **atrial flutter** (AFL) and probable *two levels* of **AVB**. 2 : 1 block in the upper level of the AVN coincides with alternating 3 : 2 and 2 : 1 block with Wenckebach periodicity in the lower level, as shown in the ladder diagram. Multiple levels of AVB within the AVN would have to be confirmed via intracardiac electrogram but are suspected when *greater* than 2 : 1 physiologic AVB occurs during AFL or atrial tachycardia, or *odd-numbered* conduction ratios are seen. Here, some level of AVB is resulting in a Wenckebach effect as conducted complexes that end short cycles do so with a longer F-R interval.

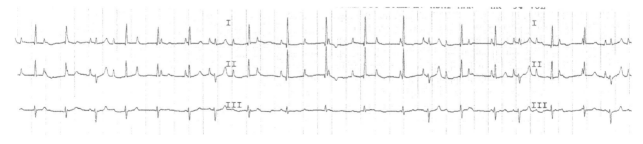

Figure 20.38 Paper speed 25 mm/s, 1 cm/mV, leads I, II, III, feline, undetermined degree AVB, the atrial rate is approximately 187 bpm, and the ventricular rate is 136 bpm. This may be incomplete AVB (high Type II second degree) since the 3rd, 7th, 13th, 16th, and 19th beats may be capture beats, with intermittent periods of *block/acceleration dissociation* between them. These capture beats also display characteristics of LAFB.

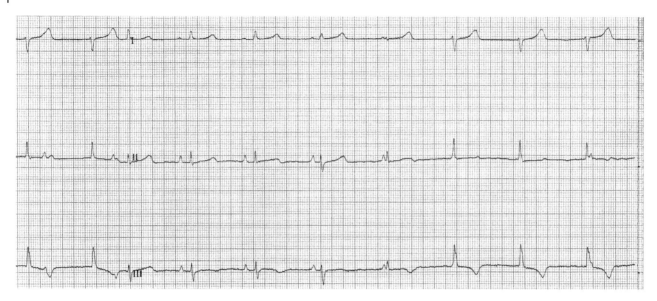

Figure 20.39 Paper speed 50 mm/s, 2 cm/mV, leads I, II, III, feline. Sinus bradycardia, atrial rate approximately 105 bpm, escape rhythm of the ventricles with similar rate ("isorhythmic dissociation with accrochage"), possible incomplete AVB (uncertain degree). The escape focus is either a slow junctional escape or accelerated ventricular escape with changing morphology of the QRS complexes. The third beat is a sinus capture, which resets the escape focus, suggesting that it is junctional by Rule of reset. However, the gradual morphology change in the QRS complexes is more likely the result of gradual ventricular *fusion* with an accelerated idioventricular rhythm, making this **block/acceleration dissociation**.

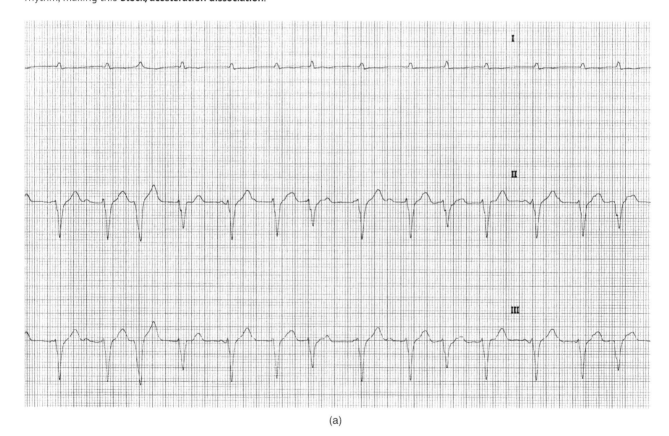

(a)

Figure 20.40a Paper speed 50 mm/s, 1 cm/mV, leads I, II, III, feline. The atrial rate is uncertain and the ventricular rhythm irregular; however, allorhythmic, so atrial fibrillation with intact AV conduction appears unlikely. Group beating is evident and suggests Wenckebach periodicity. P waves may be present after the 1st, 4th, 7th, and 10th beats (best seen in II, III), but appear dissociated as the P-R intervals are variable. The QRS complexes are prolonged, and if they are of supraventricular origin, then **bifascicular block** could explain the pattern (RBBB+LAFB).

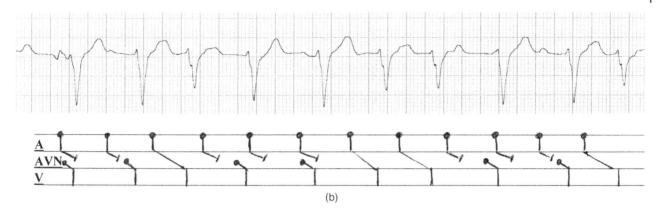

(b)

Figure 20.40b Paper speed 50 mm/s, 1 cm/mV, lead II, same cat. A ladder diagram illustrates a possible mechanism. Sinus rhythm is present and interrupted by an accelerated idiojunctional focus. Low-grade Type I second degree AVB is exposed after the fifth complex. Short periods of **block-acceleration dissociation** occur, and the junctional complexes are slightly deeper in amplitude.

Paroxysmal atrioventricular block This may create transient ventricular asystole and may result from Phase 4 block, intermittent bilateral BBB, be spontaneous or vagal in origin. Transient ventricular asystole does not fit neatly into the usual classification of AVB, as it is high grade but incomplete and not clearly of Wenckebach or Mobitz varieties. This has been postulated to be caused by enhanced Phase 4 diastolic depolarization in a diseased segment of the AVN, provoked by P-P prolongation or premature beats and is characterized by a lack of otherwise expected subsidiary pacemaker captures (i.e. "lazy escapes") often with a gradual P-Pi narrowing as the sinus node "tries" to capture the ventricle under sympathetic stimulation during ventricular asystole. The absence of otherwise expected escapes may be explained by diastolic Phase 4 depolarization not achieving threshold, bidirectional exit block of the escape focus, and repetitive concealed antegrade conduction of successively blocked sinus impulses (usually a Type I second degree AVB). Basically, sinus rhythm is followed by long periods of P waves that fail to conduct to the ventricles. This typically produces obvious syncope from so-called "Stokes-Adams attacks." An escape focus (junctional or ventricular) must come to the rescue or the patient will die of circulatory collapse. Paroxysmal AVB is probably one of the more common reasons cats with AVB present for syncope and may require pacemaker implantation.

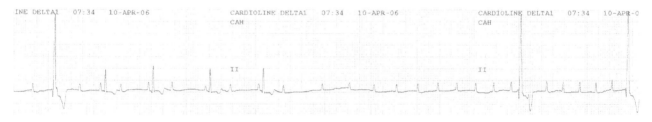

Figure 20.41 Paper speed 25 mm/s, 1 cm/mV, lead II, canine. High-grade Type II second degree AVB with **paroxysmal AVB**. This strip demonstrates that the sinus node may fire *irregularly* during AVB, confusing the examiner with sick sinus syndrome (SSS). In this case, an escape beat is followed by a short run of 2 : 1 conduction with constant/normal P-Ri, technically a ventriculophasic sinus arrhythmia. The subsequent P waves are blocked, and gradually *speed* up until an escape rhythm assumes control. This is the result of changes in autonomic tone associated with prolonged ventricular asystole. No *excessively* long sinus pauses/arrests are seen between P waves, so SSS is unlikely. A relatively longer P-P interval immediately precedes paroxysmal AVB, making Phase 4 block a likely contributor.

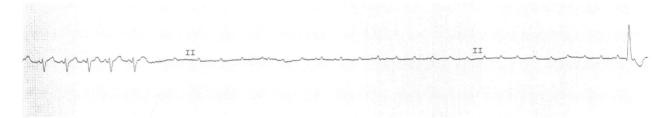

Figure 20.42 Paper speed 25 mm/s, 1 cm/mV, lead II, feline. Prolonged AVB (causing **transient ventricular asystole**) has resulted in syncope in this cat. The long period of AVB is terminated by a very late RV escape beat. This is likely from Phase 4 block, given the long P-blocked P interval.

Third degree AVB

AKA "Complete" Heart Block or third degree AVB: there is no association between the P waves and the QRS complexes (complete AV dissociation with escape by default). This is caused by bilateral bundle branch block in 90% and His bundle block in 10% in humans. Bundle branch block, high-grade AVB, and third degree AVB have been associated with cardiotoxicity with doxorubicin. Third degree AVB is often overdiagnosed and is confirmed if the following five criteria are fulfilled:

1. P waves should not only occur during the absolute refractory period of a preceding activation.
2. Isorhythmic dissociation with similar atrial and ventricular rates should not be present.
3. There must be a high enough atrial rate so all phases of the escape action potential are bombarded.
4. The escape rate must be slow enough to permit conduction of a dissociated P wave.
5. No early supraventricular QRS complexes consistent with a capture are demonstrable.

> *A Note:* Number 5 above has one possible exception – supernormal conduction. If an atrial impulse happens to occur at just the right time following an escape beat (during the so-called supernormal period), conduction may be rarely be permitted even though third degree AVB is present. These "captures" may have QRS prolongation from functional bundle branch block. However, VPCs or reciprocal complexes may commonly be coupled to escape complexes, simulating supernormal conduction. If the premature beat cannot be reliably related to a specific R-Pi (and P-R'i), then VPCs are favored.

No conduction is possible through the AVN, so the P waves (or other supraventricular foci in charge of the atria) march through the ventricular complexes which represent an escape focus. This escape focus may be junctional or ventricular in origin. Junctional escape foci are supraventricular but may have QRS prolongation secondary to concurrent fascicular or bundle branch block. Minor variation of the QRS amplitude may be present depending on AV synchrony (Brody effect). Third degree AVB may be an incidental finding in asymptomatic elderly animals, rarely may be congenital and sudden onset may cause exercise intolerance, syncope, etc. Third degree AVB is differentiated from the special term AV dissociation because the atrial rate exceeds the ventricular rate in third degree AVB. However, while third degree AVB produces complete AV dissociation, apparently complete AV dissociation may occur without third degree AVB. If the ventricular rate is consistently too low from third degree AVB, then the clinician may try injectable atropine or isoproterenol, oral sympathomimetics such as theophylline or hyoscyamine (Levsin©), but definitive treatment is a pacemaker. Pacemakers are for clinical animals ideally with little or insignificant structural heart disease, no other seriously life-limiting conditions, etc. Prolonged third degree AVB results in chronic systemic hypertension, volume overload, and a dilated heart with relatively normal contractility which mimics dilated cardiomyopathy ("bradycardia-associated cardiomyopathy"/BICM) and can lead to CHF – typically right-sided, but occasionally biventricular. This may be reversible to some degree with pacing. Patients with third degree AVB may incidentally have escape rhythms that are irregular from reciprocal

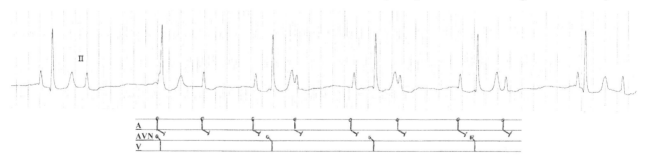

Figure 20.43 Paper speed 50 mm/s, 1 cm/mV, lead II, canine. Ventriculophasic sinus arrhythmia of the atria, junctional escape rhythm of the ventricles, apparently complete AV dissociation secondary to apparently **complete (third degree) AV block**. The ladder diagram illustrates the mechanism. The atrial rhythm is bigeminal and P-P intervals encompassing a QRS are shorter than the P-P intervals that do not. The atrial rate is approximately 120 bpm and the ventricular rate is approximately 60 bpm. Note the changing P-R intervals characteristic of AV dissociation.

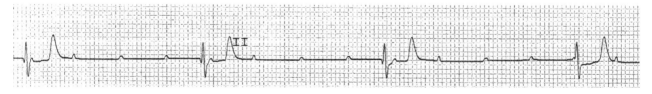

Figure 20.44 Paper speed 25 mm/s, 1 cm/mV, lead II, canine, **third degree AVB**. The atrial rate is 166 bpm, and the ventricular escape rate is approximately 28 bpm.

complexes or VPCs, commonly in bigeminy. Ventricular premature beats associated with escape complexes may rarely occur in trigeminal and quadrigeminal patterns. An important rule out for premature beats coupled to escape complexes is a supraventricular capture attributed to supernormal conduction. Atrioventricular dissociation is the rule, the atria may not be in sinus rhythm (i.e. sinus arrest, ectopic atrial rhythm, atrial tachycardia, AFL/AF), isorhythmic dissociation may occur with slow sinus rates, and escape rhythms may occasionally be usurped by accelerated foci within the junction or in the ventricles.

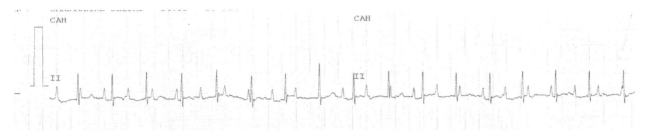

Figure 20.45 Paper speed 25 mm/s, 2 cm/mV, lead II, feline, **third degree AVB**. The atrial rate is 158 bpm, and the ventricular rate is 136 bpm from a junctional escape focus. Third degree AVB is often accompanied by a relatively fast junctional escape rhythm, and thus cats are rarely overtly symptomatic. Hyperthyroid cats with third degree AVB and junctional escape may resolve with appropriate therapy.

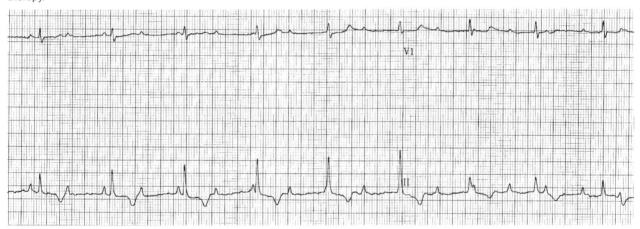

Figure 20.46 Paper speed 50 mm/Hg, 1 cm/mV, feline, leads V1 and II. **Third degree AVB**. Sinus tachycardia of the atria (atrial rate 200 bpm), junctional rhythm of the ventricles (ventricular rate 103 bpm), complete AV dissociation secondary to complete AV block. The interesting feature here is that the QRS complexes gradually increase in amplitude, but not width over the first through sixth beats. Given that the ventricular rate does not change, the QRS duration does not change, and the P-Ri has no clear relation to the QRS amplitude, and the QRS morphology/amplitude is unchanged in V1, then supraventricular influence appears to be excluded.

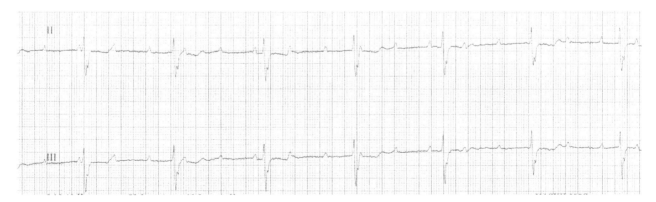

Figure 20.47 Paper speed 50 mm/s, 1 cm/mV, leads II, III, feline with CHF. **Third degree AVB**, sinus tachycardia of the atria (atrial rate approximately 220 bpm), ventricular escape rhythm (RBBB morphology, likely LV focus, ventricular rate approximately 83 bpm), with resultant complete AV dissociation.

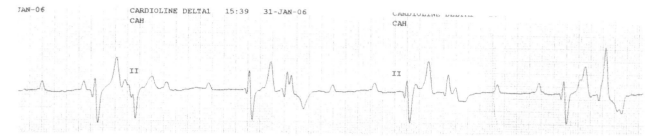

Figure 20.48 Paper speed 50 mm/s, 1 cm/mV, lead II, canine. **Third degree AVB, ventricular escape, and ventricular bigeminy**. This is a common occurrence in third degree AVB. The lengthened pauses between the escape beats, favor re-entry mechanisms, and VPCs tend to be precipitated by lengthened cycles by the Rule of bigeminy. Here, the VPCs are multiforme with irregular coupling intervals, which is unusual. They start in RBBB morphology (complex #2) and gradually *change* to a LBBB morphology (complex #8).

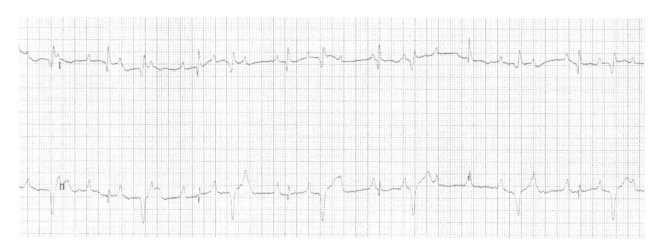

Figure 20.49 Paper speed 50 mm/s, 1 cm/mV, leads I and II, feline. **Third degree AVB, junctional escape and ventricular bigeminy**. The atrial rate is approximately 230 bpm, the junctional escape with an underlying rate of approximately 125 bpm, and VPCs in bigeminy with constant coupling intervals aside from the 11th complex.

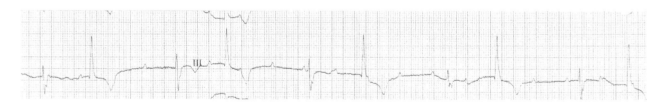

Figure 20.50 Paper speed 50 mm/s, 1 cm/mV, lead III, feline. **Third degree AVB, ventricular escape, and ventricular bigeminy**. The atrial rate is approximately 220 bpm, and the ventricular escape focus (RBBB morphology, with wide/deep S waves) is approximately 83 bpm. Ventricular premature beats (LBBB morphology) follow the escape beats in a 1:1 extrasystole with constant coupling intervals.

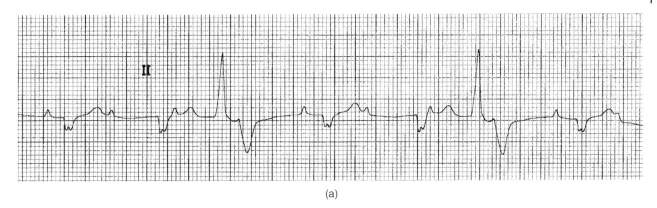

(a)

Figure 20.51a Paper speed 50 mm/s, 1 cm/mV, lead II, feline. **Third degree AVB,** *junctional escape* **with RBBB, ventricular** *trigeminy*. The atrial rate is approximately 200 bpm, the junctional escape rate (RBBB morphology) is approximately 133 bpm, complete AV dissociation is evident, and every third complex is a VPC (2 : 1 extrasystole). The underlying atrial rhythm is sinus, and AVD is evidenced by variable P-R intervals without pattern. Third degree AVB is evidenced by the rapid atrial rhythm and slower ventricular rhythm. The ventricles are controlled by a junctional escape focus with a RBBB. The instantaneous ventricular rate is 133 bpm, which is more consistent with junctional escape. The complexes are prolonged with a RBBB configuration. The VPCs here have a LBBB-like morphology.

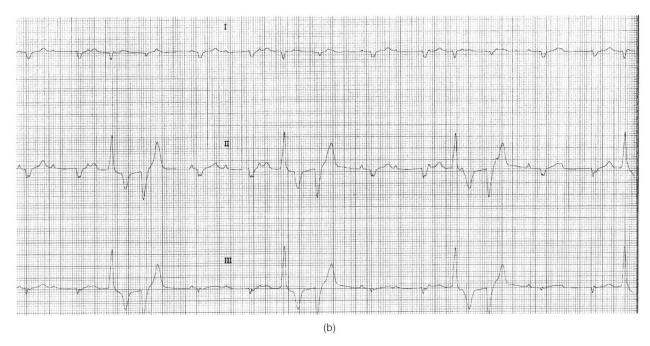

(b)

Figure 20.51b Paper speed 50 mm/s, 1 cm/mV, leads I, II, III, same feline. This unusual and complicated EKG shows complete atrioventricular dissociation secondary to **complete (third degree) AVB** with **ventricular** *quadrigeminy*. Each pair of escape beats is then followed by a pair of VPCs with alternating morphologies (LBBB-like followed by RBBB-like), suggesting alternating R and L ventricular foci (or foci within the L posterior fascicle vs. the L anterior fascicle, respectively). Another possible, but unlikely explanation could be supernormal conduction of sinus beats with P-Ri prolongation and RBBB aberrancy of the QRS following the right ventricular originating escape beats, though supernormal conduction is always a tenuous diagnosis. 2 : 2 extrasystole is rare even during sinus rhythm, much less during AVB, and bidirectional VPCs make this record unusual.

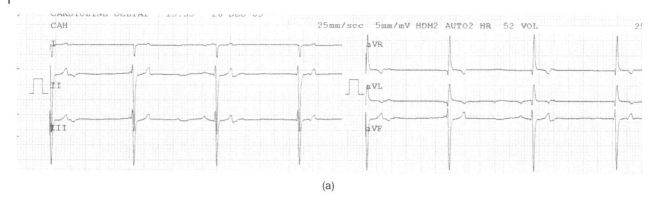

(a)

Figure 20.52a Paper speed 25 mm/s, 0.5 cm/mV, full EKG. **Third degree AVB** *and* advanced sick sinus syndrome have left this dog with an escape rhythm. The ventricular rate is approximately 59 bpm, is regular, and has narrow complexes. In of itself, this is suggestive of a junctional escape focus based on rate and QRS morphology. Severe R axis deviation (MEA approximately −100 degrees) is present, resulting in negative QRS complexes in II, III, and aVF. The atrial rate is irregular, slow, with periods of atrial asystole, suggestive of sinus nodal dysfunction.

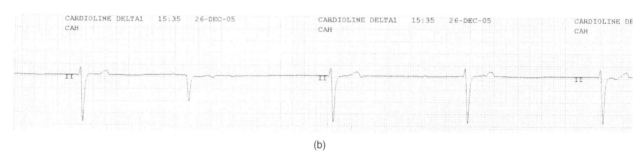

(b)

Figure 20.52b Paper speed 50 mm/s, 0.5 cm/mV, lead II, same dog. The second complex is premature and characterized by a compensatory pause. This appears to be a VPC. The junctional escape focus resumes control at exactly two R-R intervals from the first beat.

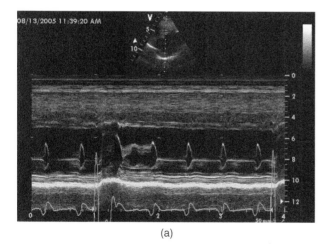

(a)

Figure 20.53a Echocardiograph of a dog with **third degree AVB**. Short-axis, right-sided view of the LV is shown in M-Mode. One ventricular complex is seen, followed by a prolonged opening and flutter of the mitral valve. The MV opens each time an atrial contraction occurs. The P waves seen are negative, followed by positive Ta waves.

When a patient is in complete (third degree) AVB, typically the atria are controlled by the sinus node. It is more technically correct to describe such an arrhythmia as "supraventricular (usually sinus) rhythm of the atria, escape (junctional or ventricular) rhythm of the ventricles, apparently complete atrioventricular dissociation by default secondary to apparently complete (3rd degree) atrioventricular block" or something to that effect. Occasionally, the atria may be controlled by another focus, i.e. ectopic atrial, or the atria may be in flutter, fibrillation, or standstill, sinus arrest, etc. As long as an escape focus has captured the ventricles, the atria can be doing anything. The trickier situations are when the atria are in flutter or fibrillation. Typically, AFL and AF result in rapid ventricular rate responses if AV conduction is intact. Normally, incomplete AVB (second degree AVB) is the rule as not all of the impulses are capable of reaching the ventricles given the normal refractoriness of the AV nodal tissue. However, if a high-grade or complete AVB develops, the ventricular rate is determined by the escape focus. A big clue to

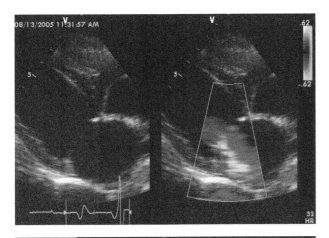

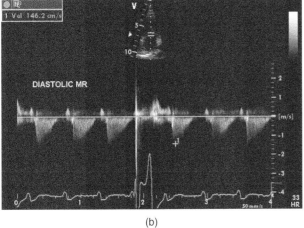

(b)

Figure 20.53b Echocardiographs of the same dog in third degree AVB. Long-axis four-chambered view from the right side. Low-velocity diastolic MR is apparent following the previous contraction of the atria without ventricular contraction. This is very common with third degree AVB, and is a manifestation of the atria contracting against a volume-loaded LV that merely sprays blood back into the LA after each atrial contraction. Note the color Doppler signal is laminar, low-velocity flow directed away from the transducer into the LA. Echocardiograph of the same dog is just below. Diastolic MR is documented in CW Doppler and is of low velocity.

high-grade Type II second degree or third degree AVB during AF or AFL is the development of a slow and regular ventricular rhythm. The complexes may appear supraventricular if coming from a junctional escape focus and ventricular in appearance if it is junctional escape with a BBB aberration or ventricular escape. The combination of AF or AFL with complete AVB has been termed Frederick syndrome. Treatment with sympathomimetics can be attempted; however, permanent pacing is often necessary for the symptomatic bradycardia associated with third degree AVB.

Atrioventricular dissociation If third degree AVB is present, then AVD is present, but AVD can be present in the absence of third degree AVB. Provided prolonged sinus arrest or atrial standstill is absent, the P wave rate (atrial rate) always exceeds the underlying ventricular escape rhythm rate in third degree AVB, and AVD is complete. The escape rhythm may be ventricular (20–45 bpm in dogs, 60–85 bpm in cats, technically originating from a bundle branch or distal Purkinje fiber) or junctional (aka "nodal" and 35–65 bpm in dogs and technically originating from the bundle of His, 80–140 bpm in cats). Escape rhythms tend to be wide and bizarre if ventricular and/or conducted with a BBB. It is imperative that the clinician to verify that the ventricular rate is consistent with that expected of a ventricular or junctional escape focus. If the ventricular rate is inconsistent with these ranges, then the diagnosis of third degree AVB should be re-evaluated or the presence of an artificial pacemaker should be considered. Occasionally, more than one escape focus can capture the ventricles making the rhythm irregular. Fusion of ventricular escape foci from opposite ventricles (or junctional escape with pre-existent BBB and fusing with a focus from the blocked ventricle) may paradoxically narrow the QRS complex. If you find third-degree AVB and the HR is exactly 100 bpm, suspect the animal has a pacemaker implanted, as most dogs cannot have a junctional escape rhythm that high,

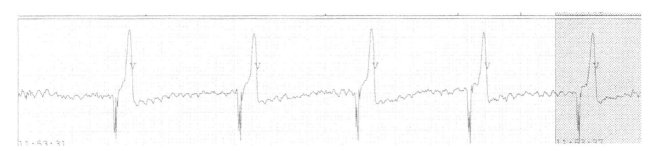

Figure 20.54 Paper speed 25 mm/s, 1 cm/mV, syncopal canine. **Atrial fibrillation (AF)** *and* **third degree AVB**. The ventricular escape rhythm is approximately 50 bpm, with QRS complexes that are regular. No P waves are evident and the baseline is undulatory, consistent with AF. Atrial fibrillation is normally typified by an irregularly irregular ventricular rate. The slow ventricular rate seen here is secondary to a *regularly* firing escape focus.

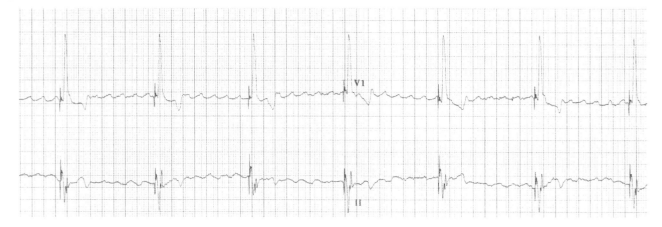

Figure 20.55 Paper speed 50 mm/s, 1 cm/mV, canine with history of third degree AVB. Post-pacemaker implantation, this dog developed biventricular failure from progressive atrioventricular valve disease. **Atrial flutter (AFL)** *and* **third degree AVB**. Type I (Typical/counterclockwise) AFL of the atria with a rate of 600 bpm, complete AVD, paced ventricular rhythm with a ventricular rate of 85 bpm. Note the pacemaker spikes preceding each ventricular complex at a rate *faster* than that expected for a typical ventricular escape focus.

and many pacemaker generators are programmed to fire at 100 bpm. Second degree AVB may display incomplete AVD if escape foci intermittently capture the ventricles.

The atrial and idiojunctional or idioventricular rhythms may occasionally become synchronized during the AVD associated with AVB. This is commonly the case if sinus bradycardia is present, or if the escape rhythm is mildly accelerated. If the period of synchronization is brief, occurring over only a few beats, the term "accrochage" is used. If the synchronization lasts for relatively long periods, then the term "synchrony" is used. Running the strips out for long periods helps the examiner determine that AV dissociation is indeed present in these cases. If the atrial and idiojunctional/ventricular rates are nearly identical, the

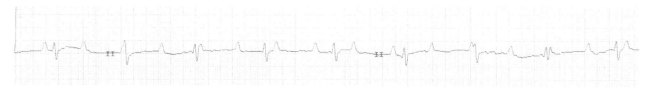

Figure 20.56 Paper speed 50 mm/s, 2 cm/mV, lead II, feline. **Third degree AVB**. Apparently complete atrioventricular dissociation is present with the atrial rate > ventricular rate.

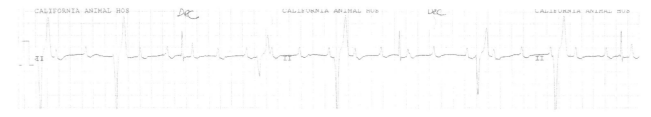

Figure 20.57 Paper speed 25 mm/s, 1 cm/mV, lead II, canine. This strip at first glance appears to show high-grade Type II second degree AVB. The P waves march through all ventricular complexes (at a higher rate) indicating **AVD**. Atrioventricular dissociation in this case appears to be incomplete, as the third and sixth complexes may well be conducted with narrow QRS complexes. The escape beats are wide, bizarre, and appear to be ventricular with a spontaneous rate of approximately 46 bpm. The fourth and seventh beats appear intermediate in waveform and are preceded by a P wave with a shorter P-R interval, suggestive of ventricular fusion beats. The escape focus, however, appears to be *reset* by the capture beats, suggesting that the escape focus is actually junctional in origin (rather than ventricular) by the Rule of reset. Ventricular fusion, however, is not possible between sinus and junctional – originating beats in the absence of an accessory pathway. Therefore, the "sinus captures" may simply be escape beats that are junctional (with narrow QRS), and the ventricular beats may be a parasystolic rhythm. The P-R intervals of the narrow complex beats are not consistent on close examination, and that is evidence of complete AVD. This strip also highlights negative Ta waves (atrial repolarization) that follow the P waves.

term "isorhythmic dissociation" is used; however, 2 : 1 synchronization (2 P waves for every 1 QRS), and higher ratios may occur as well. The mechanism of synchronization is postulated to be electromechanical in nature and similar to the phenomenon of ventriculophasic sinus arrhythmia.

The special term atrioventricular dissociation (from usurpation) and third degree AVB can coexist if two independent pacemakers are present and both are fast enough to prevent the AV node from emerging from a refractory state, though this is rare, really only occurring in the setting

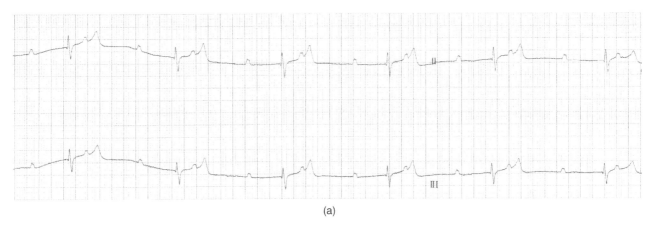

(a)

Figure 20.58a Paper speed 50 mm/s, 1 cm/mV, leads II and III, canine under anesthesia with isoflurane and fentanyl CRI. This appears to be **third degree AVB with 2 : 1 AV synchronization**. Here, the atria maintain a relatively constant rate of 130 bpm, beating twice for every (presumed) idiojunctional beat (rate 70 bpm), and appear to maintain a relatively constant relationship with the QRS complexes. Alternatively this strip could be interpreted as a high-grade Type I second degree AVB with 2 : 1 conduction. The P-R intervals, however, are changing slightly, suggesting AV dissociation. Furthermore, if the P waves preceding the QRS complexes are indeed conducting them, the P-Ri is exceedingly long at 0.28 second. Remember if isorhythmic dissociation is present, then third degree AVB cannot be diagnosed definitively.

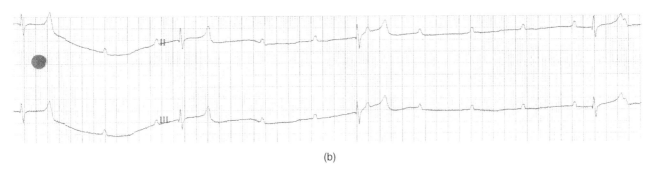

(b)

Figure 20.58b Paper speed 50 mm/s, 1 cm/mV, leads II and III, same dog still under anesthesia. Here, the ventricular rhythm is irregular, and the P-R intervals are clearly changing, *suggesting* AV dissociation and an irregular idiojunctional rhythm. Alternatively, the first two QRS complexes may actually be conducted, and the third and fourth complexes may represent an idiojunctional escape rhythm. If this were the case, however, the P-Ri of the "conducted beats" is markedly shorter than in the above strip. His bundle EKG would be required for a definitive diagnosis.

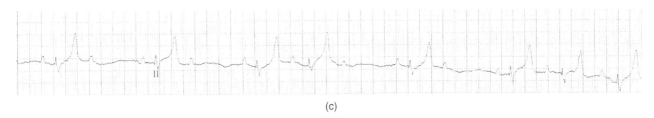

(c)

Figure 20.58c Paper speed 50 mm/s, 1 cm/mV, lead II, same dog, the next day after anesthesia. 2 : 1 Type I second degree AVB occurs at the beginning of the strip, and is followed by a typical Wenckebach period, with gradual prolongation of the P-Ri until failure of conduction occurs. Perhaps, the above strips truly represent a very high-grade Type I second degree AVB, caused by the vagomimetic influence of fentanyl and/or isoflurane. Fentanyl has marked vagal effects and may exacerbate underlying SA nodal or AV nodal disease, resulting in bradycardia.

of so-called "double tachycardia" with AVD (ventricular tachycardia and simultaneous supraventricular tachycardia – sinus, ectopic atrial tachycardia, high junctional tachycardia, AF or AFL), and the block is functional or physiologic (see Chapter 25). More commonly, an irritable focus (i.e. accelerated idioventricular or idiojunctional rhythm or junctional or ventricular tachycardia) may supercede an escape focus during uncertain second degree or third degree AVB, and the block is usually pathologic consistent with block/acceleration dissociation. Syncope may be precipitated by long asystolic periods following accelerated rhythms that result in overdrive suppression of subsidiary escape foci.

Ventriculoatrial block

Retrograde AVB (ventriculoatrial block or VA block/VAB) may rarely be seen following ventricular or junctional premature complexes, paced or escape beats with ventriculoatrial conduction (VA conduction) and is generally not seen during antegrade AVB unless escape beats have VA conduction. First degree VA block has a long R-P′ interval (values not really established, but generally in excess of what is considered to be a normal P-Ri for the species). Third degree VA block simply results in failure of all impulses to traverse the AVN and capture the atria and is not really evident on surface EKG other than to note retrograde P′ waves are always absent. This may occur even if retrograde conduction is still possible (i.e. if the atrial rhythm is more rapid than the junctional or ventricular rhythm, it will suppress VA conduction). Second degree VA block will cause irregularity of the atrial rhythm as conduction is intermittently blocked. Type I VAB (Wenckebach) is typified by gradual R′-P′ prolongation prior to failure of retrograde conduction to the atria. Type II VAB (Mobitz) is exemplified by constant R′-P′ intervals, random failure to conduct with exact

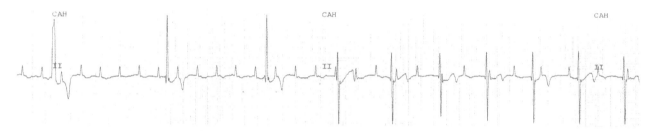

Figure 20.59 Paper speed 25 mm/s, 1 cm/mV, lead II, canine. Third degree AVB has made this patient syncopal. AVD is present throughout the strip, and initially a ventricular escape rhythm is present with a HR of approximately 38 bpm. Halfway through the strip, another focus, likely **junctional**, captures the rhythm with a ventricular rate of approximately 158 bpm.

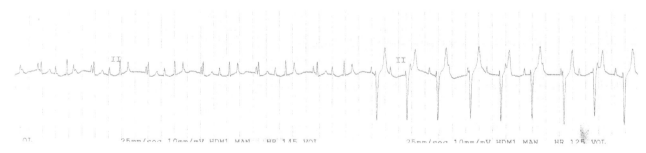

Figure 20.60 Paper speed 25 mm/s, 1 cm/mV, lead II, feline. Third degree AVB is present with a junctional escape rhythm of approximately 136 bpm. Halfway through the strip, an **accelerated idioventricular rhythm** captures the ventricles resulting in a HR of approximately 125 bpm. The junctional rhythm at the beginning is within the range of normal rates associated with junctional escape in the cat, whereas the ventricular rhythm is faster than that normally associated with ventricular escape in the cat, making it accelerated.

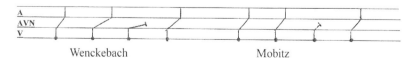

Figure 20.61 Ladder diagrams illustrating **ventriculoatrial block**. A ventricular focus with ventriculoatrial conduction is shown. Type I (Wenckebach) VAB to the left displays progressive R-P′ interval prolongation prior to failure of conduction. Type II (Mobitz) VAB to the right shows random failure of conduction with constant R-P′ intervals.

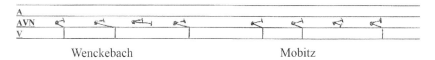

Wenckebach   Mobitz

Figure 20.62 Ladder diagrams illustrating **exit block**. A junctional focus with retrograde VA block and antegrade exit block is shown with sinus arrest. To the right, a junctional focus displays Type I (Wenckebach) exit block with progressive prolongation (of the *H-V'* interval for *His bundle* to ectopic *ventricular* myocardial depolarization) prior to failure of conduction. To the left, Type II (Mobitz) block occurs with random failure of conduction and constant H-V' (and subsequent R-R) intervals.

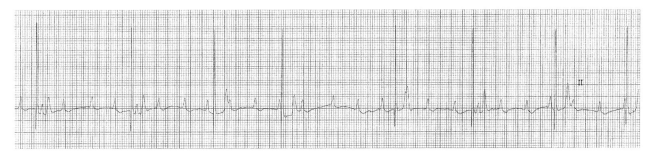

Figure 20.63 Paper speed 25 mm/s, 1 cm/mV, lead II, canine. Sinus rhythm of the atria, junctional escape rhythm of the ventricles, complete AVD secondary to complete (third degree) AVB. The junctional escape rhythm here is irregular with group beating characteristic of Wenckebach periodicity. This may be from **Type I exit block** from the escape focus. A "*respiratory junctional arrhythmia*" (variation in the junctional discharge rate due to autonomic influence/respiratory phase) seems unlikely given the lack of a concurrent respiratory sinus arrhythmia.

multiples of P'-P' intervals in between blocked complexes. If every other junctional or ventricular beat is followed by a retrograde P' wave, then 2 : 1 VA block is present.

Exit block Exit block is interruption of conduction from the tissue immediately surrounding the source of the focus in question and is most commonly associated with sinoatrial block, premature beats, junctional rhythms, accelerated ventricular rhythms or ventricular tachycardia, and rarely if ever seen during antegrade AVB. Escape rhythms are most commonly from junctional or ventricular foci and only rarely from atrial or sinoatrial regions. These may be irregular in rhythm. Most often escape rhythms may be interrupted by captures, VPCs, reciprocal complexes, or superceded by another escape focus, any of which may upset the underlying rhythm. If the escape focus is unifocal and the preceding situations excluded, the cause of sudden irregularity in ventricular rhythm may be exit block. First degree exit block is not evident on surface EKG and third degree exit block is indistinguishable from arrest/asystole. Second degree exit block is intermittent and thus evident on surface EKG if present. Type I exit block (Wenckebach) may cause group beating and is manifested by R-R intervals between blocked impulses being less than 2 R-R intervals. Type II exit block (Mobitz) is characterized by R-R intervals between blocked impulses being equal to (or some exact multiple of) two R-R intervals. It is also common for automatic foci to "ramp up" in rate at the onset of an escape rhythm, so the investigator should look for irregularities in the rhythm after an established escape rhythm has ensued for evidence of exit block. If the ectopic junctional or ventricular rhythm suddenly halves in rate, then the onset of 2 : 1 exit block is assumed.

Further reading

Carvalho, K.N., Rush, J.E., and Wemore, L.A. (2014). ECG of the month. *JAVMA* 244 (8): 902–904.

Chin, K.J. (2005). Atrioventricular conduction block induced by low-dose atropine. *Anesthesia* 60: 935–936.

Cruse, A.M., Booth, M.A., and DeFrancesco, T.C. (2008). ECG of the month. *JAVMA* 232 (4): 510–512.

Damato, A.N. and Lau, S.H. (1971). Concealed and supernormal atrioventricular conduction. *Circulation* XLIII: 967–970.

El-Sherif, N. et al. (1978). Atypical Wenckebach periodicity simulating Mobitz II AV block. *Br. Heart J.* 40: 1376–1383.

Fisch, C. and Knoebel, S.B. (2000). *Electrocardiography of Clinical Arrhythmias.* Futurama Publishing Co.

Fowler, M.M., Jesty, S.A., Gompf, R.E. et al. (2013). ECG of the month. *JAVMA* 243 (1): 52–54.

Goldberg, L.B., Levy, M.N., and Edelstein, J. (1975). The postponed compensatory pause as a manifestation of positive feedback in atrioventricular conduction. *Circulation* 52.

Kellum, H.B. and Stepien, R.L. (2006). Third-degree atrioventricular block in 21 cats (1997-2004). *J. Vet. Intern. Med.* 20: 97–103.

Kinoshita, S. and Konishi, G. (1987). Atrioventricular Wenckebach periodicity in athletes: influence of increased vagal tone on the occurrence of atypical periods. *J. Electrocardiol.* 20 (3): 272–279.

Marriot, H.J. (1956). Atrioventricular synchronization and accrochage. *Circulation* XIV: 38–43.

Marriot, H.J.L. and Conover, M.B. (1998). *Advanced Concepts in Arrhythmias*, 3e. Mosby.

Marriott, H.J. (1998). *Pearls & Pitfalls in Electrocardiography, Pithy Practical Pointers*, 2e. Williams & Wilkins.

Pick, A. and Langendorf, R. (1979). *Interpretation of Complex Arrhythmias*. Lea & Febiger.

Rosen, K.M. (1973). Junctional tachycardia: mechanisms, diagnosis, differential diagnosis, and management. *Circulation* XLVII: 654–664.

Scheinman, M. (2016). *Cardiac Electrophysiology Clinics. Interpretation of Complex Arrhythmias: A Case-Based Approach*, vol. 8. No.1. Elsevier.

Scheinman, M., Thakur, R.K., and Natale, A. (eds.) (2016). *Cardiac Electrophysiology Clinics: Interpretation of Complex Arrhythmias: A Case-Based Approach*. Elsevier.

Schmidt, M.K., Estrada, A.H., and Sleeper, M.M. (2007). ECG of the month. *JAVMA* 230 (7): 1002–1004.

Schrope, D.P. and Kelch, W.J. (2006). Signalment, clinical signs, and prognostic indicators associated with high-grade second or third-degree atrioventricular block in dogs: 124 cases (January 1, 1997-December 31, 1997). *JAVMA* 228 (11).

Schuller, S., Van Israël, N., and Else, R.W. (2007). Third degree atrioventricular black and accelerated Idioventricular rhythm associated with a Heart Base Chemodectoma in a syncopal Rottweiler. *J. Vet. Med.* 54: 618–623.

Silverman, M.E., Upshaw, C.B., and Lange, H.W. (2004). Woldemar Mobitz and his 1924 classification of second-degree atrioventricular block. *Circulation* 110: 1162–1167.

Surawicz, B. and Knilans, T.K. (2001). *Chou's Electrocardiography in Clinical Practice: Adult and Pediatric*, 5e. Sauders.

Winter, R.L. and Bright, J.M. (2011). ECG of the month. *JAVMA* 239 (8): 1060–1062.

21

Junctional Premature Systoles

CHAPTER MENU

Junctional premature complexes, 259
    Resetting, 259
    Resetting with a pause, 260
    Interpolation, 260
    Junctional bigeminy, 262
    Junctional trigeminy, 262
    Junctional premature complexes with aberrancy, 262
    Non-conducted junctional premature complexes, 263
Concealed conduction, 263
Atrial fusion, 264
Junctional reciprocal complexes, 265
Junctional parasystole, 269

Junctional premature complexes Junctional premature complexes (JPCs, junctional premature systoles/extrasystoles) arise from the so-called "junctional" area, which is the area of the atria immediately surrounding the anatomical AV node, the cristal terminalis and AVN itself. In leads II, III, and aVF, P′ wave morphology is typically negative from concentric retrograde activation of the atrial myocardium (P′ axis of −80 to −100 degrees). The P′ wave of a JPC precedes the QRS, occur during the QRS or come after the QRS. Given that most JPCs depolarize the atria, if the P′ waves are not obvious, counting one P-P interval from the post-extrasystolic sinus P wave may help identify when the atria were depolarized, helping to disclose hidden P′ waves within the QRS complex or S-T segment of the JPC. The P′-P interval will be at least one P-P interval or, if resetting with a pause occurred, the P′-P interval will be a little longer than the P-P interval. Rarely, junctional beats may be associated with positive P′ waves, and it is thought that atrial conduction proceeds over one of the internodal tracts (Bachmann's bundle) to depolarize the atria in a superior to inferior direction. Where the P′ wave is found in relation to the QRS depends on the relative rates of antegrade (to the ventricles) and retrograde (to the atria) conduction. Some authors have insisted that junctional beats must have a shorter P′-Ri than the prevailing sinus P-Ri, and thus narrow-QRS premature beats with retrograde P′ waves and a normal to long P′-Ri must be ectopic atrial rather than junctional in origin. This has been shown to not always be the case, as antegrade conduction to the ventricles may be sufficiently delayed to produce a long P′-Ri even with a junctional origin. Occasionally, retrograde activation of the atria fails completely, so no P′ is present, and the SAN is not reset. The T wave is typically oriented the same direction as sinus-originating QRS complex T waves. Typically, a narrow-QRS is present (supraventricular appearance); however, conduction abnormalities such as bundle branch block or fascicular block may prolong the QRS or slightly distort it. Junctional premature complexes may occur in bigeminal/trigeminal rhythms. Concealed conduction within the AVN may be antegrade or retrograde. Atrial fusion, reciprocal complexes, and even parasystolic foci are all possible sequelae.

Resetting Resetting occurs when the interval from the ectopic R′ wave to the post-extrasystolic R wave is exactly equal to the R-R interval. Resetting occurs because the junctional focus has depolarized the sinus node early, starting the sinus rhythm over again at a new interval.

Interpretation of the Electrocardiogram in Small Animals, First Edition. Nick A. Schroeder.
© 2021 John Wiley & Sons Inc. Published 2021 by John Wiley & Sons Inc.

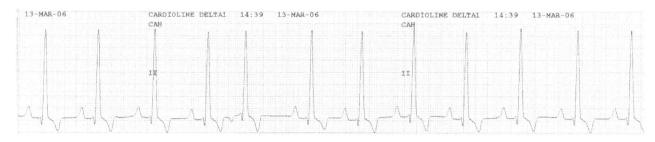

Figure 21.1 Paper speed 25 mm/s, 1 cm/mV, lead II, canine, the fifth complex is premature, has a supraventricular QRS and is preceded by a negative P′ wave consistent with a **JPC**.

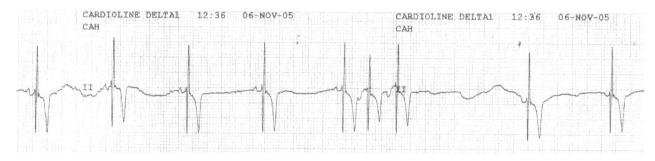

Figure 21.2 Paper speed 50 mm/s, 1 cm/mV, lead II, canine with phenylpropanalamine toxicity. The slow HR here is interrupted by the sixth complex with a couplet of **junctional premature complexes**, as evidenced by the negative P′ waves. The last two complexes may be junctional escapes, but baseline artifact may be obscuring sinus activity.

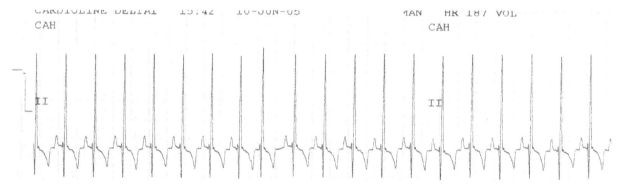

Figure 21.3 Paper speed 25 mm/s, 1 cm/mV, lead II, canine. The ninth complex is a **JPC** with no obvious P′ wave that **resets** the sinus rhythm. Careful examination of the P-P interval reveals the P′ wave of the JPC is buried within the S-T segment of the preceding sinus beat. A small notch is present on the downstroke of the T wave of the eighth complex, corresponding to the negative P′ wave of the JPC.

Resetting with a pause Resetting with a pause occurs when the interval from the ectopic R′ wave to the following sinus R wave is greater than one R-R interval, but less than two R-R intervals and is secondary to overdrive suppression of the SA node. If the JPC resets with a long enough pause, it may mimic the compensatory pause associated with VPCs (the preceding R to post-extrasystolic R interval is exactly equal to two R-R intervals).

Interpolation If the junctional focus fails to capture the atria and sinus node, then interpolation of a JPC

occurs (true extrasystole). Anterograde conduction over the His-Purkinje system may occur with concurrent retrograde block, which favors interpolation. The atrial myocardium fails to be excited by the junctional impulse, which goes on to activate ventricular myocardium. This results in a supraventricular QRS seen without an associated retrograde P′ wave. Since the sinus nodal tissue is not depolarized, the sinus node thus fires off when expected to at the next P-P interval. This is not uncommon with junctional arrhythmias. Since AV dissociation is not uncommon with junctional arrhythmias and ventricular arrhythmias, interpolated JPCs may be indistinguishable

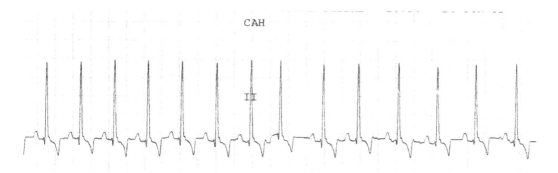

Figure 21.4 Paper speed 25 mm/s, 1 cm/mV, lead II, canine. The eighth complex is a **JPC** that causes **resetting** with a slight pause. The P′ is negative and precedes the JPC. The R-R interval is 0.4 second and the R′-R interval is 0.48 second.

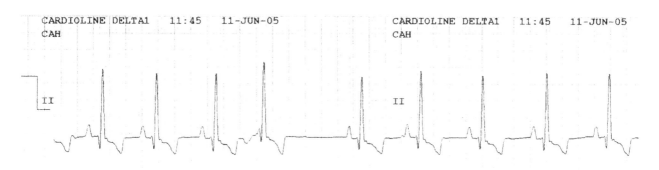

Figure 21.5 Paper speed 50 mm/s, 1 cm/mV, lead II, canine. The fourth complex is a **JPC** that resets with a long pause. The R′-R interval (0.61 second) is longer than 1 R-R interval (0.36 second), is less than 2 R-R intervals (0.72 second), and the post-extrasystolic beat is reset. This is not a fully "compensatory pause," as the interval from the beat preceding the ectopic complex to the post-extrasystolic beat (0.9 second) is not exactly equal to two R-R intervals (0.72 second). The P′ is negative and precedes the JPC.

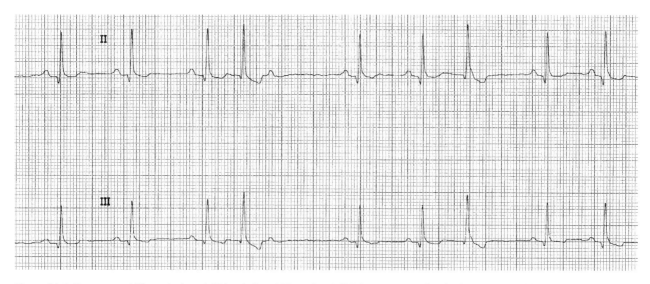

Figure 21.6 Paper speed 50 mm/s, 1 cm/mV, leads II and III, canine. Mild sinus arrhythmia with **interpolated JPCs**. The fourth complex is premature, has no associated P′ wave, and is followed by a non-conducted P wave of apparent sinus origin. The supraventricular premature QRS is thus most-likely junctional in origin and causes a functional second degree atrioventricular block of the next sinus P wave. Given that the next sinus P comes "on time," the JPC does not interfere with sinus discharge and is therefore considered interpolated. The seventh complex is another interpolated JPC and the blocked sinus P wave occurs at the end of the QRS of the JPC. Retrograde capture of the atria apparently does not occur, allowing for interpolation of these junctional complexes. The underlying sinus rhythm is not reset or reset with a pause – which is more common with atrial (and subsequent sinoatrial) capture by SVPCs.

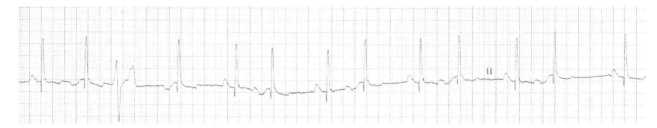

Figure 21.7 Paper speed 50 mm/s, 1 cm/mV, lead II, canine. **Junctional bigeminy**. Every other beat is a JPC that resets the sinus rhythm. The third complex is a VPC causing a compensatory pause.

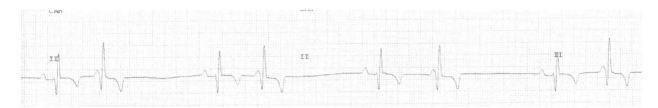

Figure 21.8 Paper speed 50 mm/s, 1 cm/mV, lead II, canine. **Junctional bigeminy**. Each sinus beat is followed by a junctional premature beat. Positive P′ waves precede each complex, but at a P′-R interval that is too narrow for a sinus or ectopic atrial complex to traverse the AVN normally and conduct to the ventricles. Occasionally, junctional foci will have *upright* P′ waves in lead II, likely due through conduction through Bachmann's bundle. Given the varied coupling intervals and constant interectopic intervals, a junctional *parasystole* is suspected and fortuitous sinus P waves occurring just before ectopic junctional beats are unlikely. Alternatively, 2 : 1 ventricular preexcitation (VPE) from Lown-Ganong-Levine (atrio-His accessory pathway) could be an alternate explanation.

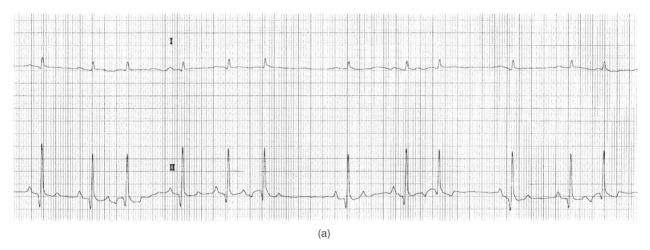

(a)

Figure 21.9a Paper speed 50 mm/s, 1 cm/mV, leads I and II, canine. **Junctional trigeminy**. One JPC follows every second sinus complex (2 : 1 extrasystole). The JPCs reset the sinus rhythm with variable pauses.

from interpolated VPCs arising from the His Bundle (which may similarly result in a narrow/supraventricular QRS dissociated from atrial activity). Rarely, JPCs may be interpolated with atrial capture and is assumed to occur due to entrance block within the SA node.

Junctional bigeminy This is a relatively uncommon occurrence where every other beat is a junctional premature complex (1 : 1 extrasystole).

Junctional trigeminy Rarely, a JPC may follow two sinus beats in an allorhythmia known as junctional trigeminy (2 : 1 extrasystole).

Junctional premature complexes with aberrancy JPCs may occasionally be conducted with aberrancy. This prolongs the QRS and mimics ventricular premature complexes. The earlier the JPC occurs, the more likely it will be non-conducted to the ventricles all together or conducted

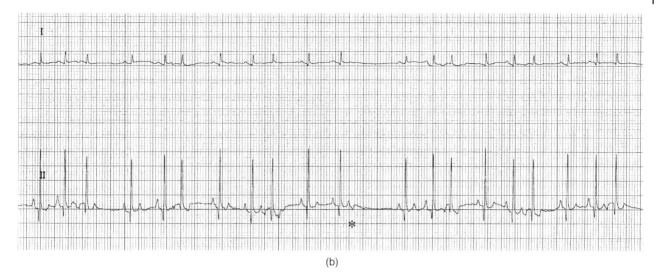

Figure 21.9b Paper speed 25 mm/s, 1 cm/mV, leads I and II, same dog. **Junctional trigeminy**. A *non-conducted JPC* (*) follows the 11th QRS causing a pause in the rhythm, but the 2 : 1 extrasystole is undisturbed.

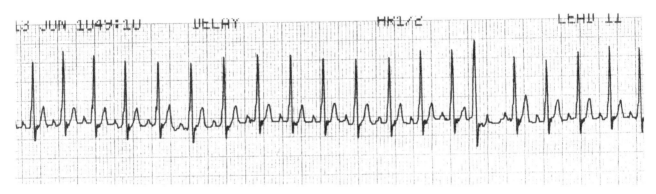

Figure 21.10 Paper speed 25 mm/s, 1 cm/mV, lead II, canine. The 15th complex is a **JPC** with a negative P′ wave that follows the QRS complex. The slightly taller ectopic QRS may be the result of a **left medial fascicular block**.

with aberrancy (usually functional right bundle branch block/RBBB). The less premature, the more likely the following QRS will be normally conducted. Not uncommonly, a left medial fascicular block may produce a narrow-QRS that is slightly taller than the sinus QRS complexes as the vector for the premature QRS becomes oriented more with lead II. An important rule out for an aberrant JPC is fusion of a JPC and simultaneous VPC.

Non-conducted junctional premature complexes Occasionally, a junctional premature beat may retrogradely capture the atria and reset the sinus node but fail to conduct anterogradely over the AVN and His-Purkinje system. This results in a pause in the sinus rhythm and a retrograde P′ without an associated QRS. The SAN is reset by the JPC. Non-conducted JPCs may not be distinguishable from atrial reciprocal complexes (atrial echo beats)

where the sinus impulse depolarizes the atria normally, turns around in the AVN to re-excite the atria retrogradely without anterograde conduction and subsequent failure to depolarize the ventricles.

Concealed conduction Evidence of concealed conduction on surface EKG is typically associated with the following: conduction delay (first degree AVB), block of P wave conduction (second degree AVB), displacement of the normal sinus pacemaker to another focus, conduction enhancement (i.e. supernormal conduction), or any combination of these. Usually, this means that if you see first or second degree AVB on post-extrasystolic beats following extrasystoles, then you can deduce that some degree of ventriculoatrial (VA) conduction exists. Clinically, these phenomena may just help you decide if premature beats are likely to be ventricular in origin or not. Concealed

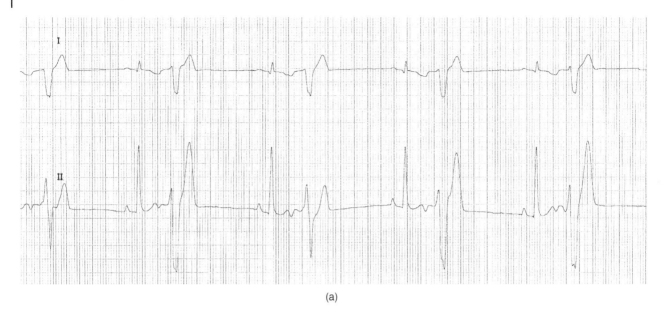

(a)

Figure 21.11a Paper speed 50 mm/s, 1 cm/mV, leads I and II, canine. At first glance, this appears to be sinus rhythm with ventricular bigeminy (1 : 1 extrasystole with ventricular premature complexes). Close scrutiny, however, reveals negative P' waves superimposed on the T waves of the sinus complexes. The QRS complexes that follow are prolonged from variable degrees of RBBB. The first and fifth QRS complexes have incomplete RBBB, while the third, seventh, and ninth complexes have complete RBBB since they are relatively more premature. This is an example of **bigeminal JPCs with aberrancy**.

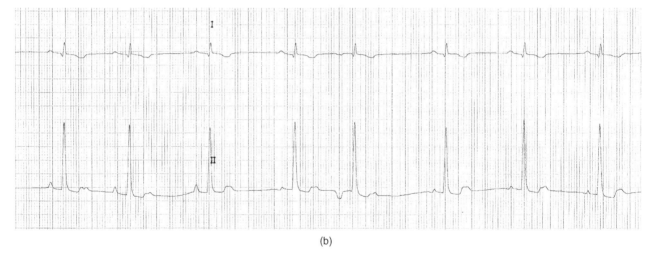

(b)

Figure 21.11b Paper speed 50 mm/s, 1 cm/mV, same dog. The fifth complex is a JPC that is not so early and is conducted normally. Note that the T waves of the sinus beats are now completely upright as superimposed retrograde P' waves are absent.

conduction is most commonly manifested on surface EKG following ventricular extrasystoles and atrial fibrillation; however, it may be noted during with JPCs as well.

Junctional premature complexes may intermittently be concealed on surface EKG. This means the focus fired, however, failed to conduct anterogradely to the ventricles (no ectopic QRS) and retrogradely to the atria (no P'). His bundle electrograms are necessary to confirm the diagnosis, but there are several clues to their presence on surface EKG.

These include abrupt and unexplained lengthening of the P-R interval, the presence of apparent Type I and II AVB in the same tracing, apparent Type II AVB in the presence of a normal QRS complex, and the presence of manifest junctional extrasystoles elsewhere in the EKG.

Atrial fusion Junctional foci may retrogradely activate the atria simultaneously with the SA node. The result is a

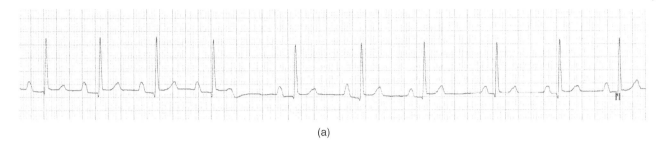

(a)

Figure 21.12a Paper speed 50 mm/s, 1 cm/mV, lead II, canine. ***Non-conducted* JPC**. A mild sinus arrhythmia is present; however, the rhythm is interrupted after the fourth beat by a non-conducted junctional premature beat. The sinus node is reset, and retrograde atrial activation is evidenced by the retrograde P′ immediately following the fourth complex. However, antegrade conduction over the AVN fails to occur, and the expected supraventricular QRS is missing.

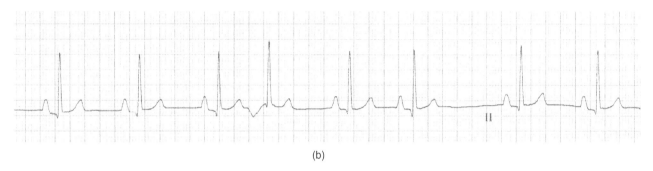

(b)

Figure 21.12b Paper speed 50 mm/s, 1 cm/mV, lead II, same dog. The fourth complex is a conducted JPC. This time, the junctional focus fires a little later, and the AVN has recovered from the previous depolarization, permitting conduction and the appearance of a supraventricular QRS. Again, the rhythm is reset by the JPC. The presence of a conducted JPC supports the diagnosis of a non-conducted JPC in the previous strip.

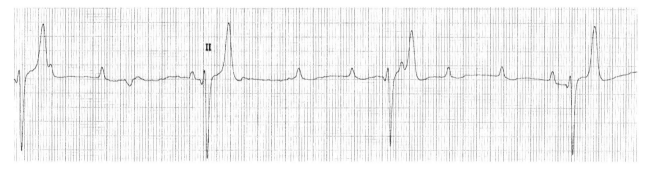

Figure 21.13 Paper speed 50 mm/s, 1 cm/mV, lead II, canine. Sinus arrhythmia of the atria, ventricular escape rhythm of the ventricles, complete AVD by default secondary to complete (third degree) AVB. The second P wave is followed by an apparently premature retrograde P′ wave that resets the rhythm consistent with either a ***non-conducted* JPC** or ***atrial reciprocal complex*** (A-V block-A sequence).

supraventricular beat with an altered P wave morphology that is intermediate between those of pure sinus origin and those of ectopic origin. These beats are neither early nor late (depending on the antegrade conduction time of the junctional focus).

Junctional reciprocal complexes Conduction delay may promote reentry, creating a reciprocal (reentrant, echo, or return extrasystole). Junctional reciprocal beats are preceded by a retrograde P′ which resets the sinus (or prevailing supraventricular ectopic) rhythm. The sequence

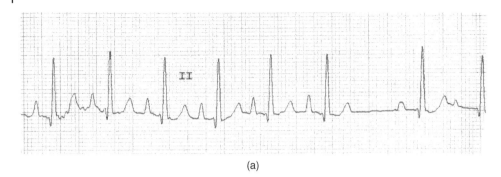

(a)

Figure 21.14a Paper speed 50 mm/s, 1 cm/mV, lead II, canine. The sinus pause between the sixth and seventh beat has resulted in a reset rhythm. A ***concealed* junctional premature beat** may have created this pause and caused the reset. The eighth complex is premature, has a positive P′ and a long P′-R interval.

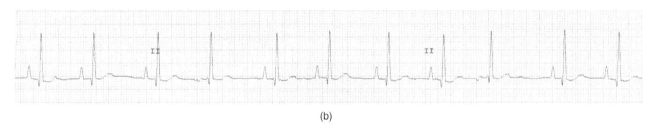

(b)

Figure 21.14b Paper speed 50 mm/s, 1 cm/mV, lead II, same dog. Manifest junctional premature beats are evident. The fourth and ninth complexes are premature, preceded by negative P′ waves, and reset the rhythm.

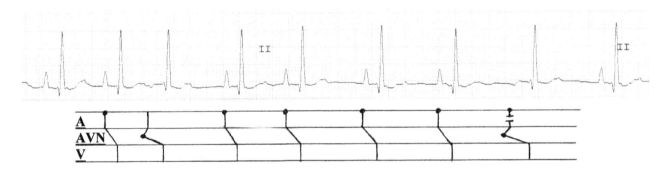

Figure 21.15 Paper speed 50 mm/s, 1 cm/mV, lead II, canine. The third complex is a JPC that resets with a pause. The eighth complex has a P wave intermediate in morphology between a sinus P and the ectopic junctional P′, consistent with an ***atrial* fusion complex**. Atrial fusion complexes may also occur with ectopic atrial premature beats.

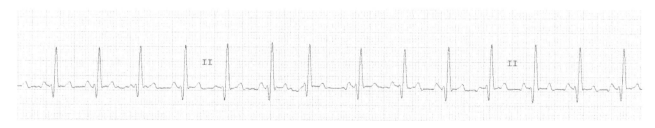

Figure 21.16 Paper speed 50 mm/s, 1 cm/mV, lead II, canine. Junctional premature beats with **atrial fusion**. The 3rd, 5th, and 11th P waves are atrial fusion complexes with morphologies intermediate between the sinus P waves and the negative P waves of the JPC (beat #7).

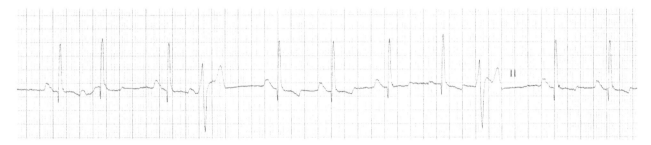

Figure 21.17 Paper speed 50 mm/s, 1 cm/mV, lead II, canine. The second beat is a JPC. The eighth complex has altered P wave morphology consistent with an **atrial fusion beat**. The fourth and ninth complexes are VPCs.

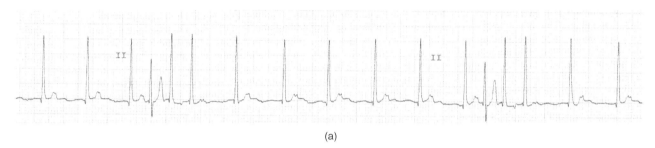

(a)

Figure 21.18a Paper speed 25 mm/s, 1 cm/mV, lead II, canine with severe CMVDz and CHF, R/O digitalis toxicity. An accelerated junctional rhythm (HR 150 bpm) is suppressing sinus nodal discharge. Presumably, retrograde P′ waves are occurring during the QRS complexes and are thus buried. The fourth complex is an interpolated VPC, which causes the following junctional QRS to reenter the atria retrogradely, which then depolarizes the ventricles normally, but early with a preceding retrograde (negative) P′ wave (seen between the fifth and sixth beats), making the sixth complex a **junctional reciprocal beat**. The junctional focus is *reset with a pause*. The pattern repeats itself after the 13th complex, another interpolated VPC, which sets up another junctional reciprocal cycle. The underlying junctional rhythm is likely the result of ***abnormal automaticity*** from digitalis intoxication; however, the interpolated VPC/junctional reciprocal cycles are secondary to ***reentry***. V-A-V sequence reciprocal cycles are one of the mechanisms creating ***allorhythmia***, a repeated arrhythmic sequence, or regularity within an irregularity.

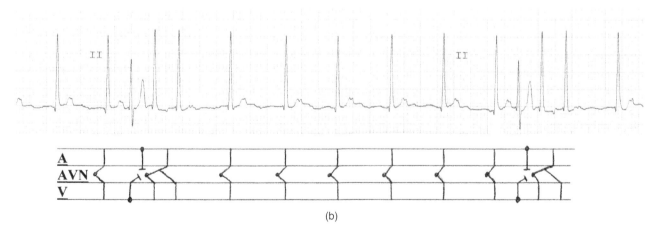

(b)

Figure 21.18b Paper speed 25 mm/s, lead II, a close-up of the same strip. A **ladder diagram** below illustrates the arrhythmia. The junctional beats originate in the AVN (indicated by the dot – the origin of the depolarization). The interpolated VPCs create junctional reciprocal beats in the proposed manner: delaying retrograde conduction to the atria, followed by a reciprocal beat.

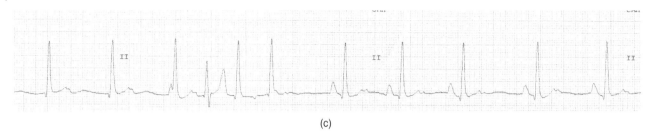

(c)

Figure 21.18c Paper speed 50 mm/s, 1 cm/mV, lead II, same dog. This strip shows transition from junctional rhythm to sinus rhythm. An interpolated VPC creates a **junctional reciprocal cycle**, but here the junctional focus was reset with a long enough pause to allow the sinus node to recapture the heart (beat #7). The third beat has a sinus P wave peeking out of the junctional QRS.

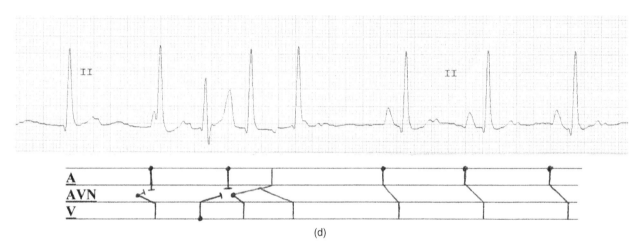

(d)

Figure 21.18d Paper speed 50 mm/s, 1 cm/mV, lead II, a close-up of the same strip. Conversion to sinus rhythm occurs following another reciprocal cycle as illustrated by the ladder diagram.

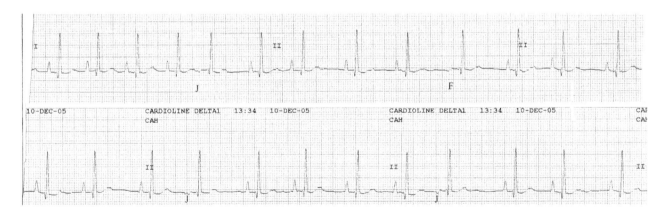

Figure 21.19 Paper speed 50 mm/s, 1 cm/mV, lead II, canine. Possible **junctional parasystole**. The 5th, 17th, and 22nd complexes are JPCs, and the 10th complex is an atrial fusion complex. Reverse coupling may occur with junctional parasystole as long as there is retrograde conduction into the atria and sinoatrial node, as evident in this strip. There is obvious lack of consistent coupling intervals with the presystolic sinus beats, which is suggestive of a parasystolic focus. The interectopic intervals are approximately 2.2 seconds.

is V-A-V. Subatrial reentry may occur (VA block) and the echo beat will not be preceded by a retrograde P′, and the sinus node will not be reset (provided sinoatrial discharge is present).

Junctional parasystole Parasystolic foci in the AV junction may persist due to entrance block. The ectopic focus discharges independent of the prevailing rhythm, atrial fusion beats may occur, and interectopic intervals have a common denominator. If retrograde conduction to the atria is present, reverse-coupling occurs, and the sinus rhythm is reset by the junctional focus.

Further reading

Fisch, C., Zipes, D.P., and McHenry, P.L. (1976). Electrocardiographic manifestations of concealed junctional ectopic impulses. *Circulation* 53: 217–223.

Marriott, H.J. (1998). *Pearls & Pitfalls in Electrocardiography, Pithy, Practical Pointers*, 2e. Williams & Wilkins.

Rosen, K.M. (1973). Junctional tachycardia: mechanisms, diagnosis, differential diagnosis, and management. *Circulation* XLVII: 654–664.

22

Junctional Tachycardia

CHAPTER MENU

Accelerated junctional rhythm, 270
 Isorhythmic dissociation, 270
Automatic junctional tachycardia, 276
Atrioventricular nodal reentrant tachycardia, 278

Accelerated junctional rhythm If a junctional focus captures the ventricles and is faster than junctional escape rhythm, but slower than junctional tachycardia, it is referred to as an accelerated junctional rhythm (if retrograde capture of the atria is present). The term accelerated idiojunctional rhythm is used if atrioventricular dissociation (AVD) is present.

> *A Note*: So-called "non-paroxysmal junctional (or atrioventricular nodal) tachycardia" is a historically used, poorly worded term and avoided here for the sake of simplicity and to avoid confusion. Most accelerated rhythms occur at a rate that is comparable to sinus rhythm. Thus, the onset and offset of these rhythms may be inapparent on physical examination since an abrupt "paroxysm" of overt tachycardia does not happen. These rhythms are neither paroxysmal nor do they constitute tachycardia per se.

Regularization of a supraventricular rhythm during atrial fibrillation is a clue to AIJR if the rate is "normal" or automatic junctional tachycardia if the rate is fast, and digoxin toxicity is highly suspected if accelerated junctional/idiojunctional rhythm or junctional tachycardia is a new arrhythmia that develops in a patient being treated with the drug.

Isorhythmic dissociation This occurs when the atrial and ventricular rates are approximately equal, though not really related to each other. This is not uncommon with AIJR, and it can be tricky to figure these EKGs out. This is certainly the case when the P waves happen to come before the QRS complexes. One mechanism of the synchronization between the atrial and ventricular rates is thought to be the result of a feedback loop. The P-R interval determines the stroke volume, which affects the blood pressure. With a

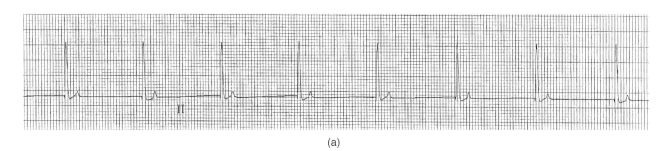

(a)

Figure 22.1a Paper speed 50 mm/s, 1 cm/mV, lead II, canine. **Accelerated junctional rhythm** with VA conduction. Retrograde P' waves are present in the S-T segment, distorting the T waves. Ventriculoatrial conduction is suppressing SA nodal discharge.

Interpretation of the Electrocardiogram in Small Animals, First Edition. Nick A. Schroeder.
© 2021 John Wiley & Sons Inc. Published 2021 by John Wiley & Sons Inc.

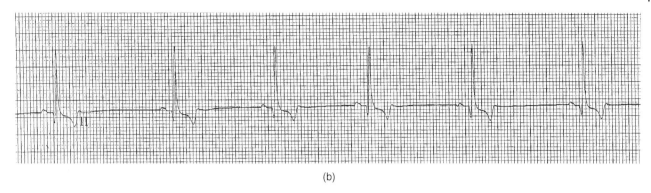

(b)

Figure 22.1b Paper speed 50 mm/s, 1 cm/mV, lead II, same dog, next day. Sinus rhythm. Note that the T waves have inverted.

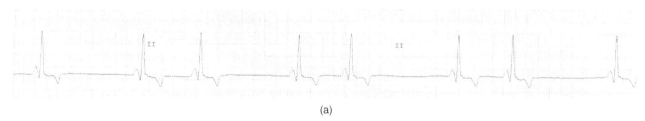

(a)

Figure 22.2a Paper speed 50 mm/s, 1 cm/mV, lead II, canine. **Accelerated junctional rhythm** with pauses (possibly 3:2 exit block). The P' waves are *upright* and *precede* the QRS complexes. The P'-R interval is too short to be physiologic conduction of an ectopic atrial or sinus beats. The bigeminal rhythm is likely secondary to exit block (3:2 Wenckebach conduction). Note the pauses are not exact multiples of the interectopic cycle length.

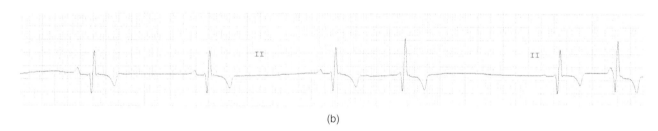

(b)

Figure 22.2b Paper speed 50 mm/s, 1 cm/mV, lead II, same dog. Here, a junctional premature beat without an obviously associated P' wave occurs after the third sinus beat. The sinus beats have normal P-R intervals, so an atrio-Hisian bypass tract (see Chapter 16) is unlikely unless intermittent anterograde block over an accessory pathway is present. The fifth complex is a junctional escape beat and is followed by a JPC with the same upright P' preceding the QRS as seen in the previous strip. This just confirms that the rhythm in the preceding strip is junctional in origin.

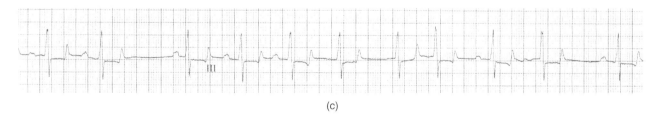

(c)

Figure 22.2c Paper speed 50 mm/s, 1 cm/mV, lead III, same dog. SA block explains the pauses, and long pause/arrest occurs after the fifth complex. The arrest is terminated by a junctional escape beat (complex #6), and a short and irregular **accelerated idiojunctional rhythm** with retrograde AVB (and AVD) ensues as evidenced by the lack of resetting of the sinus node. The ninth complex is a sinus capture.

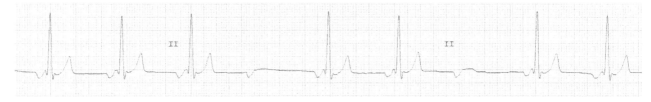

Figure 22.3 Paper speed 50 mm/s, 1 cm/mV, lead II, canine with suspect digoxin toxicity. An **accelerated junctional rhythm** is present. Occasional Type II second degree AVB occurs with retrograde atrial conduction and anterograde ventricular conduction block.

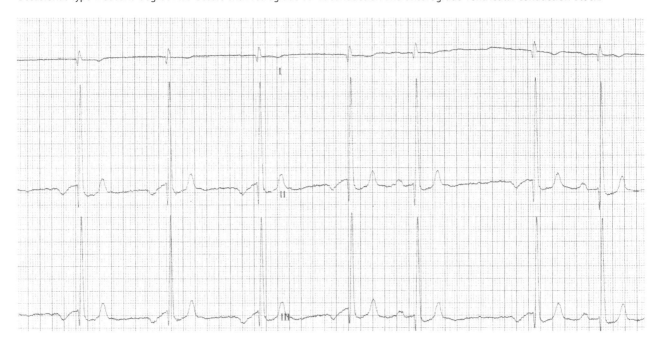

Figure 22.4 Paper speed 50 mm/s, 1 cm/mV, leads I, II, III, canine. **Accelerated junctional rhythm** (R/O **coronary sinus rhythm**) with intermittent sinus capture. The P' waves preceding the first four complexes are retrograde in the inferiors and isoelectric in I indicated a junctional or inferior RA focus, possibly from the coronary sinus. Accelerated junctional rhythms may compete for control of the HR if sinus bradycardia is present. This dog had a patent ductus arteriosus, and significant left-sided volume overload, leading to the tall R waves, consistent with LV enlargement seen here. The fifth and seventh beats are sinus captures.

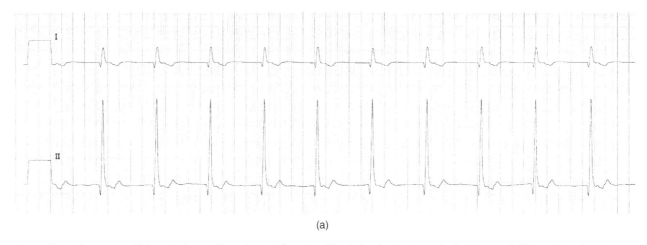

(a)

Figure 22.5a Paper speed 50 mm/s, 1 cm/mV, leads I and II, canine. This Labrador Retriever had a history of CHF and junctional arrhythmias. No P waves are clearly evident at first glance, the heart rate is normal at 120 bpm, and the QRS complexes appear supraventricular. Either atrial standstill or atrial fibrillation could explain the absence of P waves. Careful examination of the S-T segment, however, reveals retrograde P' waves following the QRS complexes and just preceding the T waves. This indicates an **accelerated junctional rhythm** with ventriculoatrial conduction with subsequent suppression of the SA node.

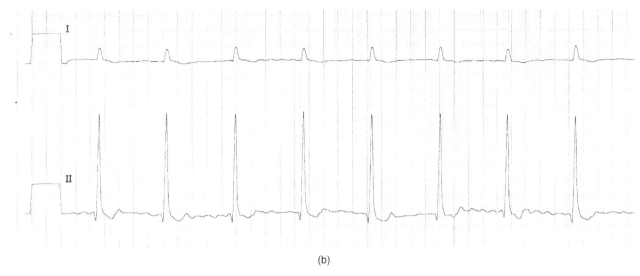

(b)

Figure 22.5b Paper speed 50 mm/s, 1 cm/mV, lead II, same dog. **Atrial fibrillation** (AF) and apparently complete **atrioventricular dissociation** (AVD) secondary to usurpation by an **accelerated idiojunctional rhythm** (AIJR). No P waves are evident, and the baseline is clearly undulating consistent with AF. The QRS complexes are mildly prolonged from left ventricular enlargement but are supraventricular with a regular rhythm suggesting AVD and rate consistent with AIJR in the presence of AF. This dog was being treated with digoxin and diltiazem prior to the onset of atrial fibrillation. In this case, while the ventricular rate is acceptable, digoxin toxicity could be a possibility. This dog had developed a pedunculated mass within the right atrium (R/O thrombus).

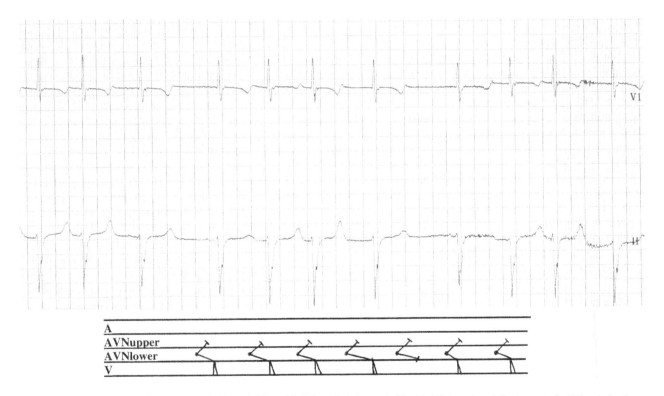

Figure 22.6 Paper speed 50 mm/s, 1 cm/mV, leads VI and II, feline. **Atrial standstill** with **idiojunctional rhythm,** *atypical* **Wenckebach periodicity,** and **rate-dependent aberrancy**. The group beating is suggestive of Wenckebach periodicity, and since the last cycle length prolongs in each series prior to failure of conduction, it is atypical. The gradual widening and peaking of the T waves at progressively shorter cycle lengths is consistent with rate-dependent aberrancy of the QRS complexes, possibly Wenckebach periodicity within the bundle branch itself. These have an atypical BBB configuration in V1. The lack of visible atrial activity is consistent with atrial standstill; however, **sinoventricular rhythm** with atypical Wenckebach and rate-dependent aberration could be a possibility. The HR is 100–187 bpm (with a concealed regular rate of 157 bpm), consistent with an accelerated idiojunctional or sinus/sinoventricular focus.

relatively normal P-R interval, the normal A-V sequence is preserved and a greater cardiac output is achieved on these beats. When the P-R interval is excessively long or short, or the atria contract just after the ventricles, then the cardiac output on these beats is decreased. The blood pressure has an inverse effect on SA nodal discharge rate via the baroreceptor reflex, and the SA nodal frequency determines the P-R interval. Thus, when the P waves precede the QRS complexes, the stroke volume is better, and blood pressure increases. This triggers the baroreceptors to decrease the frequency SA nodal discharge. Thus, the atrial and ventricular rates will regularly fluctuate around similar rates, and the P wave oscillates into and out of the QRS complex (with varying P-R and R-P intervals) in response to changes in blood pressure. The mechanism of isorhythmic dissociation involved when the P waves are consistently located within the QRS, S-T segment or before the QRS at a regular, but excessive P-R interval is unclear. Isorhythmic dissociation occurs most often in the setting of accelerated idiojunctional rhythm, since the sinus and idiojunctional rates are often similar. This is quite common in Labrador Retrievers, not uncommon in cats and rarely associated with hypothermia.

Technically, isorhythmic dissociation occurs in the setting of AVD secondary to usurpation or occasionally by default. The term usurpation refers to AVD secondary to a primary and accelerated idiojunctional/idioventricular focus that usurps control of the ventricles in the presence of a secondarily similar (usually sinus) rate. The term default refers to AVD secondary to a primary slowing of the underlying (usually sinus) rhythm (i.e. from severe sinus bradycardia, sinoatrial block, sinus arrest, or AV block) with escape of a normal and secondary idiojunctional or idioventricular subsidiary pacemaker. Thus, if an accelerated idiojunctional rhythm occurs in the setting of sinus bradycardia, the rates of the independent pacemakers may be similar. Two subdivisions of isorhythmic dissociation exist: accrochage and synchrony.

Accrochage: When the atrial rate and the ventricular rate are just slightly different, the P waves march through the QRS complexes. Accrochage typically occurs over just a *few beats*.

Synchrony: When the atrial rate and the ventricular rate are approximately equal, and the P waves periodically wander around each other (in response to changes in blood pressure and sinoatrial discharge frequency as previously

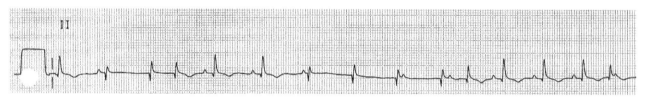

Figure 22.7 Paper speed 50 mm/s, 1 cm/mV, lead II, feline. Incomplete AVD is present in this strip, with the 1st, 5th, 6th, 11–14th beats being of sinus origin. The rest of the beats are junctional in origin (accelerated idiojunctional rhythm) and takes over when the sinus rate slows, making this an example of **accrochage** secondary to *usurpation*.

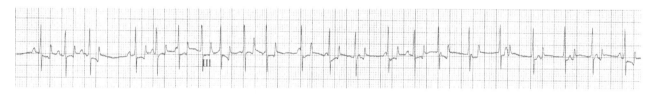

Figure 22.8 Paper speed 25 mm/s, 1 cm/mV, lead III, canine. Sinoatrial block and sinus arrest results in longer periods of accelerated idiojunctional rhythm with atrioventricular dissociation (AVD) secondary to *usurpation* and **accrochage**. The 15th complex is a sinus capture.

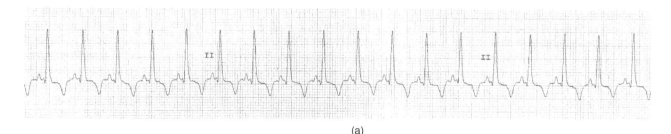

(a)

Figure 22.9a Paper speed 50 mm/s, 1 cm/mV, feline, **synchrony**. Isorhythmic dissociation is present, though the P waves precede all ventricular complexes and appear related.

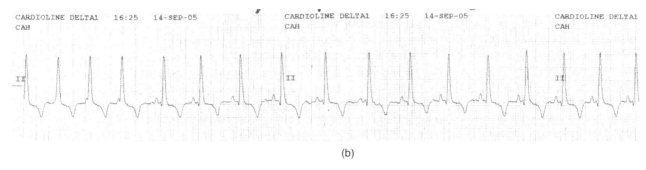

(b)

Figure 22.9b Paper speed 50 mm/s, 1 cm/mV, same cat. The rhythm reveals itself as AVD secondary to *usurpation*. The beginning of the strip shows the QRS complexes marching out from the P waves, indicating AVD. Both the atrial and ventricular rates are approximately 150 bpm. The ventricles are likely under the control of an idiojunctional conducted with LBBB aberration, though a right idioventricular focus could not be excluded on the basis of surface EKG.

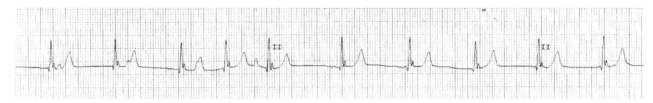

Figure 22.10 Paper speed 50 mm/s, 1 cm/mV, canine, serum digoxin 6.5 ug/dl. **Isorhythmic dissociation with synchrony** secondary to *usurpation* by an **accelerated idiojunctional rhythm**. At the beginning of the strip, the idiojunctional QRS complexes are dissociated from the P waves which appear in the S-T segment. The fifth complex appears to be a sinus capture, and the sinus rate slows again, allowing the idiojunctional focus to take over. The dissociated and synchronous P waves are probably hiding in the QRS complexes. Digoxin toxicity may produce abnormal automaticity and leads to such arrhythmias. The fourth complex may be a sinus capture with a long P-Ri secondary to a short R-Pi. The fifth complex is preceded by a long R-Pi, allowing for a shorter P-Ri.

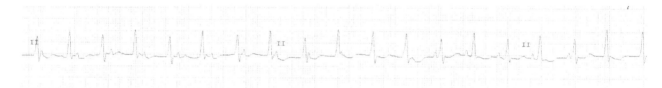

Figure 22.11 Paper speed 50 mm/s, 1 cm/mV, lead II, feline, **synchrony** secondary to AVD from *usurpation*. The idiojunctional rate is approx. 200 bpm. The P waves march through the QRS complexes because the atrial rate is slightly faster at 214 bpm.

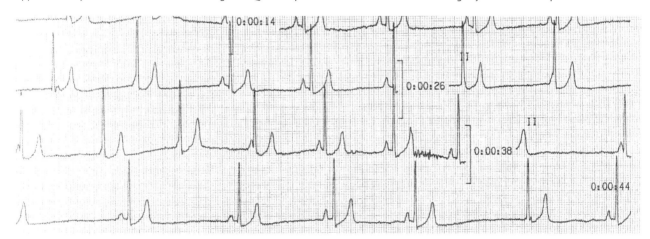

Figure 22.12 Paper speed 50 mm/s, 1 cm/mV, lead II, canine, **synchrony** secondary to AVD by *default*. The idiojunctional (escape) rate is approximately 66–92 bpm, and the atrial rate is similar. Note how the P waves wander into and out of the QRS complexes. Note that when the P waves precede the QRS complexes, the idiojunctional rate increases. Presumably, the faster ventricular rate triggers the baroreceptors as the BP rises, which then triggers a decrease in the sinus and idiojunctional discharge frequency.

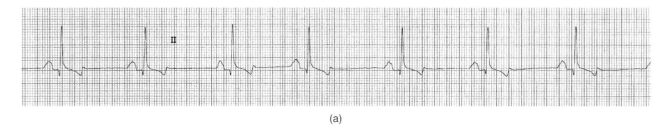

(a)

Figure 22.13a Paper speed 50 mm/s, 1 cm/mV, lead II, canine with pancreatitis. What appears to be a mild sinus arrhythmia is present with a heart rate of around 100 bpm. The P waves are markedly prolonged at 0.08 second (intra-atrial block).

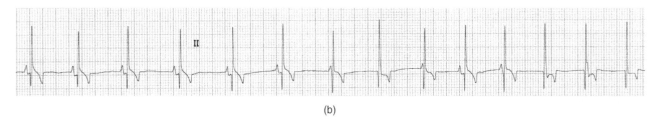

(b)

Figure 22.13b Paper speed 25 mm/s, 1 cm/mV, lead II, same dog. A longer strip reveals atrioventricular dissociation with atrial and ventricular rates similar. The P-wave march in and out of the QRS complexes. This is indicative of atrioventricular dissociation with usurpation by an accelerated idiojunctional rhythm with a rate similar to that of the underlying sinus rate. Here, retrograde VA block is evident. Since the atrial and ventricular rates are similar, this is considered **isorhythmic dissociation**.

discussed), or the P waves precede, follow, or occur within the QRS complexes, and appear to maintain a constant relationship with each other for long periods.

The easiest thing to do is run the EKG with multiple leads and for long periods to uncover the P waves. Look for sore thumbs – irregularities in the rhythm which may be capture beats which are premature. P waves are often hiding in the QRS complexes or the T waves. In addition to accelerated idiojunctional rhythm, examples of isorhythmic dissociation may include accelerated idioventricular rhythm and third degree AVB with a junctional escape rhythm and sinus bradycardia. The junctional escape rhythm can be narrow and upright in waveform, similar to sinus QRS complexes. This is a relatively common scenario in cats with third degree AVB since their junctional escape rhythms can be in the 100–130+ bpm range.

Long periods of apparent synchrony may also be explained by junctional rhythms with retrograde capture of the atria and positive P' waves that mimic those seen in sinus rhythm. The P' waves may actually be biphasic, with the terminal positive portion seen on surface EKG. The negative initial portion may not be evident, especially if it occurs within the QRS complex itself. This phenomenon has been documented in humans with apparent isorhythmic dissociation using invasive epicardial mapping and highlights the limitation of surface EKG in identifying supraventricular foci. Accelerated idiojunctional and junctional rhythms generally do not require specific therapy, but their sudden appearance during therapy with digoxin should signal the possibility of toxicity to the clinician, prompting a dosage reduction or discontinuation of the drug altogether.

Automatic junctional tachycardia Also known as ectopic junctional tachycardia, AJT originates in the AV nodal area. This SVT produces negative P' waves in II, III, and aVF that are usually hidden in the QRS complex. The onset and offset are gradual, the rhythm may be irregular, the P' waves may follow or come just before the QRS, rarely may have negative P' waves with a normal to long R-P' interval (but these SVTs are usually a coronary sinus rhythm and not worrisome). Atrioventricular dissociation is common with this form and is uncovered when vagal maneuvers are performed. If the SVT begins with a negative P', a short P' R interval, a P' following the QRS, or no P' wave, it is likely of junctional origin. If a VPC terminates a SVT, it is usually a junctional tachycardia. While automatic junctional tachycardia is generally considered a supraventricular tachycardia, atrial tissue may not actually be required for maintenance of the tachycardia, as evidenced by AVD during AJT. Automatic junctional tachycardia may be a manifestation of digoxin toxicity. So-called "incessant" or permanent junctional tachycardia may actually be circus movement tachycardia with a slowly conducting accessory pathway (R postero-septal, with retrograde and decremental conduction). Simultaneous junctional and other supraventricular tachycardia (i.e. ectopic atrial tachycardia, atrial flutter) is considered to be a "double tachycardia." Persistent and frequent junctional tachycardia may be treated with beta-blockers, calcium channel blockers, or digoxin.

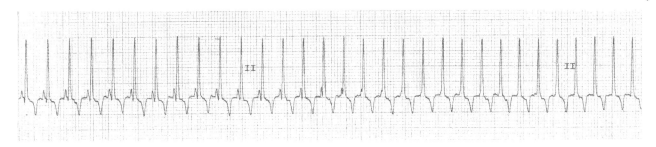

Figure 22.14 Paper speed 25 mm/s, 1 cm/mV, lead II, feline. This strip shows AJT with obvious AV dissociation. Technically, this is **isorhythmic dissociation** since the atrial and ventricular rates are similar (sinus tachycardia and junctional tachycardia). The P waves march into the QRS complexes.

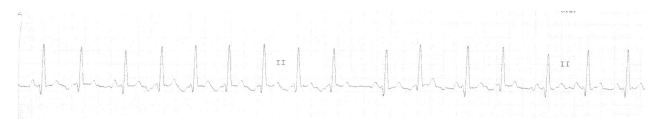

Figure 22.15 Paper speed 50 mm/s, 1 cm/mV, lead II, canine with severe LAE and CHF. The second complex is a JPC. The fourth complex starts a run of **AJT**, which is followed by a short run of junctional bigeminy and then sinus beats. Given that the P'-R interval is fairly long, this alternatively may be automatic atrial tachycardia from a focus low in the atrium, causing the negative P' waves.

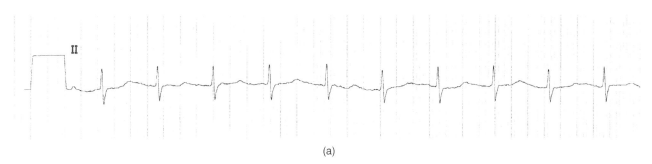

(a)

Figure 22.16a Paper speed 50 mm/s, 1 cm/mV, lead II, feline. Atrial activity is uncertain and the ventricular rate is 180 bpm. The ventricular rhythm is regular and the QRS complexes appear supraventricular, making atrial fibrillation with intact AV conduction unlikely.

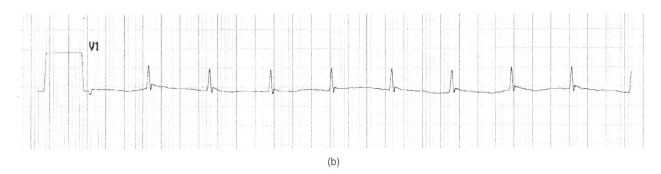

(b)

Figure 22.16b Paper speed 50 mm/s, 1 cm/mV, lead V1, same cat. P waves here appear to immediately follow the QRS complexes. The corresponding deflection is in the upstroke of the S wave in lead II. These are likely to represent retrograde P' waves, making this **junctional tachycardia** with **VA conduction**.

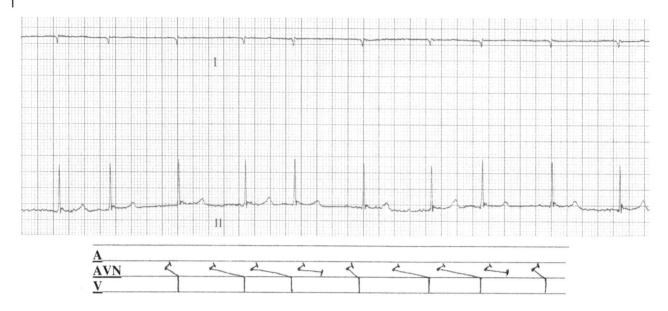

Figure 22.17 Paper speed 50 mm/s, 1 cm/mV, leads I and II, feline. **Atrial standstill** with **junctional tachycardia, exit block with Wenckebach periodicity**. The group beating is the giveaway, as illustrated by the ladder diagram. No clear evidence of atrial activity is present. The rhythm could, however, be sinoventricular with Wenckebach periodicity (4:3 conduction) as well. The HR is 136–200 bpm (with a concealed regular rate of 200 bpm), which could be consistent with a junctional tachycardia or sinus/sinoventricular.

Atrioventricular nodal reentrant tachycardia

If the AV node exhibits dual pathway physiology, atrioventricular nodal reentrant tachycardia (AVNRT) can be seen. There are actually two functional pathways in the AV node which conduct impulses. The slow pathway (alpha) and the fast pathway (beta) are present. The fast pathway has a longer refractory period but faster conduction velocity than does the slow pathway. Normally, impulses initiated in the sinus node arrive at the AVN and preferentially travel over the fast pathway, eventually proceeding into the ventricles. A supraventricular impulse may reach the AV node when the fast path is refractory, travel down the slow path and then back up (retrograde conduction) the fast path, creating a circuit that simultaneously depolarizes the ventricles and the atria. This results in P' waves that are hidden in the QRS complexes. If they are seen, they are usually negative in leads in II, III, and aVF. The P'-R interval is typically short. There is normally an abrupt onset and offset. The beginning critically has a long P-R interval. This is termed **OAVNRT** (orthodromic or "slow-fast" AVN reentry). This is the typical or common form, and you may see the P' as a "pseudo-S wave" in II, III, and aVF. If the loop conducts in the opposite direction, then **AAVNRT** (antidromic or "fast-slow" AVN reentry) develops, and the impulse goes down the fast path and up the slow path, setting up a circuit in the other direction. This is the atypical form. With AAVNRT, negative P' waves with a short P-R interval and a long R-P' interval is seen, making differentiation from circus movement due to OAVRT over an accessory pathway difficult (especially if the accessory pathway is only capable of conducting retrogradely and manifest ventricular pre-excitation is absent in sinus rhythm).

Vagal maneuvers can terminate AVNRT. If SVT terminates with a non-conducted P wave, AVNRT may be suspected, though AVNRT may terminate without AVB. Dual AV nodal pathway physiology is suggested if two discreet/consistent P-R intervals are demonstrated in the same individual. This may be unmasked following interpolated VPCs with post-extrasystolic P-Ri prolongation that persists on subsequent sinus beats. Dual AVN physiology has also been cited as the cause of transient post-extrasystolic P-Ri prolongation following interpolated VPCs. Concealed retrograde conduction into the AVN by the VPC renders the fast path refractory, but the following sinus impulse is still able to proceed antegrade over the slow path. In pseudo-interpolation where a VPC is followed by a retrograde P' wave and then a ventricular reciprocal beat, the irregularly irregular ventricular rate response during atrial fibrillation and other forms of AVNRT (i.e. "slow-slow" AVNRT) are also manifestations of dual AV nodal physiology. It should be noted the slow pathway ablation in humans can not only cure AVNRT, but can also cure atrial flutter, as the slow pathway is often involved in the macroreentrant circuit. While dual AV nodal pathway physiology has been demonstrated experimentally in the dog, atrioventricular nodal reentrant (or non-reentrant) tachycardia has yet to be proven to be a cause of naturally occurring SVT in the dog or cat.

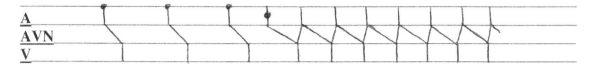

Figure 22.18 Ladder diagram illustrating the mechanism of **OAVNRT**. Sinus rhythm occurs for three beats, then an APC finds the fast pathway refractory, proceeding down the slow path, which then activates the atria retrogradely and the ventricles antegradely nearly simultaneously.

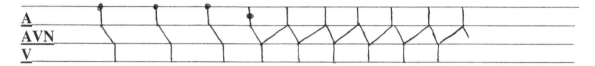

Figure 22.19 Ladder diagram illustrating the mechanism of **AAVNRT**. Sinus rhythm occurs for three beats, then an APC conducts normally over the fast pathway, but travels retrogradely across the slow pathway to activate the atria. Note that P' waves follow the QRS complexes.

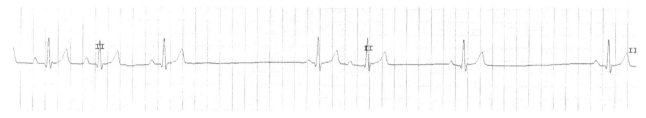

Figure 22.20 Paper speed 50 mm/s, 1 cm/mV, lead II, canine. The fifth complex is an APC with a long P'-R interval, possibly indicating that the APC conducted through the AVN via the slow (alpha) pathway. This indicates that partial recovery of the AV node has occurred, but the fast (beta) path was still refractory. Reentrant arrhythmias may result from circuits created using dual AV nodal physiology.

So-called "double-fires" can occur in such patients and "one-is-to-two" conduction may happen when depolarization over both pathways occurs simultaneously. This may be antegrade, where a single sinus/supraventricular impulse conducts twice to the ventricles over the fast and slow paths simultaneously. Sustained tachyarrhythmia may develop and is termed *non-reentrant atrioventricular nodal tachycardia* (dual atrioventricular nodal nonreentrant tachycardia/DAVNNT) where one sinus beat repeatedly double-fires to the ventricles resulting in a mildly irregular (but usually bigeminal) rhythm where the ventricular rate is double that of the atria. Seen in humans, this has yet to be documented in small animals. Conversely, this may also occur in the retrograde direction, where a single ventricular or low nodal beat conducts twice to the atria.

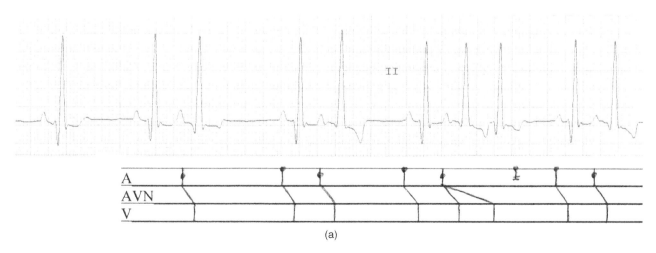

(a)

Figure 21.21a Paper speed 50 mm/s, 1 cm/mV, canine, lead II. **Atrial bigeminy with possible *one-is-to-two* conduction over dual AVN pathways**. As shown by the ladder diagram, the third APC actually may conduct twice to the ventricles: once over the fast (beta) pathway and again over the slow (alpha) pathway in the AVN.

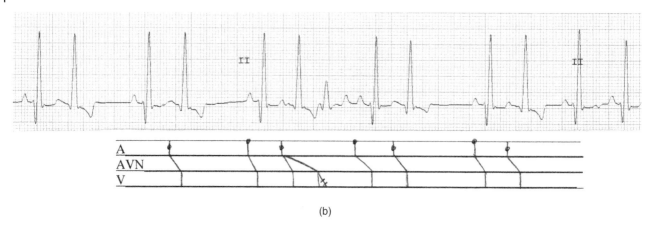

(b)

Figure 21.21b Paper speed 50 mm/s, 1 cm/mV, canine, lead II. The second conduction is aberrant (likely since the ventricles were just depolarized and the second impulse found partial refractoriness to the LBB, resulting in incomplete LBBB of the second conducted beat). The SAN fires again on schedule, indicating that the second conduction was not likely to be atrial ectopic in origin, since it failed to depolarize and reset the SAN at the expected interval. The alternative explanation is that the "second conducted beat" is actually an interpolated ventricular ectopic is unlikely, since the P-R interval of the post-extrasystolic beat is not prolonged. Since one atrial impulse conducted twice to the ventricles, it is termed "one-is-to-two" conduction or a "double-fire." Dual AVN physiology allows for these arrhythmias in addition to SVT (AVNRT).

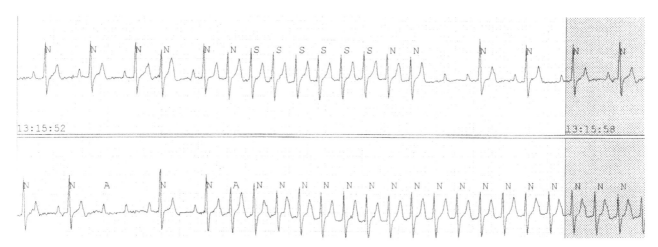

Figure 22.22 Paper speed 25 mm/s, 1 cm/mV, lead II, canine, variable periods of second degree AVB precede an SVT.

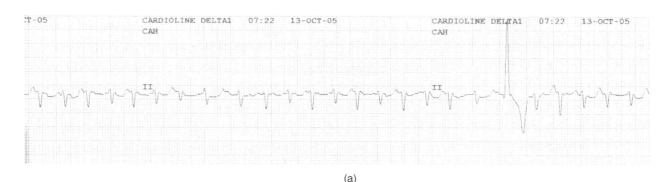

(a)

Figure 22.23a Paper speed 50 mm/s, 2 cm/mV, lead II, feline. The HR here is approximately 375 bpm, which in of itself highly suggestive of a *malignant* tachycardia of *non-sinus* origin. This cat had severe hypotension and lethargy related to this SVT. There are deep S waves of the QRS complexes, making them negative. This is because the cat has a LAFB when in sinus rhythm. The R-R interval is variable, suggesting AVB. This implies that this tachycardia may be supraventricular. The beginning of the strip shows electrical alternans, which may be suggestive of circus movement tachycardia over an accessory pathway. The P' waves appear to immediately precede the QRS complexes, though it is unclear if there is actually AVD, the presence of which would suggest VT. The RVPC toward the end of the strip is clearly different than the rest of the beats, which suggests this is really SVT. Procainamide was administered IV first without response.

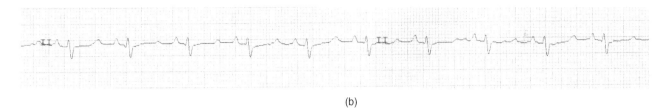

(b)

Figure 22.23b Paper speed 50 mm/s, 2 cm/mV, lead II, same cat. Following administration of IV diltiazem, the SVT broke resulting in sinus rhythm shown above. This suggests the SVT must have used the AVN as part of the circuit, since diltiazem slows conduction through the AVN. This strip clearly demonstrates the deep S waves characteristic of LAFB in lead II. The HR has slowed to 176 bpm.

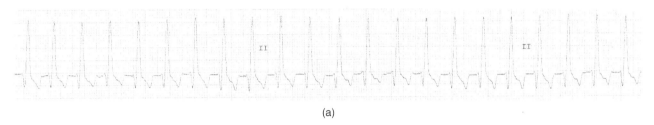

(a)

Figure 22.24a Paper speed 50 mm/s, 1 cm/mV, lead II, syncopal Standard Poodle, SVT. The HR is approximately 255 bpm. Regular, upright, and narrow QRS complexes here in lead II suggest SVT. P waves (or P' waves) are not evident in this strip.

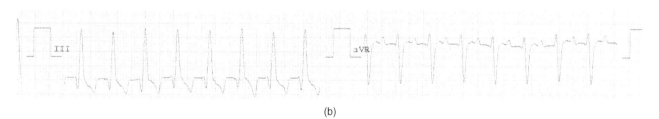

(b)

Figure 22.24b Paper speed 50 mm/s, 1 cm/mV, leads III and aVR, same dog. P' waves are seen here in lead aVR in the S-T segment between the QRS and T waves, making this a short R-P' variety of SVT.

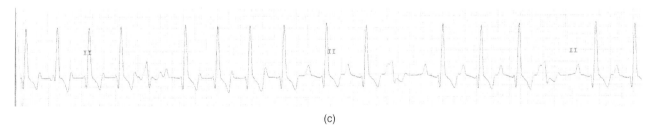

(c)

Figure 22.24c Paper speed 50 mm/s, 1 cm/mV, lead II, same dog, during administration of IV diltiazem. The HR gradually slows, and the P waves march out from the preceding T waves. First degree AVB is evident by the end of the strip. Intermittent VPCs are seen.

Further reading

Glancy, D.L., Subramaniam, P.N., Parker, J.M., and Devarapalli, S.K. (2009). Accelerated junctional rhythm, isorhythmic atrioventricular dissociation, and hidden P waves. *Proc. (Baylor Univ. Med. Cent.)* 22 (4): 371–372.

Haman, L., Praus, R., and Parizek, P. (2009). Non-re-entrant atrioventricular nodal tachycardia. *Mil. Med.* 174 (8): 866.

Karnik, A.A., Hematpour, K., Bhatt, A.G., and Mazzini, M.J. (2014). Dual AV nodal nonreentrant tachycardia resulting in inappropriate ICD therapy in a patient with cardiac sarcoidosis. *Indian Pacing Electrophysiol. J.* 14 (I): 44–48.

Levy, M.N. and Edflstein, J. (1970). The mechanism of synchronization in isorhythmic A-V dissociation. *Circulation* XLII: 689–699.

Mani, B.C. and Pavri, B.B. (2014). Dual atrioventricular nodal pathways physiology: a review of relevant anatomy, electrophysiology, and electrocardiographic manifestations. *Indian Pacing Electrophysiol. J.* 14 (1): 12–25.

Marriot, H.J.L. and Conover, M.B. (1998). *Advanced Concepts in Arrhythmias*, 3e. Mosby.

Miller, R. and Sharrett, R.H. (1957). Interference dissociation. *Circulation* 16: 803–829.

Pereira, N.J., Glaus, T., and Matos, J.N. (15, 2014). ECG of the month. *J. Am. Vet. Med. Assoc.* 244 (12): 1384–1386.

Perego, M., Ramera, L., and Santilli, R.A. (2012). Isorhythmic atrioventricular dissociation in labrador retrievers. *J. Vet. Intern. Med.* 26 (2): 320–325.

Richter, S., Sarkozy, A., de Asmundis, C. et al. (2008). Grouped beating: to couple into trouble. *Europace* 10: 1108–1109.

Rosen, K.M. (1973). Junctional tachycardia: mechanisms, diagnosis, differential diagnosis, and management. *Circulation* XLVII: 654–664.

Waldo, A., Vitikainen, K.J., Harris, P. et al. (1968). The mechanism of synchronization in isorhythmic A-V dissociation: some observations on the morphology and polarity of the P wave during retrograde capture of the atria. *Circulation* XXXVIII: 880–898.

Ventricular Arrhythmias

Ventricular arrhythmias may occur in the setting of bradycardia, normal heart rates, or tachycardia. The physical origin can loosely be determined by the morphology of the QRS on surface EKG, though this can be unreliable. The Purkinje fibers and ventricular myocytes are capable of spontaneous depolarization. Typically, diastolic Phase 4 depolarization is slower than that of sinoatrial, ectopic atrial, and junctional foci, so they tend to be the last to "escape" when superior pacemakers fail; however, ventricular escape rhythms may actually be more common in cases of canine third degree atrioventricular block given that the lesion is usually within the His bundle (or lower – i.e. bilateral bundle branch block or trifascicular block). Ventricular tachyarrhythmias ensue when these escape centers have enhanced automaticity, reentry occurs, or triggered activity allows for ectopic foci to capture the ventricles.

The morphology of ventricular beats may be helpful in localization of the origin of spontaneous depolarizations within the ventricular myocardium. The His bundle divides within the interatrial septum into right and left main bundle branches. The left bundle normally has anterior and posterior divisions; however, a medial fascicle may be present or diffuse branching can occur. Foci arising from the near or in the His bundle will produce a relatively narrow QRS, often confusing the examiner with a supraventricular origin. Those arising within the left ventricle activate the left ventricular myocardium relatively early with delayed activation of the right ventricular myocardium, resulting in a prolonged QRS with a right bundle branch block-like morphology. A left anterior fascicular origin produces an R axis, and a left posterior fascicular origin results in a superior axis. An anterior axis occurs if the origin is basilar, and a posterior axis results if the origin is apical. Foci originating from the right ventricle are marked by delayed activation of the left myocardium, producing a prolonged QRS with a left bundle branch block-like morphology. If the focus comes from the right ventricular outflow tract, then an inferior axis is present and may be slightly deviated to the left or right of +90 degrees.

The identification of ventricular tachycardia (VT) and its differentiation from supraventricular tachycardia with a prolonged QRS is of critical importance with regard to therapeutic intervention. Precordial concordance, extreme axis deviation in the limb leads, atypical bundle branch block pattern, taller left peak in V1, wide initial R wave, slurred downstroke to a late nadir, lack of RS complexes in any precordial, and extreme prolongation of the QRS all favor ventricular ectopy. Wide-complex tachycardias in general should be assumed to be VT until proven otherwise as VT is far more common than supraventricular tachycardia with aberrancy or prolonged QRS for other reasons.

Atrioventricular dissociation is commonly seen with ventricular arrhythmias and may also occur with slowing of superior pacemakers and atrioventricular block. Ventriculoatrial conduction (ventriculoatrial association) is not uncommon, resulting in a P′ wave with an axis of −80 to −100 degrees ("concentric retrograde atrial activation"). These retrograde P′ waves always follow the ventricular ectopic QRS complex. Ventriculoatrial block and exit block may occur with Type I or Type II varieties. Ventricular dissociation (double ventricular rhythms) appears to be more common with tachyarrhythmias vs. bradyarrhythmias.

Ventricular Bradyarrhythmias

Ventricular escape complexes
  Ventricular escape-capture bigeminy
Ventricular escape rhythm
Electromechanical dissociation
Asystole

Ventricular Tachyarrhythmias

Ventricular Premature Systoles

Right and left ventricular premature complexes
Compensatory pause and interpolation
  Ventricular bigeminy, trigeminy, quadrigeminy, and pentageminy

Interpretation of the Electrocardiogram in Small Animals, First Edition. Nick A. Schroeder.
© 2021 John Wiley & Sons Inc. Published 2021 by John Wiley & Sons Inc.

Concealed conduction
Ventricular fusion
Ventriculoatrial conduction/association and reciprocation
Atrial fusion
Ventricular parasystole

Ventricular Tachycardia

Accelerated ventricular/idioventricular rhythm
    Atrioventricular dissociation
        Isorhythmic dissociation
    Ventriculoatrial association
    Ventriculoatrial block
        Wenckebach vs. Mobitz
    Polymorphic and bidirectional accelerated idioventricular rhythm
Ventricular Tachycardia
    Atrioventricular dissociation with usurpation vs. ventriculoatrial association

Left ventricular tachycardia
    Fascicular ventricular tachycardia
    Bidirectional ventricular tachycardia
Right ventricular tachycardia
    Right ventricular outflow tract ventricular tachycardia
Bundle branch reentrant ventricular tachycardia
Exit block
    Wenckebach vs. Mobitz exit block
Double tachycardia
Polymorphic ventricular tachycardia
    Torsades de pointes
Ventricular flutter
    Ventricular dissociation
Ventricular fibrillation

23

Ventricular Bradyarrhythmias

CHAPTER MENU

Ventricular escape beats, 285
    Ventricular escape-capture bigeminy, 287
Ventricular escape rhythm, 287
Electromechanical dissociation, 288
Ventricular asystole, 289

Ventricular escape beats

A pause in the prevailing rhythm (i.e. due to sinus bradycardia, sinus pause/arrest, atrioventricular (AV) block, or following a tachycardia) may elicit escape beats from Purkinje fibers within the ventricular myocardium. This may occur if sinoatrial, atrial, and junctional escape centers temporarily fail to capture the rhythm. Ventricular escape beats are typically conducted with a right bundle branch block (RBBB) or left bundle branch block (LBBB)-like pattern and are thus usually wide and bizarre. Those originating in the left ventricle are typically conducted with a RBBB-like morphology, and those coming from the right ventricle are usually conducted with a LBBB-like morphology. This is the case unless fusion with a supraventricular beat occurs, in which case the QRS is intermediate in duration/morphology between those of pure supraventricular and pure ventricular origin and is always preceded by atrial activity (at a short P-R′i). Rarely, in patients with pre-existent BBB or ventricular enlargement, ventricular escape complexes originating from the blocked/enlarged ventricle may fuse with supraventricular impulses resulting in a QRS complex that is narrower and more normal in appearance. Occasionally, due to fortuitous sinus nodal discharge occurring just prior to an L ventricular escape, a deceleration-dependent RBBB may be mimicked. This is generally uncovered by variable P-R′ intervals and the presence of ventricular fusions.

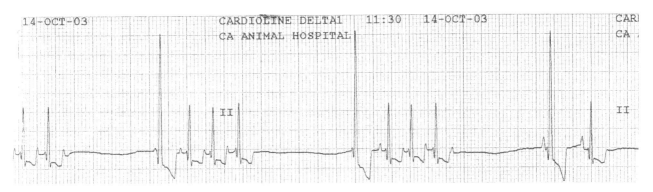

Figure 23.1 Paper speed 25 mm/s, 1 cm/mV, lead II, canine. Sinus arrests are terminated by **RV escape beats**. Short runs of SVT with Wenckebach periodicity follow the first two escape beats.

Interpretation of the Electrocardiogram in Small Animals, First Edition. Nick A. Schroeder.
© 2021 John Wiley & Sons Inc. Published 2021 by John Wiley & Sons Inc.

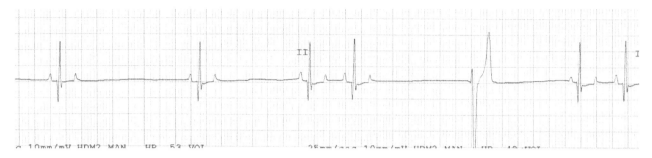

Figure 23.2 Paper speed 25 mm/s, 1 cm/mV, lead II, canine. A LV escape complex (beat #5) occurs after a pause in the rhythm.

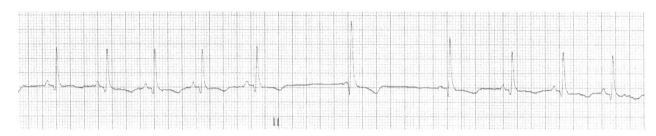

Figure 23.3 Paper speed 50 mm/s, 1 cm/mV, lead II, feline. A marked respiratory sinus arrhythmia secondary to upper airway obstruction in this cat creates pauses long enough to elicit ventricular escape beats. The sixth complex is a **ventricular escape**, and the seventh complex is a ventricular **fusion** between a sinus impulse and the ventricular focus.

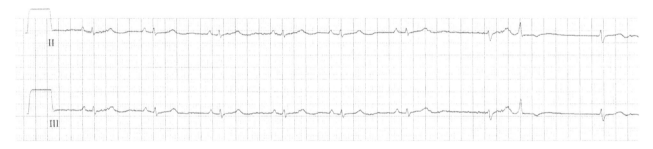

Figure 23.4 Paper speed 50 mm/s, 1 cm/mV, leads II and III, feline. Sinus arrhythmia, long Q-T interval, sinus pause, **ventricular escape**, ventricular reentry with ventricular aberrancy. A sinus pause following the sixth beat is terminated by a ventricular escape (RBBB morphology), which is immediately followed by a **reentrant (reciprocal) beat** producing a ventricular echo. This complex is conducted with a functional LBBB aberration. The pause that follows is terminated by another ventricular escape.

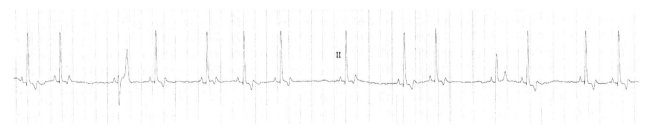

Figure 23.5 Paper speed 25 mm/s, 1 cm/mV, lead II, canine. Sinus arrhythmia with sinus pauses terminated by aberrant beats. While it is tempting to label the third complex as the result of *deceleration-dependent RBBB*, close examination of the P-R′ interval reveals it is shorter than the sinus beats. The 11th complex has a slightly longer P-R′ interval and ventricular fusion occurs. This confirms the aberrant beats are indeed left ventricular in origin.

Ventricular escape-capture bigeminy If a pause in the rhythm is terminated by a ventricular escape, which is then followed by a sinus capture in a repetitive pattern (allorhythmia), this is termed ventricular escape-capture bigeminy. The pauses may be from intermittent sinoatrial block/arrest or incomplete atrioventricular (AV) block.

Ventricular escape rhythm During severe sinus bradycardia, sinus arrest, atrial standstill, or advanced/complete AV block, failure of subsidiary pacing centers in the sinus node itself, atria or AV junction may occur, and then the inherent automaticity in the Purkinje fibers in the ventricular myocardium becomes

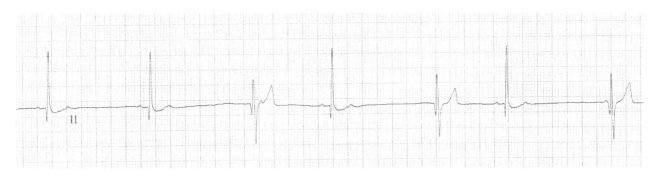

Figure 23.6 Paper speed 25 mm/s, 1 cm/mV, lead II, canine. Sinus arrhythmia with pauses eliciting ventricular escape beats in a repetitive pattern known as *ventricular* **escape-capture bigeminy**.

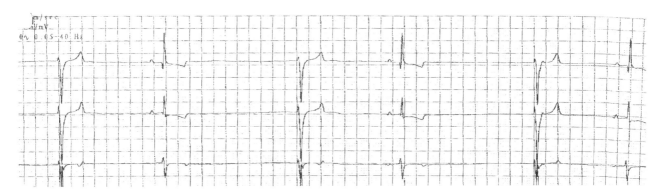

Figure 23.7 Paper speed 50 mm/s, 1 cm/mV, leads I (top), II (middle), and III (bottom), Miniature Schnauzer with sick sinus syndrome. Sinus arrest is terminated by VPCs, which are followed by a sinus capture in a repeating sequence, making a reversed-bigeminal pattern also known as **ventricular escape-capture bigeminy**. *Source: Tracing courtesy of Lynnette D'Urso.*

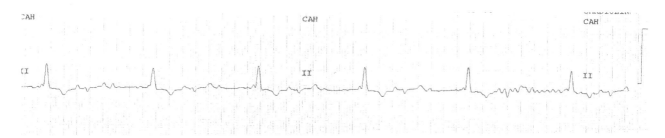

Figure 23.8 Paper speed 50 mm/s, 2 cm/mV, lead II, feline. 2:1 AVB results in a bigeminal pattern with ventricular *escape* beats. This could easily be confused with ventricular bigeminy. This is also known as *ventricular* **escape-capture bigeminy**. However, the ventricular beats here occur *following* the pause created by transient AVB, making them *escape* complexes. The escape complexes create a physiologic block of the third P wave in each series. Movement artifact is evident at the end of the strip.

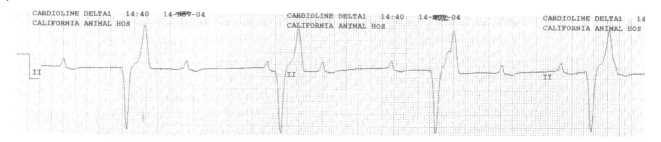

Figure 23.9 Paper speed 50 mm/s, 1 cm/mV, lead II, canine. Third degree AVB has resulted in a left **ventricular escape rhythm**. The ventricular complexes are wide and bizarre due to RBBB, indicating the focus is in the L ventricle or L bundle branch itself. The atrial rate is approximately 85 bpm, and the ventricular rate is approximately 46 bpm.

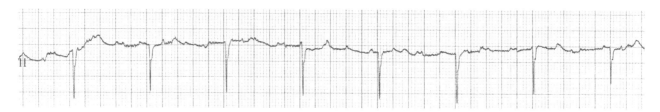

Figure 23.10 Paper speed 25 mm/s, 1 cm/mV, lead II, feline. High-grade AVB has left this cat with periods of **ventricular escape rhythm**. The atrial rate is approximately 188 bpm and the ventricular rate is approximately 60 bpm.

the last line of defense against asystole. Ventricular escape rhythms in the dog range from 20 to 50 bpm (50–80 bpm in the cat), are nonresponsive to atropine and typically have wide and bizarre complexes from effective BBB. Typically, AV dissociation occurs by default, in which a primary failure of the normal and faster pacemaker centers results in a secondary escape of a normal ventricular subsidiary pacemaker. Ventricular escape rhythms should never be suppressed. Sympathomimetics are generally ineffective and pacing is often the only treatment.

Electromechanical dissociation This occurs

when spontaneous, usually wide and bizarre ventricular complexes are seen at a slow rate on surface EKG, but no mechanical activity in the heart muscle is present, and no pulses are generated. The heart can have EMD for up to 10 minutes following circulatory collapse. The point is the clinician should feel for pulses, check with Doppler, etc. The EKG may look normal or at least as if the heart is beating when it actually is not contracting at all. One can attempt resuscitation with epinephrine, atropine, precordial thumps, electrical defibrillation, etc.; however, usually it is all over by the time one ascertains that the heart is not really beating. The most common cause for EMD is hypovolemia; however, the clinician should also rule out hypoxia, acidosis, hypothermia, hyperkalemia or hypokalemia, hypoglycemia, toxicity, cardiac tamponade, tension pneumothorax, and aortic or femoral thrombosis.

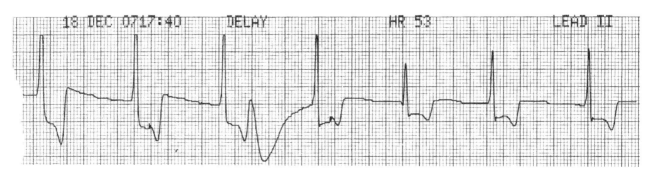

Figure 23.11 Paper speed 25 mm/s, 1 cm/mV, lead II, canine. **EMD**. This agonal dog has an apparent HR of 55 bpm. However, a lack of peripheral pulses and auscultable heart sounds indicates EMD.

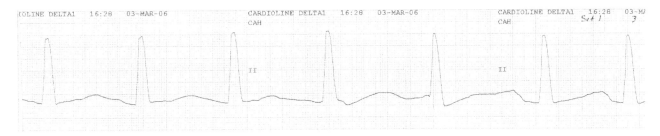

Figure 23.12 Paper speed 50 mm/s, 1 cm/mV, lead II, arresting canine. **EMD**. Wide and bizarre complexes were seen here and the patient had no pulses or auscultable heart beats.

Ventricular asystole

Ventricular asystole is defined as a flat-line EKG with no evidence of electrical activity, organized or not. The HR is zero. Defibrillation will not help, as electrical activity has ceased entirely. The patient is in complete circulatory arrest. Ventricular asystole is invariably terminal and may occur spontaneously or following electromechanical dissociation or ventricular fibrillation.

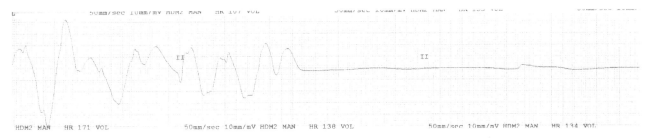

Figure 23.13 Paper speed 50 mms/s, 1 cm/mV, lead II, canine. Ventricular fibrillation followed by **ventricular asystole**. The random electrical activity of VF is followed by the flat line of asystole.

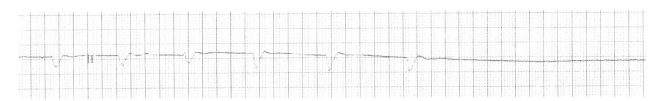

Figure 23.14 Paper speed 50 mm/s, 1 cm/mV, lead II, feline being euthanized for presumed cerebrovascular accident (CVA) secondary to thromboembolism from cardiomyopathy. **Electromechanical dissociation** followed by **ventricular asystole**.

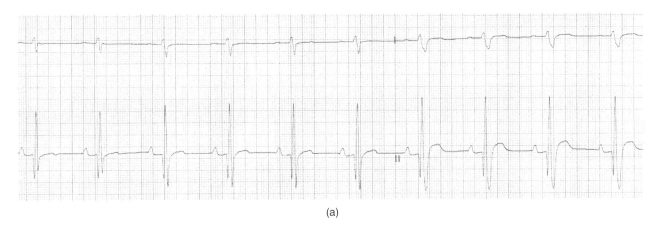

(a)

Figure 23.15a Paper speed 50 mm/s, 1 cm/mV, leads I and II, canine being euthanized with pentobarbital. Note the ventricular complexes are becoming progressively wide and bizarre.

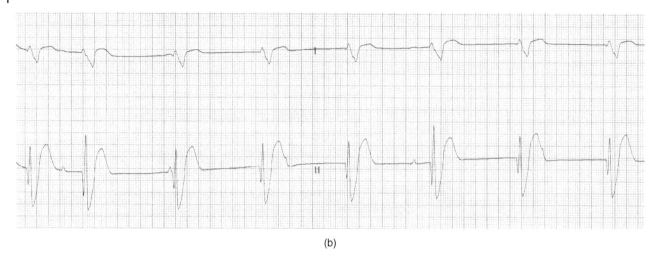

(b)

Figure 23.15b Paper speed 50 mm/s, 1 cm/mV, leads I and II, same dog. Shortly after, atrioventricular dissociation develops. The sinus rate is quite slow, irregular, and independent of the idioventricular rhythm.

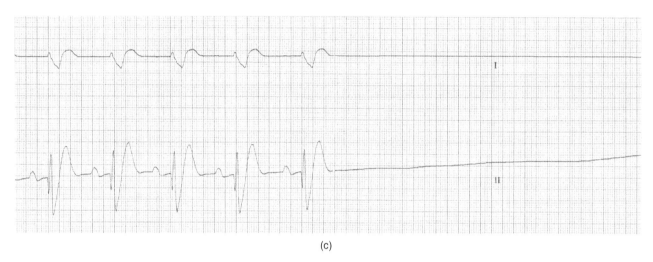

(c)

Figure 23.15c Paper speed 50 mm/s, 1 cm/mV, leads I and II, same dog. Shortly after, atrioventricular association has resumed, and is abruptly terminated by **asystole** and cardiac standstill.

Further reading

Dubin, D. (2000). *Rapid Interpretation of EKG's*, 6e. Cover Inc.

Santilli, R., Moïse, N.S., Pariaut, R., and Perego, M. (2018). *Electrocardiography of the Dog and Cat: Diagnosis of Arrhythmias*, 2e. Edna.

24

Ventricular Premature Systoles

CHAPTER MENU

Ventricular premature complexes, 291
   Right ventricular premature complexes, 292
   Left ventricular premature complexes, 292
   Compensatory pause, 293
     The "compensatory-like" pause, 295
   Interpolation, 296
     Post-extraystolic aberrancy, 298
Ventricular bigeminy, 298
   Rule of bigeminy, 298
Ventricular trigeminy, 305
Ventricular quadrigeminy, 306
Concealed conduction, 309
   Concealed ventricular bigeminy, 309
   Concealed interpolated ventricular bigeminy, 310
   Concealed ventricular trigeminy, 310
   Concealed interpolated ventricular trigeminy, 310
Ventricular fusion complexes, 311
Ventriculoatrial conduction and reciprocation, 312
Atrial fusion, 315
Ventricular parasystole, 315

Ventricular premature complexes Ventricular premature complexes (VPCs, premature ventricular contractions/PVCs, ventricular premature depolarizations/VPDs, ventricular premature beats/VPBs, ventricular premature systoles/extrasystoles) are ectopic early beats that originate from below the atrioventricular node (AVN). Those that arise higher in the interventricular septum (near or within the His bundle) have a more supraventricular-appearing waveform on EKG, and those originating further down in the ventricles have a more wide and bizarre appearance. These often do not have a P wave associated with the QRS and are thus often characterized by AV dissociation, resulting in P waves that are "interfered" with (they are blocked from conducting) because they occur when the AVN is refractory during or just after the ectopic complex. The T wave is often different than that of sinus T waves and opposite in polarity of the main QRS deflection. Ventricular premature complexes are by definition early. This means that the QRS of the VPC occurs sooner than expected and within a period clearly shorter than that of the underlying cycle length (or expected cycle length considering variation due to sinus arrhythmia, underlying atrial fibrillation, etc.). The so-called "late diastolic VPC" is one that is barely premature and should not be confused with ventricular escape complexes which occur following a long pause. Ventricular premature complexes may be mimicked by supraventricular premature complexes with aberrancy. Concealed conduction associated with ventricular extrasystoles is limited to retrograde conduction through the AVN and manifests most commonly as P-R interval prolongation following an interpolated VPC and the compensatory pause, but also includes non-conducted extrasystoles. Fusion with supraventricular foci in the ventricles or the atria may occur, and retrograde conduction, reciprocation, and parasystole are all possible.

Interpretation of the Electrocardiogram in Small Animals, First Edition. Nick A. Schroeder.
© 2021 John Wiley & Sons Inc. Published 2021 by John Wiley & Sons Inc.

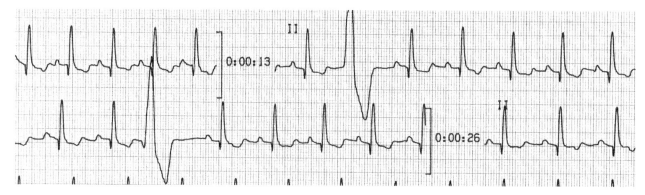

Figure 24.1 Paper speed 50 mm/s, 1 cm/mV, lead II, canine. The wide, bizarre, premature beats are upright with LBBB pattern, consistent with **RVPCs**.

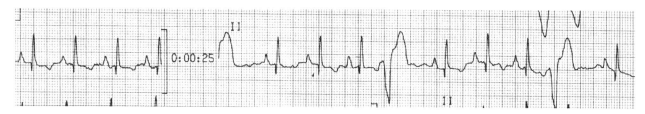

Figure 24.2 Paper speed 50 mm/s, 1 cm/mV, canine. The wide and bizarre premature beats with a RBBB pattern are consistent with **LVPCs**.

Right ventricular premature complexes These arise from the right ventricle. Typically, they are conducted with a left bundle branch block-like pattern, which result in a wide QRS complex with broad, tall R waves in lead II followed by a strongly negative T wave (mimicking LBBB, in which there is a wide QRS with a tall R wave in lead II). This is provided that the sinus QRS complexes are normal and underlying axis deviation is absent. Right ventricular premature complexes are very common in Boxers and Bulldogs with arrhythmogenic cardiomyopathy.

Left ventricular premature complexes They arise from the left ventricle. Typically, these are conducted with a right bundle branch block-like pattern, which result in a wide QRS complex with broad, deep S waves in lead II followed by a strongly positive T wave (mimicking RBBB, in which there is a wide QRS with a deep S wave in lead II). Again, this is provided that underlying axis deviation is absent. The right bundle branch typically has a longer refractory period than the left bundle branch, so premature beats are more commonly conducted with a RBBB, and LVPCs tend to be more common than RVPCs.

Ventricular premature complexes may be confused with sinus/supraventricular beats conducted with bundle branch block (BBB) and ventricular escape beats. Ventricular premature complexes are conducted with a BBB-like morphology but are "early" and often without an associated P wave (as in BBB). Escape beats occur following a pause,

making them "late," rescuing the heart from asystole. Fusion complexes are "on-time" with the supraventricular focus. Aberrant junctional extrasystoles with intact ventriculoatrial (VA) conduction with P′ waves following the ectopic QRS or VA block) may be indistinguishable from VPCs on surface EKG.

Keep in mind that the determination of site of ventricular origin based on morphology and axis of the ectopic QRS are generalizations. Studies have been done which demonstrate that a stimulus in one area of the ventricle may result in waveforms on surface EKG that vary considerably. The terms "uniforme" or unifocal VPCs arise from a single irritated focus in the myocardium, and "multiforme" VPCs have variable morphologies; however, both have constant coupling intervals suggesting a unifocal source. Multifocal VPCs arise from multiple areas in the myocardium and have variable coupling intervals. However, one focus may have varied exits and morphologies. Multifocal supraventricular complexes tend to have variable P-P′ intervals, and multifocal VPCs tend to have varied R-R′ intervals. Multifocal VPCs are thought to signify a more electrically unstable myocardium and warrant more aggressive antiarrhythmic therapy.

Relatively narrow-complex VPCs may be produced from fascicular foci within the ventricles. If the ventricular beat originates in the left posterior fascicle, it will be conducted with a RBBB+LAFB pattern and have an L axis. If the ventricular beat originates in the left anterior fascicle, it will be

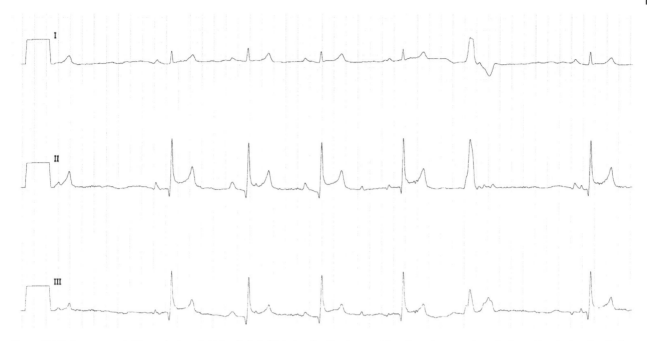

Figure 24.3 Paper speed 50 mm/s, 1 cm/mV, leads I, II, III, Labrador Retriever with pulmonic stenosis and tricuspid valvular dysplasia. Sinus arrhythmia, first degree atrioventricular block, prolongation of the QRS complexes (0.10 second), S-T segment elevation, and a ventricular premature complex (beat #5) with a so-called "**ugly QRS**." Marked prolongation of the VPC (0.12 second) and slurring of the upstroke (peak to peak 0.04 second) are evident. Presumably, ventricular hypertrophy, fibrosis, and hypoxemia all contribute to prolong the sinus QRS complexes and account for S-T segment elevation.

conducted with a RBBB+LPFB and have an R axis. Beats that originate in the His bundle itself may have a relatively normal QRS duration and MEA, since they can conduct over the normal Purkinje system. The further away from the conduction system, the more wide-and-bizarre the QRS complex becomes as depolarization occurs cell-to-cell. A narrow-complex fusion beat may occur if a patient has pre-existing BBB or ventricular enlargement (leading to prolongation of the QRS) and a VPC from the same ventricle with conduction delay fortuitously occurs, normalizing the QRS complex duration.

VPCs that have a so-called "ugly QRS" with marked prolongation, slurring of the waveforms, notching with peak separation of at least 0.04 second can warn the clinician of serious underlying heart disease. This phenomenon has been associated with a dilated, globally hypokinetic ventricle.

Exit block and ventriculoatrial block (VA block) may be seen with VPCs and can be of Wenckebach or Mobitz varieties. Exit block with Wenckebach (Type I) is suggested when gradually increasing coupling intervals are seen prior to the failure of a VPC to appear when otherwise expected. Mobitz exit block (Type II) is random failure of the VPC to appear with constant coupling intervals. Exit blocks create intermittent concealment of VPCs on surface EKG. VA block necessarily occurs when VA conduction is present and retrograde P′ waves are intermittently seen following VPCs. Wenckebach VA block (Type I) occurs when the V-P′ interval gradually increases prior to failure of retrograde conduction. Mobitz VA block (Type II) is suspected when VA conduction randomly fails and the V-P′ interval is constant. A 2 : 1 VA block occurs when every-other VPC has VA conduction. Exit and VA block may be diagnosed when VPCs occur regularly (i.e. in bigeminy, trigeminy, etc.).

Compensatory pauses and interpolation are highly suggestive of VPCs. The term is a bit confusing, as the pause really does not compensate for anything, and both occur due to transient atrioventricular dissociation. Basically, VPCs penetrate the AVN retrogradely, making it temporarily refractory for the next sinus beat, which creates a functional first or second degree AVB. The blocked P wave may or may not be evident on surface EKG. Ventricular premature complexes may temporarily accelerate the discharge of the SAN (ventriculophasic sinus arrhythmia), burying the non-conducted P wave in the T wave of the VPC. Functional first degree AVB may result on post-extrasystolic beats that follow interpolated or very late diastolic VPCs. These changes represent indirect evidence of concealed conduction into the AVN by VPCs.

Compensatory pause The interval from the sinus R preceding the ectopic beat to the next sinus R is exactly equal to two normal R-R intervals. The VPC basically replaces the sinus beat, and the sinus rhythm continues undisturbed.

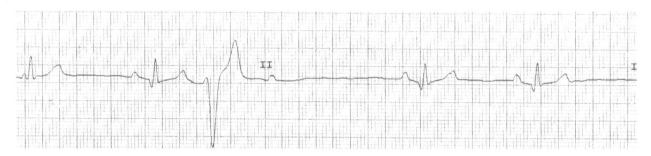

Figure 24.4 Paper speed 50 mm/s, 1 cm/mV, lead II, canine, the third beat is a VPC followed by a **compensatory pause**. The VPC creates a functional second degree AVB of the following sinus P wave, and the next P wave is conducted normally.

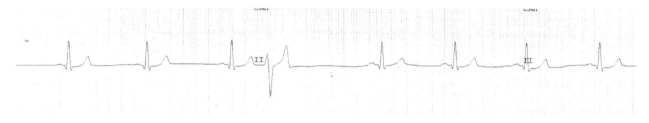

Figure 24.5 Paper speed 50 mm/s, 1 cm/mV, lead II, canine. The fourth beat is a VPC followed by a **compensatory pause**. The expected blocked sinus P following the VPC is not seen here and likely hiding in the T wave of the VPC, demonstrating how VPCs may briefly accelerate sinus nodal discharge.

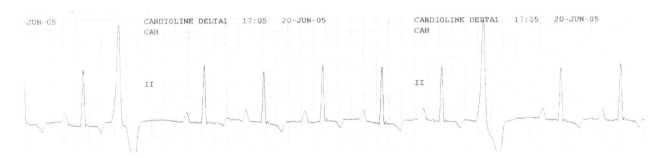

Figure 24.6 Paper speed 50 mm/s, 1 cm/mV, lead II, canine. VPCs followed by **compensatory pauses**. Here the non-conducted P waves are simply buried within the T waves of the VPCs.

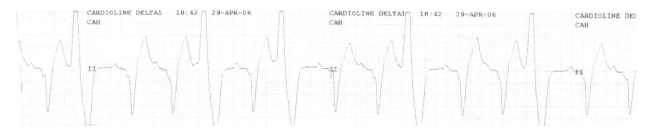

Figure 24.7 Paper speed 50 mm/s, 1 cm/mV, lead II. Bulldog with severe PS. **Complete RBBB** is present on the sinus beats. **Ventricular premature complexes** intermittently occur, creating the compensatory pauses. The QRS complexes of the sinus beats are markedly prolonged as are the ventricular beats.

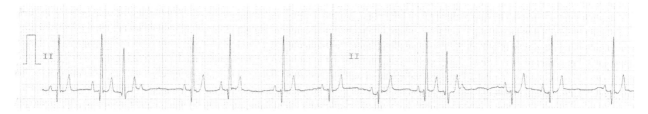

Figure 24.8 Paper speed 25 mm/s, 1 cm/mV, lead II, canine. **Fascicular VPCs**. The 3rd and 10th complexes are narrow and upright with normal-appearing T waves, suggestive of a supraventricular focus. However, careful examination reveals that these beats prevent conduction of the next sinus P wave, thus causing **compensatory pauses**. Furthermore, the initial vector of the ectopic complexes is shorter than the sinus beats. These are VPCs likely arising from a fascicular focus. The 5th and 12th complexes are APCs – note that they **reset** the underlying sinus rhythm with a pause.

The "compensatory-like" pause The concepts of compensatory pause and interpolation break down when VPCs occur during an irregular supraventricular rhythm. This may be the case during a particularly marked sinus arrhythmia and especially so during atrial fibrillation (AF). During sinus arrhythmia, examination of the R-R interval immediately preceding the VPC tends to be helpful, though somewhat inexact. Ventricular premature complexes that occur during the acceleration phase of a sinus arrhythmia commonly result in less than fully compensatory pauses. Given that no two R-R intervals are ever consistent between supraventricular beats generated by the fibrillating atria (hence the irregularly irregular rhythm of AF), the typical two R-R intervals encompassing a VPC constituting a compensatory pause and the one R-R interval encompassing an interpolated VPC can never really be demonstrated. Since the notion of what constitutes "prematurity" is unclear, some authors

consider the term "ventricular premature complex" to be inappropriate in the setting of AF and prefer "ventricular ectopic beat" or "ventricular extrasystole" as alternatives (see Chapter 18). Regardless of nomenclature, VPCs penetrate the AVN retrogradely, even during AF, often resulting in a "compensatory-like" pause because of concealed conduction. This creates a pause of substantial duration following a VPC during AF that approximates two R-R intervals.

A Note: Truly non-compensatory pauses ("less than fully compensatory pauses") are uncommonly seen following VPCs with VA conduction, those occurring simultaneously with supraventricular premature complexes, during the acceleration phase of a sinus arrhythmia, interrupting Wenckebach periodicity (Type I second degree atrioventricular block), during junctional rhythm or when the pause following the VPC is terminated by an escape complex.

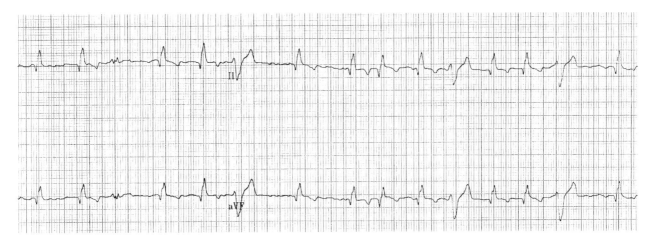

Figure 24.9 Paper speed 50 mm/s, 1 cm/mV, leads II, aVF, canine. **Atrial fibrillation** and **VPCs** followed by "*compensatory-like*" pauses. The baseline is undulating, and the rhythm is irregularly irregular with supraventricular complexes consistent with atrial fibrillation. The 6th, 11th, and 14th complexes are ventricular ectopics arising from the LV (RBBB-like morphology) and are followed by pauses comparable to two R-R intervals (though obviously inexact). The third complex is a ventricular *fusion* with a QRS complex intermediate in duration (and largely isoelectric).

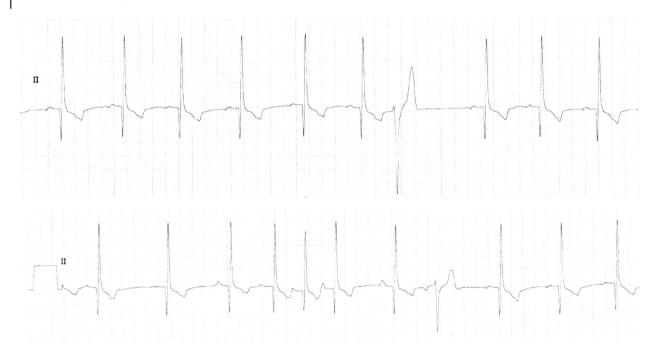

Figure 24.10 Paper speed 50 mm/s, 1 cm/mV, lead II, canine. The top strip shows a single VPC followed by a typical compensatory pause. The bottom strip shows a couplet of APCs (beats #5 and #6). Beat #8 appears to be a rare **simultaneous APC and VPC.** While it is tempting to call this an APC with aberration, careful examination shows a mildly shortened P'-Ri and the QRS is a fusion. The APC resets the sinus node, so the VPC here has a non-compensatory pause by association. The presence of VPCs and APCs in the same record supports this conclusion.

Interpolation (Interponation) The ectopic beat occurs between two normal sinus beats and does not create a pause or interrupt the underlying rhythm (true extrasystole). This is quite common with VPCs, uncommonly seen with JPCs and very rarely associated with APCs. Interpolated VPCs often partially penetrate the AVN, making it partially refractory, causing conduction of the post-extrasystolic beat to be delayed, leading to functional first degree AVB on the post-extrasystolic beat. This can be explained with dual AVN physiology (the fast path is refractory, and conduction proceeds down the slow path) and is favored if two consistent and distinct P-R intervals can be demonstrated. More commonly, variable P-R intervals are present and dependent on the coupling interval of the VPC and prevailing sinus rate. Rarely, a "postponed compensatory pause" will follow interpolated VPCs (a cause of pseudo-interpolation). The post-extrasystolic beat is conducted with P-R interval prolongation, which shortens the R-P interval to the next impulse, leading to nonconduction of the second P wave following the VPC – basically inducing a Wenckebach period. Another cause of pseudo-interpolation is ventricular reentry, also cited to be a manifestation of dual AV nodal physiology. Differentiation of the post-extrasystolic beat between one of sinus origin and a ventricular reentrant ("echo" or reciprocal) complex can be made by examining the R-R

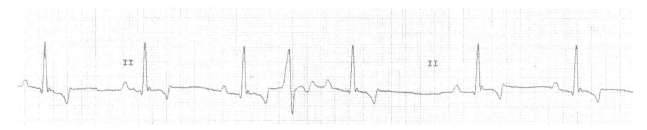

Figure 24.11 Paper speed 50 mm/s, 1 cm/mV, lead II, canine, the fourth complex is an **interpolated VPC**. There is **prolongation of the P-R interval** on the **post-extrasystolic beat** indicating the VPC partially entered the AVN, causing delayed conduction of the following sinus beat. In essence, the VPC *pushes* the QRS to the right. Interestingly, the R-R interval between the post-extrasystolic beat and the following beat (beats #5 and #6) is longer than expected. This, however, does not constitute a so-called "postposed compensatory pause," as no evidence of an AV blocked P wave is seen following the post-extrasystolic beat. Furthermore, the post-extrasystolic beat does not constitute a reciprocal complex since the R-R interval containing the VPC is the same as or slightly longer normal R-R interval and no retrograde P' wave is evident.

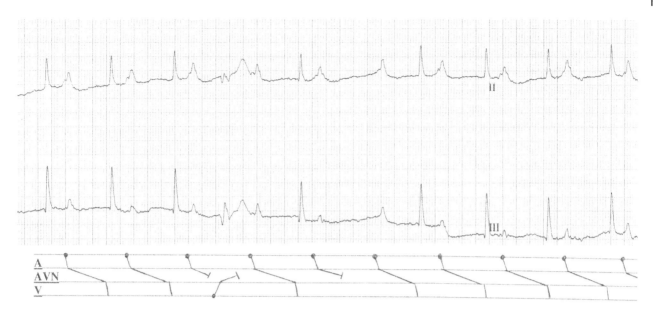

Figure 24.12 Paper speed 50 mm/s, 1 cm/mV, leads II, III, canine with severe CMVDz, CHF on digoxin. **Severe first degree AVB**, right axis deviation of the QRS, **interpolated VPC** followed by a **postponed compensatory pause**. The VPC basically initiates a Wenckebach period, causing enough further prolongation of the already prolonged P-Ri of the fifth beat, shortening the R-P interval enough to cause AV block of the following P wave.

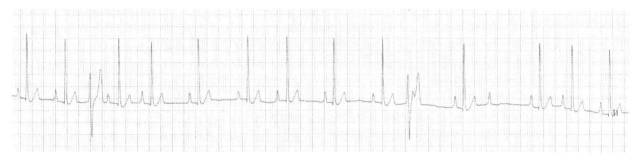

Figure 24.13 Paper speed 25 mm/s, 1 cm/mV, lead II, canine. The third complex is an interpolated VPC. Note the post-extrasystolic P-R interval prolongation on the fourth beat of sinus origin. The 11th complex is another VPC, which appears to cause a compensatory pause. Interestingly, the post-extrasystolic beat is followed by a non-conducted P wave, similar to that seen with a **postponed compensatory pause**. However, postponed compensatory pauses typically follow interpolated VPCs. Perhaps a concealed VPC prevented conduction of this beat.

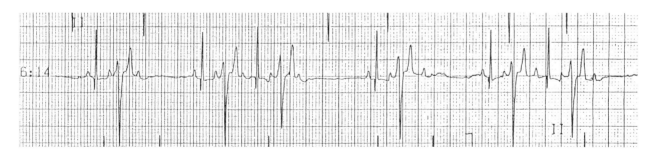

Figure 24.14 Paper speed 25 mm/s, 1 cm/mV, lead II, canine, the second complex is a LVPC that clearly prevents conduction of the following sinus beat as evidenced by the P wave without a QRS immediately following it (second degree AVB). This creates the **compensatory pause** that follows, and is also seen on the 6th, 8th, and 12th beats. The fourth complex (LVPC) is **interpolated** and causes P-R interval prolongation of the following sinus beat. The 10th beat is also interpolated and similarly causes 1st degree AVB of the 12th complex. These allorhythmic sequences are created because of R-P/P-R reciprocity. In each of the sinus-interpolated VPC-sinus-VPC with compensatory pause sequences, the interpolated VPC creates post-extrasystolic P-Ri prolongation, and the R-P interval shortens, prolonging the refractory period of the AV nodal tissue enough for the second VPC to result in a compensatory pause.

interval of the beats containing the VPC. A supraventricular (sinus) beat is favored if the R-R is equal to or longer (from concealed VA conduction by the VPC causing P-R interval prolongation) than the sinus interval. If the R-R interval containing the VPC is shorter, a reciprocal complex is favored. If the VPC during AF is interpolated, then no pause is noted and a ventricular reentry or echo beat is a rule out for the post-extrasystolic supraventricular "capture."

Post-extraystolic aberrancy Interference of subsequent conduction by VPCs is not limited to block of the post-extrasystolic P wave creating compensatory pauses or conduction delay leading to post-extrasystolic P-R interval prolongation following interpolated VPCs. Occasionally, conduction delay may transiently affect the bundle branches. Interpolated VPCs may cause post-extrasystolic aberrant ventricular conduction, mimicking polymorphic ventricular couplets. This is suspected when the post-extrasystolic QRS has a typical BBB pattern, is different than that of the morphology of the VPC, and preceding atrial activity is demonstrable or at least plausible. This may be more likely if the post-extrasystolic P-Ri is actually

not prolonged. This is the ventricular analogue to Chung's phenomenon (see Chapter 4).

Ventricular bigeminy It occurs when every other beat is premature due to 1:1 extrasystole (sinus beat, VPC, sinus beat, VPC, etc.). Ventricular bigeminy may be mimicked by supraventricular bigeminy with aberrancy and during atrial flutter with Ashman's phenomenon. Double bigeminy occurs when the ectopic complexes are alternating in morphology. This may be from competing ventricular ectopic sites or ventricular ectopy that alternates with supraventricular (usually junctional) ectopy.

Rule of bigeminy A lengthened cycle tends to precipitate a VPC. Thus, the second beat that ends a short cycle preceded by a long cycle may really be a VPC, not an aberrantly conducted APC or sinus beat. If the complex is preceded by a P' wave (at a normal or prolonged P-R interval), is of RBBB morphology, and the coupling interval to the preceding beat is variable, then this is suggestive that the anomalous QRS is really a supraventricular beat (and thus aberrant due

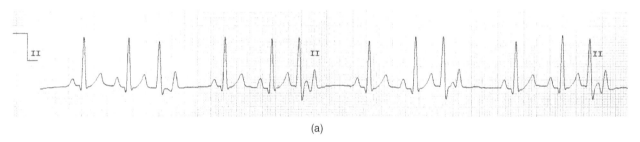

(a)

Figure 24.15a Paper speed 50 mm/s, 1 cm/mV, lead II, canine. ***Fascicular* ventricular trigeminy**. Here, the premature complexes appear to be supraventricular at first glance. However, a fully compensatory pause follows each ectopic complex. These beats did not depolarize/reset the sinus node, making them unlikely to have originated above the level of the AVN. The 6th, 9th, and 12th complexes actually show dissociated sinus P waves in the S-T segment. Remember, AVD is more common with ventricular arrhythmias. Beats arising from the His bundle or fascicles will be more supraventricular in appearance since they are conducted predominantly over the normal His-Purkinje system.

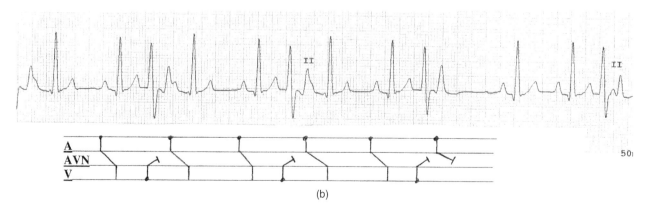

(b)

Figure 24.15b Paper speed 50 mm/s, 1 cm/mV, lead II, same dog. **Interpolated ventricular trigeminy** transitions to ventricular trigeminy with compensatory pause. A ladder diagram illustrates that the third beat is an interpolated VPC that causes post-extrasystolic P-R interval prolongation (functional first degree AVB). The next VPC prolongs the P-R interval even more, and the third VPC completely prevents conduction of the next P wave, resulting in the compensatory pause, giving a Wenckebach-like effect.

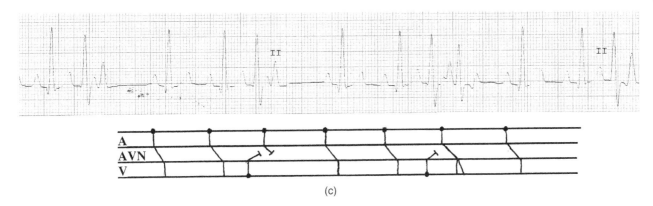

Figure 24.15c Paper speed 50 mm/s, 1 cm/mV, lead II, same dog. The first two VPCs create typical compensatory pauses. The third VPC is interpolated and creates **aberrant ventricular conduction** of the **post-extrasystolic beat**, mimicking a ventricular couplet. A ladder diagram illustrates the mechanism.

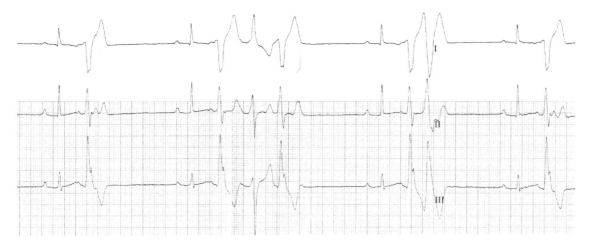

Figure 24.16 Paper speed 50 mm/s, 1 cm/mV, lead I, II, III, canine. Ventricular bigeminy is seen with **post-extrasystolic aberration** (beat #5). This gives the appearance of a multiforme/bidirectional triplet. The eighth and ninth beats appear to be a true ventricular couplet.

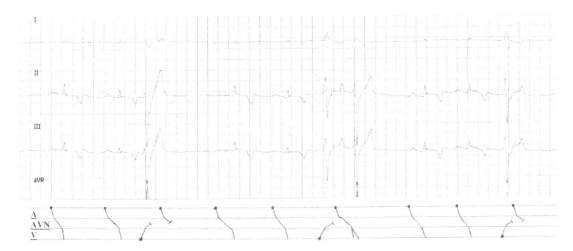

Figure 24.17 Paper speed 50 mm/s, 1 cm/mV, leads I, II, III, canine with large mediastinal mass. Ventricular trigeminy with **post-extrasystolic aberrancy**. The QRS complexes are low voltage in the large-breed dog, likely secondary to the insulating effect of the large intrathoracic mass. The third complex is a VPC creating a compensatory pause. The sixth complex appears to arise from another ventricular focus (note the slightly longer coupling interval) and is interpolated between the fifth and seventh beats. The post-extrasystolic beat (#7) appears to be another ventricular beat but may in fact be aberrantly conducted (RBBB) sinus secondary to the previous VPC. Interpolated VPCs may be followed by post-extrasystolic aberration, mimicking ventricular couplets in this manner. The last beat is another VPC from presumably the same focus, but the coupling interval is slightly longer, creating a compensatory pause.

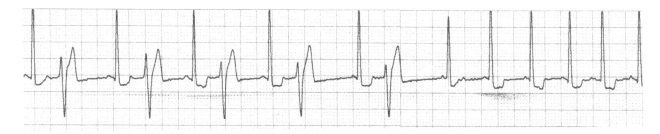

Figure 24.18 Paper speed 25 mm/s, 1 cm/mV, lead II, canine, **ventricular bigeminy**, the RBBB-like morphology suggests an L ventricular focus.

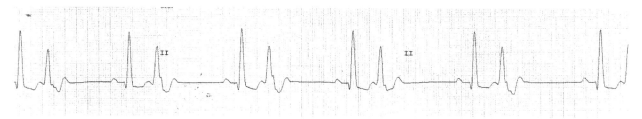

Figure 24.19 Paper speed 25 mm/s, 1 cm/mV, lead II, canine, **ventricular bigeminy**, the LBBB-like morphology suggests an R ventricular focus.

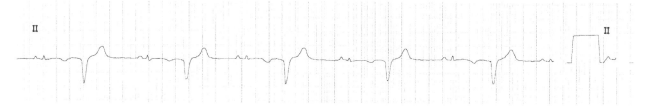

Figure 24.20 Paper speed 50 mm/s, 1 cm/mV, lead II, feline, **ventricular bigeminy**, the RBBB-like morphology suggests an L ventricular focus.

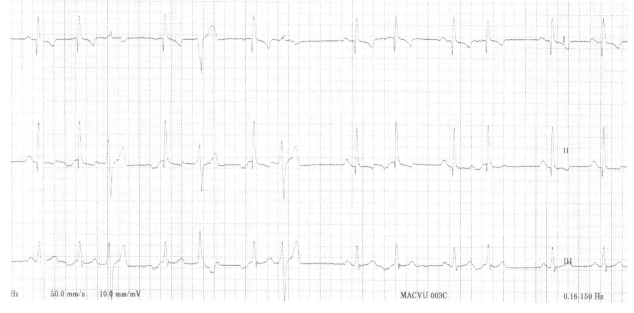

Figure 24.21 Paper speed 50 mm/s, 1 cm/mV, leads I, II, III, canine. ***Double bigeminy***. Initially, a junctional premature beat initiates a bigeminal rhythm where junctional beats are followed by VPCs in an alternating pattern. Midway through the strip, the VPCs disappear and a short run of junctional bigeminy occurs which finally terminates in sinus rhythm. Note the compensatory pauses following the VPCs gradually get longer as the VPCs occur at progressively shorter coupling intervals until the sinus node is finally able to capture. The VPCs here are multiforme, and likely multifocal, as the two different morphologies have different coupling intervals as well. The VPCs have relatively narrow QRS complexes, and the first and third VPCs have RBBB/LAFB morphology (LAD, positive in I) suggestive of a posterior fascicular origin, while the second VPC has a RBBB/LPFB (RAD, negative in I) morphology suggestive of an anterior fascicular origin.

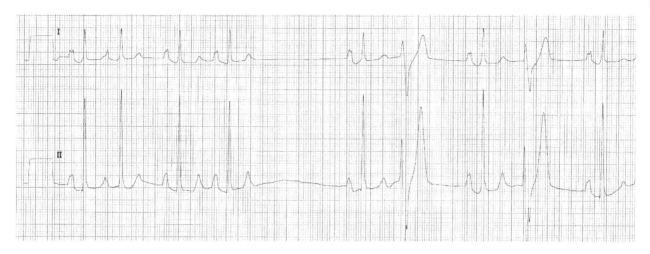

Figure 24.22 Paper speed 25 mm/s, 1 cm/mV, lead II, canine. A single VPC occurs after a lengthened cycle length and 1 : 1 extrasystole ensues, following the **Rule of bigeminy**.

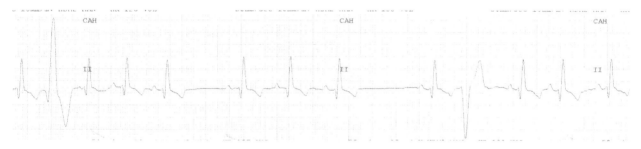

Figure 24.23 Paper speed 50 mm/s, 1 cm/mV, lead II, canine. The second complex is a single interpolated RVPC, and the 10th complex is an LVPC that occurs after a lengthened cycle, consistent with the **Rule of bigeminy**.

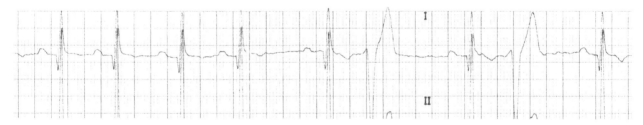

Figure 24.24 Paper speed 50 mm/s, 1 cm/mV, lead I, canine. Sinus tachycardia with an abrupt lengthening of the cycle length elicits a VPC. This, in turn, creataxses a compensatory pause, eliciting another VPC in a bigeminal rhythm consistent with the **Rule of bigeminy**.

to Ashman's phenomenon). If the premature beats cause compensatory pauses or are interpolated and are coupled to the preceding cycles by relatively fixed intervals, then this is suggestive of VPCs occurring via reentry. If the VPC produces a compensatory pause, this creates another sudden prolongation in ventricular cycle length, which in turn promotes reentry and the formation of another VPC following the post-extrasystolic beat, perpetuating a bigeminal rhythm. Though reentry is usually cited as the mechanism, early afterdepolarizations may also be implicated.

Ventricular premature complexes are commonly associated with escape beats during high grade or complete atrioventricular block, producing slow bigeminal rhythms. If the "VPCs" have opposite morphology of the escape beats

and are preceded by P waves within the S-T segment of the escape beats at a consistent interval, then supernormal conduction with aberrancy is often cited as a possibility. Most of the time supernormality is excluded based on variable P-R intervals and constant coupling intervals of the escape beats to the premature beats.

Of course, the sinus node may not always be in charge of the atria during ventricular bigeminy. The atria may be in standstill/sinoventricular rhythm, atrial tachycardia, atrial flutter, or AF. Ashman's phenomenon (long-short cycle length changes precipitating right bundle branch block aberrancy) is considered excluded if constant coupling intervals between the supraventricular captures and the ectopic beats, "compensatory-like pauses," follow the

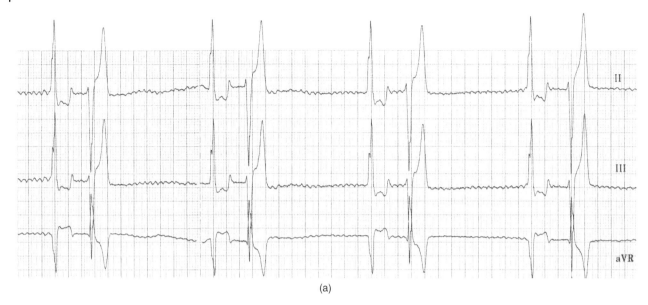

(a)

Figure 24.25a Paper speed 25 mm/s, 1 cm/mV, leads II and III, aVR, canine. **Atrial fibrillation, *high-grade* AVB, ventricular escape, and ventricular bigeminy**. High-grade atrioventricular block led to excessively slow ventricular rate response in this patient with atrial fibrillation. Ventricular escape rhythm would occasionally appear, as well as VPCs. The escape beats have a LBBB-like pattern (positive R′ in II), and the VPCs have a RBBB-like pattern (deep S′ in lead II). The VPCs tended to appear after complexes following long cycle lengths, in accordance with the **Rule of bigeminy**. Note the undulating baseline and lack of P waves, indicating atrial fibrillation. Supernormal conduction is unlikely given the constant coupling intervals.

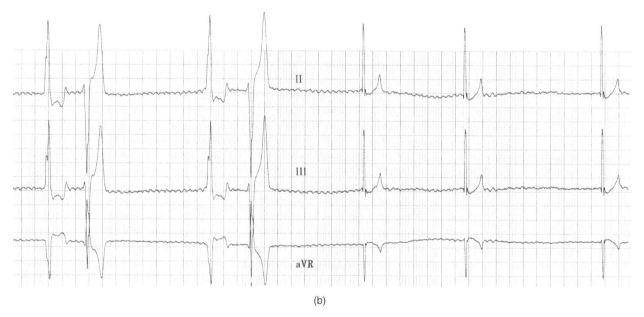

(b)

Figure 24.25b Paper speed 25 mm/s, 1 cm/mV, leads II and III, and aVR. Same dog. Ventricular escape and bigeminy terminates midway through the strip. Typical narrow, supraventricular QRS complexes appear in an irregularly irregular rhythm consistent with the fibrillating atria regaining control of the ventricles. The excessively slow ventricular rate response indicates high-grade AVB.

abnormal beats and ventricular fusion complexes can be demonstrated. A classic impostor of ventricular bigeminy is atrial flutter with alternating 2 : 1 and 4 : 1 conduction with RBBB aberrancy on short cycles (see Chapter 6).

Most of the time, VPCs in bigeminy are followed by compensatory pauses. Occasionally, they may be interpolated with post-extrasystolic P-Ri prolongation and/or aberrancy mimicking bidirectional couplets. However, VA conduction may also be evident during ventricular bigeminy. This may result in resetting of the sinus node, displacement of the pacemaker to ectopic atrial sites, and VA block and reentry are possibilities.

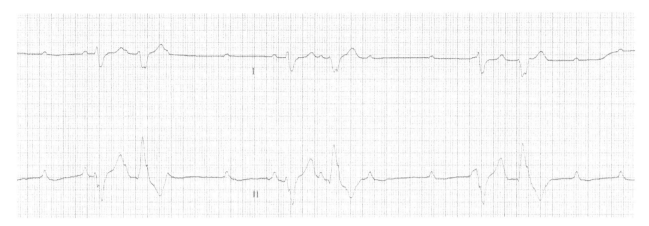

Figure 24.26 Paper speed 50 mm/s, 1 cm/mV, leads I and II, canine. **Sinus arrhythmia of the atria, ventricular escape, third degree AVB, ventricular bigeminy**. The atrial rate is slow and irregular due to sinus arrhythmia. The ventricular rate is slow (idioventricular rate of approximately 52 bpm, likely ventricular, but possibly junctional), and has a RBBB-like morphology (suggestive of a LV focus or junctional focus with RBBB). VPCs (LBBB-like morphology, suggestive of an RV focus) follow each idioventricular beat at constant coupling intervals, and the variable P-R intervals make supernormal conduction unlikely.

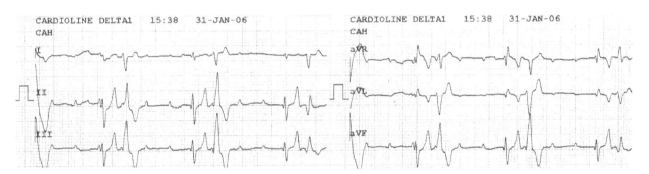

Figure 24.27 Paper speed 25 mm/s, 1 cm/mV, full EKG, canine. **Sinus rhythm of the atria, junctional escape with RBBB aberrancy, third degree AVB, ventricular bigeminy.** P waves march through the complexes at a faster rate, indicative of third degree AVB. A VPC occurs after each short cycle preceded by a long cycle, following the **Rule of bigeminy**. The VPCs (beats #1, 3, 5, and 7) are RV in origin with a LBBB-like pattern. The escape beats (#2, 4, and 6) are junctional in origin with RBBB aberrancy (the escape rhythm is approximately 66 bpm, most consistent with a junctional focus). Again, constant coupling intervals and variable P-R intervals exclude supernormality.

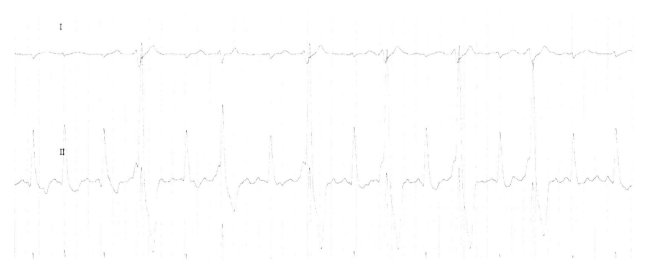

Figure 24.28 Paper speed 50 mm/s, 1 cm/mV, leads I and II, canine. **Atrial flutter with ventricular bigeminy**. Note the undulating baseline characteristic of atrial flutter. After three beats, 1 : 1 extrasystole develops. Ashman's phenomenon is excluded based on the presence of fusion (beat #5) and the LBBB-like morphology of the ectopic beats. "Compensatory-like pauses" follow the VPCs.

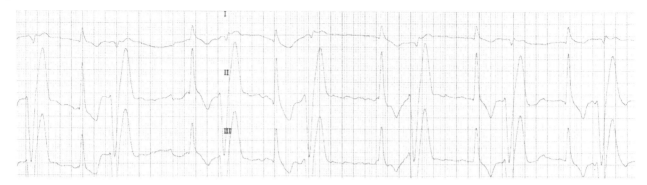

Figure 24.29 Paper speed 50 mm/s, 1 cm/mV, leads I, II, III, canine. **Atrial fibrillation, ventricular bigeminy**. Note the absence of P waves and irregular supraventricular rhythm. Every other beat is a VPC, creating "compensatory-like pauses," which create long-short sequences favorable for reentry. Note the constant coupling intervals.

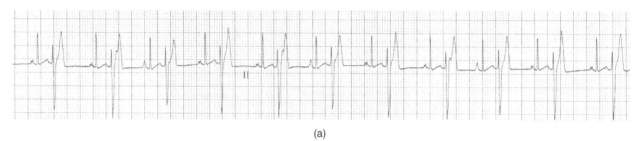

(a)

Figure 24.30a Paper speed 25 mm/s, 1 cm/mV, lead II, canine. **Ventricular bigeminy (1 : 1 extrasystole)** with **1 : 2 ectopic atrial rhythm**. In this case, one sinus beat is followed by a VPC, then an ectopic atrial (escape) beat is followed by a VPC, then another ectopic atrial beat is followed by a VPC. The sinus P waves are taller, and the ectopic atrial P′ waves are wider and notched. Then the sequence repeats itself.

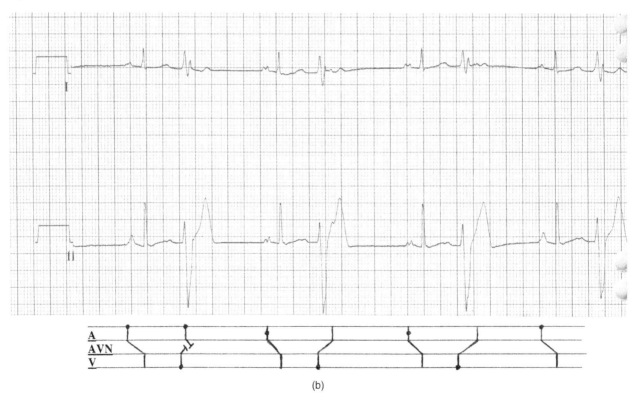

(b)

Figure 24.30b Paper speed 50 mm/s, 1 cm/mV, leads I and II, same dog. The above rhythm may be explained by **VA conduction with retrograde Wenckebach periodicity (3 : 2 VA conduction)**. When the VPC follows a sinus beat, it fails to conduct to the atria, but prevents conduction of the sinus beat. An ectopic atrial focus then captures, but then is followed by another VPC that does conduct to the atria retrogradely. The next VPC has a longer VA conduction interval, and the next VPC blocks. The retrograde P waves following the second and third VPCs are most evident in lead I. The first and fourth VPCs have retrograde conduction block.

Ventricular trigeminy

It occurs when a premature beat occurs following every second sinus beat due to 2 : 1 extrasystole (i.e. sinus beat, sinus beat, VPC, sinus beat, sinus beat, VPC, etc.). Ventricular trigeminy due to 1 : 2 extrasystole (i.e. sinus beat, couplet of VPCs, sinus beat, couplet of VPCs, etc.) can also occur and is more likely to result in VT.

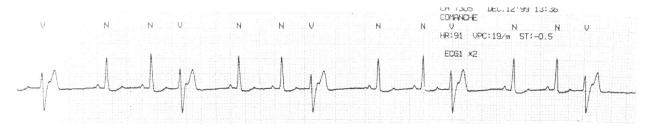

Figure 24.31 Paper speed 25 mm/s, 1 cm/mV, canine, lead II, **ventricular trigeminy (2 : 1 extrasystole)**, every third complex is a LVPC. Each VPC is followed by a compensatory pause.

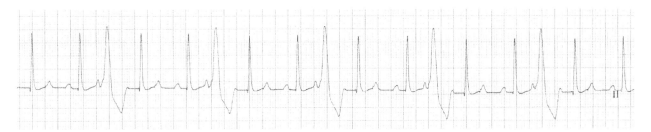

Figure 24.32 Paper speed 50 mm/s, 1 cm/mV, lead II, canine. **Interpolated ventricular trigeminy (2 : 1 extrasystole)**. Post-extrasystolic P-R interval prolongation occurs on the sinus beats following the VPCs from concealed retrograde conduction from the ventricular beats.

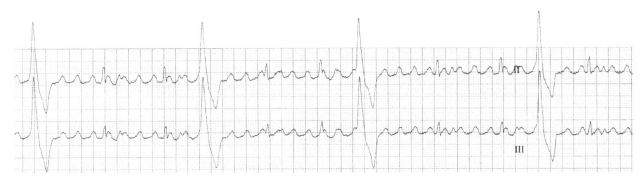

Figure 24.33 Paper speed 50 mm/s, 1 cm/mV, leads II and III, canine. **Atrial flutter, ventricular trigeminy (2 : 1 extrasystole)**. Note the regularly undulating baseline (atrial rate approximately 420 bpm) with irregular F-R intervals consistent with Type II (Atypical) atrial flutter. Every second conducted beat is followed by a VPC and a "compensatory-like" pause follows each.

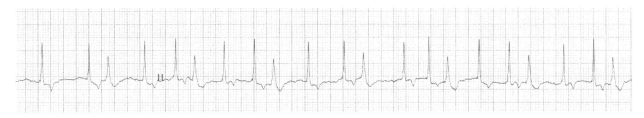

Figure 24.34 Paper speed 25 mm/s, 1 cm/mV, canine, lead II. **Atrial fibrillation, ventricular trigeminy (2 : 1 extrasystole)**. Note the irregularly irregular supraventricular rhythm, the constant coupling intervals of the VPCs, and the "compensatory-like" pauses following the VPCs.

Ventricular quadrigeminy It occurs when every fourth complex is premature if due to 3:1 extrasystole and is often a sign of concealed ventricular bigeminy. A quadrigeminal rhythm may also occur with 1:3 extrasystole, 2:2 extrasystole, or double bigeminy. Pentageminal rhythms (also known as quintageminy, 4:1 extrasystole or any number of variations, i.e. alternating bigeminy/trigeminy, etc.), and hexageminal (5:1 extrasystole) rhythms may also occur.

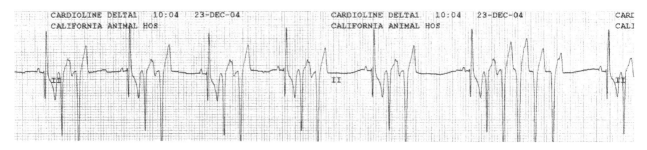

Figure 24.35 Paper speed 25 mm/s, 1 cm/mV, lead II, canine. **Ventricular trigeminy (1:2 extrasystole)** occurs before a run of non-sustained VT.

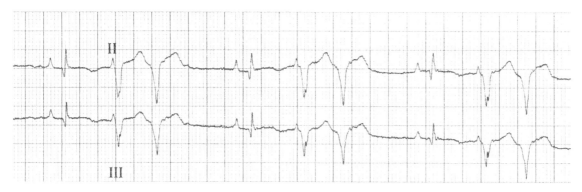

Figure 24.36 Paper speed 50 mm/s, 1 cm/mV, leads II and III, feline. **Ventricular trigeminy (1:2 extrasystole)**. This patient had a history of sustained VT and was being treated with procainamide.

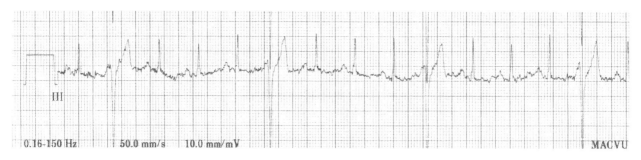

Figure 24.37 Paper speed 50 mm/s, 1 cm/mV, lead III, canine, **ventricular quadrigeminy (3:1 extrasystole)**. Every fourth complex is a VPC.

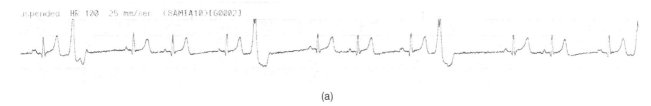

(a)

Figure 24.38a Paper speed 25 mm/s, 1 cm/mV, lead II, canine. **Ventricular quadrigeminy (3:1 extrasystole)**, possibly secondary to concealed bigeminy (odd numbers of interectopic beats, see below). However, the VPCs appear after a pause in the sinus rhythm (long-short sequence) in accordance with the **Rule of bigeminy**.

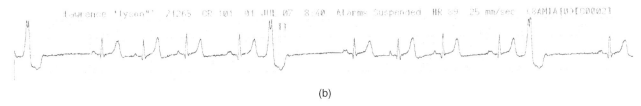

(b)

Figure 24.38b Paper speed 25 mm/s, 1 cm/mV, lead II, same dog. **Ventricular pentageminy (4 : 1 extrasystole)**. While possibly secondary to concealed bigeminy (even variant), the VPCs again appear to be coupled to late atrial escape beats that follow pauses.

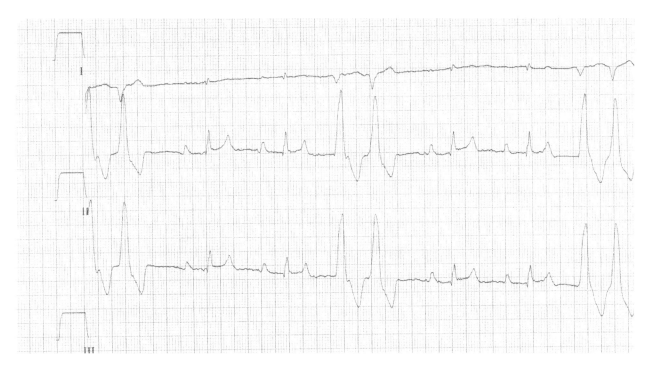

Figure 24.39 Paper speed 50 mm/s, leads I, II, III, Boxer. **Ventricular 2 : 2 extrasystole**. This creates a quadrigeminal rhythm (two sinus beats followed by two VPCs). Note the LBBB morphology of the VPCs typical of that seen in Boxers. First degree atrioventricular block is present on the sinus beats (P-Ri of 0.18 second). This patient was taking sotalol for ventricular tachycardia, and first degree AVB is a common side effect.

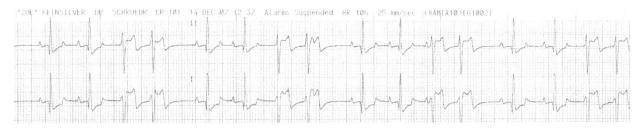

Figure 24.40 Paper speed 25 mm/s, 1 cm/mV, leads I and II, canine. **Ventricular 2 : 2 extrasystole**. A persistent ventricular quadrigeminy is present and each sequence consists of two sinus beats followed by a couplet of VPCs. Ventriculoatrial conduction (possibly retrograde VA Wenckebach with progressive R-P′ interval prolongation) is evident in the S-T segments of the VPCs.

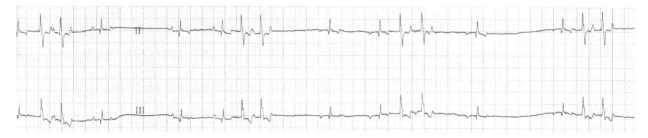

Figure 24.41 Paper speed 25 mm/s, 1 cm/mV, leads II and III, Boxer treated with procainamide. **Ventricular 2 : 2 extrasystole**. The first two beats are a couplet of VPCs. Three sinus beats intervene before another couplet of VPCs. A longer pause occurs after the second couplet, and two ectopic atrial escape beats (note the negative P′ waves) are seen before another couplet of VPC which are followed by another two ectopic atrial beats followed by a couplet of VPCs (2 : 2 extrasystole pattern).

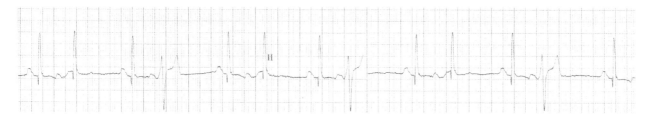

Figure 24.42 Paper speed 50 mm/s, 1 cm/mV, lead II, canine. **Double bigeminy**. In this variation, sinus beats are followed by junctional premature beats alternating with VPBs, creating a quadrigeminal rhythm (sinus-JPC-sinus-VPC repeating sequences). The JPCs have retrograde P′ waves preceding the supraventricular QRS complexes and reset the sinus node. The VPCs are wide and bizarre and create compensatory pauses. Technically, this could be considered a double *trigeminal* rhythm since the premature beats follow three preceding beats (in the case of the VPCs, one VPC follows a sinus-JPC-sinus sequence, and in the case of the JPCs, one JPC follows a sinus-VPC-sinus sequence).

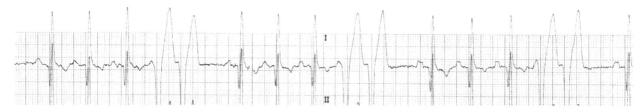

Figure 24.43 Paper speed 50 mm/s, 1 cm/mV, lead I, canine. Ventricular **pentageminy, 3 : 2 extrasystole**. Three sinus beats are followed by couplets of VPCs in a repeating pattern.

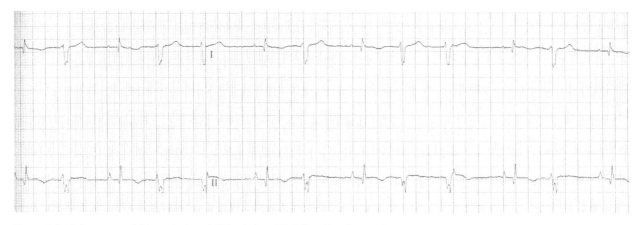

Figure 24.44 Paper speed 25 mm/s, 1 cm/mV, leads I and II, feline. Ventricular bigeminy alternating with trigeminy. There is **1 : 1 extrasystole** alternating with **1 : 2 extrasystole**, creating a **pentageminal** rhythm (sinus-VPC-sinus-VPC-VPC repeating sequence).

Concealed conduction Aside from compensatory pause and interpolation, VPCs may also show additional signs of concealed conduction. Occasionally, bigeminal and trigeminal VPCs may be intermittently concealed on surface EKG. This means the ectopic ventricular focus discharges but fails to fully propagate and capture the ventricles (and atria) secondary to exit block ("non-conducted VPCs"). Clues to the presence of concealed VPCs include periods of sinus rhythm between runs of ventricular bigeminy/trigeminy with arithmetic relationships and unexpected P-R interval prolongation of sinus beats. Verification requires intracardiac EKG.

Concealed ventricular bigeminy During ventricular bigeminy, stretches of intervening sinus rhythm may display primarily odd numbers (S = # of intervening sinus beats = $2n-1$). This is suggestive that the ventricular focus

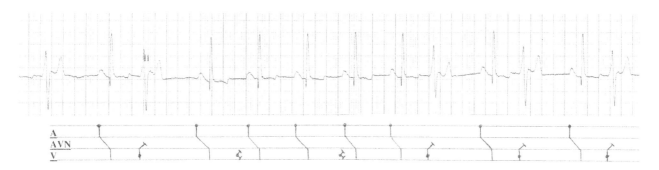

Figure 24.45 Paper speed 50 mm/s, 1 cm/mV, lead II, canine. **Concealed ventricular bigeminy**. This patient had persistent ventricular bigeminy with runs of predominantly odd numbers of intervening sinus complexes. In this case, five sinus beats are seen between runs of ventricular bigeminy. A ladder diagram illustrates where non-conducted VPCs likely occur. Coupling intervals appear to be constant, so the exit block is apparently of the **Mobitz variety.**

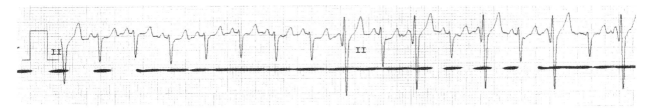

Figure 24.46 Paper speed 50 mm/s, 1 cm/mV, lead II, canine. **Concealed ventricular bigeminy**. R axis deviation is present in sinus rhythm, giving rise to the deep S waves. An odd number (in this case, seven) of intervening sinus complexes occur between bigeminal runs.

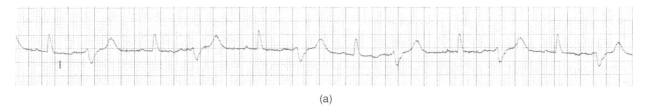

(a)

Figure 24.47a Paper speed 50 mm/s, 1 cm/mV, lead I, feline. Ventricular bigeminy. Every other beat is a VPC.

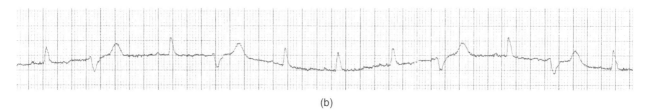

(b)

Figure 24.47b Paper speed 50 mm/s, 1 cm/mV, lead I, same cat. **Concealed ventricular bigeminy**. Here, an odd number (three) sinus beats intervene between runs of ventricular bigeminy. The coupling intervals appear to slightly lengthen prior to failure of the next VPC to appear (expected following beat #5) suggesting the exit block is of **Wenckebach variety**.

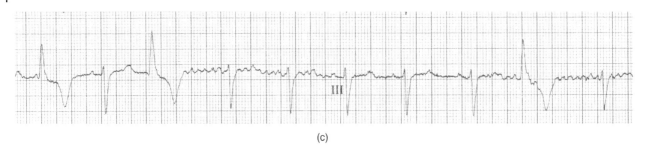

(c)

Figure 24.47c Paper speed 50 mm/s, 1 cm/mV, lead III, same cat. Concealed ventricular bigeminy. An odd number (five) of intervening sinus beats occur between runs of ventricular bigeminy. Purring artifact is seen intermittently on the baseline.

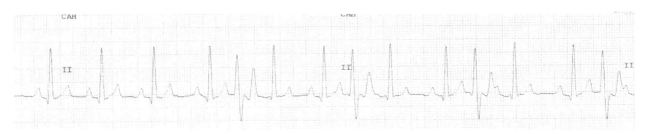

Figure 24.48 Paper speed 50 mm/s, 1 cm/mV, lead II, canine. **Concealed interpolated bigeminy** is suggested here because an even number (here two) of sinus beats intervene between interpolated VPCs.

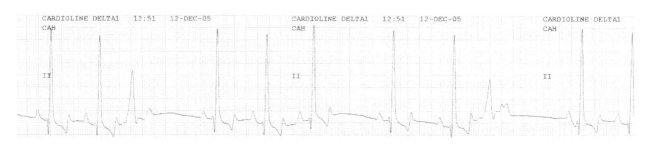

Figure 24.49 Paper speed 50 mm/s, 1 cm/mV, lead II, canine. **Concealed ventricular trigeminy** is suggested here because the number or interectopic beats is a multiple of three minus one ($6 - 1 = 5$), and most of the time this patient had ventricular trigeminy.

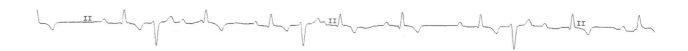

Figure 24.50 Paper speed 50 mm/s, 1 cm/mV, lead II, canine. **Concealed interpolated trigeminy**. A multiple of three (here, three) sinus beats intervene between interpolated VPCs. Careful examination of beat #8 shows that it has unexplained **P-R interval prolongation**. A concealed VPC likely occurred just before this beat, partially penetrated the AVN, making it partially refractory, causing conduction delay of the sinus beat. P-R interval prolongation is obvious on the post-extrasystolic sinus beats as well.

is concealed during these periods. Even numbered variants ($S = 2n$) have been described as well. Exit block from the ventricular focus intermittently prevents propagation of the VPCs.

Concealed interpolated ventricular bigeminy It is suggested when the number of intervening sinus beats between VPCs is even ($S = 2n$).

Concealed ventricular trigeminy It is suggested when the number of intervening sinus beats between VPCs is a multiple of three minus one ($S = 3n - 1$). Variants with $S = 3n$ or $3n - 2$ have been described.

Concealed interpolated ventricular trigeminy It is suggested when the number of intervening sinus beats between VPCs is a multiple of three ($S = 3n$).

Many other variants of concealed VPCs have been described in the human literature. The idea is that if the intervening number of sinus complexes between runs of trigeminal, quadrigeminal, etc., rhythms conforms to a simple equation, it is statistically highly suggestive of concealed beats.

Concealed quadrigeminy ($S = 4n - 1$, interpolated quadrigeminy $S = 4n$ or $4 - 2$)

Concealed pentageminy/quintageminy ($S = 5n - 1$ or $5n - 2$)

Concealed hexageminy ($S = 6n - 1$)

Ventricular fusion complexes
Also known as "Dressler beats" occur when the QRS complex is intermediate in waveform between that of the normally conducted sinus complexes and the wide and bizarre morphology of VPCs. This means a portion of the ventricles is activated over the normal His-Purkinje system and a portion of the ventricles is activated by the ventricular focus. Typically, a sinus P wave precedes the fusion QRS with a normal to short P-R' interval, and the resultant early QRS is usually narrower than the other VPCs, not as narrow as the supraventricular QRS complexes, clearly abnormal in morphology and is "on time" (meaning neither premature nor late). The longer/more normal the P-R' interval is, the more supraventricular in appearance the fusion complex will be, and the shorter the P-R' interval is, a more ventricular/ aberrant morphology will result. This is from the relative contribution of the supraventricular and ventricular foci. Ventricular fusion complexes may also arise from ventricular escape beats fusing with sinus beats during sinus pause/arrest or during incomplete (second degree) atrioventricular block.

Ventricular pre-excitation (Kent bundle type) produces a special kind of fusion complex, which is characterized by a short P-R interval and a widened QRS complex due to the presence of a delta wave (see Chapter 16). While most of the time ventricular fusion indicates ventricular ectopy, rarely, a supraventricular premature beat can fuse with a sinus beat if an accessory pathway is present (i.e. a junctional premature beat conducting down the His-Purkinje system fusing with a sinus beat conducting solely across the accessory pathway). This is an exception, in which supraventricular ectopy can result in ventricular fusion in the presence of anterograde conduction over an accessory pathway.

Ventricular fusions may result in better than expected ventricular conduction. If the patient's usual supraventricular QRS is prolonged from pre-existing complete BBB, ventricular enlargement, or ventricular pre-excitation, fusion with a VPC (or accelerated ventricular ectopic or ventricular escape) from the blocked/enlarged/pre-excited ventricle can transiently normalize the QRS duration. Schamroth famously remarked "*two wrongs can sometimes make a right*." Fusion of a VPC with a supraventricular

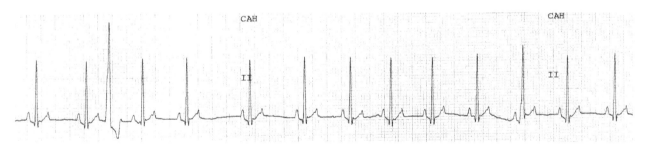

Figure 24.51 Paper speed 25 mm/s, 1 cm/mV, lead II, canine. The third complex is an interpolated VPC. Note post-extrasystolic P-Ri prolongation from concealed conduction. The 12th complex is a ventricular **fusion beat**.

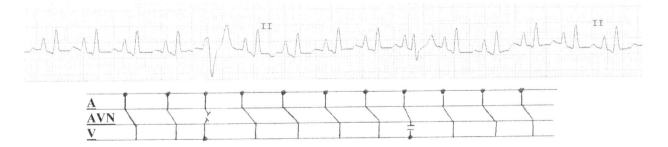

Figure 24.52 Paper speed 50 mm/s, 1 cm/mV, lead II, feline. The fourth complex is a LVPC and the ninth complex is a ventricular **fusion complex**.

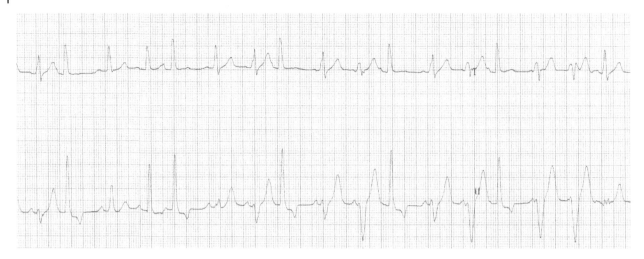

Figure 24.53 Paper speed 50 mm/s, 1 cm/mV, leads I and II, canine. This dog had many complex arrhythmias including SVT, VT, double tachycardia, SVPCs, and VPCs. **Ventricular trigeminy (1 : 2 extrasystole)** with **variable ventricular fusion** creates an interesting appearance to the groups. The 1st, 3rd, 6th, 7th, 9th, 10th, 12th, 13th, and 17th beats are ventricular fusions. The 4th beat is sinus, and the 2nd, 5th, 8th, 11th, and 14th beats are SVPCs. The 15th and 16th beats are of pure ventricular origin.

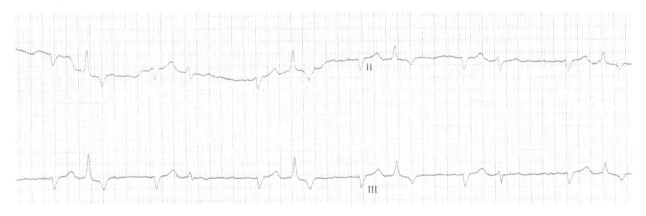

Figure 24.54 Paper speed 50 mm/s, 1 cm/mV, leads II and III, feline. **Atrial fibrillation, RBBB of the QRS, ventricular bigeminy secondary to RVPCs, ventricular fusion with normalization of the QRS**. No P waves are visible, and the interval from the premature beats to supraventricular capture is irregularly irregular, consistent with atrial fibrillation. The first beat in each pairing is prolonged from underlying RBBB. The premature beats are from the same ventricle and are conducted with a LBBB-like morphology. The 4th and 10th complexes are premature, but are narrowed, consistent with ventricular fusions. The complex is a fusion of a supraventricular impulse conducting normally down the LBB and an ectopic ventricular impulse originating in the right ventricle. Technically, it may be more appropriate to refer to the VPCs as "ventricular ectopics" given that the notion of "prematurity" during an irregularly irregular ventricular rhythm that characterizes atrial fibrillation is tenuous.

premature complex (simultaneous VPC and SVPC) simulates an SVPC with aberrancy, may occur in the absence of an accessory pathway, and usually is followed by a non-compensatory pause as the SVPC resets the sinus node. This situation is suggested by the clear demonstration of SVPCs and VPCs in the same tracing.

Ventriculoatrial conduction and reciprocation

Ventricular arrhythmias may create ventriculoatrial association or ventriculoatrial conduction (VA association vs. AV association), where the ventricular beats fully penetrate the AVN to depolarize the atria retrogradely and thus suppress the sinus node (causing resetting of the sinus node or a "non-compensatory pause"). This is in contrast to the usual situation, where ventricular arrhythmias are characterized by AV dissociation, despite partial penetration of the AVN. Retrograde P′ waves if seen, always follow the ectopic QRS and may be hidden in the T waves of the ventricular beats. Ventriculoatrial conduction results in less than fully compensatory pauses as the prevailing sinus rhythm is usually reset by the retrograde P′ wave that follows these VPCs. Ventricular premature complexes occurring during junctional rhythm commonly reset the junctional focus as well.

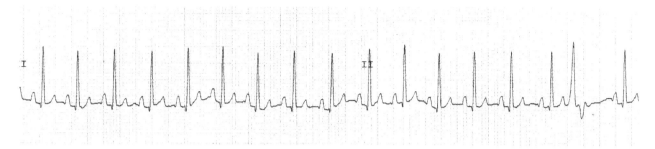

Figure 24.55 Paper speed 25 mm/s, 1 cm/mV, lead II, canine. **Ventriculoatrial conduction**. The 16th complex is a RVPC that is immediately followed by a *negative* P wave. This indicates the impulse completely penetrated the AVN to depolarize the atria retrogradely. The sinus node is then reset by the retrograde P wave.

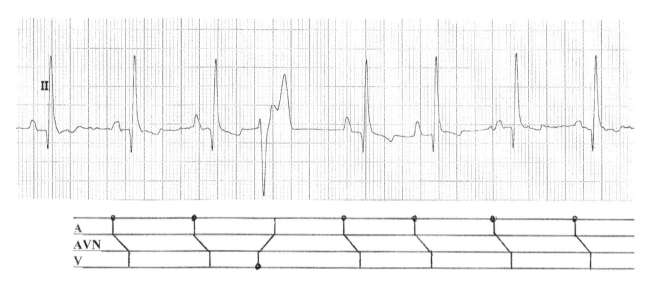

Figure 24.56 Paper speed 50 mm/s, 1 cm/mV, lead II, canine. A VPC follows the third complex and is followed by a less than fully compensatory pause (non-compensatory pause). This indicates resetting of the sinus node and implies **ventriculoatrial conduction** by the VPC. The ladder diagram illustrates the mechanism. The P'-P interval is equal to the P-Pi and the R-Ri encompassing the VPC is less than two R-R intervals.

Ventricular reciprocal complexes are possible with ventricular beats if reentry occurs in the AV node. These post-extrasystolic beats are reentrant/reciprocal complexes, "echoes," or return extrasystoles. The sequence is V-A-V. VA conduction not only permits ventricular reentry but also atrial fusion. Differentiating a reentrant/reciprocal beat following a VPC from a sinus capture following an interpolated VPC may be challenging. Typically, reciprocal beats are preceded by a negative P' wave. Given that the P wave polarity/morphology can be unreliable when the P wave occurs during the S-T segment of the preceding complex, this presents some problems for the examiner. If the P wave of the post-extrasystolic beat is clearly positive, occurs at the expected time (i.e. the P-P interval containing the VPC equals the normal P-P interval), is of normal configuration as the prevailing sinus P wave, and the P-R interval on the post-extrasystolic beat is prolonged (functional first degree AVB of the post-extrasystolic beat from

concealed conduction), then interpolation of the VPC is favored. This makes the R-R interval containing the VPC slightly longer than the normal R-R interval. If the P wave of the post-extrasystolic beat is clearly retrograde in the inferior leads, and the interval from the pre-extrasystolic beat to the post-extrasystolic beat is normal to less than one R-R or P-P interval, then ventricular reentry (reciprocation, ventricular echo) is favored. Subatrial reentry (VA block) is also possible and a negative P' wave and resetting of the SA node may not appear, but the supraventricular QRS of the ventricular reentry will. Usually the reciprocal complex will have a narrow supraventricular QRS unless pre-existent BBB or post-extrasystolic aberrancy develops.

Concealed reentry may be suspected on surface EKG during AF when VPCs are followed by particularly closely coupled supraventricular beats, which could represent ventricular echo or reciprocal beats. Definitive differentiation between a supraventricular capture following an

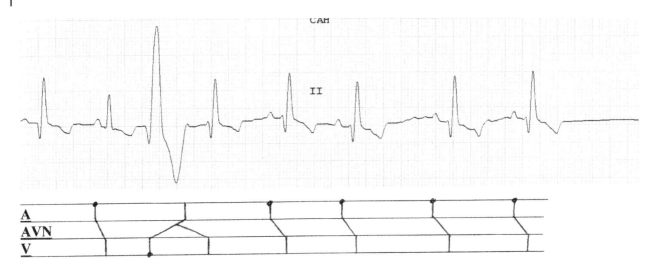

Figure 24.57 Paper speed 50 mm/s, 1 cm/mV, lead II, canine. V-A-V conduction is illustrated with a ladder diagram. The third complex is a RVPC and is followed by a *reciprocal* beat, resulting in pseudo-interpolation of the VPC. Note that the sinus to post-extrasystolic beat interval (the R-R interval containing the VPC) is shorter than the preceding R-R interval, making the beat following the VPC more likely a reciprocal complex (vs. a sinus-originating post-extrasystolic beat following an interpolated VPC). The retrograde P′ wave is visualized just following the T wave of the VPC. Furthermore, the sinus node is reset by the retrograde premature depolarization that follows the VPC.

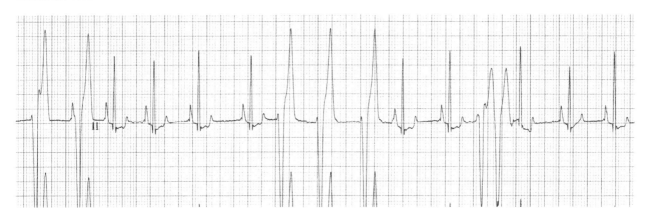

Figure 24.58 Paper speed 25 mm/s, 1 cm/mV, lead II, canine. Accelerated idioventricular rhythm appears intermittently in this patient with severe hemorrhagic gastroenteritis. The first two complexes are ventricular, followed by four of sinus origin, then three of ventricular origin. The couplet of VPCs is followed by a retrograde P wave, then a **reentrant** or "echo beat." The albeit irregular sinus rhythm is reset by the retrograde P wave. Note VA conduction with retrograde P′ waves in the S-T segments of the first and fifth VPCs.

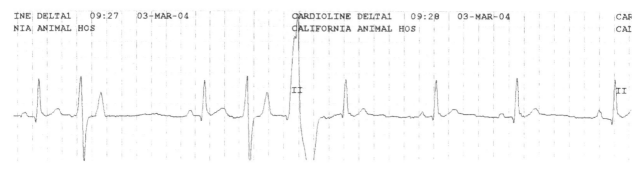

Figure 24.59 Paper speed 50 mm/s, 1 cm/mV, lead II, canine. The second complex is a LVPC followed by a compensatory pause. The fourth beat is a LVPC, is followed by a RVPC and then an "**echo beat**." The P wave of the sixth complex is negative and immediately follows the T wave of the RVPC. The negative P wave then conducts back to the ventricles through the AVN creating the normal supraventricular QRS of the sixth complex. Echo beats are also termed *reciprocal beats* or *reentrant* beats. This is an example of V-A-V conduction.

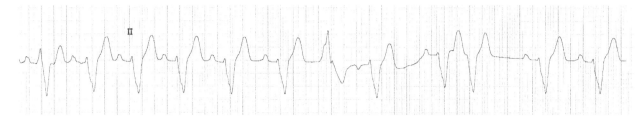

Figure 24.60 Paper speed 50 mm/s, 1 cm/mV, lead II, canine. Sinus rhythm with complete RBBB is interrupted by a VPC which is followed by a reentrant beat with RBBB. Note the retrograde P′ that follows the VPC (LBBB-like morphology). The 10th complex is a SVPC with an inapparent P′.

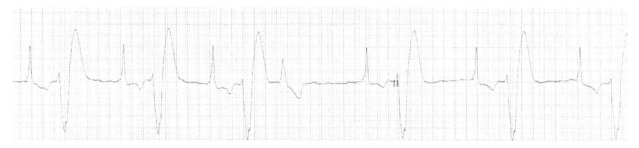

Figure 24.61 Paper speed 50 mm/s, 1 cm/mV, lead II, canine. **Atrial fibrillation, ventricular bigeminy, post-extrasystolic aberration**. The supraventricular rhythm is irregularly irregular. VPCs (RBBB morphology, likely left ventricular in origin) follow the supraventricular beats in a 1 : 1 extrasystole, and "**compensatory-like**" pauses follow the VPCs – except after the sixth complex. The seventh complex is of LBBB morphology and is likely supraventricular in origin. The sixth complex is an ***interpolated*** VPC, which causes post-extrasystolic LBBB aberration. Since the VPCs likely originate from the LV, a functional LBBB would be expected on a supraventricular stimulus occurring soon enough following the VPC. Alternatively, the seventh complex could represent a ***ventricular echo*** with LBBB aberration, though this is impossible to be certain of based on surface EKG.

"interpolated" VPC and a ventricular reentry following a VPC may be impossible on surface EKG during AF.

Atrial fusion

Atrial fusion may occur with supraventricular ectopy but can also occur with ventricular ectopy, provided intact VA conduction with retrograde activation of the atria (or portion of the atria, as is the case with atrial fusion) is present across the AV node. Ventricular fusion thus alters the morphology of the QRS complex while atrial fusion alters the morphology of the P wave.

> ***Take Home Message:*** One may get an *idea* if premature complexes that are otherwise ambiguous in waveform are supraventricular or ventricular depending on how they behave (i.e. if it resets or causes compensatory pauses). Of course, like everything in cardiology, the truth is more complicated. Due to the high frequency of sinus arrhythmia in the dog, intervals consistent with resetting or compensatory pause may be inexact resulting in non-compensatory pauses. Supraventricular premature beats may cause an apparent compensatory pause if they reset with a pause of certain duration so that the next sinus beat appears to be on time, and supraventricular complexes may rarely be interpolated from SAN entrance block. Similarly, VPCs may reset the sinus node if VA association is present and they

completely penetrate the AVN, retrogradely depolarize the atria and sinus node, with nonconduction of the retrograde P following the VPC or the production of a reentrant or echo beat (either of which will reset the SAN at a new interval, creating a non-compensatory pause). For these reasons, these described intervals can be unreliable; however, in most instances premature beats behave as described above, so these intervals remain useful.

Ventricular parasystole

Parasystole is another technically distinct form of dissociation that you may encounter. Literally, parasystole means "one heart that beats as two." The usual presentation of this is a normal sinus rhythm and a regular ectopic focus (i.e. a ventricular focus) that is spontaneously depolarized at an independent rate (uncoupled from the dominant rhythm). The two rhythms are not only independent of each other, but the ectopic focus is protected by entrance block, so that the underlying sinus rhythm never interrupts it. Atrial or junctional parasystole is quite rare and tricky to diagnose. In these cases, the supraventricular parasystolic focus resets the sinus rhythm, producing reverse coupling. Ventricular parasystole is more common and may be seen in Boxers with arrhythmogenic cardiomyopathy or in cases of hypothyroidism. Modulated parasystole is not uncommon

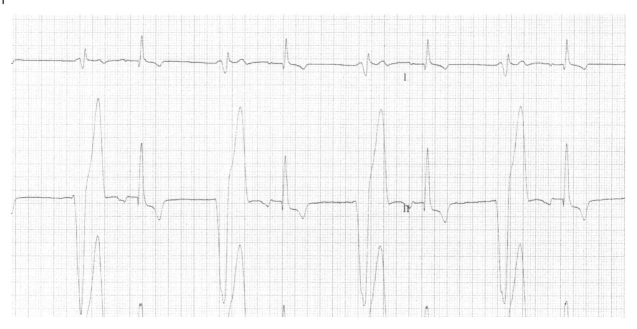

Figure 24.62 Paper speed 50 mm/s, 1 cm/mV, leads I and II, canine. **Accelerated ventricular rhythm and *reciprocal* bigeminy**. The sinus node is being suppressed by the ventricular beats, which have complete VA conduction and are each followed by a reciprocal complex in a bigeminal rhythm.

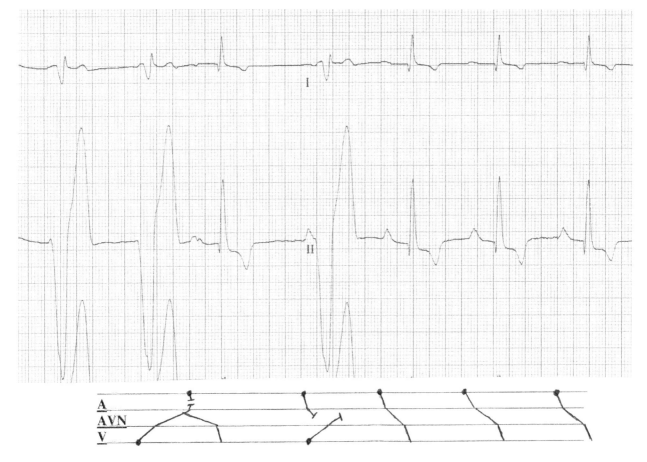

Figure 24.63 Paper speed 50 mm/s, 1 cm/mV, leads I and II, same dog. **Accelerated ventricular rhythm, ventriculoatrial conduction, reciprocation, and *atrial fusion***. Mild sinus arrhythmia is present. The second ventricular beat is followed by a complex with altered P wave morphology consistent with an atrial fusion, and a narrow QRS from ventricular reentry. Note that the P′ wave is intermediate in morphology between that of the retrograde P′ waves seen in the previous strip and the sinus P waves. This beat is followed by a VPC. Sinus rhythm ensues after the VPC.

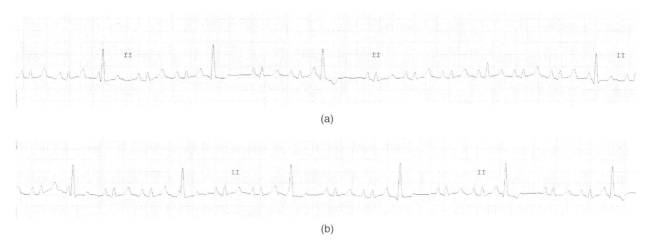

(a)

(b)

Figure 24.64 (a) Paper speed 50 mm/s, 1 cm/mV, lead II, feline. **Ventricular parasystole**. The coupling intervals between the normal and ectopic beats are variable, fusion complexes are present in the top strip (beats #13 and #16), and the interectopic intervals are all multiples of each other. The intervals between VPCs are as follows: 0.98, 0.98, 1.47, 0.98 seconds (implying the actual minimal interectopic interval is 0.49 second). (b) Paper speed 50 mm/s, 1 cm/mV, lead II, same cat. With 0.98 second between each VPC here, the interectopic intervals are constant, and there is obvious varied coupling with the sinus beats preceding the VPCs.

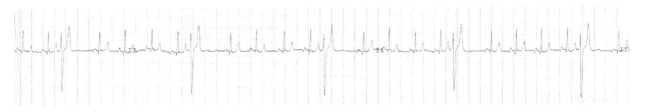

Figure 24.65 Paper speed 25 mm/s, 1 cm/mV, lead II, canine. **Ventricular pentageminy**. The left ventricular focus appears to be firing independently of the underlying sinus rhythm. This could be a parasystolic focus. However, the coupling intervals are suspiciously consistent.

and occurs when the prevailing supraventricular (usually sinus) rhythm has some effect on the parasystolic focus (despite its so-called "protection"). Multiple forms of modulated parasystole have been described and are beyond the scope of this text. There are four criteria for parasystole:

1) Coupling intervals between the normal and ectopic beats are variable.

2) Intervals that separate ectopic complexes are related to one another in a simple arithmetic relationship that is a multiple of the duration of the ectopic complexes.
3) Ventricular fusion complexes occur.
4) Parasystolic complexes appear when the heart is excitable (during pauses or slowing of the SAN, i.e. during carotid sinus massage).

Further reading

Chugh, S.N. (2012). *Textbook of Clinical Electrocardiography for Postgraduates, Residents and Practicing Physicians*, 3e. Jaypee Brothers Medical Publishers (P) Ltd.

Damato, A.N. and Lau, S.H. (1971). Concealed and supernormal atrioventricular conduction. *Circulation* XLIII: 967–970.

Denes, P. (1981). Bigeminy in ventricular interpolation. *Chest* 79: 343–345.

Ettinger, S.J. and Suter, P.F. (1970). *Canine Cardiology*. W.B. Saunders Company.

Fisch, C. and Knoebel, S.B. (2000). *Electrocardiography of Clinical Arrhythmias*. Futurama Publishing Co.

Goldberg, L.B., Levy, M.N., and Edelstein, J. (1975). The postponed compensatory pause as a manifestation of positive feedback in atrioventricular conduction. *Circulation* 52: 546–551.

Katz, L.N. and Pick, A. (1956). *Clinical Electrocardiography, Part I the Arrhythmias with an Atlas of Electrocardiograms*. Lea & Febiger.

Langendorf, R. and Pick, A. (1975). Concealed intraventricular conduction in the human heart. *Adv. Cardiol.* 14: 40–50.

Langendorf, R., Pick, A., and Winternitz, M. (1955). Mechanisms of intermittent ventricular bigeminy: I. appearance of ectopic beats dependent upon length of the ventricular cycle, the "rule of bigeminy". *Circulation* 11: 422–430.

Lerma, C. et al. (2007). The rule of bigeminy revisited: analysis in sudden cardiac death syndrome. *J. Electrocardiol.* 40: 78–88.

Mani, B.C. and Pavri, B.B. (2014). Dual atrioventricular nodal pathways physiology: a review of relevant anatomy, electrophysiology, and electrocardiographic manifestations. *Indian Pacing Electrophysiol. J.* 14 (1): 12–25.

Marriot, H.J.L. and Conover, M.B. (1998). *Advanced Concepts in Arrhythmias*, 3e. Mosby.

Marriott, H.J. (1998). *Pearls & Pitfalls in Electrocardiography, Pithy, Practical Pointers*, 2e. Williams & Wilkins.

Moulton, K.P., Medcalf, T., and Lazzara, R. (1990). Premature ventricular complex morphology: a marker for left ventricular structure and function. *Circulation* 81 (4): 1245–1251.

Pick, A. and Langendorf, R. (1979). *Interpretation of Complex Arrhythmias*. Lea & Febiger.

Santilli, R., Moïse, N.S., Pariaut, R., and Perego, M. (2018). *Electrocardiography of the Dog and Cat: Diagnosis of Arrhythmias*, 2e. Edna.

Schamroth, L. (1970). Reciprocal rhythm of ventricular origin during atrial fibrillation with complete AV block. *British Heart J.* 32: 564–567.

Scheinman, M., Thakur, R.K., and Natale, A. (eds.) (2016). *Cardiac Electrophysiology Clinics: Interpretation of Complex Arrhythmias: A Case-Based Approach*. Elsevier.

25

Ventricular Tachycardia, Flutter, and Fibrillation

CHAPTER MENU

Accelerated idioventricular rhythm, 319
   Atrioventricular dissociation, 321
   Ventriculoatrial association and ventriculoatrial block, 323
   Polymorphic and bidirectional AIVR, 325
Ventricular tachycardia, 328
   Left ventricular tachycardia, 331
      Fascicular VT, 333
      Bidirectional VT, 333
   Right ventricular tachycardia, 336
      Right ventricular outflow tract-VT, 336
   Bundle branch reentrant VT, 336
   Exit block, 338
   Double tachycardia, 340
   Polymorphic VT, 342
      Torsades de pointes, 342
Ventricular flutter, 342
Ventricular fibrillo-flutter/ventricular dissociation, 345
Ventricular fibrillation, 346

Accelerated idioventricular rhythm Ventricular rhythms that are faster than ventricular escape, but slower than classical ventricular tachycardia (HR approximately 40–180 bpm) are termed accelerated ventricular rhythms (AVR).

> *A Note*: Some authors prefer to reserve the term "accelerated" for those ectopic rhythms with rates strictly within 10% of the underlying sinus rate. Ectopic rhythms with a rate less than that (but faster than escape) may be referred to as "accelerated escape" and those faster than 10% of sinus, but less than 180–200 bpm to be "slow ventricular tachycardia." This terminology is not considered really helpful by this author given that the sinus nodal discharge has such a wide range of normal heart rates and the fact that sinus rhythm is not always present (i.e. atrial fibrillation, atrial standstill, ectopic atrial, or junctional rhythm).

Otherwise known as "non-paroxysmal ventricular tachycardia," AIVR is usually monomorphic and only rarely polymorphic, bidirectional, or associated with R on T phenomenon. The onset and offset of AIVR is often gradual and commonly associated with various degrees of ventricular fusion, occasionally confusing the examiner with multifocal ventricular arrhythmias.

> *Another Note*: So-called "non-paroxysmal ventricular tachycardia" is a historically used, poorly worded term and avoided here to avoid confusion and for the sake of simplicity. Most accelerated rhythms occur at a rate that is comparable to sinus rhythm. The onset and offset of these rhythms may not be obvious on physical examination since an abrupt "paroxysm" of overt tachycardia does not happen. These rhythms are not paroxysmal, nor do they constitute tachycardia per se.

Interpretation of the Electrocardiogram in Small Animals, First Edition. Nick A. Schroeder.
© 2021 John Wiley & Sons Inc. Published 2021 by John Wiley & Sons Inc.

The term accelerated idioventricular rhythm is used if atrioventricular dissociation (AVD) is present, and if ventriculoatrial (VA) association is present the term accelerated ventricular rhythm (AVR) is used. Most of these display AVD, and thus the prefix idio- is retained. Parasystolic AIVR is common and exposed if the prevailing supraventricular rhythm (typically sinus) fails to reset the parasystolic ventricular focus. Arguably the most overtreated arrhythmia in veterinary medicine, AIVR is quite common among patients that have gastric-dilitation volvulus (GDV), hemoabdomen from ruptured splenic or hepatic neoplasia (usually hemangiosarcoma), pericardial effusion (post-pericardiocentesis, usually secondary to ruptured right atrial mass/hemangiosarcoma), immune-mediated hemolytic anemia, or traumatic myocarditis (hit-by-car). Typically not associated with serious tachycardia or hemodynamic compromise, AIVR actually responds poorly to antiarrhythmic therapy for ventricular tachycardia (VT), is secondary to noncardiac issues, and often will resolve on its own following correction of the underlying disorder. Apparent treatment success may be wrongly attributed to medical intervention (i.e. with lidocaine) as the sinus node eventually starts taking over the rhythm. Importantly, the development of AIVR (or accelerated idiofascicular rhythm) during atrial fibrillation should alert the clinician to the possibility of digoxin toxicity.

Atrioventricular dissociation refers to the atria and the ventricle beating independently of one another. This is a broad category that involves multiple different EKG phenomena. This means that "AV dissociation" is not an electrocardiographic diagnosis, but a symptom of an underlying arrhythmic mechanism. Technically, VT, AIVR, AIJR (accelerated idiojunctional rhythm), block/acceleration dissociation, and third degree AVB all fall into this category. AVD is termed "incomplete" (aka "interference" AVD) if fusion complexes or capture beats occur. Remember, ventricular fusions do not interrupt the ventricular rhythm whereas capture beats do, provided the ectopic ventricular focus is not parasystolic. The AV node is thus capable of impulse transmission if it is not refractory. Prolonged AVD is said to be "apparently complete," as fusion/capture may not have a chance to occur for long periods. AVD is termed "complete" if no fusion complexes or capture beats occur, and so the AV node is incapable of impulse transmission (even if it is actually transected or not), which really only occurs in the setting of third degree AV block, when the AVD occurs by default.

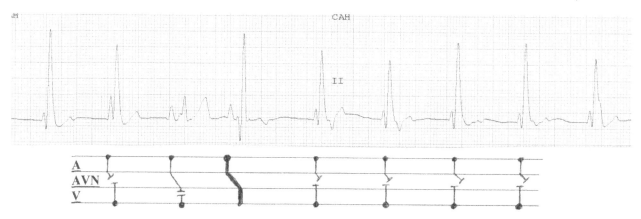

Figure 25.1 Paper speed 50 mm/s, 1 cm/mV, lead II, canine. **Accelerated idioventricular rhythm**. A ladder diagram illustrates AVD. The third complex is a **fusion beat** and the fourth complex is a **capture beat** (in bold).

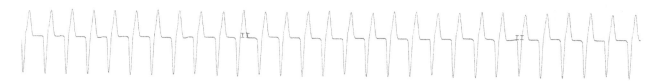

Figure 25.2 Paper speed 25 mm/s, 1 cm/mV, lead II, canine, **accelerated** *ventricular* **rhythm**. The ventricular rate is 166 bpm. P waves are not evident, but likely hiding within or just after the QRS complexes in the T waves. Since it cannot be *proven* here that AVD *is* present, this rhythm is more appropriately termed "accelerated *ventricular* rhythm (AVR)." **Ventriculoatrial conduction** very well may be present, and retrograde P′ waves could easily be hiding within the T waves. Approximately 50% of ventricular rhythms (AVR or VT) have VA conduction in people. Pulsed wave Doppler of the AV inflows via echocardiography could elucidate whether or not AVD is present. The ventricular complexes display a RBBB pattern consistent with an L ventricular focus.

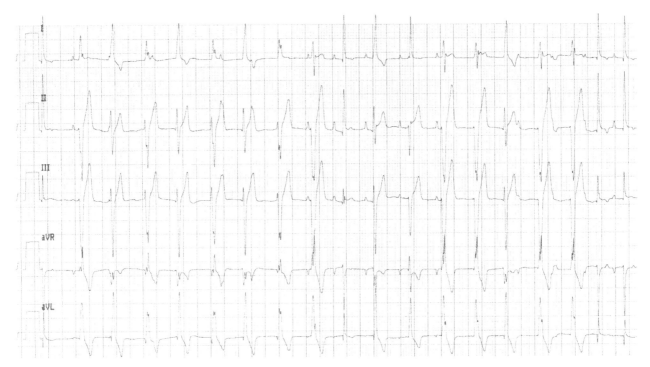

Figure 25.3 Paper speed 25 mm/s, 1 cm/mV, leads I, II, III, aVR, aVL, canine. **Parasystolic AIVR with fusion**. Sinus arrhythmia is present and the atrial rate is approximately 130 bpm. An accelerated and parasystolic idioventricular focus has captured the ventricles for the first half of the strip, and variable degrees of fusion cause an **electrical alternans** of the QRS complexes.

Atrioventricular dissociation AVD (the "proper" term) technically occurs when the ventricular rate *exceeds* the atrial rate. A rapid ventricular or junctional focus that takes control of the ventricles often results in AVD. Given that AVD encompasses other EKG phenomena (including atrioventricular block), this is more appropriately termed AV dissociation due to *usurpation,* and the sinus (atrial) rate is normal or fast, but still less than that of the ventricles. Examples include VT, automatic junctional tachycardia (AJT, a type of SVT), accelerated idioventricular rhythm (AIR/AIVR), and AIJR. Slowing of the sinus rate may result in AVD by default, and a junctional or ventricular escape rhythm may take over. An accelerated idiojunctional or idioventricular rhythm may also take over when the sinus rate is slow and a quite mild degree of AV block

is present, resulting in AVD (so-called block/acceleration dissociation). If you look carefully, P waves actually march through the QRS complexes most of the time during these arrhythmias. At high heart rates, it can often be difficult to see P waves. Running the strips at 50 mm/s can help uncover some of these P waves.

If the supraventricular (typically sinus) and idioventricular rates are quite similar, AVD is termed "isorhythmic dissociation." Isorhythmic dissociation secondary to AIVR with nearly identical sinus and idioventricular rates may lead to apparently complete AVD and long periods where the P waves appear before the idioventricular QRS complexes, resulting in a condition referred to as "synchrony." If the AVD is incomplete, the idioventricular rate is (usually) slightly faster than the sinus rate, and the P waves are

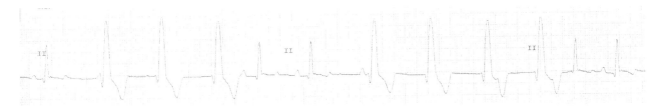

Figure 25.4 Paper speed 50 mm/s, 1 cm/mV, canine with right atrial hemangiosarcoma and pericardial effusion, **AIVR**. A right ventricular focus (LBBB pattern) captures the rhythm before the second sinus beat is conducted, resulting in an accelerated idioventricular rhythm. The fourth complex is a sinus **capture beat**, AIR resumes after the fifth beat, and the 11th beat is another capture (the P wave is hiding in the T wave of the last ventricular complex).

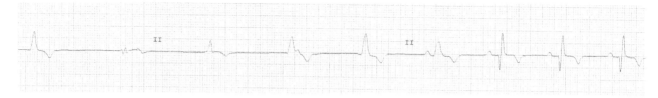

Figure 25.5 Paper speed 50 mm/s, 1 cm/mV, lead II, canine. An **idioventricular rhythm** has captured the ventricles and slowly speeds up before capture by the sinus node (beat #7). The variable morphologies of the ventricular beats are likely due to variable ventricular conduction from the same ectopic focus vs. multiple foci since the idioventricular rate is regular. The sixth complex is a **fusion beat**.

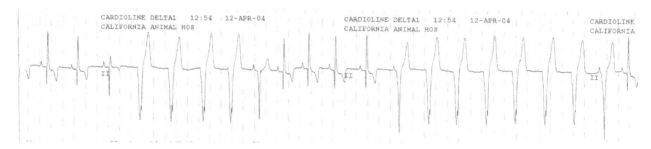

Figure 25.6 Paper speed 25 mm/s, 1 cm/mV, lead II, canine with IMHA. **AIVR.** A left ventricular focus captures the ventricles with the third complex (fusion beat). The resulting accelerated idioventricular rhythm is hemodynamically well-tolerated by the dog.

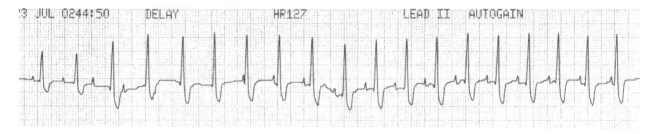

Figure 25.7 Paper speed 25 mm/s, 1 cm/mV, lead II, feline. **AIVR.** The ventricular rate is approximately 136 bpm, as is the atrial rate, technically making this an isorhythmic dissociation with accrochage. The P waves appear before the R ventricular complexes in most of the strip, which not only mimics a sinus rhythm, but may also lead to reasonably normal cardiac output since the atria contract just prior to the ventricles.

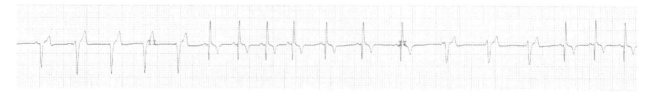

Figure 25.8 Paper speed 25 mm/s, 1 cm/mV, lead II, canine. **AIVR.** The idioventricular rhythm is interrupted by periods of sinus rhythm. This patient had a splenic infarction following a GDV/gastropexy. AIR is very common following GDV surgery, is typically well-tolerated by the patient, poorly responsive to antiarrhythmics and self-limiting. Persistent AIR and colic in this patient more than 72 hours postoperative indicated an unresolved problem. Timely splenectomy resulted in resolution of the arrhythmias.

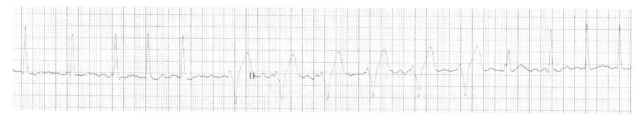

Figure 25.9 Paper speed 50 mm/s, 1 cm/mV, lead II, canine with CMVDz. **Atrial fibrillation and AIVR with fusion**. The baseline is undulating and devoid of P waves with an irregularly irregular rhythm and supraventricular QRS complexes consistent with atrial fibrillation. A pause after the fifth complex is followed by a monomorphic, accelerated idioventricular rhythm. Note the regular ventricular rate. The 12th complex is a fusion between a supraventricular impulse and an idioventricular beat, and thus has an intermediate QRS morphology.

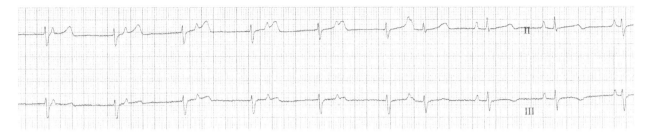

Figure 25.10 Paper speed 50 mm/s, 1 cm/mV, leads II and III, feline under anesthesia. **Sinus bradycardia**, **isorhythmic dissociation** ("**accrochage**") from **accelerated idioventricular rhythm**. Note the P waves slowly marching out from the idioventricular beats at the beginning of the strip until the sinus node is able to capture with the seventh complex. The 8th and 9th beats are sinus, and the 10th beat is a ventricular fusion. The sinus and idioventricular rates are similar (thus "isorhythmic dissociation"), leading to relatively long periods of AV dissociation. AVD was incomplete in this case, making this "accrochage."

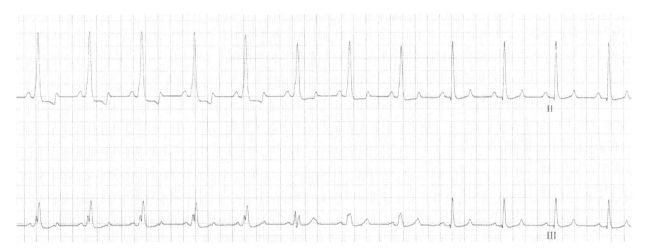

Figure 25.11 Paper speed 50 mm/s, 1 cm/mV, leads II and III, canine. **Isorhythmic dissociation** secondary to **accelerated idioventricular rhythm** with **ventricular fusion**. The sinus and ventricular rates are nearly identical. At the beginning of the strip, the P-R interval is short, and the slurred upstroke of the QRS mimicking a reversed version of the so-called "Concertina Effect" or gradual loss of *ventricular pre-excitation*. However, by the middle of the strip, the P-R intervals are lengthening and the QRS complexes normalize. The last four beats are of pure sinus origin, while the rest are ventricular fusions from an accelerated idioventricular rhythm. This is most obvious in lead III.

clearly marching into and out of the idioventricular QRS complexes, it is referred to as "accrochage" and tends to be short-lived. Isorhythmic dissociation may also occur during AIJRs with similar sinus rates, ventricular or junctional tachycardia with concurrent sinus tachycardia, or complete atrioventricular block with junctional or ventricular escape and sinus bradycardia.

Ventriculoatrial association and ventriculoatrial block
Sometimes (50% of the time) AVR or VT will result in VA conduction, resulting in P′ waves that follow the ventricular complexes, with subsequent suppression of the sinus nodal discharge (so not all AVR or ventricular tachycardias

have AVD). The impulse travels retrogradely through the AVN to excite the atria, and the P′ waves always follow the QRS with a concentric retrograde activation of the atria (P′ axis −80 to −100 degrees). The P′ waves are commonly lost in the S-T segment, manifest as a "pseudo-S wave," and multiple leads may need to be examined to uncover them. Not all ventricular impulses may penetrate the AV node, and the resultant ventriculoatrial block (VA block) may be of Type I (Wenckebach) or Type II (Mobitz) varieties. Type I VA block is manifested by gradual prolongation of the QRS-P′ interval prior to failure of conduction while Type II VA block is marked by random failure of conduction and constant QRS-P′ intervals. 2:1 VA block may be of either variety.

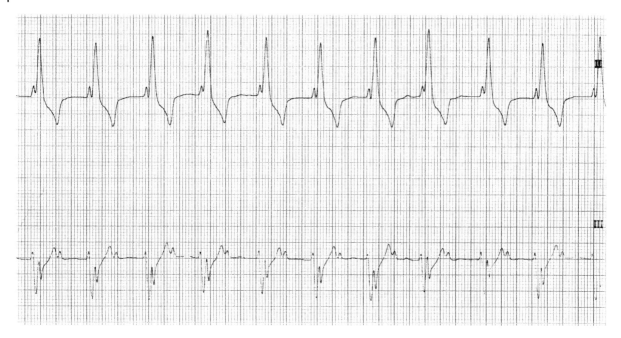

Figure 25.12 Paper speed 50 mm/s, 1 cm/mV, leads II and III, canine. **Accelerated ventricular rhythm with 1:1 VA conduction**. The ventricular rhythm is regular with a rate of 180 bpm (making this a borderline ventricular tachycardia) and retrograde P waves are visualized in III in the middle of the T waves (far less obvious in II).

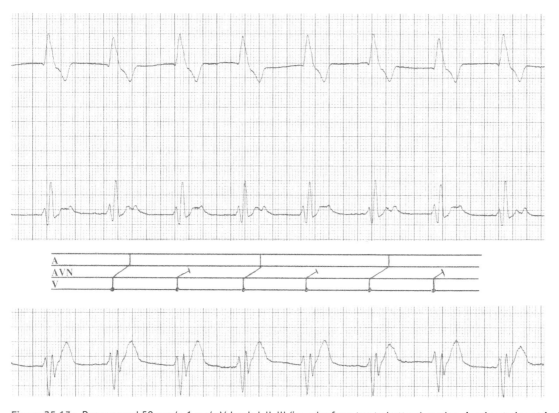

Figure 25.13a Paper speed 50 mm/s, 1 cm/mV, leads I, II, III (in order from top to bottom), canine. **Accelerated ventricular rhythm** with **2:1 VA conduction**. This patient was a post-op thorascopy for biopsies, confirmed malignant histiocytosis. The ventricular rate is approximately 140 bpm. No obviously *dissociated* P waves are seen. However, careful examination of lead II shows retrograde P' waves following every other QRS complex in the S-T segments. The QRS complexes are wide, bizarre, and have an atypical BBB pattern. Retrograde Wenckebach periodicity is possible with ventricular rhythms and VA conduction. The ladder diagram beneath lead II (in the middle) illustrates the mechanism. Since the sinus node is depolarized along with the atria, suppression of the SA nodal discharge occurs. Since VA association is present, and AV dissociation is not, this is properly termed accelerated *ventricular* rhythm (the modifier *idio-* is used only if AV dissociation occurs). Whether the VA block is *Type I (Wenckebach)* or *Type II (Mobitz)* is unclear given that successive VA conduction over more than one beat is absent.

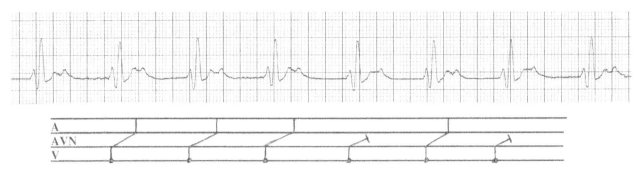

Figure 25.13b Paper speed 50 mm/s, 1 cm/mV, lead II, same dog. **AVR with VA conduction with retrograde Wenckebach periodicity**. Retrograde transmission of the ventricular impulse can gradually prolong (albeit subtly here) before failure of conduction to the atria.

Polymorphic and bidirectional AIVR Most of the time, AIVRs are monomorphic. Polymorphism is commonly mimicked by ventricular fusion at the onset and offset of AIVR. More than one morphology to the ectopic ventricular QRS, especially if the different morphologies are associated with differing rates, suggest polymorphic AIVR. Alternation of morphologies on a beat-to-beat basis produces a so-called bidirectional AIVR. This is frequently mimicked by an AIVR with VPCs in bigeminy. If the rate is lower than 180 bpm, but faster than ventricular escape, a bidirectional rhythm of ventricular origin termed accelerated bidirectional idioventricular rhythm (if AVD is present) is used. Bidirectional AIVR/VT should be distinguished from underlying ventricular rhythms (i.e. LVT, RVT, AIVR, etc.) with 1:1 extrasystole and VPCs from the opposite ventricle (ventricular bigeminy). The ventricular rhythm in bidirectional VT is regular, while AIR/VT with 1:1 ventricular extrasystole is bigeminal. Polymorphic and bidirectional AIVR may warrant antiarrhythmic therapy (sodium or potassium channel blockade) if hemodynamic compromise is evident (hypotension, collapse, etc.).

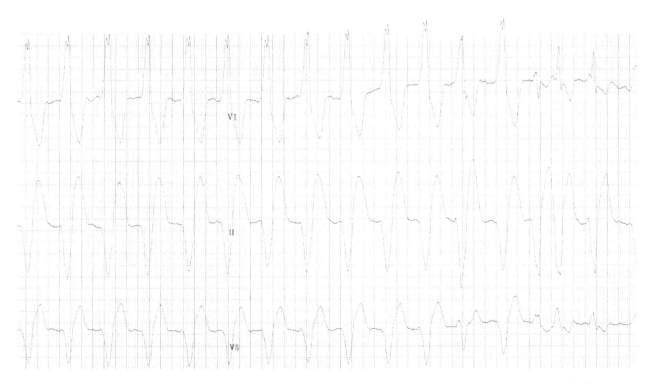

Figure 25.14a Paper speed 50 mm/s, 1 cm/mV, leads V1, II, and V5, canine treated with diltiazem and lidocaine. **Atrial fibrillation and polymorphic accelerated idioventricular rhythm/VT producing in AV dissociation**. The baseline is undulating, and no evidence of P waves (dissociated or not) are present. The rhythm is relatively monomorphic with an atypical RBBB pattern and extremely wide QRS complexes (making it more likely ventricular). Toward the end of the strip, polymorphic complexes occur at a faster and more irregular rhythm.

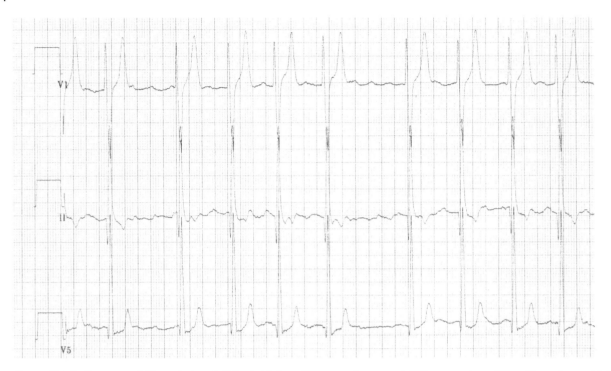

Figure 25.14b Paper speed 50 mm/s, 1 cm/mV, leads VI, II, and V5, same dog on oral diltiazem and mexilitine. The polymorphic VT has resolved completely. Atrial fibrillation with a slower ventricular rate response is present. The rhythm is irregularly irregular, and the QRS complexes are narrow and supraventricular.

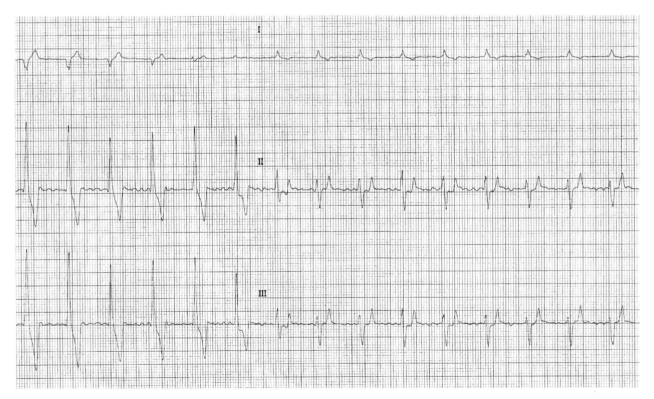

Figure 25.15a Paper speed 25 mm/s, 1 cm/mV, leads I, II, III, canine. Atrial fibrillation, apparently complete **AVD** secondary to usurpation by polymorphic AIVR. Note the QRS complexes occur at a regular rhythm indicative of AVD during AF. The complexes change morphology over a few beats.

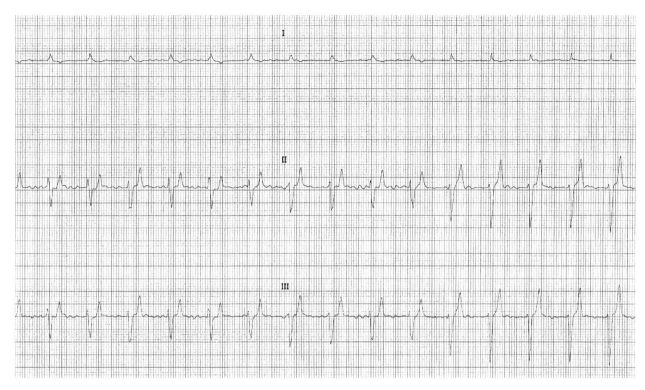

Figure 25.15b Paper speed 25 mm/s, 1 cm/mV, leads I, II, III, same dog. The ventricular focus again shifts morphology over a series of beats. Given that the rate does not change, this is consistent with a **unifocal AIVR**, albeit with exit changes resulting in polymorphism.

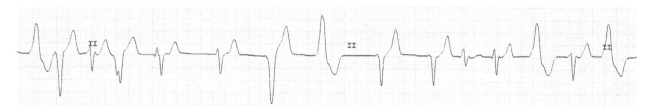

Figure 25.16 Paper speed 50 mm/s, 1 cm/mV, lead II. Canine. **Polymorphic accelerated idioventricular rhythm**. Atrial activity is uncertain, and the patient may be in atrial fibrillation with AVD and an irregular, polymorphic accelerated idioventricular rhythm has control of the ventricles. Ventriculoatrial conduction is not evident at least in this lead. The changing ventricular rates with changes in morphology are indicative of a **multifocal** ventricular arrhythmia.

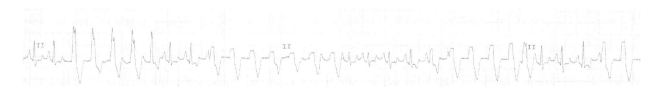

Figure 25.17 Paper speed 25 mm/s, 1 cm/mV, lead II, canine with DCM. **Accelerated idioventricular rhythm** with fusion and capture mimics the twisting around the baseline characteristic of torsade de pointes.

Ventricular tachycardia Tachycardias (usually around 180–250 bpm) arising in the ventricles are termed ventricular tachycardias. Ventricular tachycardia is defined as three or more successive ventricular beats at above 180 bpm. Ventricular tachycardia is usually characterized by AV dissociation (that is, you may see P waves wandering in and out of the complexes, but they can be tough to find at high HRs). Atrioventricular dissociation during VT is secondary to usurpation. If you see very wide/bizarre complexes that have an atypical BBB morphology, precordial concordance (the left chest leads with all positive or all negative complexes), or fusion and/or capture beats,

VT is usually the diagnosis. Capture beats may also be seen with second degree AVB and represent P waves followed by supraventricular QRS complexes – meaning the sinus node "captured" the ventricle. Occasionally (and up to 50% of the time in humans), VT will have ventriculoatrial conduction (VA conduction or VA association) with resultant suppression of the SA nodal discharge. Retrograde P′ waves may or may not be seen following the QRS complexes, and retrograde Wenckebach periodicity or 2:1 VA conduction may occur. If VT has an irregular rhythm, exit block from a unifocal VT or multifocal VT is a possibility. The atrial rhythm may be uncertain

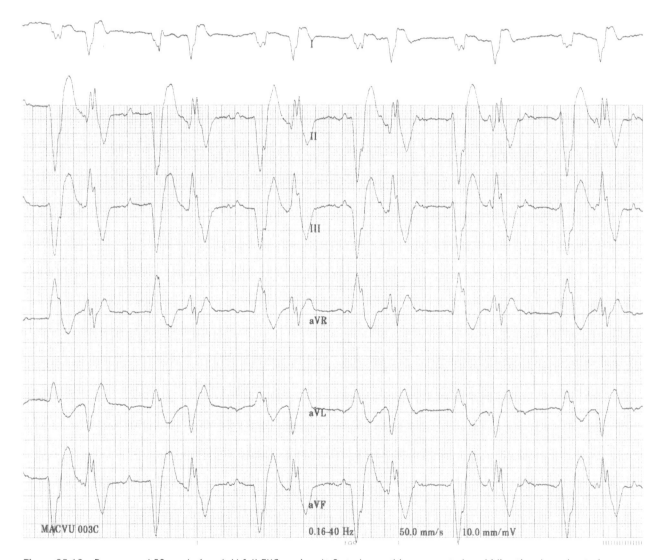

Figure 25.18a Paper speed 50 mm/s, 1 cm/mV, full EKG, canine. At first glance, this appears to be a bidirectional accelerated idioventricular rhythm. The heart rate is approximately 160 bpm. Usually, bidirectional VTs have constant R-R intervals. Here, the R-R intervals alternate, suggesting coupling of complexes, and bigeminy secondary to re-entry. Here, an underlying ventricular rhythm is present with RBBB-like morphology where every-other-beat is premature, and of LBBB-like morphology. Atrioventricular dissociation throughout suggests a ventricular origin; however, a junctional focus (with alternating aberrancy and block) or re-entry with aberrancy (V-A-V reciprocal beats with LBBB aberrancy) are possibilities. An alternate, and perhaps more appropriate term for this strip given the bigeminal rhythm could be **accelerated idioventricular rhythm with ventricular bigeminy**.

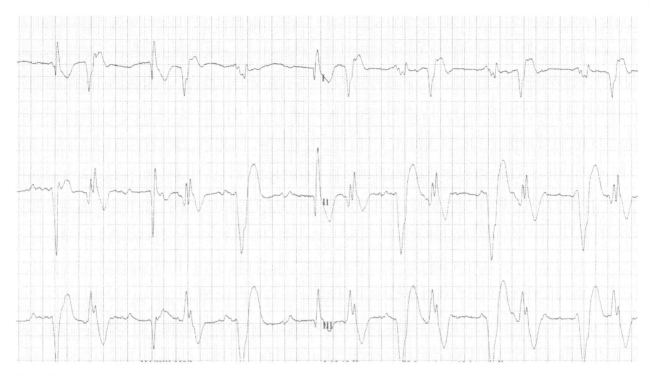

Figure 25.18b Paper speed 50 mm/s, 1 cm/mV, leads I, II, III, same dog. **AIVR/ventricular bigeminy** with **ventricular fusion**. The first and third complexes are ventricular fusions. The sixth complex is of pure sinus origin. This patient had an exceptionally long P-Ri and was being treated with digoxin. The presence of ventricular fusion argues for a ventricular origin of the ectopic rhythm. The appearance of accelerated idioventricular rhythm should lead the clinician to be suspicious of digitalis intoxication.

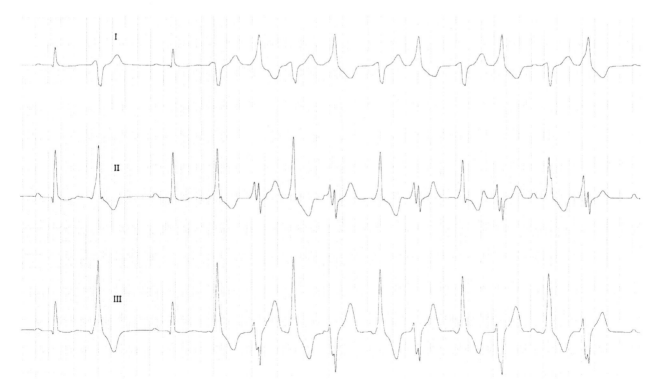

Figure 25.19 Paper speed 50 mm/s, 1 cm/mV, leads I, II, III, canine. **Bidirectional AIVR**. Ventricular premature beats in bigeminy initiates a non-sustained and bidirectional AIVR. Note the alternating axes and regular ventricular rhythm (vs. bigeminal) consistent with a single ventricular focus with alteration of morphology on a beat-to-beat basis.

during sustained VT, especially if the ventricular rate is rapid. Atrioventricular dissociation or VA conduction may not be obvious, even if multiple leads are evaluated. Rule outs for wide-complex tachycardias (WCTs) include aberrantly conducted (i.e. with BBB) SVT or AF, which, by the way, are generally uncommon (see Chapter 8). Ventricular tachycardia originating from a septal, fascicular focus, or bundle-branch re-entry will produce narrow QRS tachycardias since both ventricles are activated nearly simultaneously. If untreated, sustained VT can progress to VF and sudden cardiac death (SCD). This is an arrhythmia that had better make the clinician run for the lidocaine (procainamide is a backup) or think about starting mexilitine or sotalol. Amiodarone may be considered in refractory cases. The rhythm of monomorphic VT is usually absolutely regular! The pulses usually are inappropriately weak, however. Criteria for the treatment of VT include four things the clinician needs to know:

1) **RATE**: VT above 170–180 bpm.

2) **MULTIFORME**: or multifocal, thought to signify a more electrically unstable myocardium.

3) **R on T PHENOMENON**: when the R wave comes "on" the T wave (technically just after the peak) of the preceding complex – represents ectopic foci beginning when the myocardium has not quite finished depolarizing (the so-called "vulnerable period"), predisposing to the degeneration to VF.

4) **HEMODYNAMIC COMPROMISE**: arguably the most important criterion: i.e. is it causing the animal a problem? Low blood pressure, syncope, collapse, weakness, etc.

Many different types of VT are possible in dogs and cats. Monomorphic VTs have uniforme ventricular complexes, the axis of which in the horizontal plane often belies the ventricle of origin and are typically unifocal with regular rhythms/coupling intervals. Multimorphic VTs have variable conduction with polymorphic complexes, but still have relatively regular rhythms/coupling intervals. The ventricular focus is still unifocal, but with variable exit directions, resulting in variable waveforms. The clue is that the ventricular rate does not change along with the change in ventricular morphology, which often occurs over a series of complexes. Multifocal VTs are thus not only multiforme/polymorphic in ventricular morphology but are also characterized by irregular rhythms/coupling intervals, indicating multiple ventricular foci.

Ventricular tachycardia may occur in patients with or without underlying sinus rhythm, may be automatic, reentrant, or the result of triggered activity, be coupled to ectopic VPCs, may have a predictable exit morphology or alternatively degenerate into a chaotic rhythm. It is important for the clinician to exclude wide-complex supraventricular tachycardia from VT. Ventricular tachycardia may arise from the left or right ventricle. Those arising from the left ventricle can come from the anterior or posterior fascicles, the septum, or the apex. Double tachycardia results when a VT usurps control of the ventricles during sustained SVT, resulting in AV dissociation. Ventricular tachycardia may arise from one of the outflow tracts of the ventricles, typically producing a superior axis. Bidirectional ventricular tachycardias can arise from a reentrant circuit involving the left anterior and posterior

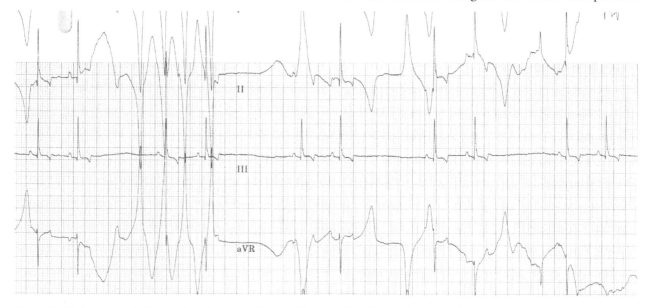

Figure 25.20 Paper speed 25 mm/s, 1 cm/mV, leads III and aVR, canine. Baseline **artifact** mimicking VT. Panting resulted in wide baseline excursions that *resemble* **ventricular tachycardia**. Lead III is still stable and shows a supraventricular bigeminal rhythm (likely Type I second degree SAB with 3:2 conduction).

fascicles while bundle-branch block reentry involves the left and right bundle branches themselves. Torsades de pointes (**TdP**) is a specific type of polymorphic VT. Ventricular flutter (VFL) is a macroreentrant circuit within the ventricles (not confined to the R and L bundle branches) that may be a manifestation of ventricular dissociation or hyperkalemia and is usually a precursor to ventricular fibrillation (VF).

Left ventricular tachycardia Typically, tachycardias originating from the left ventricular myocardium will be conducted with a RBBB-like pattern. Therefore, these are usually right-axis deviated, producing negative QRS complexes followed by positive T waves in lead II.

These often have positive precordial concordance (positive QRS in V1–V6). Similar to LVPCs, LVT may actually have varied QRS axes in the horizontal plane, and origin may require analysis of the chest leads. Idiopathic LVT occurs in the absence of structural heart disease and other predisposing causes (such as pericardial effusion, hemoabdomen, tumors, etc.). Foci arising from the left ventricular outflow tract (LVOT-VT) may be difficult to distinguish from those coming from the right ventricular outflow tract (RVOT-VT) given that both have an inferior axis. Fascicular VT arises from either the left anterior or left posterior fascicle. Alternation of conduction over the left fascicles results in bidirectional VT.

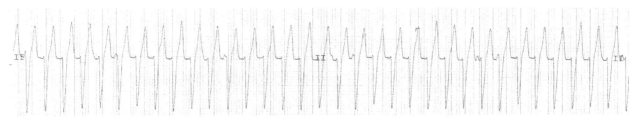

Figure 25.21 Paper speed 25 mm/s, 1 cm/mV, lead II, canine. **LVT**. The ventricular beats are wide and bizarre, negative in lead II, and AVD is present. P waves are seen intermittently dissociated from the ventricular rhythm.

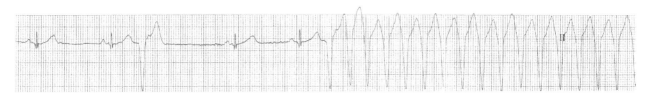

Figure 25.22 Paper speed 50 mm/s, 1 cm/mV, lead II, feline. A run of **LVT** occurs following a single VPC following a compensatory pause.

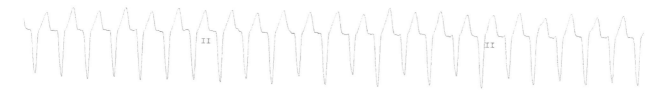

Figure 25.23 Paper speed 50 mm/s, 1 cm/mV, lead II, canine. **LVT**. No P waves are evident and are likely hiding within the QRS complexes and T waves. Toward the end of the strip, **electrical alternans** is apparent, which is common during tachycardia of any origin.

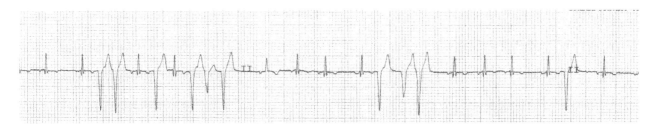

Figure 25.24 Paper speed 25 mm/s, 1 cm/mV, lead II, feline. Non-sustained **LVT**. Couplets and triplets of ventricular beats occur, some with **R on T phenomenon**.

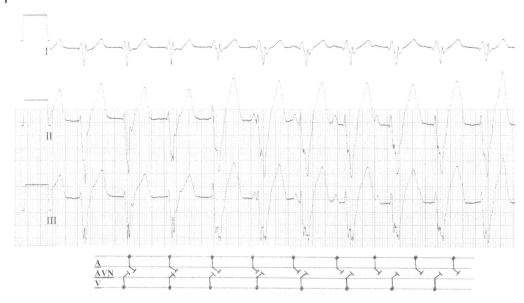

Figure 25.25a Paper speed 50 mm/s, 1 cm/mV, leads I, II, III, canine. **LVT with AVD**. A focus likely in the left ventricle produces wide and bizarre ventricular QRS complexes that have a RBBB-like pattern. P waves are clearly dissociated (marching in and out of the QRS complexes) from the ventricular rhythm, as demonstrated by the ladder diagram. **Atrioventricular dissociation** is a good indication that a wide-complex tachycardia is ventricular in origin.

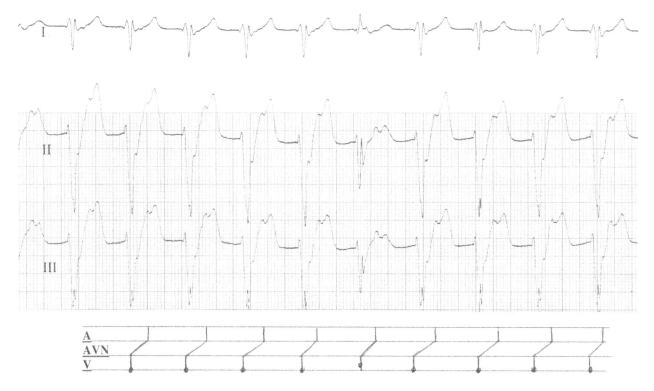

Figure 25.25b Paper speed 50 mm/s, 1 cm/mV, leads I, II, III, same dog. **LVT with VA conduction**. Seconds after the above strip, this patient developed complete **ventriculoatrial association**. Here, *retrograde* P′ waves are seen following the QRS complexes in the S-T segments. Note that we do not see any sinus P waves. This is from suppression of the SA node from ventriculoatrial conduction that occurs in ventricular tachycardias in approximately half of human cases. The sixth complex is likely an ectopic ventricular beat or multiforme complex from the same focus since the axis in I switches completely. An alternative explanation could be a ventricular fusion if the fifth beat was actually a reentrant (reciprocal beat); however, it would be unlikely for the sixth beat to have VA conduction if it were a fusion complex (V-A-F-*A* sequence). Since the sinus node is suppressed, a typical fusion (sinus +VPC) is not possible. *"All things being equal, the simplest explanation tends to be the right one."*

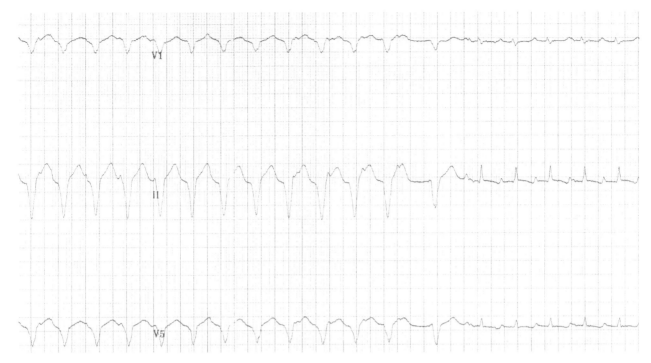

Figure 25.26 Paper speed 50 mm/s, 1 cm/mV, leads V1, II, V5, feline. This cat was weak and syncopal from LVT. Procainamide IV was bolused and the rhythm converted. The 10th–12th complexes show **VA conduction** with retrograde P′ waves following the QRS complexes within the S-T segment.

Fascicular VT Tachycardias arising from Purkinje fibers in one of the left fascicles will typically produce rather narrow-QRS complexes with oppositely directed T waves. Left anterior fascicular tachycardias will usually be right-axis deviated (i.e. conducted with a RBBB + LPFB pattern) and left posterior fascicular tachycardias will usually be left-axis deviated (i.e. conducted with a RBBB + LAFB pattern) in the frontal plane.

Bidirectional VT Rarely, the fascicles of the left bundle branch may alternately pace the ventricles on a beat-to-beat basis. The result is a relatively narrow QRS complex tachycardia with alternating axes in the horizontal plane. A focus in the AV junction or His bundle may alternatively be conducting with RBBB/LAFB alternating with RBBB/LPFB. Thus, bidirectional tachycardias may be supraventricular or ventricular in origin. Typically, the R-R intervals are fixed, but alternation of longer and shorter diastolic intervals may occur with QRS configuration changes, in which the intervals between similar complexes are equal, and the interval between dissimilar complexes is unequal. Bidirectional VT may be seen in end-stage digoxin toxicity and is typically seen immediately prior to arrest.

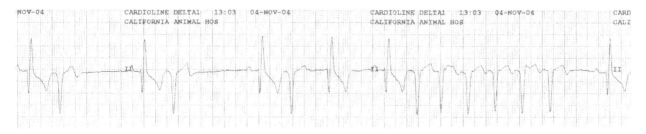

Figure 25.27 Paper speed 25 mm/s, 1 cm/mV, lead II, canine. Ventricular bigeminy precipitates a short run of **fascicular VT** with **VA conduction**. This rather narrow QRS complex VT has retrograde P′ waves that follow each of the ventricular beats. Mild electrical alternans of the ventricular QRS complexes is also evident. Tachycardias of ANY origin may display total (QRS) electrical alternans.

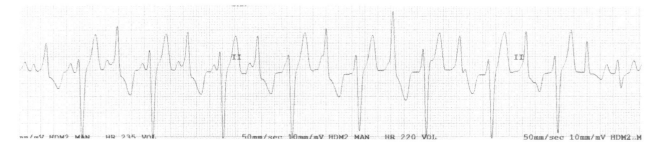

Figure 25.28 Paper speed 50 mm/s, 1 cm/mV, lead II, canine with a history of ventricular arrhythmias and acute onset of seizures secondary to an invasive frontal sinus adenocarcinoma. **Bidirectional ventricular tachycardia**. Every other beat is ventricular and oriented opposite of the previous beat. Note the regular ventricular rhythm and AVD – P waves march into the complexes by the middle of the strip. This patient fibrillated shortly after this strip and died.

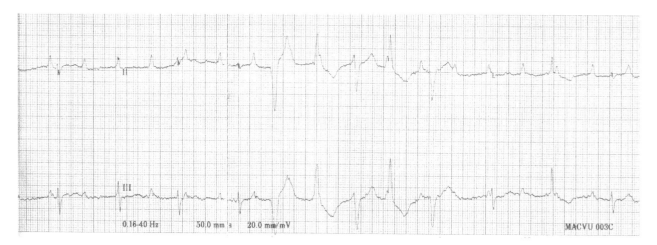

Figure 25.29 Paper speed 50 mm/s, 2 cm/mV, leads II and III, feline. **Third degree AVB**, **sinus tachycardia** of the atria (atrial rate approximately 200 bpm), **junctional escape rhythm** (ventricular rate approximately 115 bpm), and brief **bidirectional ventricular tachycardia** (ventricular rate approximately 200 bpm), which occurs following the fourth complex. Note the alternating axes of the ventricular beats and fairly regular ventricular rhythm.

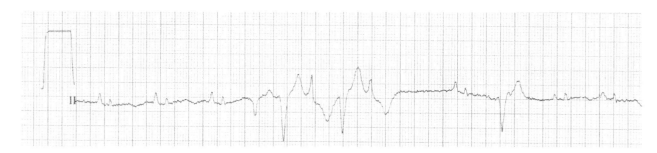

Figure 25.30 Paper speed 50 mm/s, 2 cm/mV, lead II, feline. Sinus rhythm is followed by a non-sustained run of **bidirectional VT**. A VPC follows the ninth beat. The Q-T interval is long at approx. 0.20 second.

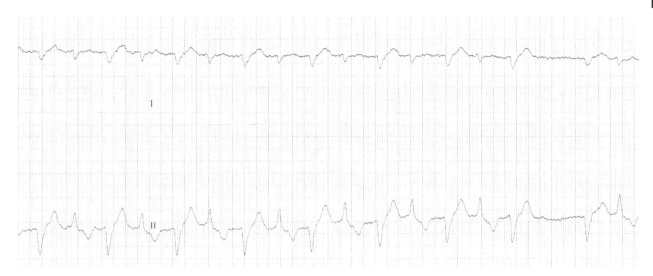

Figure 25.31 Paper speed 50 mm/s, 1 cm/mV, leads I and II, feline with history of severe unclassified cardiomyopathy, CHF, and atrial fibrillation. **Atrial fibrillation, non-sustained bidirectional ventricular tachycardia**. A pause in the rhythm toward the end of the strips reveals the undulating baseline typical of AF.

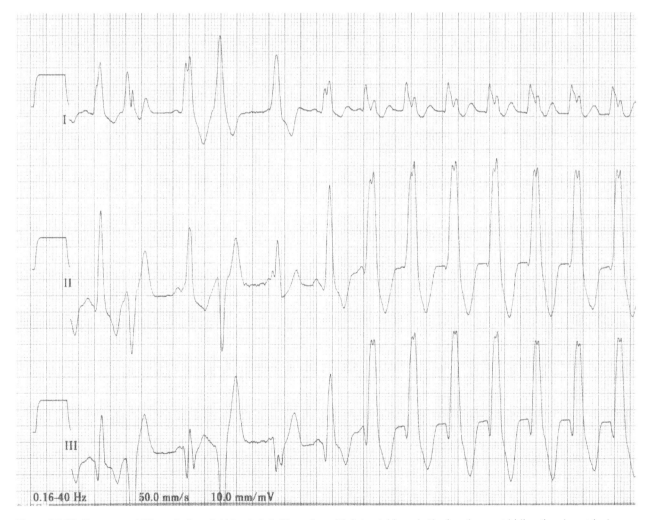

Figure 25.32 Paper speed 50 mm/s, 1 cm/mV, leads I, II, III, canine with intractable arrhythmias. *Apparent* bidirectional ventricular tachycardia is evident on the first half of the strip with the ventricular complexes alternating in axes. The rhythm converts to a monomorphic RVT midway through the strip. Note that the alternating axes are evident only in leads II and III. This patient died suddenly. Given that the RBBB-like beats are *premature*, this strip may be better termed **accelerated right idioventricular rhythm, left ventricular bigeminy, followed by right ventricular tachycardia**.

Right ventricular tachycardia Tachycardias arising from the right ventricular myocardium are typically conducted with a LBBB-like pattern, resulting in a QRS complex that is normal to left-axis deviated. Therefore, the QRS complexes are usually positive and the T waves negative in lead II. That said, analysis of the chest leads may be necessary to confirm a RV originating tachycardia (often with negative precordial concordance). Idiopathic RVT occurs in the absence of structural heart disease and predisposing causes (pericardial effusion, hemoabdomen, tumors, etc.). Ventricular tachycardia arising from the outflow tract of the right ventricle (RVOT-VT) is not uncommon in Boxers with arrhythmogenic cardiomyopathy and English Bulldogs with segmental arrhythmogenic right ventricular cardiomyopathy.

Right ventricular outflow tract-VT Tachycardias originating from the right ventricular outflow tract are quite common among Boxers or English Bulldogs with arrhythmogenic cardiomyopathy. Potentially ablatable in humans, RVOT-VTs typically have an inferior axis (usually approximately 90 degrees/vertical axis in the limb leads), are negative in VI (though this may be variable), and may be positive, negative, or isoelectric in lead I. If the QRS is positive in I, then the focus is more likely to be posterior, whereas if the QRS is negative or isoelectric, then the focus is more anterior. R wave notching in the inferior leads is apparently common with free wall foci, and aVL is typically negative if the focus is within 2 cm of the pulmonary valve.

Bundle branch reentrant VT Rarely, a macroreentrant circuit may form across the right and left bundle branches. Typically, conduction will proceed antegradely across the RBB and retrogradely across the LBB, producing a LBBB-like pattern (normal to left axis in the horizontal plane) with relatively narrow QRS complexes. Rarely,

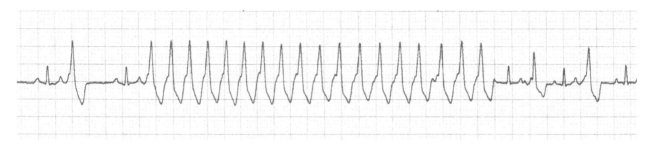

Figure 25.33 Paper speed 25 mm/s, 1 cm/ mV, lead II, canine. **RVT**. Ventricular bigeminy follows a run of VT. The R waves are positive in lead II.

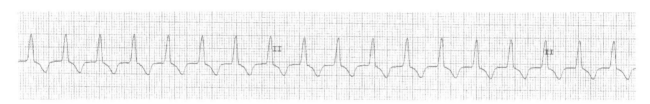

Figure 25.34 Paper speed 50 mm/s, 1 cm/mV, lead II, feline. **RVT**. The P waves are either hiding within the QRS complexes or VA conduction is present (and retrograde P′ waves are hiding within the T waves).

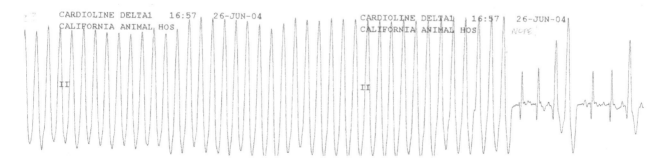

Figure 25.35 Paper speed 25 mm/s, 1 cm/mV, lead II, syncopal Boxer. **RVOT-VT**. Rapid VT occurs (nearly ventricular flutter) prior to termination.

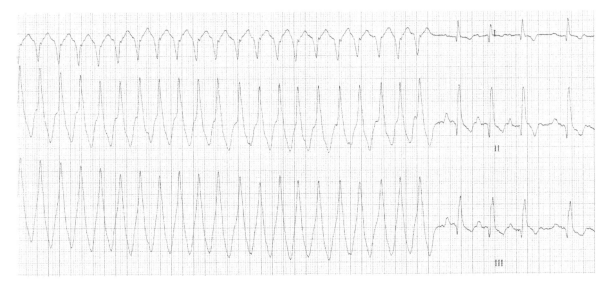

Figure 25.36 Paper speed 50 mm/s, leads I, II, III, Boxer dog. **RVOT-VT.** Note the superior axis of the ventricular beats. Lead I may be positive or negative when a ventricular focus from an outflow tract causes tachycardia. The negative QRS axis in I suggests an anterior origin within the RVOT.

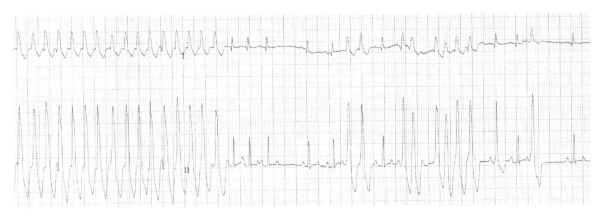

Figure 25.37 Paper speed 50 mm/s, 1 cm/mV, leads I and II, canine undergoing pericardiocentesis. **RVOT-VT.** Note the *triply postponed compensatory pause* following the initial run of VT.

conduction will proceed anterogradely across the LBB and retrogradely across the RBB, producing a RBBB-like pattern (right axis in the horizontal plane). Evidence of diffuse conduction system disease is usually present (incomplete BBB, AVB, etc.), and AVD is the rule during BBR-VT. This may be seen with advanced cardiomyopathy, suggested as a cause of VT in Boxer arrhythmogenic cardiomyopathy and is a potentially ablatable tachycardia in humans (the RBB is completely ablated, interrupting the circuit). Definitive confirmation requires an invasive electrophysiologic study.

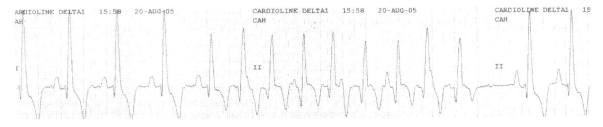

Figure 25.38 Paper speed 50 mm/s, 1 cm/mV, lead II, canine with dilated cardiomyopathy. Possible **BBR-VT.** Incomplete LBBB is present in sinus rhythm (QRS duration approx. 0.08 second, with first degree AVB (P-Ri 0.10 second) indicates conduction system disease. Paroxysmal RVT (LBBB pattern) starts with the fifth complex producing a relatively *narrow* QRS duration of approximately 0.08 second (mimicking SVT with LBBB aberration). Atrioventricular dissociation is present as well, making this more likely a *ventricular* tachycardia.

Exit block Ventricular tachycardias are typically regular in rhythm if they are unifocal. Occasionally, a monomorphic VT will become irregular. This typically occurs secondary to exit block from the irritated focus. If there are pauses in the rhythm less than twice the previous cycle length with group beating, it suggests Type I or Wenckebach exit block. If the pauses in the rhythm are exact multiples of the interectopic interval, then the block is of the Type II Mobitz variety. If the pauses are long enough, a sinus or supraventricular capture may terminate the pause. Sudden halving of the ventricular rate suggests the onset of 2:1 exit block.

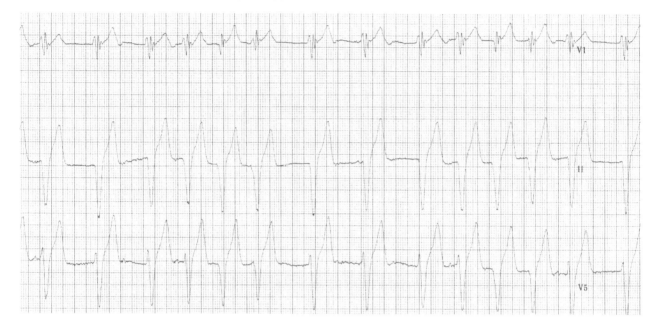

Figure 25.39 Paper speed 50 mm/S, 1 cm/mV, leads V1, II, and V5. **Irregular LVT with intermittent VA conduction and exit block**. There is clearly negative precordial concordance with a RBBB-like pattern, suggesting a left ventricular focus. The rhythm appears irregular. P waves are at first obviously dissociated at the beginning and end of the strip but disappear midway. P waves are not seen during some of the relatively longer pauses when they would be expected to, suggesting inhibition of the sinus node and at least intermittent VA conduction. The longer pauses are less than twice the previous cycle length, suggesting a **Wenckebach exit block** from the ventricular focus. Initially there appears to be 2:1 conduction, which is followed by a group with 1:1 conduction. Then, 2:1 occurs midway through the strip and is followed again by another Wenckebach period. Irregular VTs may be associated with an increased risk of sudden cardiac death (SCD).

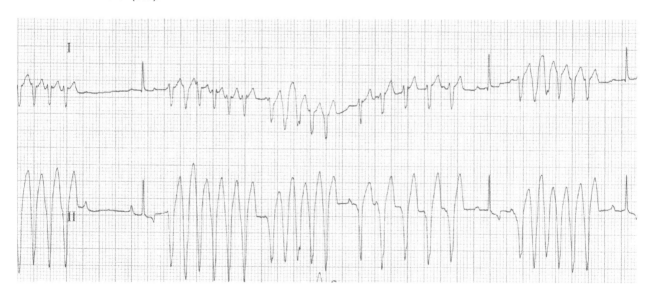

Figure 25.40 Paper speed 50 mm/s, 1 cm/mV, leads I and II, canine. **Irregular LVT** with likely **exit block**. Rapid VT with a RBBB-like pattern is suggestive of a LV focus. Halfway through the strip, the VT abruptly slows down, suggestive of 2:1 exit block. The ventricular rhythm does not obviously speed up prior to pauses, and the resultant pauses that are twice the previous cycle length suggest **Mobitz exit block**.

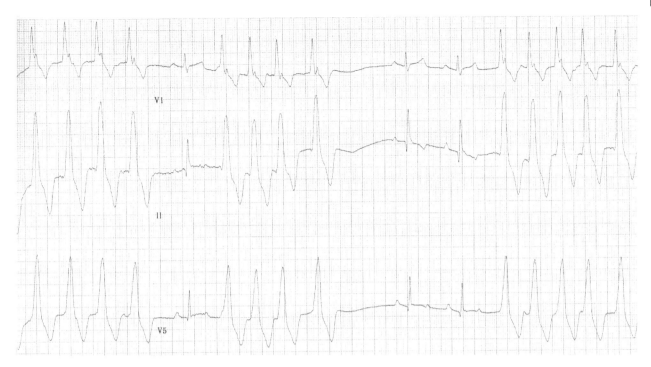

Figure 25.41 Paper speed 50 mm/s, 1 cm/mV, leads VI, II, V5, Boxer, **RVOT-VT with probable exit block**. Note that each salvo of VT shows group beating. The pattern here is suggestive of gradual prolongation prior to failure of conduction (Type I exit block). Typically, Wenckebach exit block results in group beating with R′-R′ intervals getting shorter prior to a pause, with the pauses less than 2 R′-R′ intervals. Note that the R′-R′ interval shortens before a pause between the eighth and ninth beats. Exit block may explain irregularity in the rhythm during ventricular rhythms.

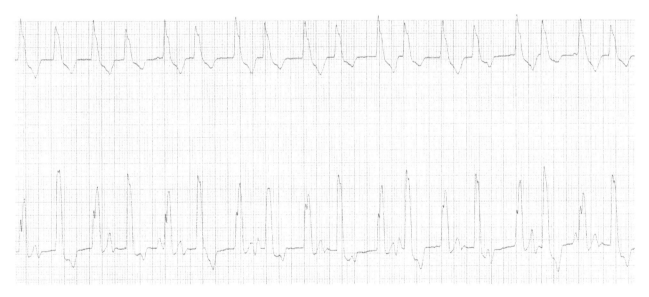

Figure 25.42 Paper speed 50 mm/s, 1 cm/mV, lead I (top) and II (bottom), canine. **RVT with group beating and total QRS-T electrical alternans**. Complete AVD is present as evidenced by the P waves marching through the ventricular complexes without relation to them. The rhythm is bigeminal and irregular. The most likely explanation is 3:2 conduction and Type I exit block. The electrical alternans is likely secondary to the tachycardia.

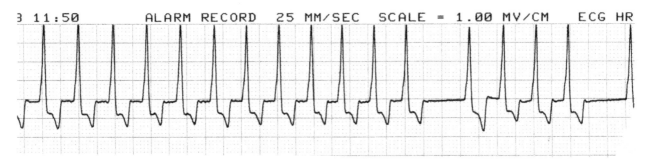

Figure 25.43 Paper speed 25 mm/s, 1 cm/mV, lead II, canine. Atrial rhythm uncertain, possibly atrial fibrillation, **RVT** with **Mobitz/Type II exit block** with pauses that are twice that of the underlying cycle length.

Double tachycardia Double tachycardia is simultaneous supraventricular and ventricular tachycardia. This is one of the rare occasions when AV dissociation from usurpation and AV block are coexistent, though the AV block during double tachycardia is physiologic. (The other situation is during block acceleration-dissociation, when the AV block is often pathologic.) Basically, atrial fibrillation, atrial flutter, atrial tachycardia, upper junctional tachycardia or sinus tachycardia (any SVT not requiring the AV node for perpetuation), and a VT occur at the same time. The AV node is rapidly depolarized from both the atria and the ventricles, effectively preventing it from emerging from a refractory state. These are dangerous arrhythmias, are generally associated with severe structural heart disease, and may be seen with digoxin toxicity. Clinical management is often unrewarding, and patients with double tachycardia frequently pass suddenly.

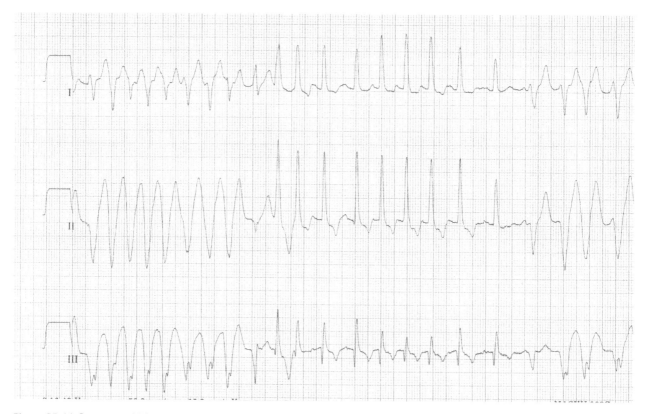

Figure 25.44 Paper speed 50 mm/s, 1 cm/mV, leads I, II, III, canine. *Double tachycardia*. LVT briefly terminates to reveal an underlying rhythm of supraventricular tachycardia. LVT resumes at the end of the strip. Simultaneous tachycardia of the atria and the ventricles is known as "double tachycardia," which can be a manifestation of digoxin toxicity. This patient was not taking digoxin at the time of this strip; however, it did suddenly die of intractable arrhythmias. This is one of the rare instances where AVB and AVD secondary to usurpation coexist, since the atria and ventricles are both beating rapidly enough to prevent the AVN from emerging from a refractory state.

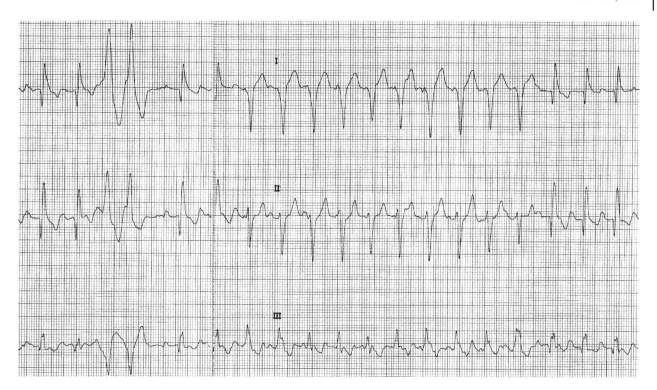

Figure 25.45 Paper speed 50 mm/s, 1 cm/mV, canine, leads I, II, III. Boxer with DCM. **Double tachycardia**. The underlying rhythm is SVT (spontaneous rate 207 bpm), which is interrupted briefly by a couplet of VPCs (LBBB-like morphology, third and fourth complexes), then resumes before usurpation by LVT (spontaneous rate 250 bpm). Atrioventricular dissociation is evident during the double tachycardia and the onset and offset are ventricular fusions (7th and 16th complexes).

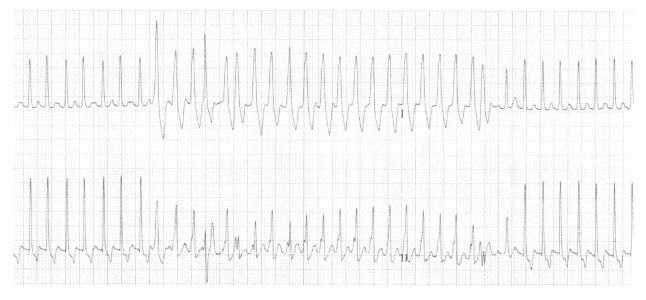

Figure 25.46 Paper speed 25 mm/s, 1 cm/mV, leads I and II, canine. **Double tachycardia**. The underlying rhythm is supraventricular tachycardia (SVT). Right ventricular tachycardia (RVT) develops a third of the way through the strip with a rate slightly faster than that of the SVT and resultant AV dissociation. SVT resumes at the end. Simultaneous tachycardia of the atria and the ventricles is known as *double tachycardia*, which may result from digitalis intoxication. This patient died suddenly of intractable arrhythmias and did not happen to be on digoxin.

Polymorphic VT Tachycardia that originates in the ventricles with variable morphologies of the QRS-T complexes and that are specifically not of the type of torsades de pointes (TdP) (see below) are termed polymorphic ventricular tachycardias. The Q-Ti of the normal sinus complexes preceding the tachycardia is normal, and the VT may or may not display phasic alternation of axes in the horizontal plane. If polymorphic VT is regular with consistent coupling intervals, it may yet be unifocal (with "multiforme" QRS complexes) but with variable exit directions resulting in changing QRS morphologies. Polymorphic VT may be grossly irregular, then considered likely to be multifocal, and is frequently a preamble to VF. German Shepherd puppies of certain lines may be predisposed to familial polymorphic VT, with 50% or greater affected puppies likely to suffer sudden cardiac death, typically secondary to VT degenerating to VF and usually when the puppy is asleep (vagal tone apparently worsens these arrhythmias). Those that survive to 18 months may live normal lives, with most of this subgroup outgrowing their arrhythmias by one year of age.

Torsades de pointes A particular form of polymorphic VT occurs in association with long Q-T syndromes and sudden death. Torsade de pointes (singular, pleural is torsades de pointes) is characterized by ventricular complexes that become taller in amplitude, then smaller/negative, then taller/positive, resulting in a pattern that makes the ventricular complexes appear to twist around the baseline (TdP literally means "twisting of the points"). Relatively rarely, TdP may degenerate into VF, making this a potentially preterminal arrhythmia. Torsade de pointes are not uncommonly preceded by a short–long–short cycle sequence that is initiated by a two-beat run of ventricular bigeminy, the second of which starts the tachycardia and falls on the T wave of the preceding sinus beat. Three criteria for TdP are often cited:

1) The rhythm immediately prior to the onset of TdP is slow, and the Q-Ti is prolonged (i.e. >0.25 second).
2) The onset of TdP involves an R on T premature beat.
3) The set of complexes following this are fast (>180 bpm), more regular than VF, but continually changing in amplitude and polarity (duration usually short at 5–10 seconds).

Although rarely seen in veterinary patients, TdP has been described a few times. The treatment of choice is magnesium sulfate. Magnesium sulfate is something the clinician should also consider using when VT is refractory to standard medications – occasionally a low serum magnesium will predispose to VT, and unless it is corrected, the VT will not go away. Check the electrolytes: low magnesium is associated with hypokalemia.

Ventricular flutter This is a macroreentrant (circus-movement entirely confined to the ventricular

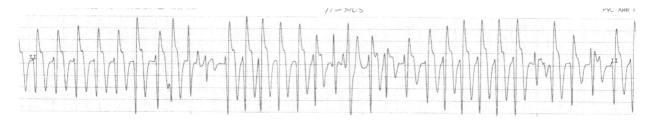

Figure 25.47 Paper speed 25 mm/s, 1 cm/mV, lead II, canine. **Polymorphic VT, likely unifocal**. AV dissociation is present throughout, and the ventricular complexes twist around the baseline in a manner similar to that seen with torsades de pointes.

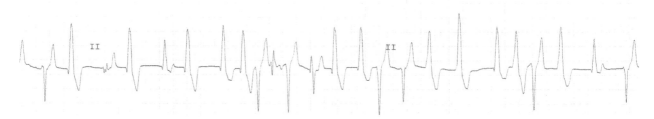

Figure 25.48 Paper speed 25 mm/s, 0.5 cm/mV, lead II, canine. **Polymorphic VT, likely multifocal**. There are varied morphologies to the ventricular complexes. The rhythm is additionally grossly irregular (absolute arrhythmia – similar to that seen with AF). A pattern is discernible one-third the way into the strip, with the complexes regularly proceeding from negative to positive polarity that repeats itself, followed by a gradual reversal of polarity. This is clearly a dangerous arrhythmia not only likely to be hemodynamically compromising, but also indicative of a very electrically unstable ventricular myocardium. Atrial activity is not evident, suggestive of VA conduction/suppression of SA nodal discharge, or atrial fibrillation and AV dissociation.

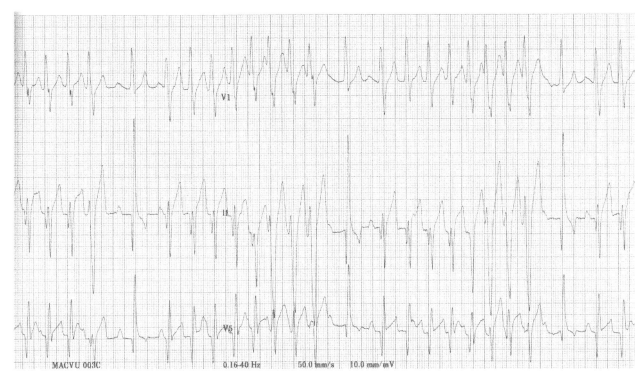

Figure 25.49 Paper speed 50 mm/s, 1 cm/mV, leads V1, II, and V5, 5-month old German Shepherd dog with familial ventricular tachyarrhythmias. **Polymorphic VT**. The 5th, 14th, and 23rd complexes are sinus. Note the P-R interval prolongation on the 14th and 23rd complexes, indicating partial penetration of the preceding ventricular impulse into the AVN with resultant secondary 1st degree AVB on the post-extrasystolic beats. AV dissociation is present during the paroxysmal tachycardia, and the morphology of the VT changes toward the end of the tachycardia.

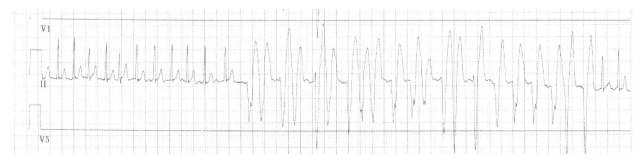

Figure 25.50 Paper speed 25 mm/s, 1 cm/mV, lead II, canine with advanced CMVDz and CHF. At the beginning of the strip, typical **AF** with a rapid ventricular rate response is present. After the 11th complex, a **polymorphic VT** takes over. The irregularity of the VT may confuse the examiner with AF and RBBB aberration. However, the ventricular complexes have an atypical pattern as shown below on the precordial leads. The serum digoxin level in this patient was low; however, the digoxin was discontinued anyway due to VT.

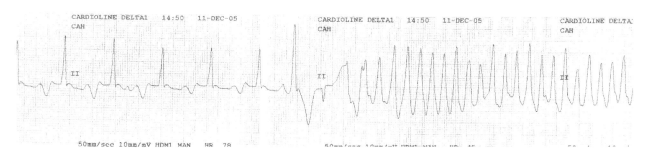

Figure 25.51a Paper speed 50 mm/s, 1 cm/mV, lead II, syncopal feline. **Torsade de pointes**. This cat had frequent bouts of syncope associated with prolonged ventricular asystole from AVB. A ventricular escape rhythm would eventually rescue the heart, followed by a slow sinus rhythm. Here, bizarre and tall sinus complexes with a long Q-Ti and slow rhythm are terminated by a fusion complex, then an R on T premature beat that results in a polymorphic VT with changing amplitudes, consistent with TdP.

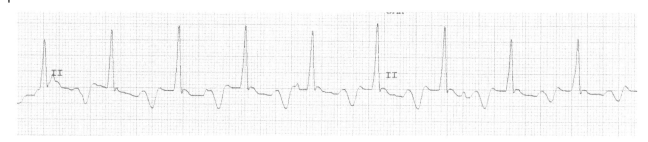

Figure 25.51b Paper speed 50 mm/s, 1 cm/mV, lead II, same cat immediately before the onset of TdP. The long Q-Ti and negative T/U waves are obvious.

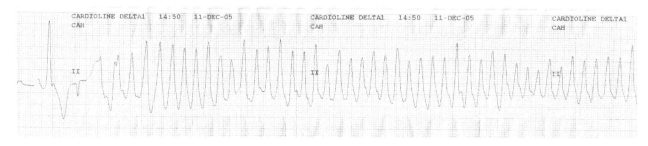

Figure 25.51c Paper speed 50 mm/s, 1 cm/mV, lead II, same cat at the onset of TdP. The twisting around the baseline is more obvious during the VT when a longer strip is analyzed. Ideally, the rest of the leads would have been run simultaneously. Often, TdP may show more dramatic undulating change in polarity in other leads.

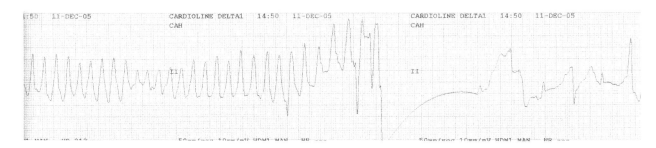

Figure 25.51d Paper speed 50 mm/s, 1 cm/mV, lead II, same cat at the offset of TdP. Chest compression is evident by the dramatic drop in baseline, and a slow, irregular ventricular rhythm rescues the heart.

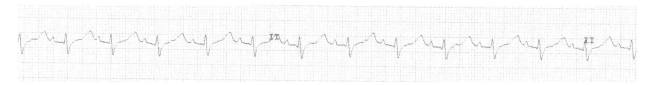

Figure 25.51e Paper speed 50 mm/s, 1 cm/mV, lead II, same cat in sinus rhythm. The Q-Ti is prolonged at approximately 0.24 second.

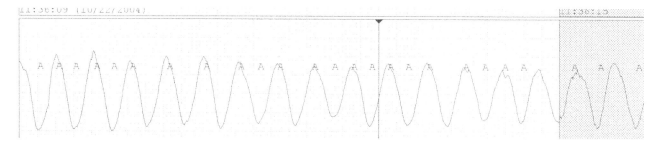

Figure 25.52 Paper speed 25 mm/s, 1 cm/mV, lead II, canine. **Ventricular flutter**. The VFL is sine-wave in appearance.

myocardium) prefibrillatory rhythm that appears as a smooth, undulating "sine-wave" on surface EKG, faster than VT usually around 250–450 bpm. No fusion or capture beats occur. Representing a transition from VT to VF, it can be associated with severe hyperkalemia, is sine-wave-like in appearance, associated with circulatory collapse, and is generally preterminal.

Ventricular fibrillo-flutter/ventricular dissociation

Generally, this is a brief transitional rhythm following organized VFL and preceding overt VF. The regular sine-wave appearance of VFL degenerates into a less-regular rhythm with nonuniform undulation of the baseline. This is generally impossible on surface EKG to differentiate from ventricular dissociation

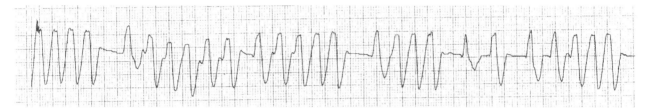

Figure 25.53 Paper speed 25 mm/s, 1 cm/mV, lead II, feline, **ventricular flutter** preceding terminal fibrillation.

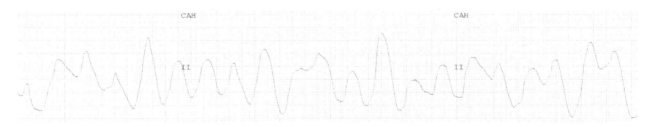

Figure 25.54 Paper speed 50 mm/s, 1 cm/mV, lead II, canine. **Ventricular fibrillo-flutter**. Here, the regular sine-wave is becoming far-less organized and is well on its way to frank fibrillation.

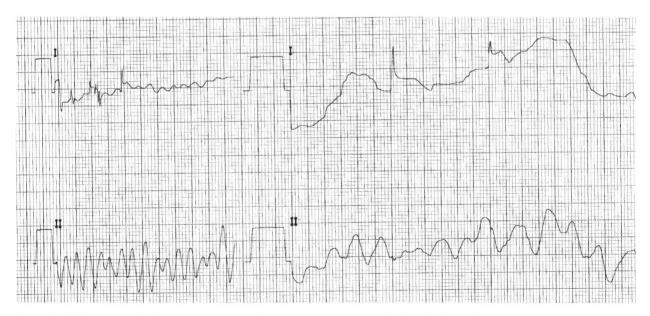

Figure 25.55 Paper speed 25 followed by 50 mm/s, 1 cm/mV, leads I and II, canine. **Ventricular fibrillo-flutter**. Note the more organized flutter at the beginning and how it quickly degenerates and becomes less organized.

(ventriculo-ventricular dissociation, double ventricular rhythms) where one ventricle is fibrillating, the other in flutter. Ventricular fibrillo-flutter is associated with circulatory collapse, is an immediate precursor of fibrillation, and as such requires cardioversion.

Ventricular fibrillation

VF occurs when the ventricles have no meaningful mechanical activity and the EKG shows an undulating baseline without identifiable complexes at a very high rate (>450 bpm). Grossly, the ventricles in fibrillation are classically described as

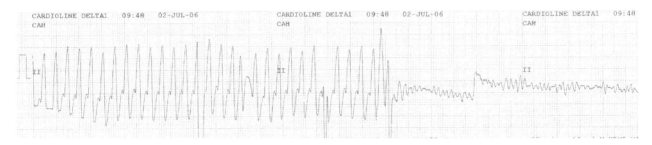

Figure 25.56 Paper speed 25 mm/s, 1 cm/mV, lead II, syncopal Boxer. Unstable rapid **VT** that degenerates into terminal **ventricular fibrillation**. Note that the VF is immediately preceded by an **R on T beat**. This patient experienced **sudden cardiac death** (**SCD**), an unfortunate risk associated with arrhythmogenic cardiomyopathy. A precordial thump (visible as the sudden upward deflection just after the onset of VF) was unsuccessful. Immediate defibrillation is the treatment of choice.

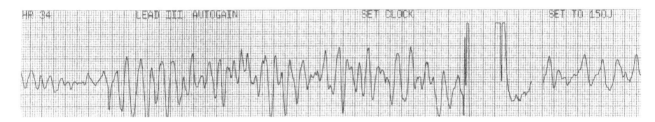

Figure 25.57 Paper speed 25 mm/s, 1 cm/mV, lead II, canine. *Coarse* **VF**. The baseline shows coarse VF with a markedly undulating baseline and no identifiable complexes. The tracing is interrupted as 150 joules of DC current is applied to the patient in a vain attempt at defibrillation.

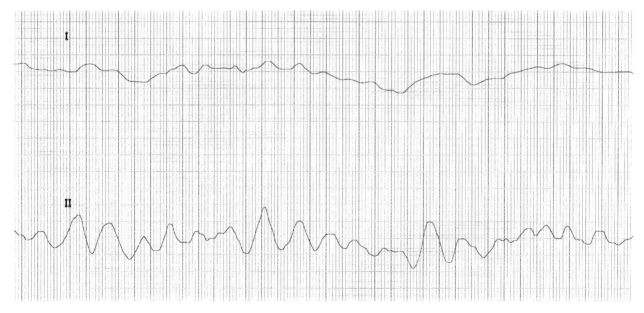

Figure 25.58 Paper speed 50 mm/s, 1 cm/mV, leads I and II, canine. **Ventricular fibrillo-flutter/coarse VF**.

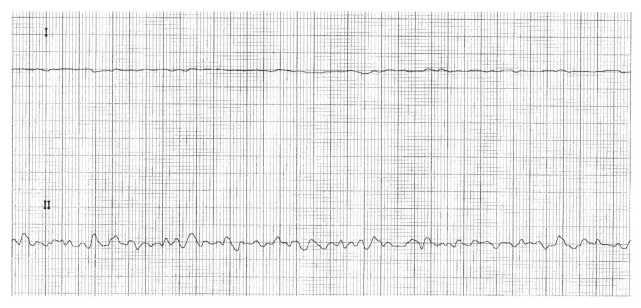

Figure 25.59 Paper speed 50 mm/s, 1 cm/mV, leads I and II, same dog. Fine **VF**. As time passes, the fibrillatory waves become lower in amplitude.

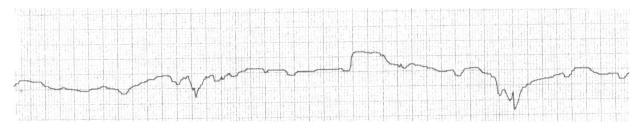

Figure 25.60 Paper speed 25 mm/s, 1 cm/mV, lead II, canine. *Fine* **VF**. Note the minimally undulating baseline. The longer VF persists, the less likely defibrillation will be successful.

having the appearance of a "bag of worms," with unco-ordinated and irregular/ineffectual mechanical activity. Associated with complete circulatory collapse, this is a preterminal event and death ensues. Treatment is generally impossible without electrical defibrillation (cardioversion), but occasionally a precordial thump stuns the myocardium and may rarely allow for the sinus rhythm to be restored. As with atrial fibrillation, both coarse and fine varieties exist (see Chapter 18). Coarse VF has an undulating baseline with wide and erratic excursions, whereas fine VF has a minimally undulating baseline.

Further reading

Chowdhry, I.H., Hariman, R.J., Gomes, J.A., and El-Sherif, N. (1983). Electrocardiogram of the month, transient digitoxic double tachycardia. *Chest* 83 (4): 686–687.

Dubin, D. (2000). *Rapid Interpretation of EKG's*, 6e. Cover Inc.

Ettinger, S.J. and Suter, P.F. (1970). *Canine Cardiology*. W.B. Saunders Company.

Fox, P.R., Sisson, D., and Moïse, N.S. (1999). *Textbook of Canine and Feline Cardiology: Principles and Clinical Practice*, 2e. W.B. Saunders Company.

Marriot, H.J.L. and Conover, M.B. (1998). *Advanced Concepts in Arrhythmias*, 3e. Mosby.

Pick, A. and Langendorf, R. (1979). *Interpretation of Complex Arrhythmias*. Lea & Febiger.

Riera, A.R.P., Barros, R.B., de Sousa, F.D., and Baranchuk, A. (2010). Accelerated idioventricular rhythm: history and chronology of the main discoveries. *Indian Pacing Electrophysiol. J.* (ISSN 0.972-6292) 10 (1): 40–48.

Sanders, R.A. and Kurosawa, T.A. (2013). ECG of the month. *JAVMA* 243 (3): 342–344.

Santilli, R.A., Bontempi, L.V., Perego, M. et al. (2009). Outflow tract segmental arrhythmogenic right ventricular cardiomyopathy in an English Bulldog. *J. Vet. Cardiol.* 11: 47–51.

Santilli, R., Moïse, N.S., Pariaut, R., and Perego, M. (2018). *Electrocardiography of the Dog and Cat: Diagnosis of Arrhythmias*, 2e. Edna.

Tilley, L.P. (1992). *Essentials of Canine and Feline Electrocardiography*, 3e. Lippincott Williams & Wilkins.

Part IV

Pacemakers

Pacemaker implantation in small animals has been performed in experimental as well as clinical settings. The very first artificial pacemaker was implanted in a dog. Dogs and cats may be recommended for pacemaker implantation for symptomatic bradyarrhythmias. Pacemakers are indicated for dogs and cats with clinical manifestations of bradycardia, usually secondary to high-grade Type II second degree atrioventricular block, third degree atrioventricular block, sick sinus syndrome, and persistent atrial standstill. Cats more commonly require pacemakers for paroxysmal atrioventricular block or symptomatic third degree atrioventricular block in which the escape rhythm is unacceptably low (which, by the way, is rare). Inherently artificial, pacemakers are less physiologic than the normal pacemaker of the heart (the sinus node) which is under the autonomic influence of the nervous system. As such, a variety of EKG abnormalities are associated with artificial pacing.

Pacemakers may be programmed in a variety of mode functions and create patterns on surface EKG associated with each modality. The pulse rate may be converted into an interval in ms by dividing it into 60 000. The modes are represented by a group of three to four letters that denotes the functionality of the pacing system. The first letter indicates the site of pacing and may be A (pacing the atrium), V (pacing the ventricle), D ("dual" pacing both the atria and ventricle), or O (none). The second letter denotes the sensing capacity of the system: A (senses atrium), V (senses ventricle), D (dual, sensing atrium and ventricle), or O (none). The third letter represents the response to the sensing and I (inhibits pacing), T (triggers pacing), D (inhibits and triggers pacing), or O (none) is used. The fourth letter indicates rate modulation, and R (rate modulation present) or O (none, often omitted) is used. The most common system used is VVIR (ventricular sensed, paced, inhibits pacing, rate modulation present) and requires a single right ventricular lead. The DDD system requires an atrial and ventricular lead, senses and paces both the right atrium and right ventricle, and

is inhibited by sensing. Biventricular pacing (RV apical lead, LV lead via coronary sinus) may be prescribed to improve atrioventricular synchrony; however, three leads (including the RA lead) are used, increasing the chance of complications such as lead dislodgement or fracture. The mode VOO is the so-called "magnet mode" and paces the ventricle through any native rhythm (i.e. no sensing), resulting in artificial parasystole.

It is important for the clinician to be able to know when a pacemaker is functioning normally and be able to suspect and diagnose pacemaker malfunction. Ventriculoatrial conduction is common, especially in patients paced for sick sinus syndrome, less so in those with antegrade atrioventricular block and notably absent in patients with atrial standstill. Atrial and ventricular fusion may occur. While pacemakers are commonly used, implantable cardioverter-defibrillators (ICDs) are not prescribed in small animals with any regularity. Algorithms for detecting tachycardia in humans tend to overinterpret the naturally quite variable rates of normal sinus nodal rhythm in dogs, resulting in inappropriate defibrillation in response to sinus tachycardia. The clinician should not only be able to identify a paced animal from surface EKG, but also should be able to diagnose if problems or malfunction of the pacing system are present.

Pacemakers: The Basics
Indications
Unipolar vs. bipolar
Modes
Endocardial/transvenous vs. epicardial leads
MEA of the paced QRS

Pacemakers: Some Abnormalities
Concealed conduction
Ventriculoatrial conduction
Paced fusion vs. pseudofusion beats
Paced reciprocal beats

Interpretation of the Electrocardiogram in Small Animals, First Edition. Nick A. Schroeder.
© 2021 John Wiley & Sons Inc. Published 2021 by John Wiley & Sons Inc.

Pacemakers: Trouble

Undersensing
Oversensing
Failure to capture

Battery depletion
Pacemaker-mediated tachycardia
Pacemaker syndrome

Further Reading

Hesselson, A.B. (2003). *Simplified Interpretation of Pacemaker ECGs*. Futura.

26

Pacemakers

The Basics

CHAPTER MENU
Indications, 351
Pacemaker polarity, 351
Modes, 351
Lead placement, 353
MEA of the paced QRS, 353

Indications Pacemaker implantation is indicated for symptomatic bradycardia that is unresponsive or refractory to medical therapy. Commonly used medications to treat bradycardia include sympathomimetic drugs such as theophylline or hyoscyamine. Most dogs that ultimately require pacing have high-grade Type II second degree atrioventricular block, third degree atrioventricular block, sick sinus syndrome, or persistent atrial standstill (see Chapters 11, 13, and 20). Most cats that require pacing have transient ventricular asystole from paroxysmal atrioventricular block (see Chapter 20). Some cats with third degree atrioventricular block and with ventricular escape rhythms and a heart rate in the 60–80 bpm range may also require pacing, but this is rare. Most cats with third degree atrioventricular block have junctional escape rhythms with ventricular rates over 100 bpm, are asymptomatic, and do not require pacing.

Pacemaker polarity Unipolar systems use the generator itself as one pole and the lead tip as the other pole, typically producing large and obvious pacing spike artifacts on surface EKG. Bipolar systems have the anode and cathode placed close to each other at the end of the lead, resulting in a small pacing spike. Usually, leads are placed transvenously through the jugular with the tip inserted into the apex of the right ventricle. This results in wide and bizarre ventricular beats with left bundle branch block (LBBB)-like morphology. The generator is typically placed in a pocket of muscle in the cervical region. Cats typically must have an epicardial lead placed with the generator placed intra-abdominally between body wall layers since transvenous lead placement is associated with a high incidence of chylothorax as a complication. Unipolar systems have a higher incidence of skeletal muscle stimulation and the voltage may need to be adjusted as a result.

Modes Most veterinary generators were historically programmed to be VVI (ventricular pacing, ventricular sensing, ventricular sensing inhibits ventricular pacing) mode. Most units are preprogrammed to keep the HR to at least 100 bpm, and now many are rate-responsive (VVIR, usually 80–140 bpm) depending on preprogramming and local muscle activity sensed by the generator. Less commonly, dual chamber (DDD, dual sensing, dual pacing, dual sensing inhibits dual pacing) or biventricular pacing (RV and LV pacing, typically dual sensing) systems may be used.

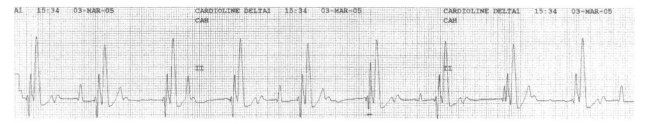

Figure 26.1 Paper speed 50 mm/s, 1 cm/mV, lead II, this canine patient had a **unipolar pacemaker** implanted for third degree AVB, **VVI**. The pacing spikes are obvious, and the LBBB of the QRS complexes is consistent with an RV apically placed lead. The HR is 100 bpm.

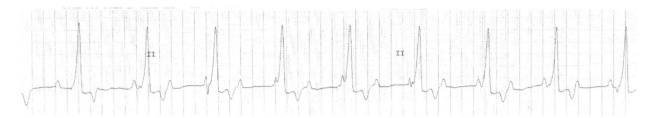

Figure 26.2 Paper speed 50 mm/s, 1 cm/mV, lead II, canine patient with a bipolar pacemaker implanted for third degree AVB, **VVI**. The pacing spikes are very small, negative deflections evident on beats three and six consistent with a **bipolar system**. The P waves obviously march through a ventricular rate of 100 bpm.

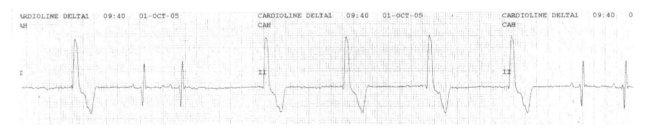

Figure 26.3 Paper speed 50 mm/s, 1 cm/mV, lead II, Miniature Schnauzer following **VVIR** bipolar pacemaker implantation for SSS. The pacemaker senses the native QRS and is inhibited from firing until a pause of 0.7 second occurs (HR dropping below 85 bpm).

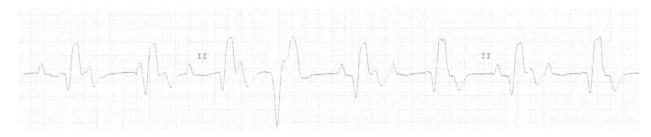

Figure 26.4 Paper speed 50 mm/s, 1 cm/mV, lead II. Third degree AVB with RV pacing. The fourth complex is a **LVPC** (RBBB morphology) that *resets* the pacemaker, which fires 0.3 second after the spontaneous ectopic complex. P waves march through the underlying paced rhythm set at 100 bpm.

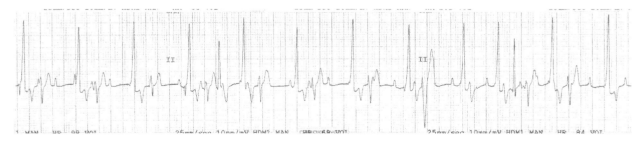

Figure 26.5 Paper speed 25 mm/s, 1 cm/mV, lead II, canine. This complicated strip shows VPCs that "reset the rhythm." The interval from the smaller, aberrantly conducted VPCs (RBBB pattern, smaller amplitude beats) to the next upright (LBBB pattern) paced beats is exactly three big boxes (15 little boxes, 0.3 second). This is because the pacemaker fires when a pause of 0.3 second occurs (it is set at 100 bpm). Occasionally, a second VPC (9th and 21st complexes) occurs and is not sensed by the pacemaker as the next pacing stimulus occurs 0.3 second after the first VPC.

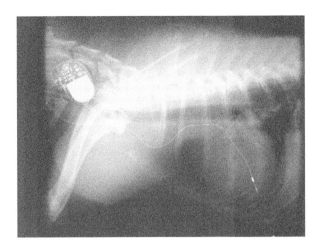

Figure 26.6 Radiograph of a Miniature Schnauzer following implantation of a transvenous pacemaker for SSS. The generator is located in a pocket in the superficial cervical musculature, and the lead travels through the R external jugular vein into the apex of the RV. This was a bipolar system, and the lead has cathode and anode near the tip of the lead in the RV.

Lead placement

Typical positioning of a transvenous ventricular lead is within the apex of the right ventricle. Active leads are screwed directly into the myocardium, and passive tined leads are tangled in the trabeculae of the right ventricular apex. Atrial leads are positioned within the right auricle. Rarely, the left ventricle may be paced by a lead positioned within the coronary sinus. Very small dogs are unable to be paced with a lead in the coronary sinus. Cats require an epicardial lead that is actively fixed by means of a small hook and sutures to the left ventricular apex.

MEA of the paced QRS

Since the lead is positioned in the RV apex with transvenous systems, changes in the QRS pattern of the paced beats can indicate problems. Most of the time, an RV apical lead creates a LBBB pattern with a normal MEA or an axis shift to the left. If lead displacement into the right ventricular outflow tract (RVOT) occurs, the paced beats will be of LBBB pattern, but the MEA may shift to the right, typically into the normal range (between 0 and 90 degrees). If the paced beats suddenly change to a RBBB pattern with a right axis shift, displacement of the lead into the coronary sinus or perforation of the lead through the IVS may have occurred. Epicardial lead placement in the LV apex normally creates paced beats with a RBBB and RAD pattern.

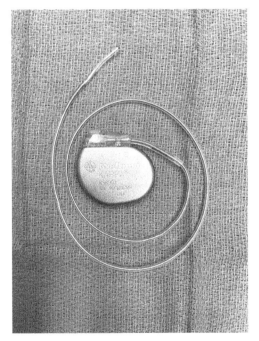

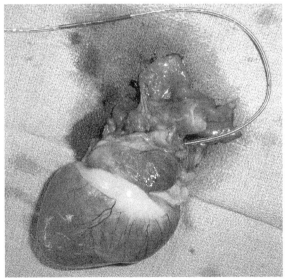

(a)

Figure 26.7a Photographs of a dog with a transvenous pacemaker. To the left, the generator has been explanted, and the lead is seen extending from the port. The excess lead is usually wrapped around the generator proximal to where it enters the R external jugular vein. To the right, the heart has been removed and the right aspect is up. The lead enters the cranial vena cava on the right to enter the right side of the heart.

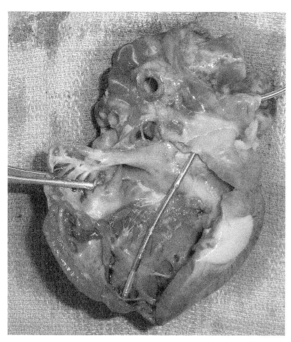
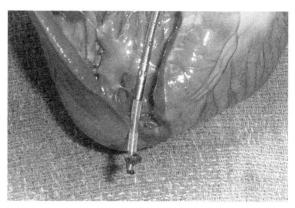

(b)

Figure 26.7b Gross specimen from the same individual. The right heart has been opened, exposing the lead coursing from the CrVC into the RA, across the tricuspid valve into the right ventricular apex. The tip of the lead is ensnared in the trabeculae of the RV apex.

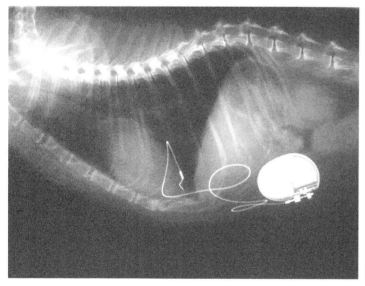
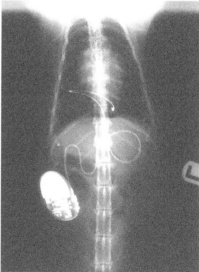

Figure 26.8 Radiographs from a cat paced for third degree AVB. An epicardial lead was implanted transdiaphragmatically, and the generator was implanted in a muscle pocket within the abdominal cavity.

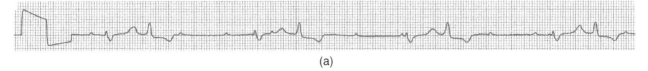

(a)

Figure 26.9a Paper speed 50 mm/s, 1 cm/mV, feline. **Third degree AVB** with **junctional escape** and **ventricular bigeminy**. Complete AV dissociation is present as evidenced by P waves marching through (and independent of) the QRS complexes with the atrial rate exceeding the ventricular rate. Ventricular bigeminy is not uncommon during third degree AVB.

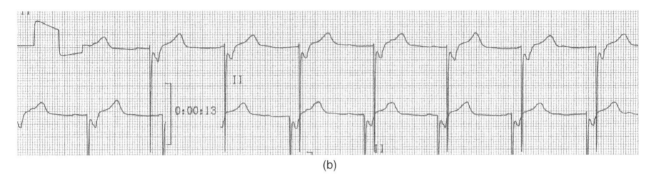

(b)

Figure 26.9b Paper speed 50 mm/s, 1 cm/mV, lead II, same cat following pacemaker implantation. The **unipolar** pacemaker (evidenced by high-voltage pacing artifacts) has been set at 100 bpm. The QRS complexes are negative in lead II consistent with a RBBB pattern.

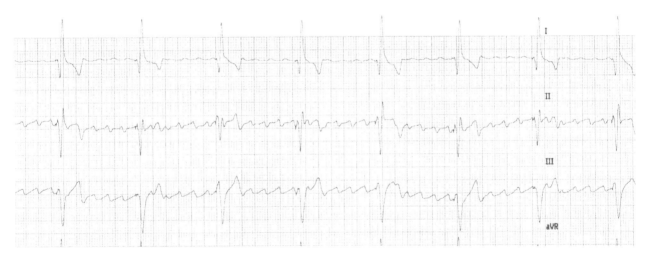

Figure 26.10 Paper speed 50 mm/s, 1 cm/mV, leads I, II, III, canine. **Atrial flutter, third degree AVB, right ventricular paced rhythm**. This VVIR unit was set with a LRL of 70 bpm. Note the sawtoothed baseline characteristic of AFL (Type I typical counterclockwise AFL with an atrial rate of approximately 600 bpm). The ventricular rhythm is independent of the atrial rhythm, indicating AV dissociation and third degree AVB. This patient had biventricular failure secondary to advanced atrioventricular valvular disease, and the atrial enlargement predisposed to atrial flutter. The QRS complexes have **a LBBB-like morphology** and **L axis deviation**.

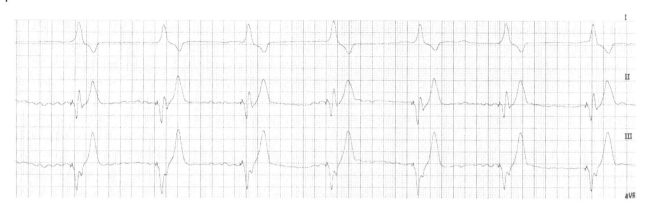

Figure 26.11 Paper speed 50 mm/s, 1 cm/ mV, leads I, II, III, canine. **Atrial fibrillation, third degree AVB, right ventricular paced rhythm**. This VVIR unit was set with a LRL of 70 bpm. Note the undulating baseline characteristic of AF, and the lack of irregularly irregular supraventricular QRS complexes. This patient had high-grade atrioventricular block and prior to pacemaker implantation and atrial fibrillation.

Further reading

Surawicz, B. and Knilans, T.K. (2001). *Chou's Electrocardiography in Clinical Practice: Adult and Pediatric*, 5e. Saunders.

27

Pacemakers

Some Abnormalities

CHAPTER MENU

Concealed conduction, 357
Ventriculoatrial conduction, 357
Paced fusion complexes, 357
Paced reciprocal complexes, 361

Concealed conduction Concealed conduction is inferred on surface EKG when unexpected pauses or delay of conduction occur. This may be seen in animals with artificial pacemakers implanted. Retrograde (ventriculoatrial conduction) from paced impulses may not fully propagate to the atria but may prolong following P-R intervals on following sinus captures in patients with some intact AV nodal conduction.

Ventriculoatrial conduction This may occur with ventricular pacing, and the atria may be retrogradely activated by the impulse generated by the pacemaker. This occurs commonly in animals paced for sick sinus syndrome as AV nodal conduction is often preserved. Animals with persistent atrial standstill by definition are incapable of ventriculoatrial (VA) conduction. If VA conduction is possible, of course so is reciprocation and ventriculoatrial block (VA or retrograde AV block). Reciprocal beats occur when the impulse turns around within the AVN to reactivate the ventricles. Ventriculoatrial block may be of two types. Wenckebach VA block (Type I) is characterized by gradual prolongation of the V-P′ interval prior to failure of retrograde conduction, and Mobitz VA block (Type II) is random with fixed V-P′ intervals. If every-other-paced beat is followed by a retrograde P′ wave, then 2:1 VA block is present. If VA conduction is present during paced rhythm, it should alert the clinician to the possibility of triggered reentrant supraventricular tachyarrhythmias.

Paced fusion complexes Paced fusion complexes occur when the heart is simultaneously stimulated by a native impulse (typically supraventricular sinus) and a paced impulse. The "concertina effect" has been coined to describe the gradual progression (or regression) of ventricular fusion and may be seen when the native sinus rhythm is similar in rate to the preprogrammed paced rate (isorhythmic dissociation). The degree of narrowing of the QRS complex depends on the relative contributions of ventricular depolarization over the normal His-Purkinje network vs. that activated by the artificial ventricular pacemaker lead. Ventricular fusions that occur between right ventricular paced beats and ectopic ventricular premature complexes from the left ventricle may narrow the QRS complex since both ventricles are activated nearly simultaneously. This idea serves as the basis for cardiac resynchronization therapy and biventricular pacing.

Paced **pseudofusion** complexes occur when the pacing spike is superimposed on a native QRS complex; the stimulus is too late to cause true fusion, and the stimulus occurs during the native refractory period of the ventricles. Fusion and pseudofusion beats may be normal or abnormal, depending on how you look at it. Pseudofusion is never abnormal in of itself, but fusion is abnormal in the sense that it indicates ectopy if supraventricular capture is excluded. It is important for the clinician to

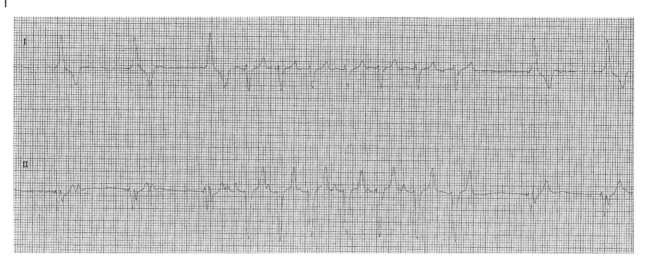

Figure 27.1 Paper speed 50 mm/s, 1 cm/mV, leads I and II, canine paced for SSS. Right ventricular paced rhythm is interrupted by SVT with aberrancy (RBBB). Initially, the QRS complexes are of LBBB-like morphology and preceded by small pacing spikes. **Ventriculoatrial conduction** is present with retrograde P′ wave in the T waves. **Supraventricular tachycardia** with alternation of P′ wave morphology on a beat-to-beat basis occurs consistent with a reentrant mechanism ensues. Following termination of the SVT, RV paced rhythm resumes.

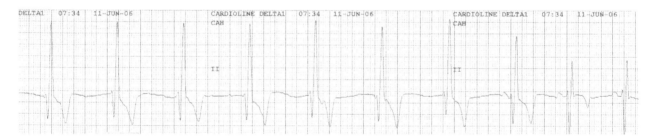

Figure 27.2 Paper speed 50 mm/s, 1 cm/mV, lead II, patient with SSS and VVIR bipolar pacing system. The first seven complexes are generated by the pacemaker with a HR of 100 bpm. The eighth complex is preceded by a sinus P wave, has a short P-R interval and a QRS intermediate in morphology between the paced beats and the following sinus beats, and is therefore a *paced fusion beat*. No atrial activity is noted prior to this complex, confirming abnormal sinus function. Paced fusion beats in VVI mode are common with SSS patients and *normal* since the atrial activity is not sensed by the device.

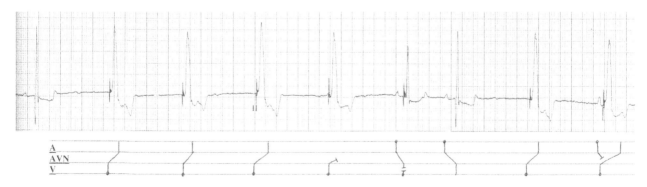

Figure 27.3 Paper speed 50 mm/s, 1 cm/mV, lead II, canine with SSS and VVIR bipolar pacing. VA conduction occurs for the first three paced beats. The fourth paced beat blocks in the AVN (*Wenckebach VA block*). The next complex (sixth) is a **paced fusion beat**. The last complex is paced but has a prolonged R′-P′ interval because a preceding sinus impulse delaying retrograde conduction through the AVN is initiated by the paced beat.

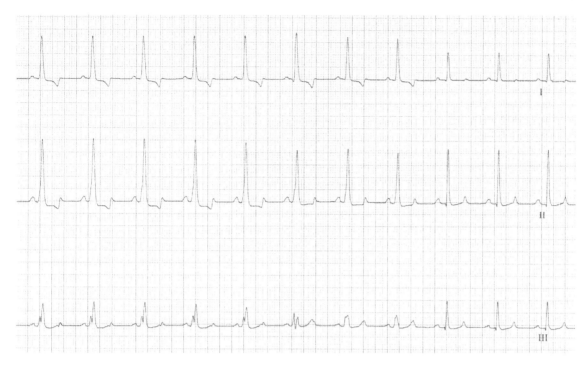

Figure 27.4 Paper speed 50 mm/s, 1 cm/mV, leads I, II, III, canine with bipolar pacemaker. Long periods of **paced fusion** resulted in complexes mimicking ventricular pre-excitation (short P-Ri, slurring of the upstroke of the R wave from the presence of a delta wave) from the so-called *concertina effect*. The sinus rate is very close to the preprogrammed LRL of the VVIR pacemaker, allowing for long periods where the sinus P waves precede the paced complexes, similar to that seen with accelerated idioventricular rhythms and isorhythmic dissociation. Note that the shorter the P-Ri, the more widened the QRS is from more activation of the ventricles by the pacemaker. The longer the P-Ri, the narrower the QRS becomes, as more of the ventricles are activated over the normal His-Purkinje system. The pacing spikes are very low amplitude. The last three complexes are entirely of sinus origin.

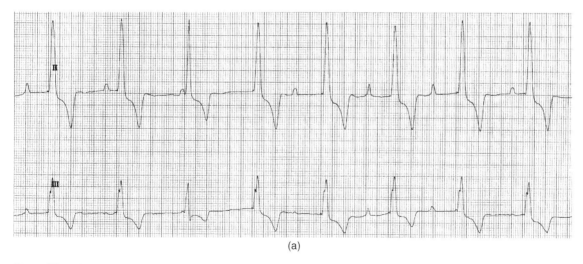

(a)

Figure 27.5a Paper speed 50 mm/s, 1 cm/mV, leads II and III, canine with bipolar pacemaker. Apparently complete AV dissociation is evident throughout the strip. The first and fourth to seventh visible P waves have plenty of time to conduct to the ventricles, but clearly fail to do so, consistent with third degree AV block. Very small pacing spikes are visible preceding each QRS complex, which are conducted with a LBBB-like morphology, consistent with an artificial pacemaker placed in the RV apex. The third QRS complex differs from the rest as it is slightly *narrower* than the rest. It *happens* to be preceded by a P wave, but at a P-Ri that is too short to indicate conduction (in the absence of an accessory pathway) and fails to interrupt the underlying ventricular rhythm, making a supraventricular capture unlikely.

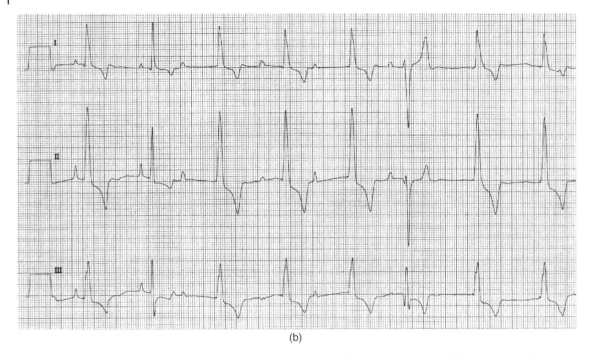

(b)

Figure 27.5b Paper speed 50 mm/s, 1 cm/mV, leads I, II, III, same dog. The second and sixth QRS complexes differ from the rest. The sixth QRS complex is premature, resets the pacemaker at the LRL (100 bpm or 0.6 second), is prolonged at 0.09 second, and is of RBBB-like morphology consistent with a VPC originating from the left ventricle. The second QRS complex is of more normal duration at 0.06 second and is "on time." This is consistent with a *ventricular fusion complex* between the focus producing the LVPC (complex # 6) and the underlying right ventricular paced rhythm. Fortuitous activation of both ventricles resulted in near-normal conduction and thus a narrow QRS complex. This indicated that the third QRS in the previous strip was also a ventricular fusion, albeit with more contribution from the artificial pacemaker than the ectopic LV focus. While it is tempting to explain these strips as a high-grade Type II second degree AVB with intermittent sinus captures and fusions with a RV pacemaker, careful examination of the P-R intervals reveals too much variation to be consistent with intermittent intact AV conduction.

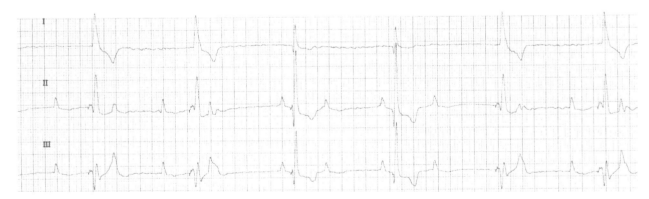

Figure 27.6 Paper speed 50 mm/s, 1 cm/mV, leads I, II, III, canine with high-grade AVB, VVIR bipolar pacing. The first two beats are paced. The third beat is sinus conducted, and a pacing spike is superimposed on the beginning of the QRS. The morphology of this QRS, however, is identical to that of the next sinus conducted beat, making this a **pseudofusion beat**. The sinus impulse immediately after the second sinus conducted beat is AV blocked, and the pacemaker takes over again.

remember that ventricular fusions are "on time" and do not interrupt the underlying ventricular rhythm whereas supraventricular captures during pacing would be expected to be premature and reset the rhythm at the lower rate limit (or at a slightly longer interval if hysteresis is in effect). Equally as important, the clinician should not mistake fusion/pseudofusion for pacemaker malfunction, especially undersensing (see Chapter 28).

Paced reciprocal complexes Intact VA conduction may permit reentry within the atrioventricular node and subsequent reactivation of the ventricular myocardium over the normal His-Purkinje system. The sequence is V-A-V. This is only possible if some AV nodal conduction is intact, so it is uncommonly seen in patients with antegrade AV block, and more likely in those with sick sinus syndrome.

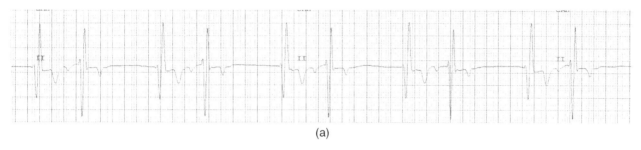

(a)

Figure 27.7a Paper speed 50 mm/s, 1 cm/mV, lead II, **VA conduction with** *reciprocal* **bigeminy**. Each paced beat is followed by a negative P′ wave and a reentrant or reciprocal beat (VAV conduction). The pacing spikes are not apparent due to bipolar pacing. The impulse originates in the RV apex, penetrates the AVN retrogradely to depolarize the atria as evidenced by the negative P′ waves. The impulse then reenters the AVN in an anterograde fashion to depolarize the ventricles again as evidenced by the narrower QRS complexes. VA conduction is more common in patients with SSS, which is what this patient had and may predispose to pacemaker syndrome.

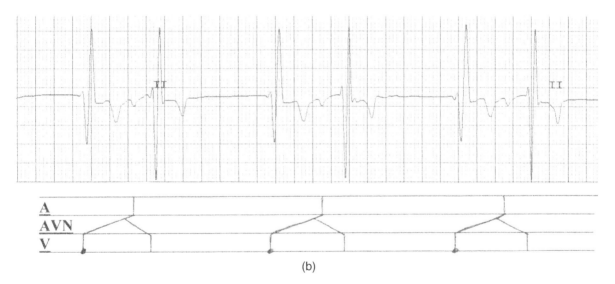

(b)

Figure 27.7b Paper speed 50 mm/s, 1 cm/mV, lead II, ladder diagram of the same patient, illustrating the reentrant mechanism of the reciprocal beats. The VAi is approximately 0.24 second which would be expected to constitute *first degree ventriculoatrial block* – though normal VA conduction times in small animals are not really established. A long VAi promotes reentry, resulting in reciprocal complexes here as seen.

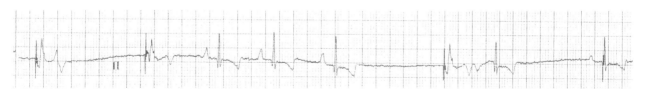

Figure 27.8 Paper speed 50 mm/s, 1 cm/mV, lead II, canine paced for SSS. The first beat is paced with a native P wave superimposed (and not conducted) within the S-T segment. The second beat is paced, followed by three sinus beats. The sixth beat is paced, is followed by a retrograde P′ wave, and a reciprocal beat follows.

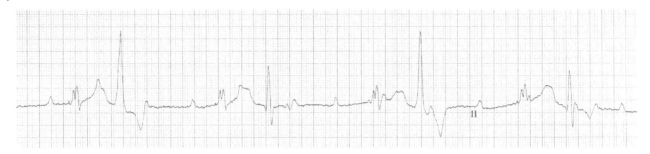

Figure 27.9 Paper speed 50 mm/s, 1 cm/mV, lead II, canine paced for third degree AVB. Sinus rhythm of the atria is interrupted and reset by reciprocal beats, R ventricular paced rhythm of the ventricles, **reciprocal bigeminy with** *alternating* **aberrancy**. The first complex is paced, which is followed by a retrograde P′ wave within the T wave and is then followed by a QRS with LBBB aberrancy. The third beat is again paced, but this time it is followed by a reciprocal beat with normal duration. The sixth beat has less aberrancy than beat #2. The earlier the reciprocal QRS is, the more likely BBB is. This is an example of phase 3 or acceleration-dependent BBB. Despite the fact that this patient has anterograde complete AVB, retrograde conduction is intact, and the formation of reciprocal beats is possible occasionally in such patients.

Further reading

Barold, S.E., Linhart, J.W., and Samet, P. (1968). Reciprocal beating induced by ventricular pacing. *Circulation* XXXVIII: 330–340.

28

Pacemakers

Trouble

CHAPTER MENU

Undersensing, 363
Oversensing, 363
Failure to capture, 363
Battery depletion, 367
Pacemaker-mediated tachycardia, 367
Pacemaker syndrome, 367

Malfunctions of pacemaker systems include abnormal pacing rates/rhythms from under/oversensing, loss of capture, and battery depletion. Complications of pacing itself also include the so-called pacemaker syndrome and pacemaker-mediated tachycardia (PMT). External interference of pacing systems may occur with transthoracic electrical cardioversion, electrocautery, and magnetic resonance imaging. Ringing (or ring) artifact creating fine oscillations where sharp transitions happen (usually in the S-T segment) may occur from notch filters used to remove 50 or 60 Hz noise and tends to be worse on EKG monitoring equipment used during surgery. Pacemaker-mediated tachycardia typically occurs with oversensing retrograde P′ waves from ventriculoatrial conduction or tracking of atrial tachyarrhythmias in dual-chamber pacemakers (DDD mode) and is thus uncommon in small animals. Pacemaker syndrome results from chronic loss of atrioventricular synchrony.

Undersensing

Undersensing occurs when the pacing system fails to respond to native complexes appropriately and may occur with native QRS electrograms of low amplitude, lead displacement, low-voltage ventricular ectopics, electrolyte imbalance, lead or insulation fracture, inappropriate programming, component failure, or drug effects. The blanking period is typically set at 25–100 msec after a pacing spike in which no events are deliberately sensed.

Oversensing

Oversensing is a major cause of intermittent pauses and is due to automatic delay from inappropriate inhibition. T-waves, muscle fasciculations, atrial depolarization in association with right ventricular outflow tract lead displacement, etc., may all be sensed inappropriately as native QRS complexes, inhibiting firing of the pacemaker. Oversensing was most common in association with unipolar pacing systems. Loose connections or partial lead fractures may be to blame. The refractory period is programmed to adjust to the patient's Q-T interval. If it is too long, the unit would not sense premature beats and may sense the T waves. Oversensing is not uncommon in the immediate period following pacemaker implantation and typically resolves following recovery from anesthesia.

Failure to capture

Loss of capture or failure to capture may be identified on EKG as regular pacing spikes at the correct interval without expected paced QRS complexes and may occur due to exit block, elevation of pacing threshold, lead displacement, unstable lead position, and/or myocardial perforation. Lead dislodgement may not always result in failure to capture as displacement into the right atrium may be associated with atrial pacing. "Hysteresis" (also known as Wedensky's effect) is a function of many units. Testing is done from capture to the loss of capture (vs. the other way around). It requires greater energy to regain capture. This is a feature of some pacemakers that give the heart "a chance" if the R-R interval falls below that of the preprogrammed lower rate limit, only occurs after a sensed ventricular event, and lengthens battery life. It is important for the clinician not to confuse hysteresis with failure to capture. Hysteresis is typically

Interpretation of the Electrocardiogram in Small Animals, First Edition. Nick A. Schroeder.
© 2021 John Wiley & Sons Inc. Published 2021 by John Wiley & Sons Inc.

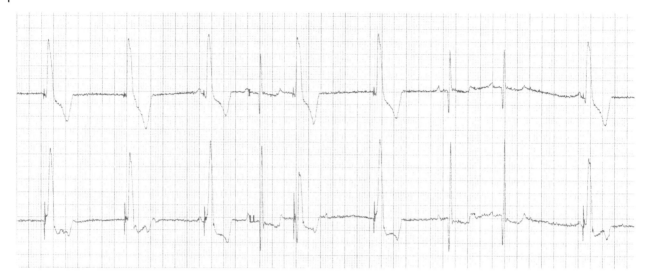

Figure 28.1 Paper speed 50 mm/s, 1 cm/mV, leads I and II, canine implanted with a VVIR (80–140 bpm) bipolar pacemaker. **Undersensing**. The fourth complex is sinus and apparently not sensed by the pacemaker. The fifth complex is a paced beat, and it occurs exactly at the same interval following the previous paced beat. The instantaneous HR between the fourth and fifth complexes is approximately 150 bpm – over the upper rate limit (URL) of the pacemaker. The morphology of the fifth complex is slightly different than that of the other paced beats likely secondary to the preceding (and not sensed) sinus beat. The lead in this dog was not in the RV apex and likely tangled in the chordae tendinae of the tricuspid valve, possibly contributing to intermittent and insignificant contact failure, since the pacemaker is able to capture the ventricles as programmed.

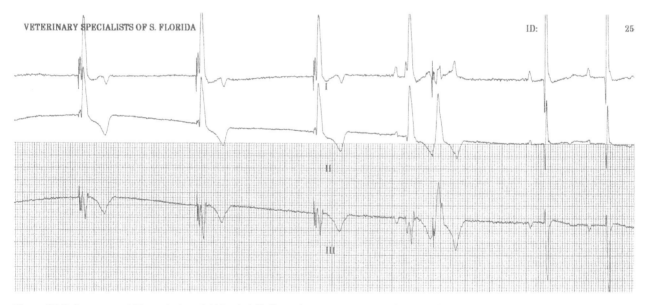

Figure 28.2 Paper speed 50 mm/s, 1 cm/mV, leads I, II, III, canine post-pacemaker implantation for SSS, mode VVIR. The first three beats are paced. The fourth complex is preceded by a sinus P wave, has a short P-R interval, and a wide/bizarre complex consistent with a ventricular **fusion beat**. The pacemaker fires right after this on time with the preceding paced beats, indicating that the unit *failed* to sense the ectopic beat. The resultant ventricular complex (#5) is different than the previous paced complexes (likely due to aberrant conduction induced by the preceding VPC). This manifestation of **undersensing** is not likely to be a problem since it occurred following an unusual beat. The last two complexes are sinus captures.

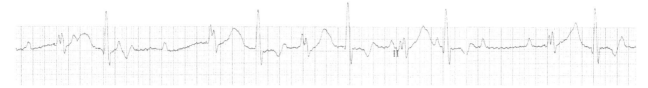

Figure 28.3 Paper speed 50 mm/s, 1 cm/mV, lead II, canine. Right ventricular paced rhythm and reciprocal bigeminy. **Undersensing** of the reciprocal beats occurs after the fourth complex and resolves spontaneously after the eighth complex.

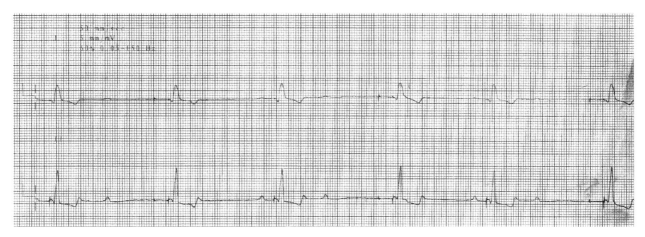

Figure 28.4 Paper speed 50 mm/s, 0.5 cm/mV, leads I and II, canine with dual leads (RA and RV leads), DDD. **Undersensing** *and* **failure to capture**. The first complex is VPaced, followed by an unsensed native P wave (not followed by a preprogrammed VPace), which is then followed by an atrial spike with failure to capture the atria. This is followed by a VPaced beat (beat # 3) at a preprogrammed P-Ri. Failure to capture the atrial myocardium suggests lead dislodgement (common with atrial leads) and the undersensing of native atrial depolarization is likely associated.

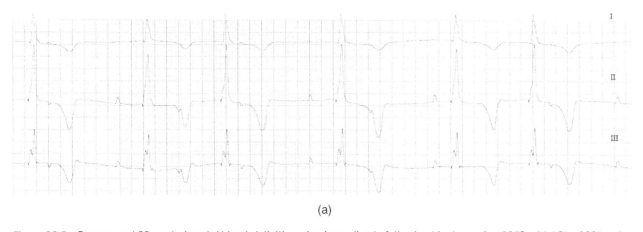

(a)

Figure 28.5a Paper speed 50 mm/s, 1 cm/mV, leads I, II, III, canine immediately following bipolar pacing (VVIR with LRL of 90 bpm). **Oversensing**. The irregular rhythm is secondary to the unit oversensing the T waves. The longer pauses are caused by resetting of the pacemaker from the deeper T waves. Note the incredibly long Q-Ti (0.45 second) with deep T waves that are at least 2 mV in amplitude (in precordial leads). The generator was preprogrammed with a sensing amplitude of 1.5 mV. These changes to the QRS were anesthesia-associated. Note **VA conduction** with retrograde P' waves following the paced QRS complexes. Whenever a sinus impulse occurs before a paced impulse, VA conduction is *delayed* (beats #2 and #4) or even *blocked* altogether (beat #5, consistent with *possible* retrograde Wenckebach block – progressive R-Ri prolongation prior to failure of conduction associated with progressive T wave amplitude increase and subsequent VA block). The tallest T waves (QRS-T complexes with the longest R-P' interval) are oversensed as a native QRS, delaying the following ventricular pacing stimulus, creating group beating and a trigeminal ventricular rhythm.

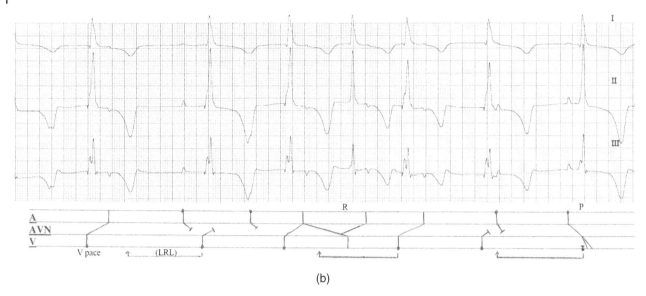

(b)

Figure 28.5b Paper speed 50 mm/s, 1 cm/mV, leads I, II, III, same dog. The ladder diagram illustrates an alternative mechanism of oversensing. The LRL (lower rate limit) period indicates the generator is sensing the first and third complex's T waves. The first and third complexes also have VA conduction, producing a **reciprocal beat** (fourth beat, narrow QRS labeled "R"), which is not recognized by the generator (**undersensing**). The next paced beat should have occurred following the predetermined LRL after the reciprocal complex. The last complex (labeled "P") is a pseudo-fusion beat (native beat with LBBB aberration with superimposition of the pacing spike on the QRS). True fusion is unlikely given the absence of a pacing spike right before the QRS complex. The pacemaker appears to have been oversensing the terminal portion of the QRS of sixth complex (coincidentally with the native P wave), since the delay before the next impulse is longer than expected for the LRL.

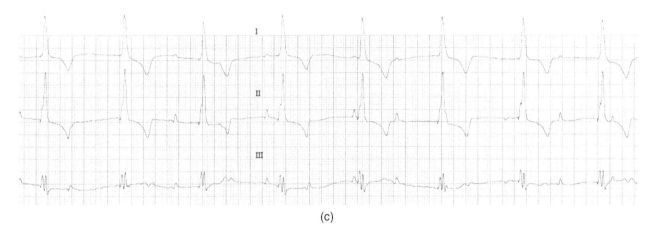

(c)

Figure 28.5c Paper speed 50 mm/s, 1 cm/mV, leads I, II, III, same dog following recovery. AV dissociation, AV block, and ventricular paced rhythm at 90 bpm (LRL). No oversensing is occurring. Note the Q-Ti has shortened, and the T waves are not as deep. No adjustments to the pacemaker were ultimately necessary.

used in patients with some native capture (i.e. incomplete high-grade second degree AVB or sick sinus syndrome with intact AV conduction). Some terms are important to understand regarding pacing capture. Rheobase is the lowest voltage that results in capture at an infinitely long pulse duration. Chronaxie is pulse width required to stimulate the heart at twice the rheobase voltage (approximates the point of minimum threshold energy). Thresholds are performed at pacemaker interrogation in order to determine this minimum threshold energy. Rising thresholds may lead to failure to capture, may be encountered for a short period immediately following pacemaker implantation from myocardial inflammation/fibrosis, and can be ameliorated by using steroid-eluting lead tips.

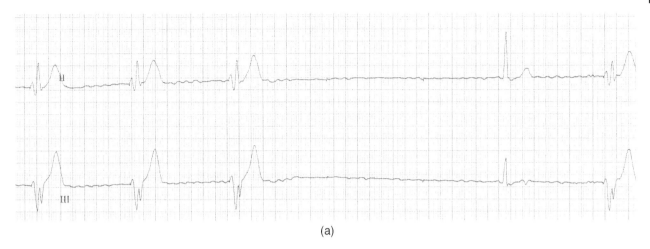

(a)

Figure 28.6a Paper speed 50 mm/s, 1 cm/mV, leads II and III, canine paced for high-grade second degree AVB. **Failure to capture**. Atrial fibrillation is evident on the baseline. The first three complexes are paced. A long pause in the rhythm is caused by failure to capture. A supraventricular capture terminates the pause, and the pacemaker again captures the ventricles with the last complex. This dog had concurrent pancreatitis and the inflammation presumably traversed the diaphragm, affecting the ventricle, thus interfering with the pacing system. Interestingly, this dog also had mild pleural effusion and no overt echocardiographic evidence of right-sided congestive heart failure (giving more weight to the suggestion that inflammation from the pancreatitis was the underlying issue vs. a lead dislodgement).

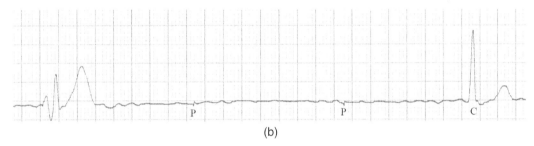

(b)

Figure 28.6b Paper speed 50 mm/s, 1 cm/mV, lead II, same dog. Close-up of the same strip. Loss of capture is evidenced by the presence of two very small pacing spikes without an associated ventricular QRS (labeled P). The pause is terminated by a native supraventricular capture beat (labeled C).

Battery depletion Abnormal pacing rates may occur with end of battery life (reversion to a lower pacing interval) or the deliberate application of a magnet (return to VVO pacing). This is rare in paced small animals as the likelihood of a dog or cat outliving expected battery life of an implanted pacemaker tends to be low.

Pacemaker-mediated tachycardia This may rarely occur in patients paced with DDD systems and AV sequential pacing. If the patient has intact ventriculoatrial conduction, which is more common in patients paced for sick sinus syndrome, then the atrial lead may sense retrograde P′ waves and trigger a ventricular paced beat following a predetermined interval, setting up a circuit (antidromic reentry). Rarely, atrial sensing of ventricular pacing may result in orthodromic reentry. Programming

appropriate postventricular atrial refractory period intervals can prevent this. If the patient has a dual chamber pacing system (DDD) and subsequently develops an irregularly irregular rhythm, then tracking of atrial fibrillation should be suspected. Mode switching option may not be activated, which is exacerbated by atrial undersensing. Though this is not technically a malfunction, the system should be reprogrammed to VVIR as chronic pacing at the upper rate limit may occur.

Pacemaker syndrome This occurs from decreased cardiac output and blood pressure that usually result from the loss of AV sequential pacing and is exacerbated by VA conduction. It may be contributed to by increased pulmonary arterial and venous pressures. Pacemaker syndrome is diagnosed if clinical signs of congestive heart failure resolve with restoration of AV sequential pacing. In humans, the diagnosis is implied if a greater than 20 mmHg drop in blood pressure occurs with the onset of ventricular pacing. The diagnosis is suspected in dogs if the blood pressure drops immediately with ventricular pacing and persists after 30 seconds. The ideal treatment is implantation of a dual chamber pacemaker. If the atrial and ventricular rates are similar despite the complete AVD seen with third degree AVB following pacing, then pacemaker syndrome is expected to be unlikely.

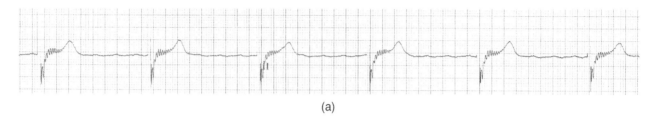

(a)

Figure 28.7a Paper speed 50 mm/s, 1 cm/mV, lead II, previously paced feline presented with acute lethargy. **Third degree AVB, atrial flutter or focal atrial tachycardia, and ventricular paced rhythm** of approximately 63 bpm, indicative of **battery depletion**. The lower rate limit (LRL) of this cat's pacemaker was originally set at 100 bpm, and a decrease in rate is a programmed signal designed to occur when the battery is low. Fine, sawtoothed undulations of the baseline at approximately 400 bpm indicate atrial flutter or tachycardia, which was confirmed on echocardiography (see below).

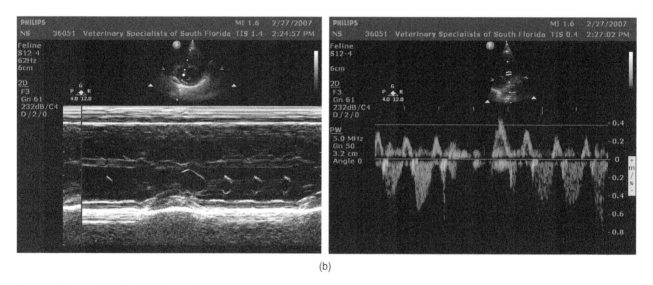

(b)

Figure 28.7b Echocardiographs of the same cat. To the left, M-mode of the LV and mitral valve shows repetitive diastolic opening of the mitral valve coincident with atrial systole. To the right, pulsed wave of the mitral inflow shows discreet A waves occurring at a spontaneous rate of approximately 336 bpm, consistent with AFL. Atrial flutter, due to the presence of atrial contractions, may put the patient at slightly less risk of thromboembolism than those with atrial fibrillation. One large E wave is seen in the middle of the tracing (following ventricular systole initiated by the pacemaker). Diastolic mitral regurgitation occurs following each atrial systole as well (common with third degree AVB).

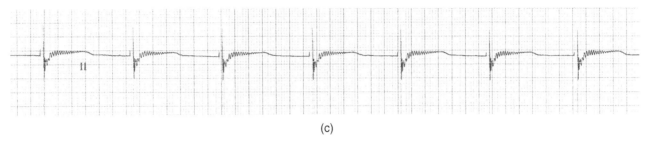

(c)

Figure 28.7c Paper speed 50 mm/s, 1 cm/mV, lead II, same cat following generator replacement. The ventricular rate is now 90 bpm, and the **Q-T interval** is long due to anesthesia.

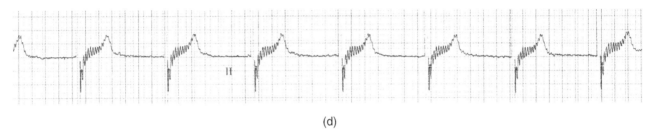

(d)

Figure 28.7d Paper speed 50 mm/s, 1 cm/mV, lead II, same cat, the day after reimplantation. The Q-T interval has improved. **60-cycle interference ("ringing") artifact** is present within the S-T segment.

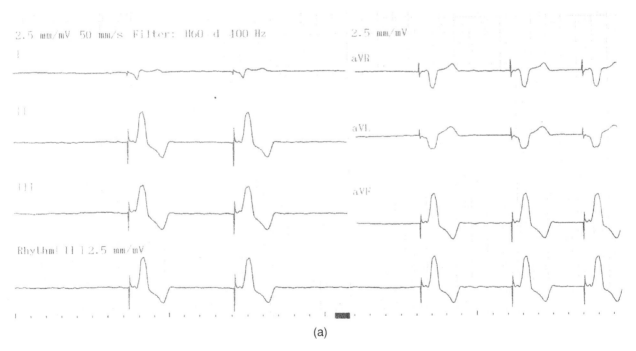

(a)

Figure 28.8a Paper speed 50 mm/s, 0.25 cm/mV, full EKG, canine. **Tracking of atrial fibrillation**. This patient had a DDD system with atrial sensing. The ventricular rhythm is irregularly irregular and fine undulations of the baseline consistent with atrial fibrillation are present.

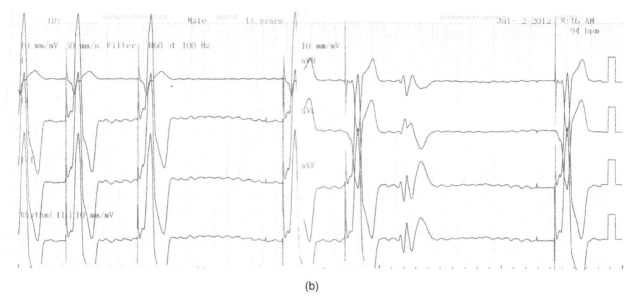

(b)

Figure 28.8b Paper speed 50 mm/s, 1 cm/mV, full EKG, same dog. The increased sensitivity here reveals atrial undersensing and failure to capture as the atrial lead apparently fails to sense fibrillatory waves and vainly attempts to pace the atria. A small atrial pacing spike is visualized immediately preceding the fourth and seventh complexes, which are Vpaced. The sixth complex is a VPC. The slower ventricular rate here and evidence of at least intermittent atrial undersensing show that the tracking of atrial fibrillation in this individual was incomplete. This patient's pacemaker was subsequently reprogrammed to V'VIR.

Further reading

Alasti, M., Machado, C., Rangasamy, K. et al. (2018). Pacemaker-mediated arrhythmias. *J. Arrhythmia* 34 (5).

Hesselson, A.B. (2003). *Simplified Interpretation of Pacemaker ECGs*. Futura.

Moses, H.W., Miller, B.D., Moulton, K.P., and Schneider, J.A. (2000). *A Practical Guide to Cardiac Pacing*, 5e. Lippincott Williams & Wilkins.

Rishniw, M., Brownell, L.D., Jetton, J. et al. (2014). ECG of the month. *JAVMA* 244 (11): 1258–1259.

Surawicz, B. and Knilans, T.K. (2001). *Chou's Electrocardiography in Clinical Practice: Adult and Pediatric*, 5e. Saunders.

Thomason, J.D., Fallaw, T.L., and Calvert, C.A. (2008). ECG of the month. *JAVMA* 233 (9): 1406–1408.

Index

a

aberrancy **43–92**
  atrial 43–50, 52, 54
  rate-dependent 43, 45, 55, 60, 61,
    64, 67, 69–71, 83, 89, 95, 133,
    159, 160, 166, 202, 273
  ventricular 43, 47, 55, 59–61, 69,
    80, 85, 87–89, 94, 96, 131, 133,
    139, 140, 151, 157–159, 193,
    196, 201–204, 206, 212, 213,
    219–221, 224, 251, 259,
    262–264, 273, 283, 286, 291,
    298, 299, 301–303, 312, 313,
    328, 362
absolute ventricular arrhythmia *96*,
  196, 197
accelerated atrial rhythm 106, 139,
  158, **166**, 167
accelerated junctional rhythm 240,
  267, **270**–273, 275, 282
  accelerated idiojunctional rhythm
    94, 205–207, 224, 270, 271,
    273–276, 320
accelerated ventricular rhythm 257,
  316, 319, 320, 324
  accelerated idioventricular rhythm
    68, 178, 205, 219, 246, 256, 258,
    276, 284, 314, **319**–323, 325,
    327–329, 347, 359
    bidirectional **325**, 328
    polymorphic **325**, 327
accrochage 220, 226, 227, 246, 254,
  258, 274, 322, 323
albuterol 28
allorhythmia *8*, *96*, 112, 141, 213,
  223, 246, 262, 267, 287, 297
amiodarone 330
amplitudes **7**
anemia 38, 320
antidromic 87, 95, 111, 119, 140, 164,
  180, 186, 204, 210, 212, 278
aortic stenosis 23

arborization block 44, 77, **86**
arrhythmogenic cardiomyopathy 68,
  292, 315, 336, 337
artifact
  baseline 3, 8, 105, 155, 160, 172,
    174, 194, 260, 330
  60-cycle interference 369
  double QRS 221
  panting 105, 108, 127, 194, 242,
    330
  purring 78, 84, 145, 194, 195, 310
  ringing 194, 363, 369
Ashman's phenomenon 44, **55**,
  57–59, 61, 67, 140, 157, 158,
  168, 180, 187, 188, 193, 196,
  201–203, 244, 298, 301, 303
asthenic habitus 17, 78, 80
asystole 79, 81, 93, 94, 96, 97, 100,
  101, 103, 111, **114**–116, 123,
  126, 128, 132, 148, 205, 208,
  229, 247, 252, 257, 283, 285,
  288, **289**, 290, 292, 343, 351
atenolol 70, 215
atrial dissociation 166, **171**–174, 188,
  200
atrial fibrillation 12, 34, 36, 38, 40,
  46, 59, 60, 70, 75, 79, 83, 87,
  94–96, 123, 126, 128, 130, 140,
  141, 147, 153, 159, 173, 174,
  181, 187, 188, 192, **196**–**209**,
  231, 245, 246, 253, 264, 270,
  272, 273, 277, 278, 291, 295,
  302, 304, 305, 312, 315,
  318–320, 322, 325–327, 335,
  340, 342, 347, 356, 367, 369, 370
  aberrancy 91, **201**–207
atrial flutter 46, 47, 59, 84, 90, 95, 96,
  105, 123, 127, 129, 130, 140,
  166, 171, 172, **187**–**195**, 197,
  200, 208, 236, 244, 245, 254,
  276, 278, 298, 301–303, 305,
  340, 355, 368

  atypical 188
  reverse typical ("true atypical")
    140, 188, 191, 194
  Type I 187, 189, 190, 192, 193
  Type II 188, 192
  typical atrial flutter 187
atrial muscular dystrophy 139, 141,
  145, 148
atrial premature complexes **151**–**165**
  aberrant atrial premature
    complexes 157
  left atrial premature complexes
    151
  multifocal atrial premature
    complexes 153
  right atrial premature complexes
    151
atrial septal defect 55
atrial standstill 8, 27, 28, 33, 96, 117,
  123, 126, 130, 139, **141**, 143,
  145, 147–149, 216, 219, 253,
  272, 273, 278, 287, 319, 349,
  351, 357
atrioventricular block 27, 32, 47, 92,
  93, 100, 103, 112, 115–117, 123,
  124, 127, 129, 135, 139, 140,
  144, 154, 166, 169, 187, 193,
  197, 211–213, 216, 218, 219,
  223, 224, 227, **228**–**258**, 261,
  283, 293, 301, 302, 307, 311,
  321, 323, 349, 351, 356
  antegrade 228, 349
  complete 197, 207, 218, 221, 224,
    227, 228, *248*, 251, 252, 254,
    301, 323
  first degree 27, 32, 112, 124, 127,
    129, 135, 139, 154, 212, 228,
    229, 293, 307
  high grade 129, 217, 228, **235**, **241**,
    256, 302
  incomplete 228, *231*, 287
  low grade **231**, **240**

Interpretation of the Electrocardiogram in Small Animals, First Edition. Nick A. Schroeder.
© 2021 John Wiley & Sons Inc. Published 2021 by John Wiley & Sons Inc.

atrioventricular block (*contd.*)
  paroxysmal   212, 228, 229, **247**, 349, 351
  retrograde   229, 256, 271
  second degree   96, 115, 117, 212, 216, 218, 219, 223, 224, **231**, 258, 261, 283, 295, 311, 349, 351
  third degree   47, 216, 218, 223, 224, 228, **248**, 258, 283, 349
  2:1   103, 116, **234**, **240**
atrioventricular dissociation   27, 87, 94–*96*, 100, 103, 104, 139, 140, 196, 197, **204**, 205, 207, 211, 212, 216, 218, 221, 224, 227, 228, 249, 251, 252, **253**–255, 270, 273, 274, 276, 282–284, 290, 293, 319, **320**, **321**, 328, 330, 332, 337, 341
atrioventricular nodal reentrant tachycardia   95, 175, 212, 270, **278**, 279, 281
  antidromic atrioventricular nodal reentrant tachycardia   212, 278
  orthodromic atrioventricular nodal reentrant tachycardia   212, 278
atrioventricular reentrant tachycardia   38, 95, 140, 162, 175, **179**, 182
  antidromic atrioventricular reentrant tachycardia   180
  orthodromic atrioventricular reentrant tachycardia   179
atrioventricular septal defect (see also *endocardial cushion defect*)   77, 83
automatic atrial tachycardia   139, **166**, 167, 169, 197, 277
  left atrial tachycardia   139, 166
  multifocal atrial tachycardia   139
  right atrial tachycardia   166
automatic junctional tachycardia   212, 270, **276**, 277, 321

b

Bartonella,   38
battery depletion   350, 363, **367**, 368
Bayés syndrome   26, 46, 54
biatrial abnormality   1, 16, **19**
bifascicular block   21, 23, 44, 62, 77, **79**, 80–82, 178, 246
bigeminy   *95, 96*

atrial   56, 88, 96, 103, 110, 117, 139, 141, 142, 151, **156**, 159, 163, 167, 214, 279
  double   298, 300, 306, 308
  escape-capture bigeminy   96
    atrial   125, 126, 139, **141**–143, 156
    junctional   211, **213**, 215, 216, 232
    sinoatrial   100, 103, **112**, 113, 119
    ventricular   283, 285, **287**
  escape-echo bigeminy   22, 96, 223, 277
  junctional   212, 259, **262**, 277, 300
  sinoatrial/sinus   69, 100, 103, **112**, 113, 117, 119, 133–135, 138
  ventricular   47, 59, 73, 177, 187, 203, 243, 245, 250, 264, 283, 287, 291, **298**, 299–306, 308–310, 312, 315, 318, 325, 328, 329, 333, 335, 336, 342, 355
bilateral bundle branch block   68, 77, **79**, 241, 248, 283
biventricular enlargement   1, 9, 16, **23**, 199
Bix rule   187–189
block/acceleration dissociation   219, 220, 228, **242**, 245, 246, 256, 320, 321
brachycephalic syndrome   105, 231
Brody effect   38–40, 95, 213, 214, 248
Brugada syndrome   36, 41, 174
bundle of Kent   175, 176, 209

c

capture   *94*
chemodectoma (also see *heart-based mass*)   36, 155, 189, 258
chronic mitral valvular disease   16, 18, 28, 32, 39, 90, 91, 129, 193, 197, 201
chronic tricuspid valvular disease   21
Chung's phenomenon   44, 45, **47**–51, 53, 54, 58, 95, 141, 298
compensatory-like pause   70, 83, 188, 203, 208, 291, **295**, 301, 303–305, 315
compensatory pause   64, 95, 108, 154, 155, 160, 233, 252, 257, 260–262, 283, 291, **293**, 294–299, 301, 305, 309, 312–315, 317, 331, 337
complete atrioventricular block   197, 227, 301, 323

complete left bundle branch block   23, 44, 67, **68**, 69, 71, 73, 75
complete right bundle branch block   21, 44, 55, **62**, 63, 65
concealed conduction   52, 93, 96, 140, 151, 154, 158, 161, 188, 196, 201, **207**, 208, 212, 233, 259, **263**, 284, 291, 293, 295, **309**, 311, 313, 349, **357**
  concealed junctional extrasystoles   96, 238, 266, 269
  concealed ventricular bigeminy   291, 306, **309**, 310
  concealed ventricular trigeminy   291, **310**
concertina effect   177, 186, 323, 357, 359
congestive heart failure   19, 39, 86, 104, 128, 129, 131, 136, 175, 181, 197, 198, 202, 208, 237, 243, 248, 249, 267, 272, 277, 297, 335, 367
cor pulmonale   19
Cushing's response/CNS ischemic response   27, 31, **34**

d

defibrillation   116, 288, 289, 346, 347, 349
delta wave   6, 7, 90, 175, 176, 178, 179, 182, 259, 311
dextrocardia   13
dextropositioning   13, 14
Dietz-Marques phenomenon   172
digoxin
  effects   1, 27, **32**
  toxicity   32, 33, 59, 121, 166, 172, 202, 203, 205, 207, 223, 230, 271–273, 275, 276, 320, 333, 340
dilated cardiomyopathy   23, 40, 68, 79, 86, 90, 181, 201, 248, 337
diltiazem   34, 130, 171, 172, 181, 183, 187, 189–191, 205, 207, 273, 281, 325, 326
double nodal rhythms   223, 224, 226
double tachycardia   207, 256, 276, 284, 312, 319, 330, **340**, 341, 347
doxorubicin   248
Dressler's beats   311

e

early afterdepolarization   93, 301
early repolarization   1, 16, **24**–26, 30, 36

Ebstein's anomaly 17, 90, 179, 181

echo beat 133, 163, 269, 298, 314, 315

electrical alternans 2, 27, **38**–41, 170, 180, 181, 184, 189, 199, 227, 230, 280, 321, 331, 333, 339

electromechanical dissociation 255, 283, 285, **288**, 289

endocardial cushion defect (see also *atrioventricular septal defect*) 77, 83

epsilon wave 6, 7

escape beats 47, 60, 62, *94,* 103, 105, 106, 108, 118, 119, 141–143, 193, 205, 208, 213–215, 217, 219, 223, 231, 236, 244, 250, 251, 254, 256, 285–287, 292, 301–303, 307, 308, 311

    atrial 49, 118, 119, 124, 126, **141**–143, 241, 307, 308

    junctional 104, 177, **213**, 214, 222, 223, 237, 271

    sinoatrial **112**

    ventricular 60, 80, 108, 115, 124, 208, **285**–287, 292, 311

escape rhythm 28, 33, 46, 47, 50, 52, 79, 81, 82, 84–86, 96, 104, 107, 108, 114, 118, 124, 125, 127, 130, 134, 141, 143, 144, 148, 149, 166, 194, 197, 205, 206, 211, 213, 216–221, 223–226, 242–249, 252–257, 265, 270, 276, 283, 285, 287, 288, 302, 303, 321, 334, 343, 349

    atrial 50, 107, 124, 139, **141**, 143, 166

    junctional 33, 82, 104, 148, 194, 205, 206, 211, 213, **216**–224, 226, 248, 249, 253, 256, 257, 270, 276, 334

    ventricular 28, 47, 79, 81, 84, 86, 108, 114, 125, 127, 148, 149, 194, 205, 206, 216, 219, 225, 243, 245, 249, 253, 256, 265, 283, 285, **287**, 288, 302, 321

exit block 94, 100, 117, 121, 123, 126, 128, 131, 139, 171, 172, 208, 211, 212, 217, 223, 228, 229, 247, **257**, 271, 278, 283, 284, 293, 309, 310, 319, 328, 338–340, 363

extrasystole 95

f

failure to capture 350, **363**, 365–367, 370

false poling 1, 3, **12**, 13

fascicular premature complexes 156, 292, 295

fascicular tachycardia **333**

fibrillo-flutter

    atrial 188, 200

    ventricular 319, 345, 346

first degree atrioventricular block 27, 32, 46, 61, 62, 67–69, 75, 84, 86, 94, 95, 109, 110, 112, 118, 124, 127, 129, 134, 135, 139, 154, 155, 170, 212, 218, 228, **229**–233, 236–239, 263, 281, 293, 296–298, 307, 313, 337

first degree bundle branch block 43

first degree exit block 257

first degree interatrial block 18, 45

first degree sinoatrial block 117, 154

Frederick syndrome 194, 253

fusion complexes *94*

    atrial fusion complexes 45, 47–51, 54, 106, 139, 151, 153, **162**, 163, 165, 171, 212, 259, 264, 266–269, 284, 291, 313, 315, 316

    paced fusion complexes 349, **357**–359

    paced pseudofusion complexes 349, **357**, 360, 361

    ventricular fusion complexes 61, 64, 67, 68, 72, 73, 87, 113, 139, 157, 175, 178–180, 204, 220, 246, 254, 257, 284, 286, 291, 295, 302, **311**, 312, 315, 317, 319, 323, 325, 329, 332, 349, 360, 364

g

gap phenomenon 159, 234

group beating 43, 93, *96,* 117, 118, 189, 231, 232, 234, 246, 257, 273, 278, 338, 339, 365

h

Hay 240

heart-based mass (also see *chemodectoma*) 36, 155, 189, 258

heartworm 19, 220

hemangiosarcoma 63, 320, 321

horizontal axis 1, 3, 16, **23**, 24

hypercalcemia 28, 30

hyperkalemia **28**–30, 77, 103, 104, 139, **141**, 144, 147, 288, 331, 345

hypermagnesemia 29

hypertrophic cardiomyopathy 23, 77, 84, 175, 223

hypocalcemia 29, 30, 40

hypokalemia 1, 6, 17, 27, **28**, 29, 40, 288, 342

hypomagnesemia 28, 29

hypothermia 1, 6, 27, 29, 32, 197, 274, 288

hypoxia 5, 6, 35, 36, 127, 243, 288

i

incomplete left bundle branch block **67**, 68, 70, 78, 85, 90, 223, 280, 337

incomplete right bundle branch block **55**, 56–59, 61, 62, 66, 90, 207, 264

indeterminate axis **24**

interatrial block **18**–20, 26, **45**–47, 53, 54, 93, 124, 126

interatrial reentrant tachycardia **171**

interference 96, 194, 282, 298, 320, 363, 369

interpolation/interponation 27, 56, 100, 133, 139, 151, **154**, 203, 259, **260**, 261, 278, 283, 291, 295, **296**, 309, 313–315, 317

intervals 1, 3, **5**, **6**

interventricular conduction disturbance 19, 23, 28, 43, **90**–92, 199, 201

intra-atrial block 18, 26, 44–46, 54, 95, 276

ischemia 4, 6, 27, 29, 33–37, 41, 202

isorhythmic dissociation 94, 104, 211, 212, 220, 221, 246, 248, 249, 255, 270, 274–277, 284, 321–323, 357, 359

j

James bundles/fibers (Atrio-His) 175, 178, 262, 271

J-point 24, 35, 36, 41

junctional dissociation 211, 213, **223**–226

junctional premature complexes 94, 96, 131, 157, 204, 212, 256, **259**–**269**

junctional tachycardia 47, 206, 212, 227, 240, 256, 258, 269, **270**–**282**

k

Kent bundle   175, 176, 311
Killip's rule   197, 198

l

late afterdepolarization   93
leads   1, **3**, 4
left anterior fascicular block   23, 40,
        44, 67, **77**, 78–83, 85, 86, 136,
        176, 178, 203, 220, 221, 245,
        246, 280, 281, 292, 300, 333
left atrial abnormality   1, 16, **17**
left axis deviation   9, 12, 16, 21, 23,
        28, 77, 78, 81–83, 144, 146, 200
left bundle branch block   23, 28, 44,
        46, 53, 55, 56, 62, **67–76**, 80, 81,
        83–85, 87–90, 115, 130, 149,
        157, 159, 160, 202–204, 206,
        217, 219, 223, 231, 250, 251,
        275, 280, 283, 285, 286, 292,
        300, 302, 303, 307, 312, 315,
        321, 328, 336, 337, 341,
        351–353, 355, 358, 359, 362, 366
left medial fascicular block   40, 60,
        77–79, 157, 213, 214, 263
left posterior fascicular block   21, 44,
        55, 62, 64, 77, **78**–83, 85, 109,
        226, 293, 300, 333
left ventricular enlargement   1, 9, 11,
        13, 16, **22**, 28, 40, 67, 111, 124,
        168, 197, 201, 273
left ventricular hypertrophy   12, 20,
        22–24, 29–31, 66–68, 80, 83, 145
Legenere's disease   228
Leishmania   38
Lev's disease   228
long Q-T interval   6, 28–32, 40, 106,
        120, 126, 286, 342, 343–345
Lown-Ganong-Levine syndrome   82,
        175, 178, 179, 186, 262
low-voltage QRS   1, 27, **38**, 39, 41, 363
lymphoma/lymphosarcoma   30, 230

m

magnesium   1, 28, 342
Mahaim fibers   176
Marfan's syndrome   191
marijuana   148, 214
masquerading bundle branch block
        44, 70, 73, 77, **80**, 82
mean electrical axis   1, 3, **10**, 11, 80,
        94, 99
medetomidine   39, 46, 120, 230
metoprolol   237

mexiletine   326, 330
Mobitz   43, 45, 62, 67, 73, 77, 79, 81,
        86, 93, 100, 178, 211, 212, 228,
        231, 234, 235, 238, 240, 241,
        247, 256–258, 284, 293, 309,
        323, 324, 338, 340, 357
myocardial infarction   1, 4, 24, 37, 77,
        87, 90, 117, 157, 201

n

non-conducted atrial premature
        complexes   96, 103, 110, 139,
        156, **159**
non-conducted junctional premature
        complexes   212, 259, **263**, 265
non-conducted ventricular premature
        complexes   **309**
non-paroxysmal idioatrial tachycardia
        166
non-paroxysmal idiojunctional
        tachycardia   166, 270
non-paroxysmal ventricular
        tachycardia   166, 319
notch   90, 157, 175, 176, 201, 260, 363

o

obesity   38
orthodromic   60, 95, 140, 179,
        182–184, 186, 212, 278, 367
Osborn wave   6, 26, 32
overcompensatory pause   154
overdrive suppression   87, 101, 116,
        123, 126, 128, 130, 132, 133,
        153, 154, 161, 162, 188, 207,
        213, 219, 222, 256, 260
oversensing   350, **363**, 365, 366

p

pacemaker   8, 17, 22, 33, 45, 49, 52,
        61, 87, 93–96, 99, 100, 103,
        105–108, 114, 116, 118, 122,
        123, 128, 134, 139, 141, 142,
        145, 148, 158, 162, 167, 193,
        194, 205, 228, 234, 240, 244,
        247, 248, 253, 254, 263, 274,
        288, 302, **349–371**
pacemaker-mediated tachycardia   87,
        350, 363, **367**, 371
pacemaker syndrome   36, 350, 363,
        367, 368, 369
paper speeds   1, 3, **8**, 9
parasystole   *94*, 96, 97, 101, 133–136,
        138, 139, 151, 157, 163, 165,

        172, 212, 259, 262, 268, 269,
        284, 291, 315, 317, 349
    atrial   134, 139, 151, 157, **163**, 165,
        172
    junctional   212, 259, 262, 268, **269**,
        315
    sinoatrial   101, 133, **134**, 135, 136,
        138
    ventricular   284, 291, **315**, 317
patent ductus arteriosus   23, 272
p biatriale   1, 16, **19**, 21, 153, 161, 237
p congenitale   16
pentageminy   283, 307, 308, 311, 317
pentobarbital   289
pericarditis   1, 27, 36, **38**, 41
pleural effusion   38, 367
p mitrale   1, 16, **17**–19, 24, 25, 45, 46,
        53, 59, 124, 126, 131, 137, 172,
        197
pneumothorax   38, 288
P on Ta   192, 197, 198
post-extrasystolic aberrancy   47, 49,
        209, 313
post-extrasystolic atrial aberrancy
        44, 45–54
post-extrasystolic potentiation   95
post-extrasystolic P-R interval
        prolongation   65, 95, 135, 151,
        154, 155, 233, 278, 297, 298,
        302, 305, 311
post-extrasystolic revelation of
        rate-dependent bundle branch
        block   70, 95
post-extrasystolic T wave   29, 33, 95
postponed compensatory pause   155,
        257, 296, 297, 317, 337
p pseudo-biatriale   1, 16, **19**, 21
p pseudo-mitrale   1, 16, 18, **19**
p pseudo-pulmonale   1, **16**, 18
p pulmonale   1, 15, **16**, 17, 26, 127,
        131
precordial thump   88, 346, 347
premature systole
    atrial   139, **161–165**
    junctional   212, **259–269**
    sinoatrial   101, 112, 113, **133–135**
    ventricular   **291–318**
P-R interval   3, **5**–7, 28, 36, 39, 53, 56,
        60, 61, 64, 68, 72–74, 81, 82, 84,
        85, 95, 99, 110, 112, 113, 121,
        124, 133, 134–136, 139, 151,
        155, 156, 159, 161–164, 175,
        176–179, 185, 211, 213, 214,
        218–221, 228–236, 238,

240–244, 246, 251, 254, 255, 264, 270, 271, 274, 278, 281, 285, 286, 291, 296–298, 303, 305, 309–311, 313, 323, 343, 357, 358, 360, 364

procainamide   87, 117, 181, 183, 280, 306, 308, 330, 333

pseudo-atrial dissociation   172, 174

pseudo-electrical alternans   **38**, 39, 40

pulmonary hypertension   19, 21, 71, 172

pulmonic stenosis   20–22, 293

pulseless electrical activity (*see electromechanical dissociation*)

P wave   **5**, 7

q

QRS complex   **6**, 7

Q-T interval   3, **6**, 7, 24, 27–32, 34, 35, 38, 67, 104, 106, 120, 126, 221, 286, 334, 363, 369

quadrigeminy   95, 251, 283, 291, **306**, 307, 311

Q wave   5, **6**, 7, 37, 75, 99, 229

r

rate dependent bundle branch block   67, 159, 202

rate dependent left bundle branch block   **67**, 69, 70, 160

rate dependent right bundle branch block   55, **60**, 61, 64, 202

reciprocal complexes
  atrial   85, 139, 151, **162**, 163–165, 175, **179**, 180, 182, 263
  junctional   212, 248, 257, 259, 263, **265**, 267
  paced   357, **361**
  sinoatrial   101, **133**, 135
  ventricular   278, 286, **313**, 315

renal failure   28–30, 32, 40, 109, 121, 145–147

resetting   47, 56, 85, 100, 118, 123, 133–135, 139, 151, **153**–156, 159, 163, 212, 219–222, **259**, 260, 261, 271, 302, 312, 313, 315, 365

resetting with a pause   118, 123, 133, 139, 151, **153**, 154, 212, 219, 259, **260**

reversed bigeminy (*see escape-capture bigeminy*)

right atrial abnormality   1, **16**

right axis deviation   9, 14, 17, 21, 55, 78, 79, 129, 198, 297

right ventricular enlargement   1, 11, 16, **19**–21, 28, 55, 79

right ventricular hypertrophy   19, 21, 24, 78, 80, 83

R on T   197, 319, 330, 331, 342, 343, 346

Rule of bigeminy   201, 203, 243, 244, 250, 291, **298**, 301–303, 306, 318

Rule of reset   85, 130, 211, 213, **219**, 221, 223, 246, 254

R wave   5, **6**, 7

s

Salvador Dali sign   32

second degree atrioventricular block   35, 61, 62, 68, 72, 73, 79, 94–96, 109–111, 113, 115, 117, 120, 126, 127, 129, 131, 134, 135, 142, 154, 159, 161, 194, 204, 212, 215, 216, 218, 219, 228, 230, **231**–**247**, 252, 254, 255, 258, 261, 263, 272, 280, 293–295, 311, 328, 349, 351, 360, 366, 367

second degree bundle branch block   62, 67, 86

second degree exit block   257

second degree interatrial block   45–47

second degree sinoatrial block   31, 100, 112, **117**–121, 126, 133, 135

second degree ventriculoatrial block   256

sick sinus syndrome   30, 33, 96, 101, 103, 115, 117, 121, **123**–**132**, 148, 194, 204, 213, 226, 228, 247, 252, 287, 349, 351–353, 358, 361, 364, 366, 367
  bradycardia variant   101, 123, **126**, 127
  tachycardia-bradycardia variant   **128**, 129, 131, 132

sinoatrial block   30–32, 68, 69, 93, 96, 100, 112–114, **117**–**122**, 123, 126, 127, 133, 135, 141, 142, 148, 154, 156, 160, 213, 216, 222, 241, 257, 274, 287, 330

sinoventricular rhythm   28, 29, 139, 141, 144–148, 206, 273, 301

sinus arrest   33, 100, 103, **114**–117, 120, 123–127, 130, 131, 145, 148, 216, 217, 222–226, 249, 252, 253, 257, 274, 285, 287

sinus arrhythmia   8, 10, 18, 22, 24, 26, 33, 38–40, 45, 61, 65, 74, 91, 96, 99, 100, 103, **105**–112, 114, 116–118, 121, 127, 129, 133, 134, 145, 154–156, 159–161, 174, 177, 213, 215–217, 230, 233–239, 243, 247, 248, 255, 257, 261, 265, 276, 286, 287, 291, 293, 295, 303, 315, 316, 321

sinus bigeminy   69, 100, 103, **112**, 113, 117, 119, 133–135, 138

sinus bradycardia   29, 30–32, 35, 39, 40, 96, 100, **103**, 104, 114, 120, 123, 126, 129, 132, 156, 159, 213, 214, 216, 217, 220, 222–226, 229, 239, 246, 252, 272, 274, 276, 285, 287, 323

sinus nodal dysfunction   101, 111, 121, **123**–125, 252

sinus nodal reentrant tachycardia   95, 101, 133, **137**

sinus pause   61, 96, 100, 103, **114**, 117, 123, 126, 127, 132, 133, 135, 141, 160, 213, 214, 218, 230, 241, 247, 266, 285, 286, 311

sinus tachycardia   10, 17, 27, 38, 39, 41, 64, 71, 72, 93, 95, 100, 101, 105, 108, 115, 124, 133, **136**–138, 180, 187, 197, 218, 228, 230, 239, 249, 277, 301, 323, 334, 340, 349

situs inversus   1, 3, 12, **13**

slur   90, 91

sotalol   205, 307, 330

Spodick's sign   41

S1-S2-S3 pattern   19, 21

stork-leg sign   41

S-T segment   1, 3–5, **6**, 7
  depression   **35**–37, 127, 243
  elevation   1, 4, 24, 27, **35**–37, 41, 120, 293

subaortic stenosis   58

supernormal conduction   60, 94, 96, 162, 165, 205, 234, 244, 248, 249, 251, 263, 301–303

supernormal exciatation   139, 151, **159**, 160

supracompensatory pause (*see overcompensatory pause*)

supraventricular tachycardia 20, 38, 41, 43, 44, 59, 60, 78, 87–90, 92, 94, *95*, 96, 128, 131, 136, 138, 139, 153, 166, 175, 182, 186, 187, 197, 256, 276, 283, 330, 340, 341, 358

S wave **6**, 7

synchrony 94, 225, 226, 248, 254, 274–276, 321, 363

systemic hypertension 23, 29, 35, 123, 145, 248

t

Ta wave **5**, 7, 8, 16, 27, 46, 108, 136, 192, 197, 198, 230, 236, 252, 254

Tetralogy of Fallot 59

third degree atrioventricular block 29, 47, 79, 81, 82, 86, 108, 109, 193, 194, 204, 212, 216–218, 220, 221, 223, 224, 228, 231, 242, 244, **248**–258, 265, 276, 283, 288, 303, 334, 349, 351, 352, 354–356, 362, 368

third degree bundle branch block 43

third degree exit block 257

third degree interatrial block 45–47

third degree sinoatrial block 117, 122

third degree ventriculoatrial block 256

thwarts 96, 97, 118, 127, 214

torsades de pointes 29, 40, 126, 284, 319, 327, 331, **342**, 343

transition of a pacemaker 49, 94, 139, 141, 158, 167

tricuspid dysplasia 17, 20, 21, 90, 192

trifascicular block 43, 44, 61, 62, 67, 68, 77, **81**, 83–86, 283

trigeminy 95
  atrial 78, 147, 151, 156, **157**, 158, 159, 165
  junctional 259, **262**, 263
  ventricular 53, 54, 64, 251, 291, 298, 299, **305**, 306, 310, 312

T wave **6**, 7

Type I 2nd degree atrioventricular block 6, 35, 61, 111, 117, 126, 127, 129, 161, 219, 228, 230, **231**, 232–237, 239, 247, 255, 295

Type I 2nd degree bundle branch block 43, 62, 67

Type I 2nd degree exit block 257, 271, 278, 293, 309, 330, 338, 339

Type I 2nd degree sinotatrial block **117**, 118, 120, 122, 127, 330

Type I 2nd degree ventriculoatrial block 211, 256, 293, 323, 357, 358, 365

Type II 2nd degree atrioventricular block 72, 73, 120, 215, 218, 219, 228, 232–235, 238, **240**–244, 247, 254, 272, 349, 351, 360

Type II 2nd degree bundle branch block 43, 62, 67

Type II 2nd degree exit block 257, 293, 338, 340

Type II 2nd degree sinoatrial block **120**

Type II 2nd degree ventriculoatrial block 211, 256, 293, 323, 357

u

unclassified cardiomyopathy 184, 203, 335

undersensing 350, 361, **363**–367, 370

unipolar 3, 349, 351, 352, 355, 363

U wave **6**, 7, 27, 31–33, 344

v

vagal maneuver 95, 137, 179, 235, 276, 278

vagotonia 105, 228, 230, 236, 239

ventricular dissociation 283, 284, 319, 331, **345**, 346

ventricular fibrillation 4, 94–96, 181, 197, 284, 289, 319, 331, **346**

ventricular flutter 284, 319, 331, 336, **342**–345

ventricular pre-excitation 6, 77, 78, 82, 90, 139, **175**–180, 182–186, 278, 311, 323, 359

ventricular premature complexes 32, 37, 47, 56, 75, 87, 88, 94, 100, 111, 115, 154, 156, 166, 201. 203, 217, 233, 262, 264, 283, **291**–**318**
  left ventricular 64, 88, 283, 291, **292**, 297, 301, 305, 311, 314, 331, 352, 360
  multifocal 292
  right ventricular 56, 75, 280, 291, **292**, 301, 313, 314

ventricular septal defect 23, 90, 179

ventricular tachycardia 40, 43, 47, 87, *95*, 96, 123, 126, 131, 166, 181, 197, 201, 205, 207, 231, 256, 257, 283, 284, 307, **319**–**348**
  bidirectional 284, 330, **333**–335
  bundle branch reentrant 284, 319, **336**, 337
  left 201, 284, 319, 325, **331**, 332, 333, 338, 340, 341
  polymorphic 40, 126, 284, 319, 326, 331, 342, **342**, 343
  right 284, 319, 335, **336**, 337, 339–341
  right ventricular outflow tract 283, 284, 319, 331, 336

ventriculoatrial association 95, 283, 284, 312, 319, **323**, 332

ventriculoatrial block 93, 94, 211, 212, 228, 229, **256**, 283, 284, 293, 319, 323, 357, 361

ventriculoatrial conduction 5, 47, 93–96, 100, 123, 129, 131, 148, 162, 180, 217, 256, 270, 272, 283, 284, 291, 307, **312**, 313, 316, 320, 327, 328, 332, 349, 357, 358, 363, 367

ventriculophasic junctional arrhythmia 211, 213, **226**

ventriculophasic sinus arrhythmia 61, 100, 103, **108**–111, 116, 117, 127, 156, 159, 235, 236, 239, 247, 248, 255, 293

vertical axis 1, 16, **24**, 336

w

wandering pacemaker 22, 33, 45, 61, 96, 99, 100, 103, **105**–107, 118, 141, 142, 234

waveforms 3, **5**, 7

Wenckebach 1, 45, 61, 62, 67, 93, 96, 100, 110, 112, 117, 118, 120, 126, 133, 135, 155, 159–164, 178, 193, 211, 212, 218, 228, **231**–238, 245–247, 255–258, 271, 273, 278, 284, 285, 293, 295–298, 304, 307, 309, 323–325, 328, 338, 339, 357, 358, 365

wide QRS complex supraventricular tachycardia **87**

Wolff-Parkinson-White syndrome 77, 175, 176, 186